Dinophysis Toxins

Dinophysis Toxins: Distribution, Fate in Shellfish and Impacts

Special Issue Editors

Beatriz Reguera
Juan Blanco

MDPI • Basel • Beijing • Wuhan • Barcelona • Belgrade

MDPI

Special Issue Editors
Beatriz Reguera
Spanish Institute of Oceanography (IEO)
Oceanographic Centre of Vigo
Spain

Juan Blanco
Marine Research Centre (CIMA)
Spain

Editorial Office
MDPI
St. Alban-Anlage 66
4052 Basel, Switzerland

This is a reprint of articles from the Special Issue published online in the open access journal *Toxins* (ISSN 2072-6651) from 2018 to 2019 (available at: https://www.mdpi.com/journal/toxins/special_issues/Dinophysis_toxins)

For citation purposes, cite each article independently as indicated on the article page online and as indicated below:

LastName, A.A.; LastName, B.B.; LastName, C.C. Article Title. *Journal Name* **Year**, *Article Number*, Page Range.

ISBN 978-3-03921-363-4 (Pbk)
ISBN 978-3-03921-364-1 (PDF)

Cover image courtesy of VGOHAB (IEO): https://vgohab.com/

Contents

About the Special Issue Editors . . . . **ix**

Beatriz Reguera and Juan Blanco
Dinophysis Toxins: Distribution, Fate in Shellfish and Impacts
Reprinted from: *Toxins* **2019**, *11*, 413, doi:10.3390/toxins11070413 . . . . **1**

Rafael Salas and Dave Clarke
Review of DSP Toxicity in Ireland: Long-Term Trend Impacts, Biodiversity and Toxin Profiles from a Monitoring Perspective
Reprinted from: *Toxins* **2019**, *11*, 61, doi:10.3390/toxins11020061 . . . . **5**

Sarah C. Swan, Andrew D. Turner, Eileen Bresnan, Callum Whyte, Ruth F. Paterson, Sharon McNeill, Elaine Mitchell and Keith Davidson
Dinophysis acuta in Scottish Coastal Waters and Its Influence on Diarrhetic Shellfish Toxin Profiles
Reprinted from: *Toxins* **2018**, *10*, 399, doi:10.3390/toxins10100399 . . . . **24**

Raúl Fernández, Luz Mamán, David Jaén, Lourdes Fernández Fuentes, M. Asunción Ocaña and M. Mercedes Gordillo
Dinophysis Species and Diarrhetic Shellfish Toxins: 20 Years of Monitoring Program in Andalusia, South of Spain
Reprinted from: *Toxins* **2019**, *11*, 189, doi:10.3390/toxins11040189 . . . . **44**

Lincoln A. Mackenzie
A Long-Term Time Series of *Dinophysis acuminata* Blooms and Associated Shellfish Toxin Contamination in Port Underwood, Marlborough Sounds, New Zealand
Reprinted from: *Toxins* **2019**, *11*, 74, doi:10.3390/toxins11020074 . . . . **72**

Hazel Farrell, Penelope Ajani, Shauna Murray, Phil Baker, Grant Webster, Steve Brett and Anthony Zammit
Diarrhetic Shellfish Toxin Monitoring in Commercial Wild Harvest Bivalve Shellfish in New South Wales, Australia
Reprinted from: *Toxins* **2018**, *10*, 446, doi:10.3390/toxins10110446 . . . . **90**

Alex Alcántara-Rubira, Víctor Bárcena-Martínez, Maribel Reyes-Paulino, Katherine Medina-Acaro, Lilibeth Valiente-Terrones, Angélica Rodríguez-Velásquez, Rolando Estrada-Jiménez and Omar Flores-Salmón
First Report of Okadaic Acid and Pectenotoxins in Individual Cells of *Dinophysis* and in Scallops *Argopecten purpuratus* from Perú
Reprinted from: *Toxins* **2018**, *10*, 490, doi:10.3390/toxins10120490 . . . . **107**

Catharina Alves-de-Souza, José Luis Iriarte and Jorge I. Mardones
Interannual Variability of *Dinophysis acuminata* and *Protoceratium reticulatum* in a Chilean Fjord: Insights from the Realized Niche Analysis
Reprinted from: *Toxins* **2019**, *11*, 19, doi:10.3390/toxins11010019 . . . . **115**

Patricio A. Díaz, Beatriz Reguera, Teresa Moita, Isabel Bravo, Manuel Ruiz-Villarreal and Santiago Fraga
Mesoscale Dynamics and Niche Segregation of Two *Dinophysis* Species in Galician-Portuguese Coastal Waters
Reprinted from: *Toxins* **2019**, *11*, 37, doi:10.3390/toxins11010037 . . . . **138**

Thiago Pereira Alves and Luiz Laureno Mafra Jr.
Diel Variations in Cell Abundance and Trophic Transfer of Diarrheic Toxins during a Massive *Dinophysis* Bloom in Southern Brazil
Reprinted from: *Toxins* **2018**, *10*, 232, doi:10.3390/toxins10060232 . . . . **159**

Han Gao, Mengmeng Tong, Xinlong An and Juliette L. Smith
Prey Lysate Enhances Growth and Toxin Production in an Isolate of *Dinophysis acuminata*
Reprinted from: *Toxins* **2019**, *11*, 57, doi:10.3390/toxins11010057 . . . . **178**

Han Gao, Chenfeng Hua and Mengmeng Tong
Impact of *Dinophysis acuminata* Feeding *Mesodinium rubrum* on Nutrient Dynamics and Bacterial Composition in a Microcosm
Reprinted from: *Toxins* **2018**, *10*, 443, doi:10.3390/toxins10110443 . . . . **194**

Jorge Hernández-Urcera, Pilar Rial, María García-Portela, Patricia Lourés, Jane Kilcoyne, Francisco Rodríguez, Amelia Fernández-Villamarín and Beatriz Reguera
Notes on the Cultivation of Two Mixotrophic *Dinophysis* Species and Their Ciliate Prey *Mesodinium rubrum*
Reprinted from: *Toxins* **2018**, *10*, 505, doi:10.3390/toxins10120505 . . . . **215**

Hajime Uchida, Ryuichi Watanabe, Ryoji Matsushima, Hiroshi Oikawa, Satoshi Nagai, Takashi Kamiyama, Katsuhisa Baba, Akira Miyazono, Yuki Kosaka, Shinnosuke Kaga, Yukihiko Matsuyama and Toshiyuki Suzuki
Toxin Profiles of Okadaic Acid Analogues and Other Lipophilic Toxins in *Dinophysis* from Japanese Coastal Waters
Reprinted from: *Toxins* **2018**, *10*, 457, doi:10.3390/toxins10110457 . . . . **237**

Ryoji Matsushima, Hajime Uchida, Ryuichi Watanabe, Hiroshi Oikawa, Izumi Oogida, Yuki Kosaka, Makoto Kanamori, Tatsuro Akamine and Toshiyuki Suzuki
Anatomical Distribution of Diarrhetic Shellfish Toxins (DSTs) in the Japanese Scallop *Patinopecten yessoensis* and Individual Variability in Scallops and *Mytilus edulis* Mussels: Statistical Considerations
Reprinted from: *Toxins* **2018**, *10*, 395, doi:10.3390/toxins10100395 . . . . **251**

María Verónica Prego-Faraldo, Luisa Martínez and Josefina Méndez
RNA-Seq Analysis for Assessing the Early Response to DSP Toxins in *Mytilus galloprovincialis* Digestive Gland and Gill
Reprinted from: *Toxins* **2018**, *10*, 417, doi:10.3390/toxins10100417 . . . . **266**

Cheng Chi, Sib Sankar Giri, Jin Woo Jun, Sang Wha Kim, Hyoun Joong Kim, Jeong Woo Kang and Se Chang Park
Detoxification- and Immune-Related Transcriptomic Analysis of Gills from Bay Scallops (*Argopecten irradians*) in Response to Algal Toxin Okadaic Acid
Reprinted from: *Toxins* **2018**, *10*, 308, doi:10.3390/toxins10080308 . . . . **292**

Aifeng Li, Meihui Li, Jiangbing Qiu, Jialiang Song, Ying Ji, Yang Hu, Shuqin Wang and Yijia Che
Effect of Suspended Particulate Matter on the Accumulation of Dissolved Diarrhetic Shellfish Toxins by Mussels (*Mytilus galloprovincialis*) under Laboratory Conditions
Reprinted from: *Toxins* **2018**, *10*, 273, doi:10.3390/toxins10070273 . . . . **309**

Juan Blanco, Gonzalo Álvarez, José Rengel, Rosario Díaz, Carmen Mariño, Helena Martín and Eduardo Uribe
Accumulation and Biotransformation of *Dinophysis* Toxins by the Surf Clam *Mesodesma donacium*
Reprinted from: *Toxins* **2018**, *10*, 314, doi:10.3390/toxins10080314 . . . . **322**

Juan Blanco
Accumulation of *Dinophysis* Toxins in Bivalve Molluscs
Reprinted from: *Toxins* **2018**, *10*, 453, doi:10.3390/toxins10110453 . . . . **335**

About the Special Issue Editors

Beatriz Reguera is a Research Professor at the Harmful Microalgae group (VGOHAB) of the Spanish Institute of Oceanography (IEO) in Vigo. This group was established in 1977 following a major paralytic shellfish poisoning outbreak in Europe, and is dedicated to the study of toxic microalgae with socioeconomic impacts on public health, aquaculture, and tourism. Its multidisciplinary approach, in line with the UNESCO program on Harmful Algal Blooms (GlobalHAB), pursues research on the taxonomy, genetics, lifecycle strategies and ecophysiology, and on the environmental factors which control harmful algae populations in the field. Reguera is author and co-author of more than 100 international publications in international journals in addition to book chapters and edition of manuals and conference proceedings, and past Chair and long-standing member of the ICES-IOC WG on HAB Dynamics, the UNESCO IOC Intergovernmental Panel on Harmful Algal Blooms (IPHAB), and the International Society for the Study of Harmful Algae (ISSHA). In 2016, Reguera was awarded the IOC 50th Anniversary Commemorative Medal for outstanding cooperation to HAB program activities and, in 2018, the ISSHA Yasumoto Lifetime Achievement Award for her contributions to the biology, population dynamics, and monitoring of toxin-producing microalgae, in particular, of *Dinophysis* species.

Juan Blanco is head of the Toxic Episodes Team at the Centre for Marine Research (CIMA) of the Galician government (Xunta de Galicia). The aim of CIMA is to achieve efficient, scientifically based management of marine renewable resources. Blanco started his professional career in the Spanish Institute of Oceanography (IEO) where, jointly with the University of Santiago de Compostela, he prepared a PhD thesis on dinoflagellate cysts. His research at CIMA has focused on the relationship between phytoplankton populations and filter feeding bivalves, with special attention to the accumulation and depuration of marine toxins. His research topics range from the study of physiological mechanisms to modeling toxin uptake and fate in shellfish, and the development of analytical methodologies. The author of numerous articles and supervisor of PhD theses, Blanco has also served as coordinator of two marine research programs of the Galician government. He has also served as adviser to the Xunta de Galicia in the field of toxic phytoplankton and phycotoxin-related issues—including the design and implementation of the marine environment monitoring system currently carried out by INTECMAR—and to the European Commission on the implementation of European Directives on HAB monitoring and regulation of marine toxins in shellfish.

toxins

MDPI

Editorial

Dinophysis Toxins: Distribution, Fate in Shellfish and Impacts

Beatriz Reguera [1,*] and Juan Blanco [2,*]

1 Instituto Español de Oceanografía (IEO), Centro Oceanográfico de Vigo, Subida a Radio Faro 50, 36390 Vigo, Spain
2 Centro de Investigacións Mariñas, Xunta de Galicia, Pedras de Corón S/N, 36620 Vilanova de Arousa, Spain
* Correspondence: beatriz.reguera@ieo.es (B.R.); juan.carlos.blanco.perez@xunta.gal (J.B.)

Received: 9 July 2019; Accepted: 11 July 2019; Published: 16 July 2019

Several planktonic dinoflagellate species of the genus *Dinophysis* produce one or two groups of lipophilic toxins: (i) okadaic acid (OA) and its derivatives, the dinophysistoxins (DTXs), and (ii) pectenotoxins (PTXs) [1–3]. The OA and DTXs, known as diarrhetic shellfish poisoning (DSP) toxins, are acid polyethers that inhibit the protein phosphatase and have diarrheogenic effects in mammals [4,5]. The PTXs are polyether lactones, some of which are hepatotoxic to mice by intraperitoneal injection [6]. The toxicity of pectenotoxins has been questioned since they are not toxic when ingested orally [7]. Filter feeding bivalves retain toxic planktonic microalgae and other suspended matter, acting as vectors of the toxins through the food web. Bivalves contaminated with DTXs are a threat to public health. Shellfish resources exposed to DTXs and other toxic syndromes need to be monitored for early detection of the toxins and their causative agents and subjected to regulations aimed to protect public health.

Forty years after the identification of *Dinophysis fortii* as the causative agent of severe gastrointestinal outbreaks in Japan [1], toxins produced by a few species of *Dinophysis* have been recognized, in terms of persistence and distribution, as the main threat to intensive shellfish exploitation in western Europe, eastern Japan, and to a lesser extent in southern Chile and New Zealand. Recently, *Dinophysis* events have emerged in traditionally "DSP-toxin free" areas (e.g., eastern and north-western USA, the Pacific coast of Mexico, South China Sea). Increased monitoring and regulation may explain certain cases, but some models include *Dinophysis* as a potential winner in global warming scenarios [8], although without taking into account species-specific requirements [9].

The monitoring of *Dinophysis* species and their toxins in shellfish started in the early 1980's. The old standard mouse bioassay detected and quantified, as okadaic acid equivalent (OA eq.) units, a "cocktail" of lipophilic toxins, and needed 24 to 48 h observation of the experimental animal. The high performance liquid chromatography (HPLC) method developed by the group of Yasumoto [10] and its adaptation to analyse picked cells of *Dinophysis* [11] revealed that species of this genus produced two groups of toxins with different chemical structures and toxic effects: (i) okadaates (OA and dinophysistoxins) and (ii) pectenotoxins—only the former have diarrhetic effects, while the latter are not even regulated in some countries. Other lipophilic toxins, such as yessotoxins and azaspiracids, and even non-toxic fatty acids causing false positives, were co-extracted with *Dinophysis* toxins, leading to complex matrices for the analyses. The next breakthrough was the development of liquid chromatography coupled to mass spectrometry (LC-MS). During his plenary talk at the 8th International Conference on Harmful Algae, Vigo, 1997, Mike Quilliam forecasted this new analytical tool would replace all the other methods [12]. Two years earlier he had shown how the extraction procedure of the time led to toxin profiles of hydrolized precursors of the OA and DTXs [13]. In the same period, Maestrini [14] identified the main gaps in knowledge concerning the biology and population dynamics of *Dinophysis* species. These gaps included questions about the life cycle, nutrition (including the inability to grow *Dinophysis* in laboratory cultures), and the physical-biological interactions explaining their patchy populations.

Twenty year after these advances, considerable progress has been gained through: (i) the use of sampling strategies which follow the cell cycle and dynamics of low-density and patchy field populations of *Dinophysis* spp. [15,16]; (ii) the application of single-cell manipulations coupled to new molecular and analytical techniques, and finally (iii) the successful establishment of mixotrophic cultures of *Dinophysis* fed the ciliate *Mesodinium rubrum* [17]. Still the main problems faced to monitor *Dinophysis* spp and their toxins are: (i) taxonomic uncertainties with traditional methods, to identify species which are morphologically similar but with different toxic potential; (ii) large differences in toxin profiles and cellular content found between strains of the same species, even in the same location; (iii) to improve predictive capabilities of the occurrence of *Dinophysis* species and their toxins in shellfish; (iv) to develop cost-efficient monitoring systems for the control of shellfish toxins in different molluscs with their specific metabolic responses. Despite these uncertainties, a "*Dinophysis* trigger level" based on cell densities is still widely used in monitoring systems. Different toxins from *Dinophysis* cells/fragments, their grazers, and detritus derived from faecal pellets are ingested by shellfish, affecting their absorption, transformation and elimination in a species-specific manner, and a large proportion are released into the water [18–20]. All these processes, which play key roles in the impact of toxic outbreaks on shellfish resources, are poorly known, in particular from a metabolic and genomic point of view. Further, the direct effects of *Dinophysis* toxins on the growth and survival of shellfish species feeding on them have received little attention.

This special issue contains original contributions that advance our knowledge of the distribution and impact of *Dinophysis* toxins on the shellfish industry worldwide. A wide range of topics are covered, from monitoring and regulation of DSP toxins to *Dinophysis* population dynamics, laboratory cultures and the kinetics of uptake, transformation and impact of the toxins in shellfish. Four papers present long (>20 years) times series of monitoring data from regions in Europe and Oceania suffering blooms of *D. acuminata*/*D. acuta* every year. The impact of DSP events in Ireland, Scotland and Spain, with strains with toxin profiles dominated by OA and DTXs, contrasts with their lower impact in New Zealand, with strains with profiles dominated by PTXs. Results from these countries confirm the need for a shellfish species-specific strategy to control the impact of DSP outbreaks, and a site-specific analysis of the response of *Dinophysis*-related outbreaks to climate variability. A paper with the first report of *Dinophysis* toxins in Perú, from LC-MS analyses of individually isolated cells, shows that classification problems persist within the "*D. acuminata* complex". This problem is also pointed out in the paper from southwest Spain. Two articles deal with the population dynamics, autoecology and the concept of niche segregation for co-occurring toxic species in Reloncaví fjord, southern Chile and the Galician Rías, northwest Spain, and a paper from Brazil describes interactions between *Dinophysis* and its ciliate prey, as well as toxin transfer through the food web during an exceptional bloom of the "*D. acuminata* complex". Interactions with the prey *Mesodinium rubrum*, its effects on growth and toxin production in mixotrophic laboratory cultures, and considerations/suggestions to optimize mass cultures of *Dinophysis* are dealt with in three contributions.

Contributions from Japan, the pioneer country with the longest records of detection of *Dinophysis* toxins, include a review of the toxin profiles of different *Dinophysis* species with current analytical tools, as well as statistical considerations on DSP toxin monitoring and their anatomical distribution in shellfish. The effects of DSP toxins on shellfish are explored with advanced molecular techniques, RNA sequencing analysis and transcriptomics. Finally, different aspects of the kinetics of DSP toxin accumulation and depuration in shellfish, including predictive models, are investigated in a full review and in contributions about metabolic changes in shellfish and the effect of suspended particulate matter in toxin accumulation.

Acknowledgments: The editors are grateful to all the authors who contributed to this special issue. They are also appreciate the rigorous evaluation of the submitted manuscripts by expert peer reviewers. The valuable contributions, organization, and editorial support of the MDPI management team and staff are greatly appreciated.

References

1. Yasumoto, T.; Oshima, Y.; Sugawara, W.; Fukuyo, Y.; Oguri, H.; Igarashi, T.; Fujita, N. Identification of *Dinophysis fortii* as the causative organism of diarrhetic shellfish poisoning. *Bull. Jpn. Soc. Sci. Fish.* **1980**, *46*, 1405–1411. [CrossRef]
2. Yasumoto, T.; Murata, M.; Oshima, T.; Matsumoto, C.; Clardy, J. Diarrhetic shellfish poisoning. In *Seafood Toxins*; Ragelis, E.P., Ed.; ACS Symposium: Washington, DC, USA, 1984; pp. 207–214.
3. Reguera, B.; Riobó, P.; Rodríguez, F.; Díaz, P.; Pizarro, G.; Paz, B.; Franco, J.; Blanco, J. *Dinophysis* Toxins: Causative Organisms, Distribution and Fate in Shellfish. *Mar. Drugs* **2014**, *12*, 394–461. [CrossRef] [PubMed]
4. Murata, M.; Shimatani, M.; Sugitani, H.; Oshima, Y.; Yasumoto, T. Isolation and structural elucidation of the causative toxin of diarrhetic shellfish poisoning. *Bull. J. Soc. Sci. Fish.* **1982**, *48*, 549–552. [CrossRef]
5. Bialojan, C.; Takai, A. Inhibitory effect of a marine-sponge toxin, okadaic acid, on protein phosphatases. Specificity and kinetics. *Biochem. J.* **1988**, *256*, 283–290. [CrossRef] [PubMed]
6. Terao, K.; Ito, E.; Yanagi, T.; Yasumoto, T. Histopathological studies on experimental marine toxin poisoning. I. Ultrastructural changes in the small intestine and liver of suckling mice induced by dinophysistoxin-1 and pectenotoxin-1. *Toxicon* **1986**, *24*, 1141–1151. [CrossRef]
7. Miles, C.O.; Wilkins, A.L.; Munday, R.; Dines, M.H.; Hawkes, A.D.; Briggs, L.R.; Sandvik, M.; Jensen, D.J.; Cooney, J.M.; Holland, P.T.; et al. Isolation of pectenotoxin-2 from *Dinophysis acuta* and its conversion to pectenotoxin-2 seco acid, and preliminary assessment of their acute toxicities. *Toxicon* **2004**, *43*, 1–9. [CrossRef] [PubMed]
8. Gobler, C.J.; Doherty, O.M.; Hattenrath-Lehmann, T.K.; Griffith, A.W.; Kang, Y.; Litaker, R.W. Ocean warming since 1982 has expanded the niche of toxic algal blooms in the North Atlantic and North Pacific oceans. *Proc. Natl. Acad. Sci. USA.* **2017**, *114*, 4975. [CrossRef] [PubMed]
9. Pitcher, G.C. Harmful algae—The requirement for species-specific information. *Harmful Algae* **2012**, *14*, 1–4. [CrossRef]
10. Lee, J.S.; Yanagi, T.; Kenma, R.; Yasumoto, T. Fluorometric determination of diarrhetic shellfish toxins by high-performance liquid chromatography. *Agric. Biol. Chem.* **1987**, *51*, 877–881.
11. Lee, J.S.; Igarashi, T.; Fraga, S.; Dahl, E.; Hovgaard, P.; Yasumoto, T. Determination of diarrhetic shellfish toxins in various dinoflagellate species. *J. Appl. Phycol.* **1989**, *1*, 147–152. [CrossRef]
12. Quilliam, M.A. Liquid chromatography-mass spectrometry: A universal method for analysis of toxins. In *Harmful Algae*; Reguera, B., Blanco, J., Fernández, M.L., Wyatt, T., Eds.; Xunta de Galicia & Intergovernmental Oceanografic Comission of UNESCO: Santiago de Compostela, CA, USA, 1998.
13. Quilliam, M.A.; Hardstaff, W.R.; Ishida, N.; McLachlan, J.L.; Reeves, A.R.; Ross, N.W.; Windust, A.J. Production of diarrhetic shellfish poisoning (DSP) toxins by *Prorocentrum lima* in culture and development of analytical methods. In *Harmful and Toxic Algal Blooms*; Yasumoto, T., Oshima, Y., Fukuyo, Y., Eds.; IOC of UNESCO: Sendai, Japan, 1996; pp. 289–292.
14. Maestrini, S.Y. Bloom dynamics and ecophysiology of *Dinophysis* spp. In *Physiological Ecology of Harmful Algal Blooms*; Anderson, D.M., Cembella, A., Hallegraeff, G., Eds.; Springer: Berlin/Heidelberg, Germany, 1998; pp. 243–266.
15. Reguera, B.; Velo-Suárez, L.; Raine, R.; Park, M. Harmful *Dinophysis* species: A review. *Harmful Algae* **2012**, *14*, 87–106. [CrossRef]
16. Berdalet, E.; Bernard, S.; Burford, M.A.; Enevoldsen, H.; Kudela, R.; Magnien, R.; Roy, S.; Tester, P.A.; Urban, E.; Usup, G. GEOHAB 2014. Global Ecology and Oceanography of Harmful Algal Blooms. *GEOHAB Synth. Open Sci. Meet.* **2014**, *30*, 12–21.
17. Park, M.G.; Kim, S.; Kim, H.S.; Myung, G.; Kang, Y.G.; Yih, W. First successful culture of the marine dinoflagellate *Dinophysis acuminata*. *Aquat. Microb. Ecol.* **2006**, *45*, 101–106. [CrossRef]
18. MacKenzie, L.; Beuzenberg, V.; Holland, P.; McNabb, P.; Selwood, A. Solid phase adsorption toxin tracking (SPATT): A new monitoring tool that simulates the biotoxin contamination of filter feeding bivalves. *Toxicon* **2004**, *44*, 901–918. [CrossRef] [PubMed]

19. Fux, E.; Bire, R.; Hess, P. Comparative accumulation and composition of lipophilic marine biotoxins in passive samplers and in mussels (*M. edulis*) on the West Coast of Ireland. *Harmful Algae* **2009**, *8*, 523–537. [CrossRef]
20. Pizarro, G.; Moroño, A.; Paz, P.; Franco, J.M.; Pazos, Y.; Reguera, B. Evaluation of Passive Samplers as a Monitoring Tool for Early Warning of Dinophysis Toxins in Shellfish. *Mar. Drugs* **2013**, *11*, 3823–3845. [CrossRef] [PubMed]

toxins MDPI

Review

Review of DSP Toxicity in Ireland: Long-Term Trend Impacts, Biodiversity and Toxin Profiles from a Monitoring Perspective

Rafael Salas * and Dave Clarke

Marine Environment and Food Safety, Marine Institute, Rinville, Oranmore, H91 R673 Galway, Ireland; dave.clarke@marine.ie

* Correspondence: Rafael.salas@marine.ie; Tel.: +353-91-387-241

Received: 17 December 2018; Accepted: 18 January 2019; Published: 22 January 2019

Abstract: The purpose of this work is to review all the historical monitoring data gathered by the Marine Institute, the national reference laboratory for marine biotoxins in Ireland, including all the biological and chemical data from 2005 to 2017, in relation to diarrheic shellfish poisoning (DSP) toxicity in shellfish production. The data reviewed comprises over 25,595 water samples, which were preserved in Lugol's iodine and analysed for the abundance and composition of marine microalgae by light microscopy, and 18,166 records of shellfish flesh samples, which were analysed using LC-MS/MS for the presence and concentration of the compounds okadaic acid (OA), dinophysistoxins-1 (DTX-1), dinophysistoxins-2 (DTX-2) and their hydrolysed esters, as well as pectenotoxins (PTXs). The results of this review suggest that DSP toxicity events around the coast of Ireland occur annually. According to the data reviewed, there has not been an increase in the periodicity or intensity of such events during the study period. Although the diversity of the *Dinophysis* species on the coast of Ireland is large, with 10 species recorded, the two main species associated with DSP events in Ireland are *D. acuta* and *D. acuminata*. Moreover, the main toxic compounds associated with these species are OA and DTX-2, but concentrations of the hydrolysed esters are generally found in higher amounts than the parent compounds in the shellfish samples. When *D. acuta* is dominant in the water samples, the DSP toxicity increases in intensity, and DTX-2 becomes the prevalent toxin. Pectenotoxins have only been analysed and reported since 2012, and these compounds had not been associated with toxic events in Ireland; however, in 2014, concentrations of these compounds were quantitated for the first time, and the data suggest that this toxic event was associated with an unusually high number of observations of *D. tripos* that year. The areas of the country most affected by DSP outbreaks are those engaging in long-line mussel (*Mytilus edulis*) aquaculture.

Keywords: dinophysis; DSP; toxins; OA; DTX-2; PTXs

Key Contribution: There were no clear trends with respect to the increase/decrease of DSP events in Ireland over the studied period. *D. acuminata* is generally the dominant species in the water samples; however, the highest DSP toxicity has been found in the years when *D. acuta* becomes dominant, affecting shellfish species not generally associated with DSP toxicity, such as king scallops and oysters. The dominance of these species also has a geographical component. *D. acuta* is more prevalent below 52.5° N latitude, above which *D. acuminata* becomes the most observed species. Because the analysis of PTXs commenced in 2012, concentrations of such toxins have rarely been found in shellfish tissues; however, in 2014, high levels of these toxins were found in shellfish corresponding with the largest number of observations of *D. tripos* in any year since such monitoring began. Another feature of DSP events in Ireland is that hydrolysed OA and DTX-2 esters are more prominent than the parent compounds in shellfish tissues. This causes an 'overwintering effect' of toxins during high toxicity years, where low concentrations of toxins, below the regulatory level, remain in the shellfish for longer periods of time, sometimes extending into the spring cycle.

1. Introduction

The study of marine biotoxins is an important area of scientific research that is mainly driven by poisoning incidents in humans who consume bivalves. Diarrheic shellfish poisoning (DSP) was first recorded in the Netherlands in the 1960s, when cases of a form of gastroenteritis linked to mussel consumption were identified [1,2]. In Japan, a similar event occurred in the late 1970s [3,4].

The recording of DSP toxicity events in Ireland and the rapid development of the shellfish industry seem to have taken place in parallel. One of the first DSP toxicity events ever recorded in Ireland took place in 1984, which coincided with the start of marine biotoxin monitoring. DSP toxins were first detected by using a DSP rat bioassay (1990–1996) [2], by which samples of hepatopancreas tissue from shellfish were orally fed to rats and the consistency of the resultant faeces was rated from dry to liquid. In the 1980s, only summer closures were enforced; however, in 1994, toxins were detected by LC-MS/MS outside of the months during which there was commonly believed to be a greater risk of toxic events. DSP toxicity (OA equivalents) in mussel hepatopancreas reached a high of 13.5 $\mu g \cdot g^{-1}$ in August of 1994, and dinophysistoxins-2 (DTX-2) concentrations remained above the regulatory limits until February of 1995 (>2 $\mu g \cdot g^{-1}$). This toxic episode was associated with high cell densities of *Dinophysis acuta* (20,000 cells$\cdot L^{-1}$) observed in Bantry Bay [5] and identified the need for a year-round biotoxin monitoring programme. The incident also highlighted that the rat bioassay was not a method fit for this purpose, because it was considered to be too subjective; as a result, the rat bioassay was eventually replaced by the more sensitive mouse bioassay.

The DSP mouse bioassay was used for several years (1997–2011) [3], but in 2000, chemical characterisation via LC-MS became more widely used [3,6]. In 2002, a hydrolysis step was introduced into the LC-MS/MS method to account for the total toxin equivalent of the main toxins and to allow for the detection of the acyl derivatives of okadaic acid (OA) and other toxins in that group [7]. During the 2000s, both the mouse bioassay and the LC-MS DSP method were run in parallel until the mouse bioassay was finally discontinued in 2011. Today, the European Union (EU) harmonised LC-MS/MS protocol [8] is used as the reference method. The main toxins responsible for DSP incidents in Ireland are OA [9], DTX-2, their hydrolysed esters [10] and the non-diarrheic pectenotoxin (PTX) group [6,11]. These polyether compounds are potent phosphatase inhibitors [12] that cause intestinal illness, except for PTXs, which are hepatotoxic [13]. In this work, only the chemical data produced through LC-MS/MS analysis from 2009 to 2017 for the OA and DTX-2 parent compounds and from 2011 to 2017 for their hydrolysed esters were used.

The phytoplankton monitoring programme commenced in 1986, and originally, the main interest was in counting the high biomass phytoplankton species only. It was believed that many cells were needed in a sample to produce shellfish toxicity. Only a limited number of species were counted per sample, and limited data were recorded about the sample and how it was collected. This continued until 1995, when the first phytoplankton database, 'Fytobase', was developed by the Marine Institute. Fytobase was the first Microsoft Access database, and it was a definite improvement from the previous system. It included a standardised phytoplankton species list and unlimited space for species entry. Additionally, sample data collection, including the methodology employed, sample depth, and latitude/longitude coordinates, were recorded.

In 2002, Fytobase was superseded by the Harmful Algal Blooms database (HABs). HABs was decommissioned in 2018 and replaced by a new Windows-based system, HABs2. This new system differs from the previous one in that it is a fully automated, digitalised platform, which allows the Marine Institute to publish phytoplankton results in close to real time, and it is fully open to the public. The phytoplankton results can be plotted over a timeline to show the trends of the main toxic species, and these can be compared against the toxin results for the same area. These figures can give near real-time information and serve as an early warning system of an impending toxic event for the shellfish industry.

The biological data used in this review were collected from all the shellfish and finfish production areas in Ireland between 2005 and 2017 as part of the monitoring programme. The datasets from this time period are much more comprehensive and reliable than previous ones, as the monitoring programme has been improving, culminating in the accreditation of the Utermöhl test method [14] in 2004 to the ISO standard of 17,025. The monitoring programme comprises samples from over 80–90 shellfish production sites weekly, although not all these sites are active year-round.

The data for the purpose of this study was organised into larger geographical regions rather than individual sites or bays along the coast in order to obtain realistic values and achieve some proportionality among the regions. The rationale for this was to be able to objectively compare the coastal areas that are not as heavily influenced by shellfish production. For example, the eastern region along the Irish Sea only accounts for eight production areas as compared with the 64 production areas in the western region.

The observations of *Dinophysis* spp. in the water column in Ireland typically occur in the summer months and in the thermally stratified waters along the shelf front [15] in all the coastal locations, particularly in the southern and southwestern areas. Here, the oceanography can be quite complex, as the continental shelf is less than 100 m deep and can be highly stratified in the summer. *Dinophysis* populations can develop quite quickly and be advected into bays by prevailing winds. This advection depends on the position of the shelf front [5]. This exchange can be accentuated due to the orientation of the bays in the southwest relative to the prevailing winds [16].

The average sea surface temperatures for the western and southern waters of Ireland range between 8–10 °C in the winter and 14–17 °C in the summer [17] and tend to be several degrees higher compared with the eastern waters due to the Gulf stream current modulating the temperatures in western Ireland. In the winter, the Irish coastal waters are well mixed, with no differences between the bottom and surface temperatures, but in the summer, as the waters stratify, there can be a 5–6 °C difference between the surface and the bottom [18]. It is in the area between the coastal mixed waters and stratified offshore waters marked by a tidal front that *Dinophysis* populations are found. The transport mechanism in the southern and southwestern regions is well studied and explained by the Irish Coastal Current (ICC) [19]. This is a strong jet-like fast current moving in a clockwise direction around the south and southwest of Ireland, and it can be modulated by the shelf front due to wind forcing [16]. This transport mechanism is believed to be essential to the delivery of *Dinophysis* into these bays [20].

2. Results

2.1. Phytoplankton Records from the HABs Database

Between 2005 and 2017, a total of 25,595 phytoplankton samples were analysed, containing 346,186 phytoplankton records, of which 5315 were *Dinophysis*. During this period, 10 different species of the genus *Dinophysis* were observed in the samples (Table 1), which is a consistent measure of the diversity of this genus in Irish waters. The most observed species, without a doubt, were *Dinophysis acuminata* and *Dinophysis acuta*. The third most observed species after that was *Dinophysis tripos*, followed by a small number of observations for *D. caudata*, *D. norvegica*, *D. hastata*, *D. fortii*, *D. ovum* and *D. odiosa* and only one record of *D. nasuta*.

Our data shows that the DSP outbreaks around the Irish coast fluctuated between years of high toxicity (1994 and 1995; 2000 and 2001; 2012, 2014 and 2015) and years of low or no toxicity (1997 and 1998; 2002, 2016 and 2017). The periods of high toxicity were associated with a high number of observations of *D. acuta* and *D. acuminata* and vice versa. Other *Dinophysis* species were also present in the water with *D. tripos*, which was the next most recorded species. Up to 10 different species of this genus were recorded by the monitoring programme during this period, albeit most of them only a handful of times, so their association to toxicity in Ireland is limited.

Table 1. Total number of observations of the *Dinophysis* species in Irish waters between 2005 and 2017 by geographical area (Note: *D. dens* is included here as synonym for *D. acuta*).

	Geographical Areas						
Species Name	**East**	**South East**	**South**	**South West**	**West**	**North West**	**Total Number of Observations**
Dinophysis acuminata	160	103	126	1417	737	555	3098
Dinophysis acuta	109	51	141	1241	277	119	1938
Dinophysis tripos	0	2	9	151	13	46	221
Dinophysis caudata	0	0	1	12	1	3	17
Dinophysis norvegica	3	3	0	4	0	0	10
Dinophysis odiosa	0	0	0	10	0	0	10
Dinophysis fortii	0	0	1	7	1	0	9
Dinophysis hastata	0	0	0	0	6	1	7
Dinophysis ovum	0	0	0	3	1	0	4
Dinophysis nasuta	0	0	1	0	0	0	1

Table 2 shows the normalised, estimated number of observations of *D. acuminata* and *D. acuta* from 1500 records in each geographical area. The southern region had the least total number of samples of all the areas during the studied period, with only 1500 samples collected between 2005 and 2017. The reason for this is that the southern region also had the smallest number of active sampling sites (5). Proportionally, 1937 samples were collected during the same period in the southwest, and 1621 samples were collected in the western region, which corresponded to an average of 40 and 32 samples per year, respectively (data not shown).

Table 2. Normalised data from 1500 samples per region.

Normalised, Estimated Number of Observations by Geographical Area			
Regions	*D. acuminata*	*D. acuta*	Ratio *D. acuminata*/*D. acuta*
East	134	91	0.68
Southeast	73	36	0.49
South	158	190	1.20
Southwest	345	288	0.83
West	196	73	0.37
Northwest	190	44	0.23

The data shows that the areas with the largest number of observations for both species were in the southern and southwestern regions in comparison to the Irish Sea (east and southeast) and the western and northwestern Atlantic areas. Moreover, the ratios between *D. acuminata* and *D. acuta* in the south and southwest were different than in other regions. In the northwestern and western regions, *D. acuminata* was clearly the most observed of the two species, with ratios of 4:1 and 5:1. In the east and southeast, this tendency was not as obvious, with *D. acuminata* still being the most dominant at ratios of 3:2 and 2:1, respectively. There was a much closer ratio of 4:3 in the southwestern region and a ratio favourable to *D. acuta* in the south (5:6). This seems to indicate that *D. acuta* has larger influence in the lower latitudes (below 52° north), while *D. acuminata* clearly dominates in the west, northwest, southeast and east above 52–52.5°. The data also showed an east to west axis, influenced by seasonal circulation patterns in the Celtic Sea, where the western Irish continental shelf follows a continuous anti-clockwise circulation pattern around the west of Ireland, which would support the idea that the *Dinophysis* species were moving from the south and towards the southwestern areas rather than towards the Southeast.

Figure 1 shows the overall patterns of the two main species in Ireland during the study period. *D. acuminata* appeared to be the dominant species most years, in 11 out of 13 years, but especially in 2005, 2012 and 2013, when the differences between the recorded species were quite significant. Interestingly, this pattern was reversed in 2014 and 2015, when the *D. acuta* records nearly double those of *D. acuminata*. This data agreed well with the toxin profile for the year, as DTX-2 was the principal toxin found in the shellfish. Moreover, although not shown in Figure 1, in 2014, *D. tripos* was also a dominant species, and it was recorded in 107 samples, which was significant taking into consideration that there have only been a total of 221 recorded samples for *D. tripos* since 2005. Thus, nearly 50% of all the records for *D. tripos* were observed in 2014, which coincides with the finding of quantifiable concentrations of pectenotoxins in shellfish in 2014 (data not shown here).

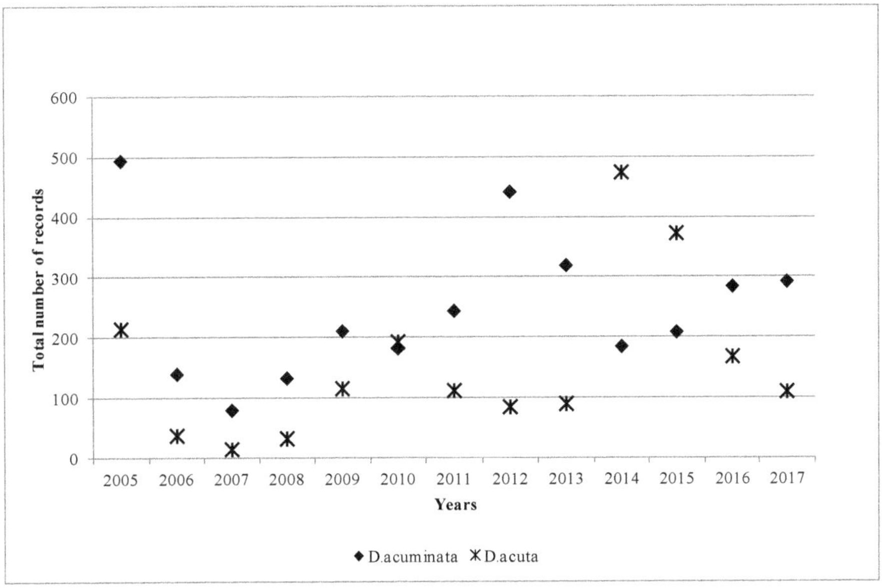

Figure 1. Number of observations of *Dinophysis acuminata* and *Dinophysis acuta* in Ireland by year between 2005 and 2017.

The seasonality trends of these three species are shown in Figure 2. *D. acuminata* appeared first in the water column and always peaked in the early summer months of June and July, while *D. acuta* generally appeared later in the summer and peaked a month later in July and August. *D. tripos* (data not shown in Figure 1) peaked in the late summer and early autumn months, in August and September, but the number of observations of this species was limited compared with the other two. Cells of these species were observed throughout the year, even during the winter months, but *D. acuminata*, in particular, can be observed in early spring, during March and April, in milder winters.

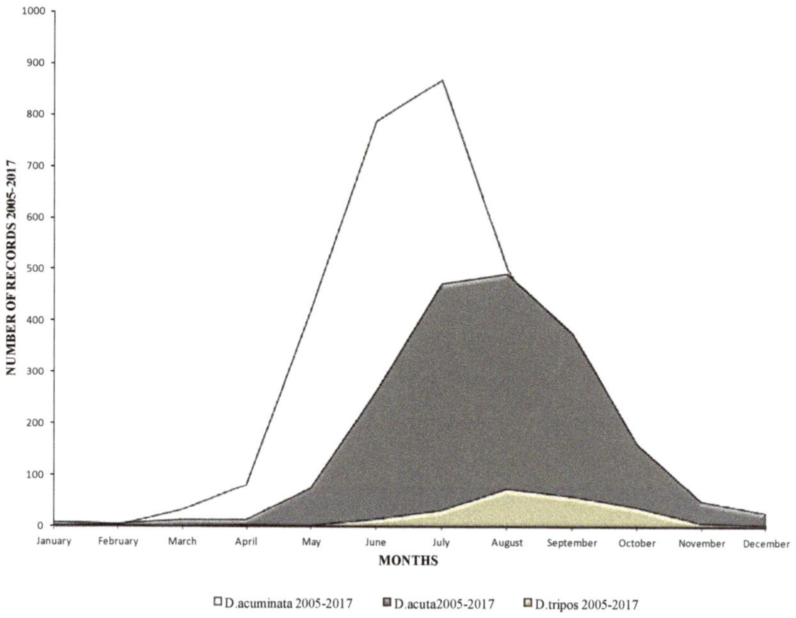

Figure 2. Seasonality of the species *D. acuta, D. acuminata* and *Dinophysis tripos* in Irish waters between 2005 and 2017.

2.2. Shellfish Toxicity Data

DTX-2 was detected on an annual basis, and it was often observed above regulatory levels, particularly in mussels in the southwest. In 1994, prolonged closures of mussel harvesting areas were observed for the first time throughout the winter months into 1995. The persistence of a toxic event over the winter period and the next spring was not unusual, and it was determined by the timing and intensity of the toxic event. Figure 3 shows the concentrations of DTX-2 above the regulatory levels for the period from 2009 to 2017. Most years, DTX-2 concentrations were observed in late summer to early autumn and remained in shellfish tissues into the next spring, generally below the regulatory levels. The high DTX-2 amounts in 2014 and 2015 can be explained by the shift in dominance in the water column from *D. acuminata* to *D. acuta* (see Figure 1), when the trends were reversed from previous years. During years of low toxicity (for example, 2012, 2013 and 2017), DTX-2 was no longer present in shellfish tissues, and this data agreed with evidence of a decline of *D. acuta* observations in the water samples. The highest observed DTX-2 concentration was 7.63 $\mu g \cdot g^{-1}$ in August 2010 in blue mussels (*Mytilus edulis*). DTX-2 above the regulatory levels has also been found in remainder tissues of king scallops (*Pecten maximus*) and Pacific oysters (*Crassostrea gigas*) (Table 3).

Table 3. Highest DSP toxin values observed in shellfish species in 2009–2017 expressed in $\mu g \cdot g^{-1}$.

Species Name	Common Name	DTX-2 $\mu g \cdot g^{-1}$	HY-DTX-2 $\mu g \cdot g^{-1}$	OA $\mu g \cdot g^{-1}$	HY-OA $\mu g \cdot g^{-1}$
Mytilus edulis	Blue mussel	7.63	7.84	1.74	2.77
Pecten maximus	King scallop	0.27	7.1	0.28	1.92
Crassostrea gigas	Pacific oyster	0.36	0.29	<RL	<RL
Cerastoderma edule	Common cockle	<RL	0.75	<RL	0.34
Spisula solida	Surf clam	<RL	0.16	<RL	0.22

HY = Hydrolysed ester of the parent toxin; OA = okadaic acid; RL = Regulatory Level.

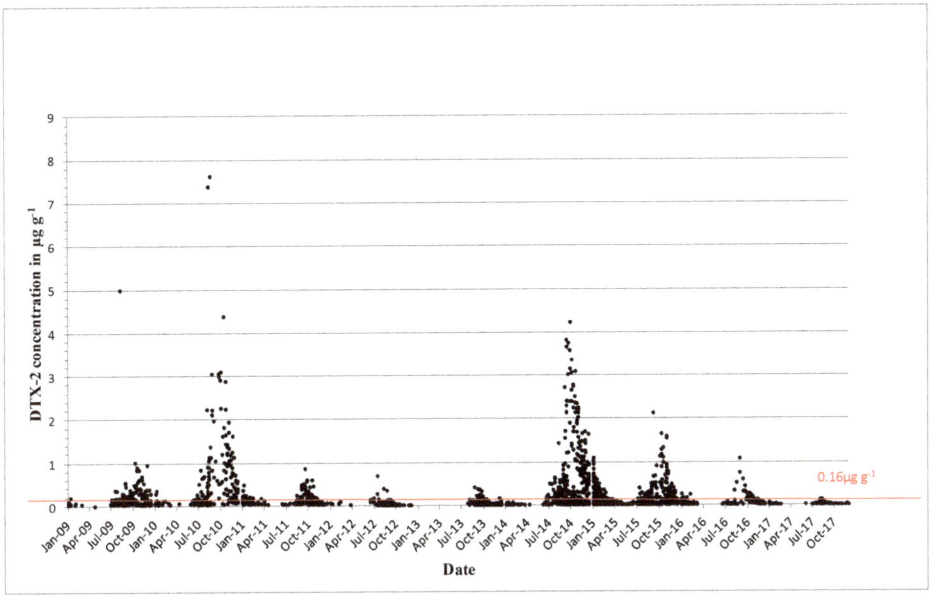

Figure 3. Dinophysistoxins-2 (DTX-2) quantifiable concentrations in μg·g^{-1} found in shellfish between 2009 and 2017. The red line equals the closure level for diarrheic shellfish poisoning (DSP) toxin equivalents 0.16 μg·g^{-1}.

DTX-2 acyl derivatives were also found in the shellfish samples (Figure 4), and their concentration in the shellfish tissues was generally higher than that in the parent compound in the same sample, as comparisons between Figures 3 and 4 would suggest. The highest ever observed hydrolysed DTX-2 concentrations were 7.84 μg·g^{-1} in blue mussels and 7.1 μg·g^{-1} in the remainder tissues of king scallops in October of 2014 (Table 3). Interestingly, DTX-2 esters have also been found to be above regulatory levels when converted back to their parent compounds through hydrolysis in samples of surf clams (*Spisula solida*) and cockles (*Cerastoderma edule*) (Table 3), even though the parent toxin has never been recorded for these species.

In summary, DTX-2 and its acyl derivatives were the predominant toxin compounds in Irish shellfish and were responsible for extended and prolonged closures during the winter months following the toxicity events when the highest concentrations (generally >1.5 μg·g^{-1}) occurred in September/October in extremely toxic years. When the highest concentrations (generally <1.5 μg·g^{-1}) occurred in August, this generally meant that there was no carry-over above the regulatory levels through to the following spring. Geographically, the southwest fared the worst with respect to harvesting closures, although this was not exclusive to this region, and other areas in the southern, western and northwestern coasts (Figure 5) were affected to a lesser extent. There is an inherent DSP toxicity bias towards the southwestern coast because of the predominance of longline rope mussel aquaculture production.

OA is found predominantly in blue mussels, where quantifiable concentrations were usually observed from May onwards and had generally increased to above the regulatory levels by June (Figure 6). These concentrations usually decreased below the regulatory levels by October–November, and the toxin was normally absent from the shellfish samples by the end of the year. The highest OA concentrations above the regulatory levels were observed in blue mussels (1.74 μg·g^{-1} in June 2012) and in the remainder tissues of king scallops, 0.28 μg·g^{-1} (Table 3). OA acyl derivatives were also present in shellfish (Figure 7) and followed the same concentration and seasonality patterns as the parent compound; however, acyl derivatives tended to stay longer in shellfish tissues during years of high toxicity. OA and its acyl derivative were predominant in the southwestern coast of Ireland (Figure 8).

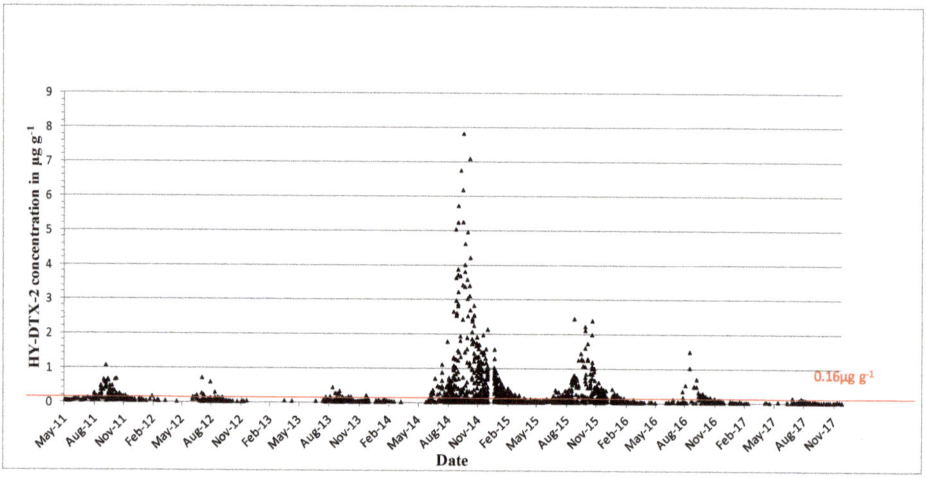

Figure 4. Hydrolysed DTX-2 quantifiable concentrations in $\mu g \cdot g^{-1}$ found in shellfish in 2011–2017. The red line equals the closure level for DSP toxin equivalents 0.16 $\mu g \cdot g^{-1}$.

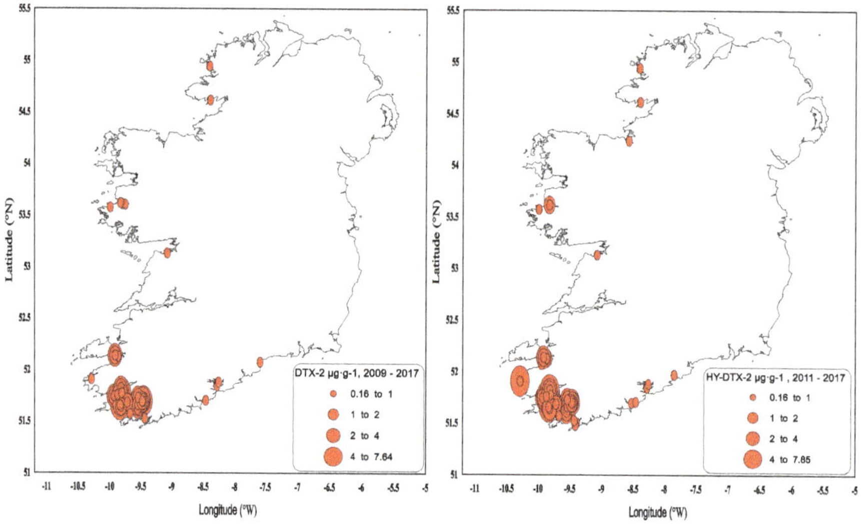

Figure 5. DTX-2 and hydrolysed DTX-2 values above the regulatory limit by geographical area in 2009–2017.

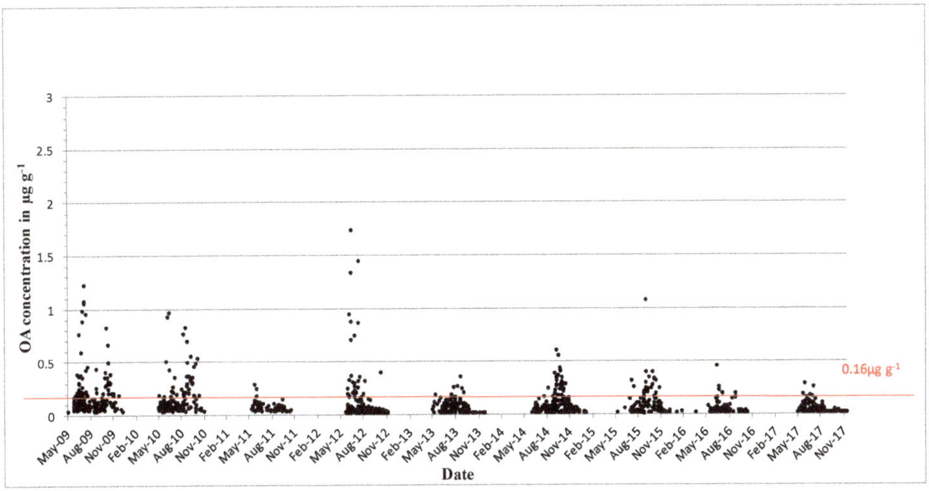

Figure 6. Quantifiable okadaic acid concentrations in μg·g^{-1} found in shellfish in 2009–2017. The red line equals the closure level for DSP toxin equivalents 0.16 μg·g^{-1}.

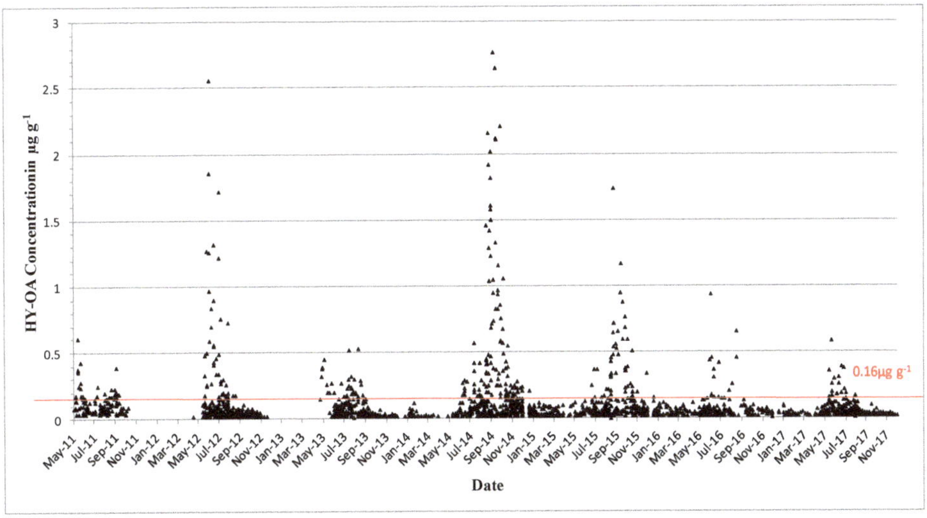

Figure 7. Hydrolysed okadaic acid quantifiable concentrations in μg·g^{-1} found in shellfish in 2011–2017. The red line equals the closure level for DSP toxin equivalents 0.16 μg·g^{-1}.

In summary, OA and its esters resulted in concentrations above the regulatory levels on an annual basis and generally occurred earlier in the year than DTX-2 and its esters. The presence of OA and its accumulation in shellfish was normally associated with the presence of *Dinophysis acuminata* cells in the water column.

Since 2012, the lipophilic method was modified to include the detection and quantification of PTX-1 and PTX-2, where the overall result is expressed as PTX equivalents μg·g^{-1} (Figure 9). Since the monitoring began, quantifiable concentrations were rarely seen, and no PTX equivalent values have been observed above the regulatory levels. The highest value observed to date was 0.13 μg·g^{-1} in the remainder tissues of king scallop. Interestingly, most of the quantified PTX equivalent values in the form of PTX-2 occurred in 2014 (from June–October). This coincided with high concentrations of DTX-2, DTX-2 esters and OA esters in shellfish, whilst PTX concentrations are recorded as being produced by *D. acuta*, *D. acuminata*, *D. fortii*, *D. caudata* and *D. norvegica*, and these phytoplankton species were occasionally observed in Irish waters. PTXs have more recently been thought to be produced by *D. tripos* [21,22], especially PTX-2. The 2014 data shows the largest number observations of *D. tripos* recorded since 2005 and the highest cell densities. The data strongly supports that *D. tripos* may have been responsible for PTXs being recorded in Irish shellfish samples for the first time since the monitoring of the PTX group began.

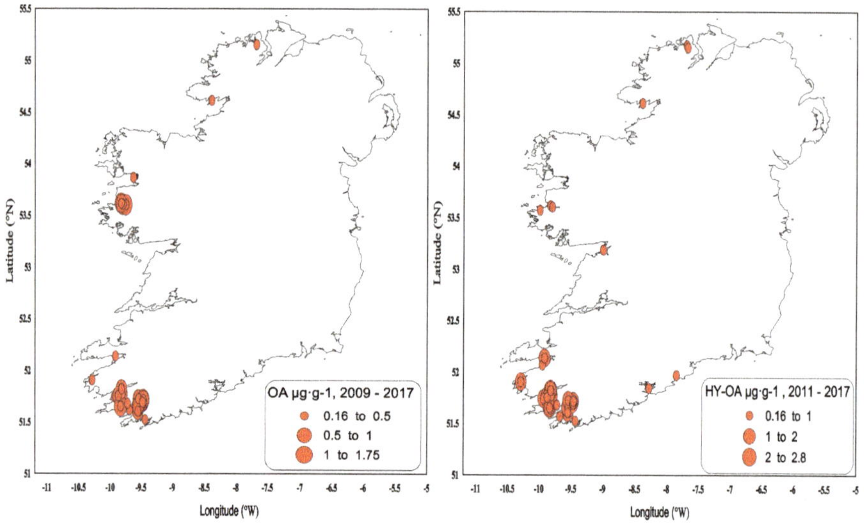

Figure 8. OA and hydrolysed OA values above the regulatory limit by geographical area in 2009–2017.

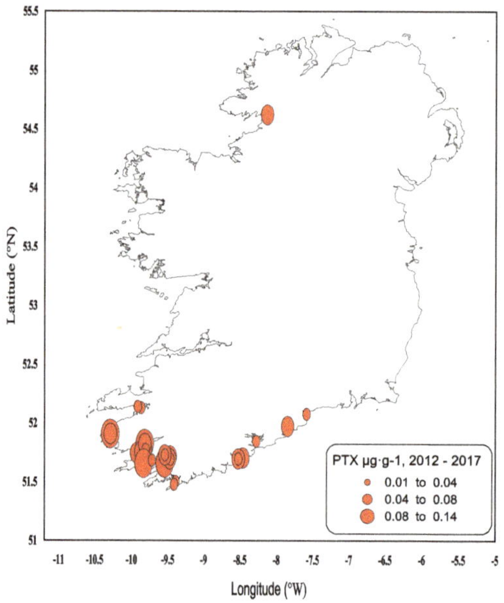

Figure 9. Quantifiable Pectenotoxin (PTX Equivalents) concentrations in shellfish in 2012–2017.

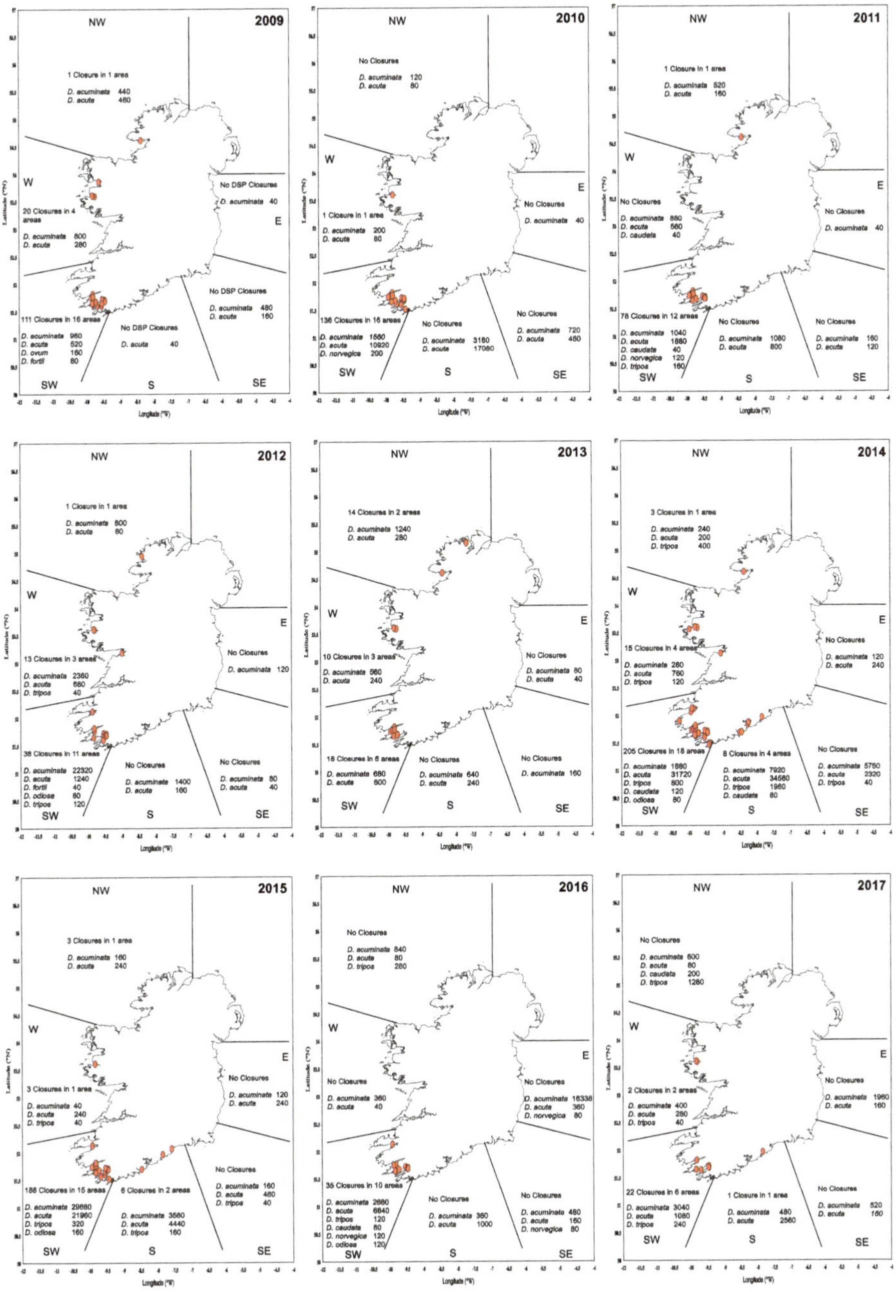

Figure 10. DSP Closure plots (2009–2017) by geographical area, *Dinophysis* diversity and maximum cell concentrations (cells·L^{-1}). Red dot (•) indicates a closure in a production area due to DSP detected above regulatory levels. NW: northwest; W: west; E: east; SW: southwest; S: south; and SE: southeast.

Maps of closures for harvesting per region during the period of 2009–2017 (Figure 10) suggest that the largest number of closures due to DSP incidents occurred in the southwest. In particular, the periods of 2009–2010 and 2014–2015 were exceptionally difficult, with protracted closures and high toxicity. These periods were related to the relative dominance of *D. acuta* in the water column, except for 2009, when more *D. acuminata* observations were made. The toxicity in these two periods showed toxic 'overwintering' (Table 4), especially in 2015 with 56 closures in January, 16 in February and 3 in March. During this time, there were no closures in the eastern and southeastern regions, and a small number of closures in the south, west and northwest. Figure 11 shows the total number of harvesting closures and the highest toxin OA equivalent recorded per year. As can be observed, 2014 and 2015 have been the worst two consecutive years for DSP toxins in Ireland since 2009 and 2010.

Table 4. Number of harvesting closures by region.

Years	Southwest											
	Jan.	Feb.	Mar.	Apr.	May	Jun.	Jul.	Aug.	Sep.	Oct.	Nov.	Dec.
2009	-	-	-	-	-	14	15	16	25	22	16	3
2010	2	-	-	-	4	13	16	28	15	20	28	10
2011	-	-	-	-	7	12	2	13	21	19	2	-
2012	-	-	-	-	-	12	15	9	2	-	-	-
2013	-	-	-	-	-	-	4	8	6	-	-	-
2104	-	-	-	-	-	10	12	23	49	34	41	36
2015	56	16	3	-	-	1	8	16	20	22	30	16
2016	4	-	-	-	-	8	4	5	6	8	-	-
2017	-	-	-	-	3	10	5	3	-	-	-	-
Years	West											
	Jan.	Feb.	Mar.	Apr.	May	Jun.	Jul.	Aug.	Sep.	Oct.	Nov.	Dec.
2009	-	-	-	-	-	5	13	2	-	-	-	-
2010	-	-	-	-	-	1	-	-	-	-	-	-
2011	-	-	-	-	-	-	-	-	-	-	-	-
2012	-	-	-	-	-	3	8	1	1	-	-	-
2013	-	-	-	-	-	-	1	6	3	-	-	-
2104	-	-	-	-	-	-	-	2	6	5	2	-
2015	-	-	-	-	-	-	-	3	-	-	-	-
2016	-	-	-	-	-	-	-	-	-	-	-	-
2017	-	-	-	-	-	-	-	2	-	-	-	-
Years	Northwest											
	Jan.	Feb.	Mar.	Apr.	May	Jun.	Jul.	Aug.	Sep.	Oct.	Nov.	Dec.
2009	-	-	-	-	-	-	-	-	1	-	-	-
2010	-	-	-	-	-	-	-	-	-	-	-	-
2011	-	-	-	-	-	-	1	-	-	-	-	-
2012	-	-	-	-	-	-	-	1	-	-	-	-
2013	-	-	-	-	-	7	3	4	-	-	-	-
2104	-	-	-	-	-	-	-	1	2	-	-	-
2015	-	-	-	-	-	-	-	-	-	-	-	-
2016	-	-	-	-	-	-	-	-	-	-	-	-
2017	-	-	-	-	-	-	-	-	-	-	-	-

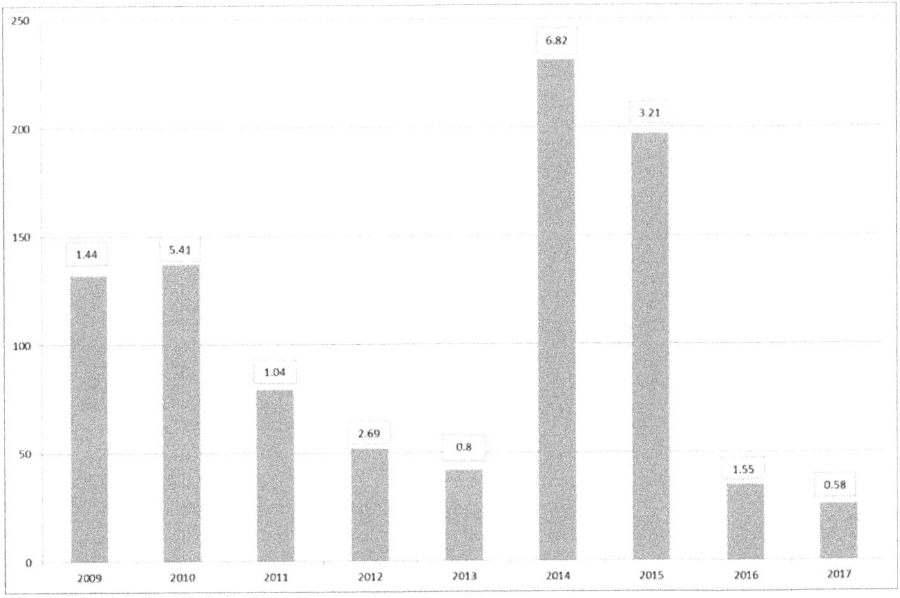

Figure 11. Number of harvesting closures due to DSP toxicity per year and maximum OA equivalents in each year in $\mu g \cdot g^{-1}$ per year.

3. Discussion

There is no doubt about the impact of the *Dinophysis* species and their associated toxins on the shellfish industry in Ireland over the years. The *Dinophysis* species, even at small cell concentrations in the water, can cause prolonged closures for the harvesting of bivalves in many areas of the country. The two main species associated with toxic events in Ireland are *Dinophysis acuminata* and *Dinophyis acuta*, although, as this review suggests, more diversity has been observed in the sampling areas, and in 2014, a toxic event in the south and southwest of the country also included another species, *Dinophysis tripos*, which was associated with the highest quantifiable concentration of pectenotoxins recorded. Pectenotoxins in Ireland have only been measured since 2012, and therefore, there is limited data for comparison, so this could be a case of increased monitoring rather than an increase in HAB events. In any case, future monitoring data will allow us to review this trend appropriately. This also highlights the importance of Phytoplankton monitoring, which through the proper identification of toxin-producing algae, can act as a valid warning system for the different toxin groups.

In 2014 and 2015, the biological data show a shift from *D. acuminata*-dominated samples to *D. acuta* domination, and this signalled a shift in the intensity and type of toxic compounds found in the shellfish for these years. DTX-2 became the dominant toxin in the shellfish, and this biological shift brought about the highest such toxin levels ever found in shellfish samples in Ireland.

An interesting aspect of DSP episodes in Ireland is the 'overwintering' effect of toxins, especially in mussels, where there is a carry-over of toxins from one year into the next. Generally, these amounts are well below the regulatory level as winter approaches and tend to disappear completely during the spring bloom. This effect is more pronounced in the hydrolysed esters both for OA and DTX-2 than in the parent compound. DTX-1 is not a concern in Ireland, it has never been measured in any quantifiable amounts by LC-MS. Although we observe *Prorocentrum lima* in our samples, this benthic dinoflagellate has never been known to cause any toxic events in Irish waters.

DSP toxins are widely distributed in the country, as our harvesting closure plots suggest, but are particularly prevalent in the southwest. There are various reasons for this disparity between the regions; the prevalent oceanographic and weather conditions in the southwest and the movement of the Irish Coastal Current clockwise around the south and southwest of Ireland allow for dinoflagellates to aggregate inside the bays. Moreover, *D. acuta* is the dominant *Dinophysis* species in the south and southwest coasts compared to other areas, and it is more toxic than *D. acuminata*. Ultimately, longline rope mussels aquaculture are the most affected production areas in Ireland.

Mussels seem to be a good biological toxin indicator in monitoring programmes, as they accumulate high levels of toxins, and according to our data, it appears to depurate slower than other bivalves. In other areas, for example the southeast (razor clams) and east (bottom mussels, razor clams, clams and cockles), there were no closures over this period. So, even after taking into consideration the differences in the number of sampling sites and shellfish species grown in the different regions, we can conclude with certainty that the southwest is the most affected region for DSP harvesting closures in the country.

In conclusion, this review indicates that DSP is a prevalent toxin in shellfish that occurs on a regular basis in Ireland and causes huge economic loss to the industry; however, harvesting closures are required to protect human health. The data do not indicate a trend towards an increase or decrease of DSP events, but rather point more towards a cyclical trend of years with high toxicity interspersed with years with low toxicity, which can be clearly tracked through biological observations in terms of number of observations. The years with the highest toxicity are related to *D. acuta* dominance in the water column rather than *D. acuminata*, although *D. acuminata* is also involved in toxic episodes regularly. Sometimes, there is a combined effect of both species, especially in the southwest, where the ratio between these two species is similar. *D. acuta*, however, appears to be the more prominent of the species in the southwestern and southern region up to the 52–52.5° N in an east–west axis, with *D. acuminata* being dominant above this latitude in the east (Irish Sea) and west of the northwest region (Atlantic area), but *D. acuminata* is significantly stronger in the west of the northwest region. The aforementioned pectenotoxin event is probably an effect of increased monitoring and surveillance by the monitoring programme rather than an increase in HAB events.

4. Materials and Methods

4.1. Biotoxin National Monitoring Programme

4.1.1. Sample Collection, Delivery and Lab Receipt

Samples of different species of marine bivalve molluscs are collected from aquaculture-classified production areas on a regular basis. The frequency is dependent on a number of parameters and can be increased or decreased due to the type of shellfish species, the time of year, the presence of known causative toxin producing phytoplanktonic species in the same or adjacent areas and the observation of quantifiable toxin concentrations observed in other shellfish species within the same production area. Generally, the frequency is weekly for mussels (*Mytilus edulis*), fortnightly for king scallops (*Pecten maximus*) and monthly for all other species (pacific oyster/*Crassostrea gigas*, flat native oyster/*Ostrea edulis*, surf clam/*Spisula solida*, razor clam/*Ensis siliqua* and cockles/*Cerastoderma edule*).

The majority of mussels produced in Ireland are done so through suspended longline rope mussel cultivation in the southwest and west. Bottom mussel cultivation also occurs to a lesser extent in a number of production areas in each of the different geographical regions. Oyster production is mainly via mesh bags on trestle tables and is mainly located along the southern, western and northwestern coasts. Razor clams are dredged mainly in the east and southeast. Dredged king scallops from classified production areas are mainly seasonal (October–March) in the southwest and harvested to a lesser extent in the west and northwest. There is a large, offshore scallop industry all around the coast of Ireland, as these scallops do not originate from classified production areas; the results from this dataset have been excluded from this review.

A minimum number of individuals of specific sizes for each shellfish species are collected, bagged, labelled and submitted to arrive at the Marine Institute laboratories the day after sample collection. Upon laboratory receipt, the sample details are logged into the HABs database, the shellfish are dissected to obtain the whole flesh (except scallop species) from each individual, which are pooled together and homogenised to obtain a whole flesh tissue homogenate weighing between 100–120 g. The sample homogenate is forwarded for toxin extraction and analysis, usually on the day of laboratory receipt. On occasions where analysis is not possible, the sample homogenate is either stored, refrigerated or frozen depending on when the analysis can be conducted. Scallop species originating from classified production areas are subjected to a different testing regime, in which the following tissues are dissected and pooled together from three different compartments: gonad (roe), posterior adductor muscle and the remainder tissues.

4.1.2. LC-MS/MS Methodology

The method described here involves sample extraction with 100% methanol. A 2 g subsample of homogenate is twice extracted with 100% methanol (2 × 9 mL) and centrifuged. Free OA, free DTX-1, free DTX-2, PTX-1 and PTX-2 are determined by reverse phase liquid chromatography (LC) coupled with mass spectrometry (MS). A gradient method is applied to separate and elute the toxins in a single chromatographic run. A number of esters of the OA group are also analysed in this method, including 7-O-acyl esters and diol-esters. To determine these esters, an alkaline hydrolysis step is performed from 1 mL of the methanolic extract prior to analysis by LC-MS/MS. The step involves the addition of 125 µl NaOH, heating in a water bath to 76 °C for 20 min, and the addition of 125 µl HCl. This hydrolysis step converts any esters of the OA group toxins back to the original parent toxins OA, DTX-1 and DTX-2, which can then be quantitatively measured. Both pre and post hydrolysis extracts are analysed by LC-MS/MS. In recent years, the Marine Institute has validated the method to run on ultra-performance (UP) LC-MS/MS instruments. The UPLC tandem mass spectrometry method has been optimised and adapted from the methodology developed and validated by Dr. Arjen Gerssen [8]. The major changes to the published method are that the column used in this method is an Acquity BEH C18 2.1 × 100mm 1.75µm particle size, and the mobile phase B is not pH adjusted to 11. These changes were introduced to improve peak shape and repeatability.

4.1.3. Sample Results and Reporting

The lipophilic results for the DSP toxin group are usually available the day after sample receipt and are published on the HABs website (https://webapps.marine.ie/habs). The DSP results are reported as total OA equivalents in $\mu g \cdot g^{-1}$ total tissue, which is the overall calculated hydrolysed result for OA and DTX-2 parent compounds. To calculate the results, a toxin equivalence factor of 0.6 is applied to DTX-2, a correction factor based on the % recovery of OA in certified reference material is applied to OA, and a dilution factor of 1.25 is applied to the calculation due to the hydrolysis step conducted on the sample.

For scallop samples, individual total OA equivalent results are reported for the individual dissected tissues: the gonad (roe), posterior adductor muscle and remainder (including the hepatopancreas) tissues. A calculated result for the whole tissue is also reported for scallop samples.

4.1.4. Chemistry Data Review and Result Interpretation

For the purposes of this review, the data was extracted from the Marine Institute's Harmful Algal Blooms (HABs) SQL Server database, which been in operation since 2001 and was used to record both bioassay (up to 2011) and chemical results for all the toxin groups for all the samples submitted for biotoxin analysis. The SQL queries were designed and run through a Microsoft Access front-end application developed in-house. For the purposes of this review, only the results from samples submitted from classified production areas have been reviewed and presented here. Sample results from offshore areas have been excluded from this review.

In total, for the years 2009–2017, 129,324 records were retrieved from HABs, where each record is an individual analysis for one of the compounds within the DSP group of toxins. This number of records equates to all the DSP analyses conducted on the 18,166 samples submitted in this time frame, which is just over 2000 samples per annum tested for DSP. The records from 2009–2017 were reviewed for OA, DTX-1 and DTX-2. Records for the esters of these parent compounds were available from May 2011–2017. For the PTX group, 33,699 records were retrieved, which equates to 11,079 samples analysed for PTX-1 and PTX-2, expressed as PTX equivalents.

The records were reviewed to observe the seasonal occurrence and geographic distribution of the individual DSP isomers. All the toxin concentrations are expressed as $\mu g \cdot g^{-1}$, and only quantifiable concentrations have been plotted in our figures. Any samples assigned values of <limit of detection or <limit of quantification have not been included in this review.

From an overall monitoring perspective and to assess the number of sites closed, data were also extracted from HABs to show the total number of samples that were above the regulatory levels, the site and species being assigned a 'closed status', and their geographic region during 2009–2017 to observe if the number of closures were increasing over this time period. These closure records only relate to the presence of DSP above the regulatory levels (>0.16 $\mu g \cdot g^{-1}$ total OA equivalents) and do not include the closures in place during 2009–2017 attributed to the presence of other toxin groups Azaspiracid shellfish poisoning (AZP), Paralytic Shellfish poisoning (PSP) and Amnesic shellfish poisoning (ASP).

4.2. *Phytoplankton National Monitoring Programme in Ireland*

4.2.1. Sample Collection, Transport and Delivery

Water samples are collected weekly for phytoplankton analysis in all shellfish production areas around the country. The Sea Fisheries Protection Agency (SFPA) is the governmental agency responsible for the coordination of sampling in these areas.

The samples are collected using a variety of methods, depending on the sampling site, tides and the type of shellfish grown in the area. Our preferred sampling method is the integrated sample using Lund tubes, but other techniques are also allowed, such as surface and discrete depth sampling using Niskin bottles. Generally, areas growing mussels on longline ropes use integrated sampling to sample the whole water column whereas in tidal sites with shallow depths and growing shellfish on the seabed, a surface or discrete depth sample is more pertinent at high tide. The Marine Institute furnishes samplers with all the required materials for collecting samples and training them on how best to take these and how to preserve, label and transport them safely. The Marine Institute in Ireland receives the samples generally one day after the sample collection.

4.2.2. Sample Analysis

The Irish Phytoplankton programme uses 25 mL volume sedimentation chambers for water sample analysis, using the Utermöhl test method [14]. At least 12 h of settlement is necessary for this volume before the analysis commences. The Marine Institute uses inverted light microscopy with a range of objectives and optical properties to identify and enumerate the species found.

The full phytoplankton community analysis is carried out in over 40 sampling sites for a total of 85, covering all the bays around the country. The other 40–45 samples are analysed for toxic only species and the presence/absence of non-toxic ones. This means that all the toxic species, including all the *Dinophysis* genera, are identified in all the samples.

4.2.3. Sample Results and Reporting

The samples are analysed within a day of sample settlement, and the results are reported regularly in our publicly available Harmful Algal Bloom (HAB) database. The results are available online within the same day of analysis. The cell densities are reported in cells per litre, and the genus *Dinophysis* is identified to the species level.

4.2.4. Harmful Algal Bloom (HAB) Database Phytoplankton Data Extraction

The HAB database was commissioned in November 2002, and for this review, the data from the period of 2005 to the end of 2017 was used. There is previous phytoplankton data available for Ireland in different formats before this date, going as far back as 1985 in previous databases.

The database was queried through Microsoft Access software and exported to Microsoft Excel spreadsheets. This review used data from 25,595 samples analysed and 346,186 species recorded during this period, 5980 of which were *Dinophysis* spp.

In order to review all the data, the country was divided into different geographical areas: east, southeast, south, southwest, west and northwest in a clockwise direction instead of studying individual sites or bays.

The eastern region extends to the north at Carlingford Lough (Cranfield House) in the frontier between the Republic and Northern Ireland in the Irish Sea, extends south to just above Wexford Harbour and includes the counties of Louth, Dublin and Meath. The southeast region starts at Cahore Point in Wexford bay and extend south towards the Celtic Sea to Wexford harbour, Rosslare, Waterford Harbour and Dungarvan to Helvick Head. The southern region extends from Helvick Head in Waterford to the west to Beacon Point to the Baltimore production area. This is mainly South County Cork including Youghal Bay, Cork Harbour, Oysterhaven, Kinsale and Roscarberry. The southwestern region starts in Baltimore and includes the southwest of Ireland, Counties Cork, Kerry and ends at Ballylongford. The western region starts at the Shannon Estuary in County Clare and extends northwards to Bellmullet Head at Dunanieran Point in Broadhaven North. The northwestern region commences here in North Mayo and extends northwards and eastwards to Lough Foyle in County Derry, on the border with Northern Ireland.

The biological data shown here has been normalised to account for the differences in the number of sites per geographical area, the sampling frequency and the number of years that samples have been collected. The best sites collect samples weekly all year-round and have been active since 2005, the starting point of our historical review. These conditions are not met by all the sites as these have a tendency to change overtime, where new sites start operating and others discontinue after many years.

The east (8 sites), southeast (8 sites) and south (7 sites) have only a small number of production areas compared with the southwest (46 sites), west (60 sites) and northwest (38 sites). So, only the top sampling sites (5–10 sites) for each region, based on the conditions above, were chosen to compare the total number of observations and the ratios of *D. acuminata* and *D. acuta* for each area.

To make this comparison, we first calculated the total number of samples per site by multiplying the average number of samples per year by the total number of years. The sum of all the samples collected over this period in the southern region sites was 1500, the lowest number in all the regions. The rule of three was used to calculate the total number of observations of *D. acuminata* and *D. acuta* in each region by multiplying 1500 by the total number of observations and dividing by the total number of samples for that region. Then, the ratio between the species was calculated using these values.

Author Contributions: R.S. was the main writer and editor of the paper. He was also involved in the data extraction, the harvesting of the original data, the investigation, the analysis of all the biological data and the creation of the figures and tables for the biological data. D.C. was involved in the data harvesting, the investigation of all the chemistry data, the writing of the Materials and Methods and Results Sections pertaining to all the chemistry data and the creation of the map surfer plots and chemistry figures.

Funding: This research received no external funding.

Acknowledgments: The authors wish to acknowledge the Marine Institute staff, students and their associated contractors, past and present, who have been affiliated and involved with the testing of both shellfish and water samples for the National Monitoring Programme for Biotoxins. The authors also acknowledge the samplers, producers, processors and the relevant agencies and authorities that have been involved in the sampling and the submitting of samples for these programmes.

Conflicts of Interest: The authors declare no conflicts of interest.

References

1. Kat, M. The occurrence of Prorocentrum species and coincidental gastointestinal illness of mussel consumers. In *Toxic Dinoflagellate Blooms, Developments in Marine Biology*; Taylor, D.L., Seliger, H.H., Eds.; Elsevier/North-Holland: New York, NY, USA, 1979; Volume 1, pp. 215–220.
2. Kat, M. *Dinophysis acuminata* blooms in the Dutch coastal area related to diarrhetic mussel poisoning in the Dutch Waddensea. *Sarsia* **1983**, *68*, 81–84.
3. Yasumoto, T.; Oshima, Y.; Yamaguchi, M. Occurrence of a new type of shellfish poisoning in the Tohoku District. *Bull. Jpn. Soc. Sci. Fish* **1978**, *44*, 1249–1255. [CrossRef]
4. Yasumoto, T.; Oshima, Y.; Sugawara, W.; Fukuyo, Y.; Oguri, H.; Igarashi, T.; Fujita, N. Identification of *Dinophysis fortii* as the causative organism of diarrhetic shellfish poisoning. *Bull. Jpn. Soc. Sci. Fish* **1980**, *46*, 1045–1411. [CrossRef]
5. McMahon, T.; Silke, J.; Nixon, E.; Taffe, B.; Nolan, A.; McGovern, E.; Doyle, J. Seasonal variation in diarrhetic shellfish toxins in mussels from the southwest coast of Ireland in 1994. In *Irish Marine Science 1995;* Keegan, B.F., O'Connor, R., Eds.; Galway University Press: Galway, Ireland, 1995; pp. 417–432.
6. Yasumoto, T.; Murata, M.; Oshima, Y.; Sano, M.; Matsumoto, G.K.; Clardy, J. Diarrhetic shellfish toxins. *Tetrahedron* **1985**, *41*, 1019–1025. [CrossRef]
7. Quilliam, M.A.; Hess, P.; Dell' Aversano, C. Recent developments in the analysis of phycotoxins by liquid chromatography–mass spectrometry. In *Mycotoxins and Phycotoxins in Perspective at the Turn of the Millennium*; De Koe, W.J., Samson, R.A., van Egmond, H.P., Gilbert, J., Sabino, M., Eds.; Wageningen Academic Publishers: Wageningen, The Netherlands, 2002; pp. 383–392.
8. Gerssen, P.P.J.; Mulder, M.A.; McElhinney, J.B. Liquid chromatography–tandem mass spectrometry method for the detection of marine lipophilic toxins under alkaline conditions. *J. Chromatogr. A* **2009**, *9*, 1421–1430. [CrossRef] [PubMed]
9. Murata, M.; Shimatani, M.; Sugitani, H.; Oshima, Y.; Yasumoto, T. Isolation and structural elucidation of the causative toxin of the diarrhetic shellfish poisoning. *Bull. Jpn. Soc. Sci. Fish* **1982**, *48*, 549–552. [CrossRef]
10. Hu, T.; Marr, J.; de Freitas, A.S.W.; Quilliam, M.A.; Walter, J.A.; Wright, J.L.C.; Pleasance, S. New diol esters isolated from cultures of the dinoflagellate *Prorocentrum lima* and *Prorocentrum concavum*. *J. Nat. Prod.* **1992**, *55*, 1631–1637. [CrossRef]
11. Yasumoto, T.; Murata, M.; Oshima, Y.; Matsumoto, K.; Clardy, J. Diarrhetic shellfish poisoning. In *Seafood Toxins, ACS Symposium Series*; Ragelis, P., Ed.; American Chemical Society: Washington, DC, USA, 1984; pp. 207–214.
12. Bialojan, C.; Takai, A. Inhibitory effect of a marine-sponge toxin, okadaic acid, on protein phosphatases. Specificity and kinetics. *Biochem. J.* **1988**, *256*, 283–290. [CrossRef]
13. Draisci, R.; Lucentini, L.; Mascioni, A. *Seafood and Freshwater Toxins: Pharmacology, Physiology, and Detection*; Botana, L.M., Ed.; Marcel Dekker, Inc.: New York, NY, USA, 2000; pp. 289–324.
14. Utermöhl, H. Zur Vervollkomnung der quantitativen phytoplankton-Methodik. *Mitt. Int. Ver. Limnol.* **1958**, *9*, 1–38.
15. Raine, R.; O'Mahoney, J.; McMahon, T.; Roden, C. Hydrography and phytoplankton of waters off South-west Ireland. *Estuar. Coast. Shelf Sci.* **1990**, *30*, 579–592. [CrossRef]
16. Edwards, A.; Jones, K.; Graham, J.M.; Griffiths, C.R.; MacDougall, N.; Patching, J.P.; Richard, J.M.; Raine, R. Transient Coastal Upwelling and Water Circulation in Bantry. *Estuar. Coast. Shelf Sci.* **1996**, *42*, 213–230. [CrossRef]
17. Elliott, A.J.; Clarke, T. Seasonal stratification in the northwest European shelf seas. *Cont. Shelf Res.* **1991**, *11*, 467–492. [CrossRef]
18. Raine, R.; McMahon, T. Physical dynamics on the continental shelf off southwestern Ireland and their influence on coastal phytoplankton blooms. *Cont. Shelf Res.* **1998**, *18*, 883–914. [CrossRef]
19. Fernand, L.; Nolan, G.D.; Raine, R.; Chambers, C.E.; Dye, S.R.; White, M.; Brown, J. The Irish coastal current: A seasonal jet-like circulation. *Cont. Shelf Res.* **2006**, *26*, 1775–1793. [CrossRef]
20. Raine, R.; McDermott, G.; Silke, J.; Lyons, K.; Nolan, G.; Cusack, C. A simple short range model for the prediction of harmful algal events in the bays of southwestern Ireland. *J. Mar. Syst.* **2010**, *83*, 150–157. [CrossRef]

21. Rodriguez, F.; Escalera, L.; Reguera, B.; Rial, P.; Riobó, P.; de Jesús da Silva, T. Morphological variability, toxinology and genetics of the dinoflagellate *Dinophysis tripos* (Dinophysiaceae, Dinophysiales). *Harmful Algae* **2012**, *13*, 26–33. [CrossRef]
22. Fabro, E.; Almandoz, G.O.; Ferrario, M.; Tillmann, U.; Cembella, A.; Krock, B. Distribution of *Dinophysis* species and their association with lipophilic phycotoxins in plankton from the Argentine Sea. *Harmful Algae* **2016**, *59*, 31–41. [CrossRef] [PubMed]

toxins

MDPI

Article

Dinophysis acuta in Scottish Coastal Waters and Its Influence on Diarrhetic Shellfish Toxin Profiles

Sarah C. Swan [1,*], Andrew D. Turner [2], Eileen Bresnan [3], Callum Whyte [1], Ruth F. Paterson [1], Sharon McNeill [1], Elaine Mitchell [1] and Keith Davidson [1]

1 Scottish Association for Marine Science, Scottish Marine Institute, Oban, Argyll PA37 1QA, UK; callum.whyte@sams.ac.uk (C.W.); ruthflo.paterson@gmail.com (R.F.P.); sharon.mcneill@sams.ac.uk (S.M.); elaine.mitchell@sams.ac.uk (E.M.); keith.davidson@sams.ac.uk (K.D.)

2 Centre for Environment, Fisheries & Aquaculture Science, The Nothe, Barrack Road, Weymouth, Dorset DT4 8UB, UK; andrew.turner@cefas.co.uk

3 Marine Scotland Science, Marine Laboratory, 375 Victoria Road, Aberdeen AB11 9DB, UK; eileen.bresnan@gov.scot

* Correspondence: sarah.swan@sams.ac.uk; Tel.: +44-(0)1631-559-000

Received: 21 August 2018; Accepted: 26 September 2018; Published: 28 September 2018

Abstract: Diarrhetic shellfish toxins produced by the dinoflagellate genus *Dinophysis* are a major problem for the shellfish industry worldwide. Separate species of the genus have been associated with the production of different analogues of the okadaic acid group of toxins. To evaluate the spatial and temporal variability of *Dinophysis* species and toxins in the important shellfish-harvesting region of the Scottish west coast, we analysed data collected from 1996 to 2017 in two contrasting locations: Loch Ewe and the Clyde Sea. Seasonal studies were also undertaken, in Loch Ewe in both 2001 and 2002, and in the Clyde in 2015. *Dinophysis acuminata* was present throughout the growing season during every year of the study, with blooms typically occurring between May and September at both locations. The appearance of *D. acuta* was interannually sporadic and, when present, was most abundant in the late summer and autumn. The Clyde field study in 2015 indicated the importance of a temperature front in the formation of a *D. acuta* bloom. A shift in toxin profiles of common mussels (*Mytilus edulis*) tested during regulatory monitoring was evident, with a proportional decrease in okadaic acid (OA) and dinophysistoxin-1 (DTX1) and an increase in dinophysistoxin-2 (DTX2) occurring when *D. acuta* became dominant. Routine enumeration of *Dinophysis* to species level could provide early warning of potential contamination of shellfish with DTX2 and thus determine the choice of the most suitable kit for effective end-product testing.

Keywords: *Dinophysis*; HAB monitoring; DSP toxins; aquaculture; shellfish toxicity; human health; time-series; seasonality; Scotland

Key Contribution: Long-term variation in seasonality and abundance of *Dinophysis* spp.; association with specific toxins in bivalve shellfish and potential impact on industry.

1. Introduction

Naturally occurring harmful algal blooms (HABs) are known to have an adverse effect on shellfish industries worldwide, with toxic contamination of shellfish from these events potentially resulting in both human illness and a detrimental impact on the often-fragile economies of rural areas [1]. Despite regulatory monitoring, the accumulation of toxins in shellfish has led to occasional reports of sickness, with relatively infrequent outbreaks of phytoplankton-generated Diarrhetic Shellfish Poisoning (DSP) around Europe and elsewhere since it was first reported from The Netherlands in the 1960s [2–4]. In the UK, DSP was associated with the ingestion of imported mussels (*Mytilus* spp.) in 1994 and with UK common (blue) mussels (*Mytilus edulis*) obtained from an unauthorised site in 1997 [5–7]. Common (blue) mussels harvested in Scotland were also linked to 159 cases of DSP in 2006 [8,9] and a further 70 reported cases in 2013 [10]. While these events are relatively few in number, their impact on consumer confidence and industry sustainability is significant.

To mitigate the risk of human illness caused by the consumption of contaminated shellfish, European Union regulations require EU Member States to have regulatory programmes in place to monitor the presence of both marine biotoxins in shellfish production areas and the causative phytoplankton [11]. In the UK, toxin testing of shellfish tissue is supported by the analysis of seawater samples for the presence of toxin-producing phytoplankton and results delivered by the monitoring programmes are used to make decisions regarding the opening and closure of classified shellfish harvesting areas. In Scotland, this information is also used by the aquaculture industry to make informed decisions, following guidance issued to harvesters by Food Standards Scotland (FSS) in 2014 [12], which may lead to either an increase in end-product testing to ensure the safety of shellfish placed on the market, or a voluntary cessation of harvesting.

Between 2012 and 2017, an average of over 2700 tests have been carried out each year on bivalves, around 70% of which were common (blue) mussels, collected from approximately 80 classified shellfish harvesting areas in Scottish coastal waters. One of the main causes for concern is the presence of lipophilic toxins, some of which cause DSP. The accumulation of these toxins in shellfish is a major problem for the aquaculture industry in Scotland. Since routine monitoring for these toxins began in 1998 using the mouse bioassay (MBA) [13], extensive harvesting closures that can last for several months in some areas have been enforced. The DSP toxins include okadaic acid (OA) and the dinophysis toxins, dinophysistoxin-1 (DTX1) and dinophysistoxin-2 (DTX2), henceforth referred to as the OA group toxins. The group collectively known as DTX3 are derivatives of OA, DTX1 and DTX2, esterified with saturated and unsaturated fatty acids [9] and the chemical structure of these toxins is described in detail elsewhere [9,14]. The relative potency of the toxins within the OA group differs, with the toxic potential of DTX1 being similar to that of OA, although both are more toxic than DTX2 [9]. Hence, a Toxicity Equivalency Factor of 0.6 is used for DTX2. The use of the MBA method meant that individual OA group toxins could not be routinely identified and previous information on the presence of these toxins came from research studies using LC-MS [13,15]. The introduction of LC-MS/MS methodology into the regulatory toxin testing in July 2011 provided the scope to assess the presence of this toxin group on a regional and temporal scale [16]. The OA group toxins are responsible for most of the toxin contamination in Scottish bivalves and the maximum permitted level (MPL) in harvestable shellfish is 160 µg okadaic acid equivalent per kg shellfish flesh (OA eq./kg) [9]. The percentage of shellfish tissue samples with OA group toxicity reported above the regulatory limit fluctuates by year [16] and between 2012 and 2017, it varied between 2.2% (in 2017) and 11.5% (in 2013), with annual maximum amounts of total OA group equivalent toxicity ranging from 694 µg OA eq./kg in 2017 to 4993 µg OA eq./kg in 2013. The exceptionally high toxin maximum from a production area in the Shetland Islands in 2013 resulted in an outbreak of DSP [10].

A number of causative phytoplankton species are associated with lipophilic toxins and those connected with the OA group toxins belong to the order Dinophysiales and include the genera *Dinophysis* Ehrenberg and *Phalacroma* Stein. Algal cells in this order are routinely identified using light microscopy in regulatory monitoring programmes. In Scottish waters they are currently reported as total *Dinophysis* spp. with an 'alert' threshold set at 100 cells/L, to ensure testing of shellfish for the presence of biotoxins. The species concept within *Dinophysis* is not clearly defined [17,18] and a certain amount of gradation in character traits can lead to morphological ambiguity. Differences in cell shape and size have been attributed to geographic variation, environmental selection, feeding behaviour and life cycle [19]. Stern et al. [18] examined the genetic sequences of cells from Scottish coastal waters with morphologies that appeared to belong to the *D. acuminata* complex and identified the presence of both *D. acuminata* Claparéde & Lachmann and *D. ovum* and also confirmed the dominance of *D. acuminata* during late spring/summer. The other main species observed is *D. acuta* Ehrenberg but with considerable interannual variability in abundance [1]. Blooms dominated by *D. acuta* have occasionally been recorded, as was the case for 2001 and 2002 in Scapa Bay in Orkney [13]. *Dinophysis dens* is sometimes observed at low concentrations in blooms of *D. acuta* and is now regarded as a life-stage of *D. acuta* [20,21]. *Phalacroma rotundatum* is also regularly detected around the Scottish coast but again at low concentrations rarely exceeding 100 cells/L. Although it has been found to contain toxins, there is some evidence that it may not be a toxin-producer itself but may instead act as a vector [22].

Another known producer of diarrhetic shellfish toxins (DSTs) is the benthic dinoflagellate *Prorocentrum lima*. This species is detected more often in the sandy sediments of shallow bays where oyster cultivation takes place, although it can also grow epiphytically [23]. *Prorocentrum lima* is recorded sporadically in integrated water column samples but cell counts are likely to be underestimated using this method and it is generally more frequently observed in samples obtained by bucket. Analysis of the data obtained through the Scottish monitoring programme failed to establish a clear link between the presence of DSP toxins in bivalve molluscs and the abundance of *P. lima* (Scottish Association for Marine Science (SAMS) unpublished data). Hence this study is focused on the apparent link between DSTs in shellfish and the presence of *Dinophysis*.

In order to understand variability within the *Dinophysis* population and its influence on toxin accumulation in bivalve molluscs, this study was undertaken to investigate the annual and seasonal variation of *Dinophysis* spp. and associated toxins in two important shellfish harvesting regions on the west coast of Scotland, Loch Ewe and the Firth of Clyde (Figure 1). Hence, the risks to human health associated with changes in species composition of blooms can be evaluated.

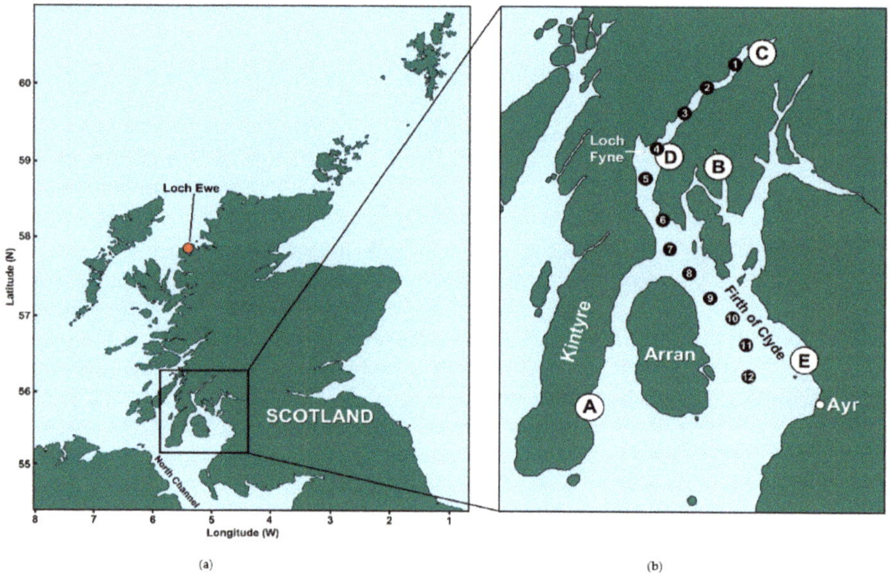

Figure 1. Maps of Scotland (**a**) and the study area showing the location of the Firth of Clyde and the official control monitoring sites for phytoplankton and shellfish (**b**), indicated by the white circles (A = Campbeltown Loch, B = Loch Striven, C = Loch Fyne: Ardkinglas, D = Loch Fyne: Otter Ferry and E = Barassie). Mussels are harvested at sites A, B and C, Pacific oysters at site D and razor clams at site E. The black circles (numbered 1 to 12) show the location of the additional phytoplankton samples obtained from the research survey conducted in early September 2015. The location of the long-term monitoring site at Loch Ewe is indicated in (**a**).

2. Results

2.1. Loch Ewe

2.1.1. *Dinophysis* Abundance

The abundance of *Dinophysis* in Loch Ewe between 1996 and 2017 varied considerably by month and between years. *Dinophysis acuminata* was recorded during the phytoplankton growing season (spring/summer) every year and in some instances during the winter months as well. Counts at or exceeding the 'alert' threshold that triggers shellfish toxin testing (100 cells/L) were obtained from March to November but the species was typically most abundant between May and August (Figure 2a). By contrast, *D. acuta* was never recorded between January and March, was detected above the 'alert' threshold from May to September but was most abundant between July and September (Figure 2b), with *D. acuminata* cells often present in the community at the same time. Bloom densities were not consistent between years, with *D. acuminata* typically recorded at maximum annual densities of less than 3000 cells/L but with some notable blooms in 2003, 2015 and 2016, when cell densities reached 4940 cells/L, 9540 cells/L and 24,340 cells/L, respectively. *Dinophysis acuta* was generally much less abundant, apart from an increase in cell densities between 1999 and 2002, including an exceptional bloom of 8040 cells/L recorded in August 2000.

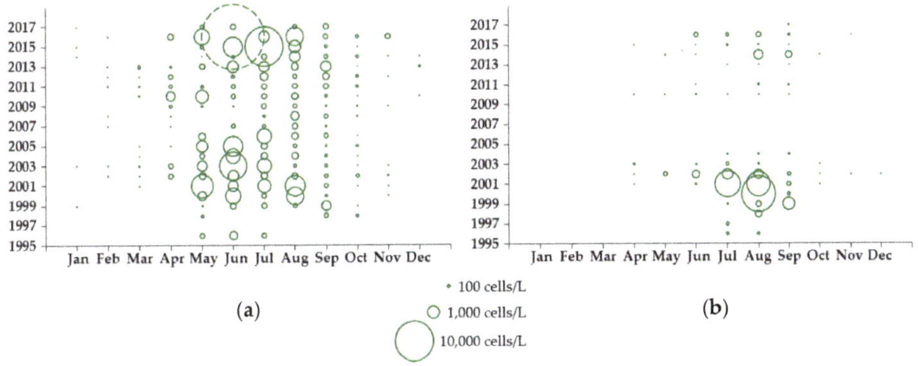

Figure 2. Maximum abundance by month for (**a**) *D. acuminata* and (**b**) *D. acuta* in phytoplankton samples obtained from Loch Ewe (NW Scotland) between 1996 and 2017, based on the analysis of 1797 records. The dashed circle in (**a**) represents a dense bloom of *D. acuminata* recorded in Loch Ewe in 2016 (24,340 cells/L).

2.1.2. Toxin Concentration in Shellfish

LC-MS analysis was carried out on samples of common mussel tissue obtained from Loch Ewe in 2001 and 2002, coinciding with blooms of *Dinophysis*. For the 2001 investigation, DTX1 and DTX2 were recorded as being either present or absent, although OA was quantified. Weekly sampling occurred in 2001 and OA group toxins were detected in mussels, with the concentration of OA reaching a maximum value of 141 μg/kg in early June (week 22), associated with a bloom of *D. acuminata* of density 2980 cells/L in the preceding week (Figure 3). DTX2 was recorded as absent until early August (week 31), following a bloom of *D. acuta* at a density of 3900 cells/L in mid July (week 29). DTX1 was only detected on one occasion, also in week 31. In 2002 the sampling frequency in Loch Ewe was increased to twice a week. Both species of *Dinophysis* were less abundant, although *D. acuminata* levels began to increase from around mid May, reaching a maximum value of 573 cells/L in mid June (week 25), whereas *D. acuta* reached a maximum abundance of 447 cells/L in early August (latter half of week 31) (Figure 4a). Okadaic acid was detected in mussels in every week continuously from late May until mid October but DTX1 was infrequently detected and mostly occurred in June when *D. acuminata* was the dominant species (Figure 4b). DTX2 was more associated with *D. acuta* (Figure 4d) and was absent until mid July (latter half of week 28), reaching a maximum value of 186 µg/kg one week after the *D. acuta* bloom peak of 447 cells/L. The apparent delay in toxin accumulation in the mussels following the *Dinophysis* blooms (Figure 4c,d) was investigated using a non-parametric Spearman's Rank-Order Correlation. The relationships between the individual toxins, OA and DTX2 and the abundance of both *D. acuminata* and *D. acuta* were explored over time, with lags of between 0 and 3 weeks at half-weekly intervals. A strong positive correlation was identified between *D. acuminata* and OA throughout the bloom period, reaching a maximum value with a two-week lag ($r_s = 0.815$, $p < 0.001$). We found no significant correlation between *D. acuminata* and DTX2. A strong positive correlation was also identified between *D. acuta* and OA throughout the bloom period but as both *D. acuminata* and *D. acuta* were present at the same time throughout most of the summer, it is difficult to discriminate the toxin contribution from each individual species. However, *D. acuta* was significantly correlated with DTX2, reaching a maximum value with a lag of 1.5 weeks ($r_s = 0.569$, $p < 0.001$).

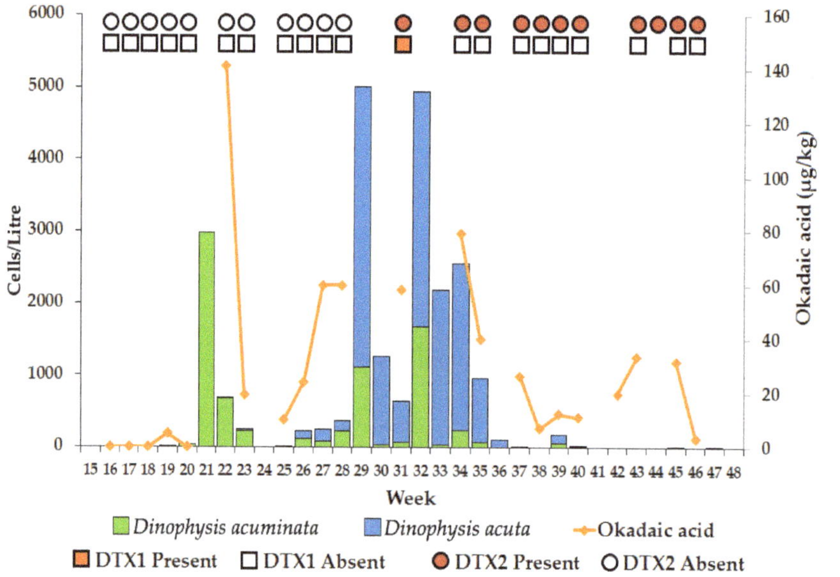

Figure 3. Stacked bar chart showing the abundance of *D. acuminata* and *D. acuta* and okadaic acid in common mussels from Loch Ewe during 2001. Cell counts were averaged for triplicate sub-samples every week. DTX1 and DTX2 were recorded as being either present or absent and are indicated by symbols.

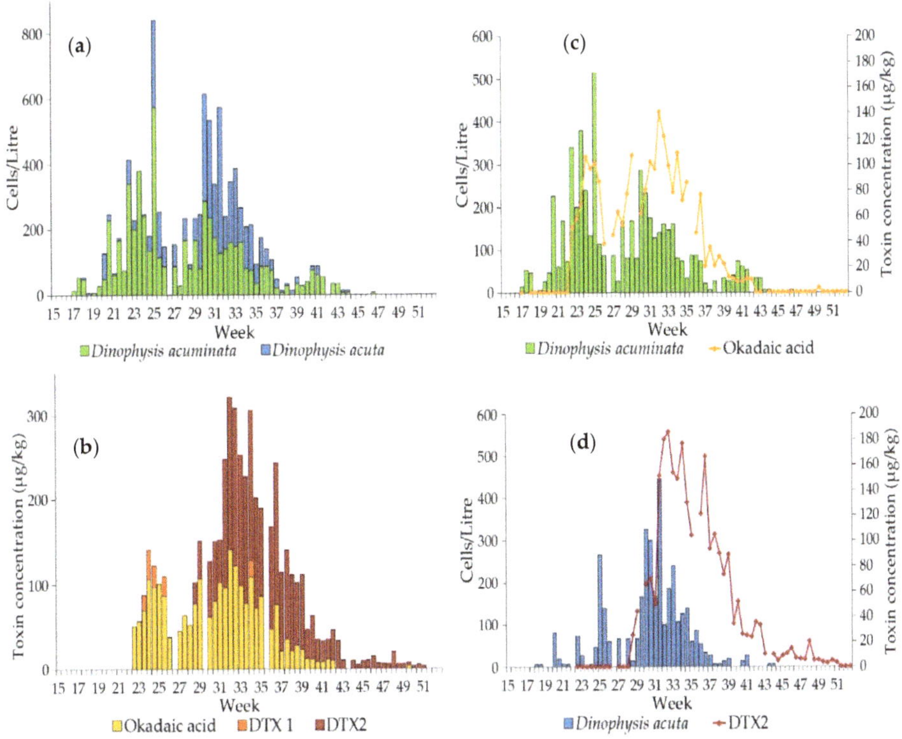

Figure 4. Abundances of *D. acuminata* and *D. acuta* in Loch Ewe during 2002 are shown in (**a**). Cell counts were averaged from triplicate sub-samples collected twice a week. Toxin concentrations in common mussels for the corresponding weeks are shown in (**b**). The relationships between *D. acuminata* and OA and between *D. acuta* and DTX2 are shown in (**c**,**d**), respectively.

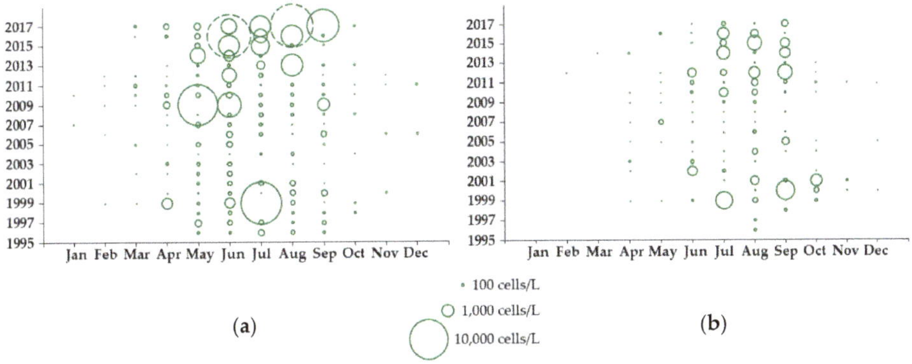

Figure 5. Maximum abundance of (**a**) *D. acuminata* and (**b**) *D. acuta* recorded at monitoring sites around the Firth of Clyde between 1996 and 2017, based on the analysis of 1001 records from eight sampling locations. The dashed circles in (**a**) represent dense blooms of *D. acuminata* observed in Loch Fyne: Ardkinglas (Site C in Figure 1b) in 2016 (85,760 cells/L) and 2017 (180,289 cells/L).

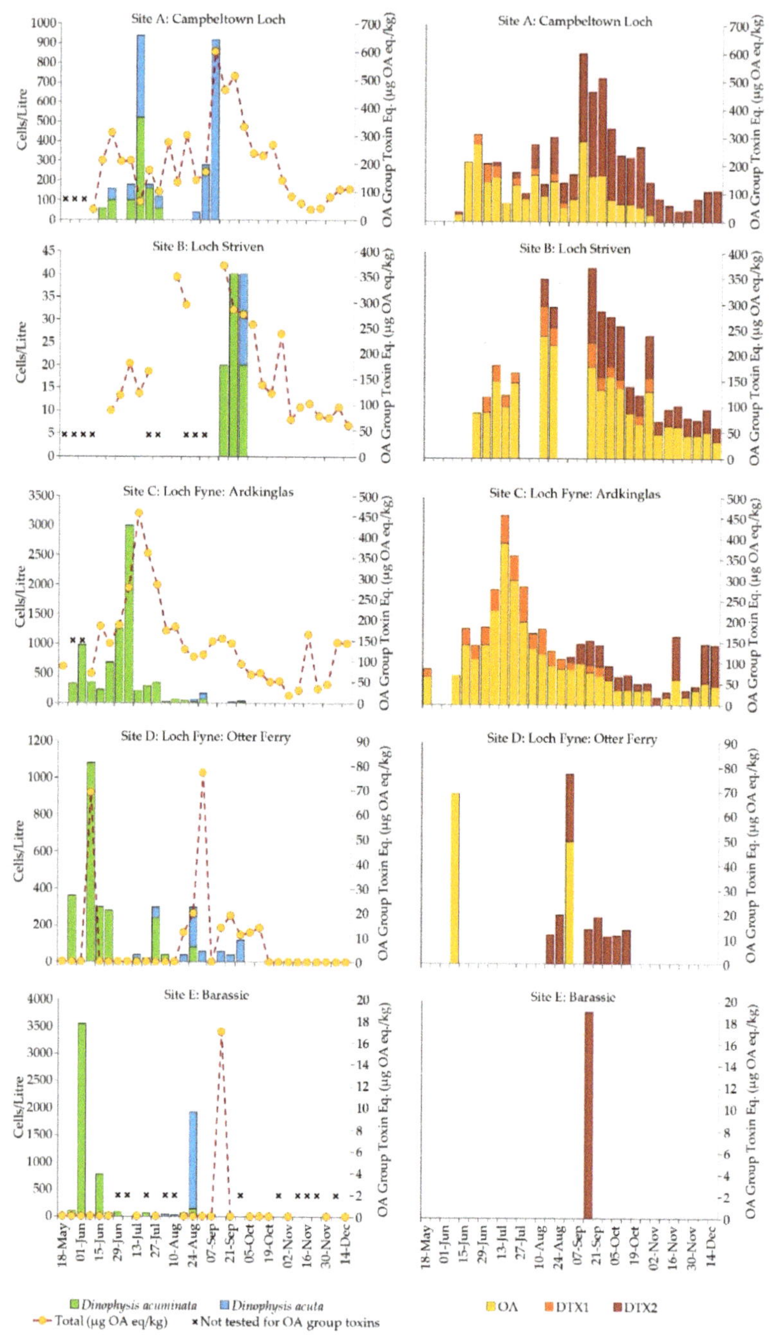

Figure 6. Left hand column shows the abundance of *D. acuminata* and *D. acuta* at official control monitoring sites and total OA group toxin equivalent (yellow circles) detected in shellfish between May and December 2015. Right hand column shows the contribution of OA, DTX1 and DTX2 (including esters) to the total OA group value (Toxicity Equivalency Factor of 0.6 applied to DTX2). No testing for lipophilic toxins was performed in late May and early June at the three mussel sites (A, B and C) due to the presence of paralytic shellfish toxins above the regulatory limit.

2.2. Firth of Clyde

2.2.1. *Dinophysis* Abundance

Time-series data collected between 1996 and 2017 from eight sampling locations around the Firth of Clyde and associated sea lochs showed a greater variability in *D. acuminata* abundance (Figure 5a). As in Loch Ewe, this species was detected in every month of the year, although this was not the case for every year and with above 'alert' threshold events from March to October. Some exceptionally dense blooms were observed in 1999, 2009, 2016 and 2017, with recorded cell densities of 13,860 cells/L, 13,260 cells/L, 85,760 cells/L and 180,289 cells/L, respectively. Apart from the 1999 bloom recorded in Loch Striven (Figure 1b, site B), the other dense blooms were all detected in upper Loch Fyne: Ardkinglas (Figure 1b, site C). *Dinophysis acuta* in the Firth of Clyde (Figure 5b) showed a similar profile to that in Loch Ewe, with cell counts also highest between July and September. Interannual variability was evident, with the densest *D. acuta* blooms occurring between 1999 and 2002 and again between 2012 and 2016, coinciding with an increase in *D. acuta* blooms further north in Loch Ewe.

A detailed examination of data obtained from the regulatory monitoring sites around the Firth of Clyde in 2015 also showed distinct patterns of abundance and seasonality for *D. acuminata* and *D. acuta* (Figure 6). Phytoplankton counts identified a bloom of predominantly *D. acuminata* widespread throughout the area from late May into mid July 2015. The highest recorded densities were 3540 cells/L at Barassie (Site E) on 2 June, 1080 cells/L at Loch Fyne: Otter Ferry (Site D) on 9 June and 2980 cells/L further up Loch Fyne at Ardkinglas (Site C) on 7 July. During this early part of summer at most of the sites, the *Dinophysis* population was exclusively *D. acuminata*. However, a mixed bloom of *D. acuminata* and *D. acuta* was observed in Campbeltown Loch (Site A) on 13 July, with cell abundances of 520 and 420 cells/L, respectively. Subsequently, *D. acuta* dominated the *Dinophysis* in Campbeltown Loch, reaching a maximum of 920 cells/L on 7 September. An increase in the abundance of *D. acuta* was also noted at all the other monitoring sites from around mid August, with a maximum bloom density of 1780 cells/L detected at Barassie on 25 August. Although regulatory phytoplankton monitoring did not begin in Loch Striven (Site B) until 15 September and *Dinophysis* counts throughout the whole area were relatively low by this time, many empty *D. acuta* theca were observed, indicating that the bloom had extended into Loch Striven in the preceding weeks.

Data from the September 2015 research cruise in the Firth of Clyde were consistent with the phytoplankton data from the regulatory monitoring sites. Figure 7a shows that *D. acuminata* was not particularly abundant in the samples from the cruise transect, with a maximum density of 200 cells/L recorded at Stations S7 and S11, to the seaward side of a marked temperature front between stations S6 and S7 [24]. The front was characterized by a body of cooler water located between Stations S4 and S6, with temperatures either side of the front being, on average, approximately 1 °C higher. By contrast, densities of *D. acuta* were more than ten times greater, with a peak abundance of 2840 cells/L at Station S7 near the mouth of Loch Fyne. There were no depth-related trends for either species but the highest densities of *D. acuta* were found in Stations S7 and S8 (Figure 7b), also coincident with the temperature front and on the seaward side. Abundance of *D. acuta* did not exceed 140 cells/L within Loch Fyne itself (Stations S1–S6).

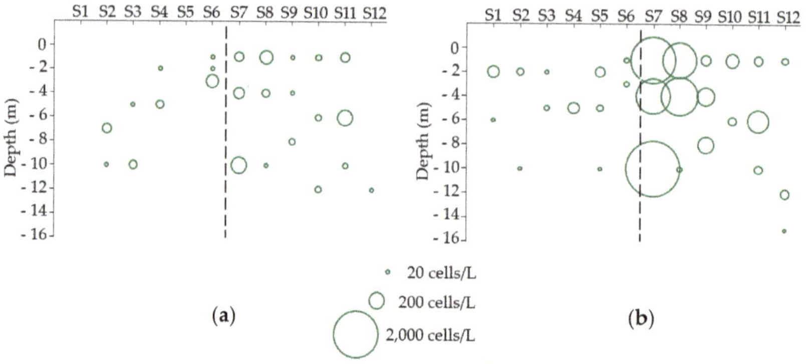

Figure 7. Abundance of (**a**) *D. acuminata* and (**b**) *D. acuta* in phytoplankton samples obtained from the research survey in early September. Stations S1 to S6 are in Loch Fyne and stations S7 to S12 are the more open waters of the Firth of Clyde (see Figure 1b). The temperature front between stations S6 and S7 is represented by a dashed line.

2.2.2. Okadaic Acid Group Equivalent Toxicity and Toxin Concentration in Shellfish

Figure 6 shows the variability in overall OA group toxicity in shellfish tissue collected from the regulatory monitoring sites around the Firth of Clyde between May and December 2015. The highest total toxin equivalent levels were recorded in mussels, with a value of 601 μg OA eq./kg reported in samples collected from Campbeltown Loch (Site A) on 7 September, coinciding with the peak abundance of *D. acuta* recorded at this site. A value of 457 μg OA eq./kg was reported, also in mussels, from Loch Fyne: Ardkinglas (Site C) a week after the dense bloom of 2980 cells/L of *D. acuminata* on 7 July. Okadaic acid group equivalent toxicity was lower in Pacific oysters and razor clams and the period of contamination was shorter, compared with that of the mussels. Two distinct OA group peaks were observed in Pacific oysters from Loch Fyne: Otter Ferry (Site D), the first peak of 69 μg OA eq./kg coinciding with the *D. acuminata* bloom of 1080 cells/L on 9 June and the second peak of 77 μg OA eq./kg on 1 September, following an increase in *D. acuta* in the preceding week. The maximum reported OA group equivalent toxin value in razor clams from Barassie (Site E) was much lower than in other shellfish species. Okadaic acid group toxicity at 17 μg OA eq./kg was detected in a razor clam sample collected on 14 September, three weeks after a bloom of density 1980 cells/L that was composed of about 90% *D. acuta*. The earlier *D. acuminata* bloom at this site of 3540 cells/L recorded on 2 June did not appear to have any associated toxin contamination of shellfish. The detection of OA group toxins in mussels, including those from other biotoxin monitoring sites around the Firth of Clyde, continued for an extended period throughout autumn and into the winter months despite the absence of any causative organism by this time.

The proportion of each toxin analogue within the OA group changed over time for the three mussel sites A, B and C (Figure 8a). June mussel samples contained approximately 83% OA in both free and ester form, which decreased over time but was still present in December samples, contributing approximately 18% to the total OA group toxins by this time. Low levels of DTX1 were also recorded, with a maximum contribution of about 23% during May, declining to below the reporting limit by November. Concentrations of total OA and total DTX1 were detected at maximum values of 389 μg/kg and 85 μg/kg, respectively from mussels collected at Loch Fyne: Ardkinglas in mid and late July 2015 (Figure 6). These elevated levels of OA and DTX1 appeared to follow the bloom of *D. acuminata* of density 2980 cells/L in early July. The DTX2 contribution increased from approximately 1% of the total OA group toxins in June to almost 82% by December (Figure 8a). The highest recorded amount of DTX2 was 581 μg/kg (with Toxicity Equivalency Factor value of 349 μg/kg), detected in mussels from Campbeltown Loch in late September 2015 (Figure 6). A greater proportion of the OA detected between May and July was in ester form (Figure 8b), with a ratio of 2:1 for esters:free but more similar proportions of free OA and OA esters were present in samples between August and October. Both DTX1 and DTX2 were detected mostly in free forms, except in May when DTX1 was all in ester form. Although low levels of pectenotoxins (PTXs) have previously been detected in mussels from Loch Fyne in 2009 during a bloom of predominantly *D. acuminata* [25], none were found in this study.

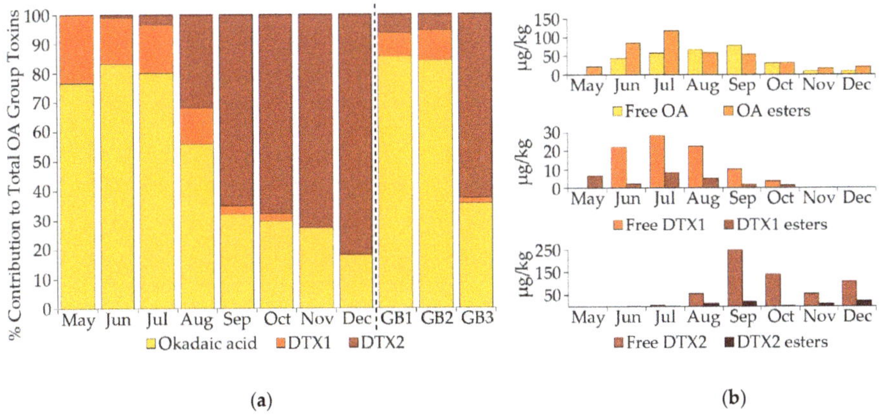

Figure 8. Mean percentage contribution of OA analogues and derivatives to total OA group toxins in mussels from sites A, B and C in the Firth of Clyde between May and December 2015 (**a**). For comparative purposes, the typical profiles obtained for mussels from Great Britain (GB1, GB2 and GB3) in the study by Johnson et al. [26] are also shown. (**b**) shows the proportion of free and esterified forms of each OA group toxin detected in the Firth of Clyde mussels.

3. Discussion

3.1. Environmental Influences on Seasonality and Abundance of Dinophysis

Both *Dinophysis acuminata* and *D. acuta* are regularly detected in the coastal waters of the North East Atlantic and the presence of these species, even at relatively low concentrations, results in a high incidence of shellfish contaminated with DSP toxins along the European Atlantic coast [2,27,28]. In Scottish coastal waters, maximum bloom densities of *Dinophysis* surveyed through the official control regulatory monitoring programme over the past 20 years have typically been in the region of 2000–10,000 cells/L, with infrequent observations of much denser patches, often in relatively enclosed areas. *Dinophysis* tends to be most abundant between May and September, prior to a late autumn decrease in line with the reduction in light levels associated with winter in temperate latitudes. The greatest *Dinophysis* cell densities in Scottish waters that usually occur between June and August are mainly composed of cells belonging to the *D. acuminata* complex. *Dinophysis acuta* blooms are observed less frequently than those of *D. acuminata* and tend to occur later in the year, typically from July onwards.

Our detailed analysis of the Clyde Sea sites and Loch Ewe conducted here concurs with the above qualitative assessment, indicating a dominance of *D. acuminata* in spring/summer with, in some years only, a switch to *D. acuta* dominance in late summer or autumn. Such temporal patterns have been observed elsewhere, for example along the Iberian shelf where the development of *D. acuminata* blooms usually begin in early March with the growth season extending until the autumnal transition from upwelling to downwelling [27–29]. In this region, *D. acuta* tends to occur in late summer-early autumn, although not every year, and has been associated with exceptionally hot summers [30] followed by a brief period of upwelling activity, leading to highly stratified conditions [2,21,28,31]. Blooms of *D. acuta* occurred between 1999 and 2002 in both Loch Ewe and around the Firth of Clyde with further occurrences in the Clyde and, to a lesser extent, Loch Ewe between 2014 and 2016. While the patterns of upwelling/downwelling that occur in Iberia are not a characteristic of Scottish waters, *D. acuta* blooms typically occur when seasonal stratification of the water column is likely [32,33].

Long-term variation in *Dinophysis* may be linked to climate [34,35]. Based on a modelling study, Gobler et al. [36] proposed that ocean warming had increased the growth rate and duration of the bloom season of *D. acuminata* over the period 1982–2006 in the North East Atlantic around the UK. However, following analysis of data from the Continuous Plankton Recorder (CPR) from the region, Dees et al. [37] did not find any increase in the number or annual duration of *Dinophysis* blooms. While the greatest number of *D. acuminata* above threshold counts occurred in each of the last three years (2015–2017), our results (Figures 2 and 5), albeit over a shorter timescale than that modelled by Gobler et al. [36], concur with the conclusion that there is no clear temporal increase in *D. acuminata* blooms. Our results for *D. acuta* also lead to a similar conclusion for this species.

In 2015 *Dinophysis* in the Firth of Clyde followed the typical pattern of an increase in *D. acuminata* through early summer, followed by a rise in the abundance of *D. acuta* in late summer and early autumn. Our boat-based field survey identified a pronounced temperature front between Stations S6 and S7 near the mouth of Loch Fyne. A substantial drop in nutrient concentrations across the front was also observed [24]. Fronts are known to be associated with dinoflagellate blooms [38–40] and in this case, we observed a separation of the phytoplankton community structure into distinct populations on either side of the front [24] with the largest concentrations of *D. acuta* at Stations S7 and S8 to the seaward side of the front (Figure 7), indicating that the front promoted the bloom or at least allowed wind-blown cells to accumulate against it. Such behaviour is consistent with the conceptual model of Smayda and Reynolds [41], who suggest that *Dinophysis* spp. are a transitional life form along the onshore-offshore mixing nutrient gradient, seeming to prefer areas of less pronounced turbulence. While they tolerate coastal upwelling sites and form modest blooms during periods of upwelling relaxation, they are common in areas where there is greater seasonal stratification and lower nutrients. Given that *D. acuta* blooms occurred in the same years in the geographically distinct Clyde Sea and Loch Ewe, local processes do not appear to control the bloom/non-bloom dynamics of this species but are likely to govern the specific location of events and their magnitude. Similar behaviour has also been reported from Irish waters with Raine et al. [42] noting that *D. acuta* mainly occurred in stratified shelf waters in late summer and hypothesizing that *D. acuta* populations developed rapidly close to tidal fronts where productivity is high. It is important to note that *D. acuminata*, although present during our 2015 survey, did not bloom nor aggregate near the frontal region, confirming the species-specific response to environmental forcing of the genus.

Other oceanographic conditions are also thought to be important in influencing *Dinophysis* transport and bloom formation. For example, coastal jets have been linked to movement of *Dinophysis* around the south-west of Ireland [40,43], with blooms being advected into coastal embayments through wind-driven exchange of water masses [40]. Such advection may result in large toxic blooms through physical accumulation rather than in situ growth [10,44]. Particle tracking model simulations by Paterson et al. [24] suggested that *D. acuta* was advectively transported into the Clyde Sea from the open sea of the North Channel. The model also predicted significant interannual differences in advection are likely in the area, with the potential for cells to be more readily exchanged between the outer waters of the Firth of Clyde and the enclosed waters of Loch Fyne (where aquaculture is concentrated) in the absence of a front.

3.2. Dinophysis and Toxin Profiles

Our results demonstrate that transition from a *D. acuminata* to a *D. acuta* dominated community in both the Clyde and Loch Ewe occurred on a number of occasions and influenced OA group toxicity detected in a range of bivalve shellfish species collected during the bloom periods. The relationship between *Dinophysis* abundance and accumulation of OA group toxins in shellfish can vary considerably and there are many factors that will determine the amount of toxin ingested by the shellfish and the rate of toxin depuration. These include the availability of other non-toxic phytoplankton species for filter feeding [45], the ingestion of other potentially toxic vector species and the location of the bivalve in the water column, whether suspended from a raft or occupying the intertidal zone [46]. Bivalve contamination will also depend on the response of the shellfish to a specific phytoplankton species or toxin [47,48] and the toxic potential of individual cells ingested, which may vary temporally, geographically and in response to life stage and nutrient availability [2,49,50]. Toxin content can vary within the same species collected from the same location at different times [51,52] and even between cells of a single species within a daily cycle [51]. Different shellfish species are also known to metabolize diarrhetic shellfish toxins differently [4,53] and mussels have been found to accumulate higher levels of diarrhetic shellfish toxins than other species when exposed to the same algal bloom conditions [4,53–58]. Consistent with this, the rope-grown mussels obtained from the Firth of Clyde in 2015 showed the highest level of OA group contamination. However, toxins in both Pacific oysters and razor clams remained below the MPL throughout the *Dinophysis* bloom period.

Dinophysis has a worldwide distribution but separate species have been associated with the production of different analogues of the OA group toxins, depending on geographic locality. The relative timing and size of *D. acuminata* and *D. acuta* blooms is therefore of considerable significance to the toxic contamination of shellfish that will likely result. Pectenotoxins have been identified as a dominant component of the toxin profile in *D. acuminata* from New Zealand [59], Japan [60,61], Chile [62,63], Argentina [64] and North America [49,63], with smaller amounts of OA and DTX1 also present. In European waters, *D. acuminata* is more associated with the production of OA. Okadaic acid has been linked to *D. acuminata* on the Swedish west coast [65] and in Denmark only OA and OA esters were identified in blue mussels during a bloom of *D. acuminata* [66]. However, a further study on Danish isolates showed strains of *D. acuminata* to produce only PTX2 and no OA or DTX [67]. Further south, OA was identified in *D. acuminata* samples collected in 1998 from north-west Spain and cells obtained in September were found to have an OA concentration of more than double that of June cells [68]. Blooms of *D. acuminata* in Portugal have also been associated with OA [69], as was a bloom in the Bay of Seine (northern France) [70]. Our study is consistent with the geographical patterns described above in demonstrating that *D. acuminata* blooms in Scottish coastal waters are associated with toxin profiles in shellfish dominated by OA, with a smaller contribution from DTX1.

Pectenotoxins also dominated the toxin profile of *D. acuta* from New Zealand waters [59], with a small amount of OA found but no DTX2. By contrast, various studies from around Spain, Portugal and Ireland have associated the presence of *D. acuta* with DTX2. Both OA and DTX2 at an approximate ratio of 3:2 were found in *D. acuta* collected from north-west Spain in 1997 [68] and DTX2, OA and PTX2 were also present in isolates of *D. acuta* from the same area in 2005-6, with a fairly constant ratio of 3:2 for OA:DTX2 [51] but with variations in toxin cell quota in different months [51]. Increased levels of DTX2 in Portuguese shellfish during late summer and early autumn of 1994 and 1995 also were associated with blooms of *D. acuta* [69]. Both DTX2 and OA in varying proportions were found in *D. acuta* obtained from the Celtic Sea and the south coast of Ireland [71,72]. A further study in the same area reported that *D. acuta* related concentrations of DTX2 and PTX2 were greater than OA in all the samples analysed [73]. Further north, during a bloom of predominantly *D. acuta* off the north-east coast of England in September 2002, mussels were found to contain 76% DTX2, 15% OA and 9% PTX2 [74]. Johnson et al. [26] also identified a toxin profile for mussels collected around Great Britain between 2011 and 2015 that contained DTX2 at 63%, with OA at 35% and a small amount of DTX1 (<2%).

Our investigation of the Firth of Clyde 2015 event showed that the proportion of toxins contributing to the OA group varied throughout the year, with more OA and DTX1 detected in shellfish between May and August followed by an increase in DTX2, such that it was the dominant toxin by early September. The increase in the abundance of *D. acuta* and its replacement of *D. acuminata* as the dominant species contributed to a greater proportion of DTX2 contamination of shellfish in both the Clyde in 2015 and Loch Ewe in 2001 and 2002. Some studies have hypothesized that blooms of *D. acuta* may result in extended periods of toxic contamination of shellfish. Vale, 2004 [54], examined the elimination rates of OA and DTX2 in both mussels and oysters and concluded that DTX2 was eliminated at a slower rate than OA in mussels, although the elimination rate of DTX2 in cockles was similar to that of OA. Mussels from Loch Ewe (this study) remained contaminated with both DTX2 and OA into the winter of 2001, although only DTX2 was still present in mussels during winter 2002. In the Clyde mussel samples, the proportion of free OA to esterified OA increased throughout the summer months and DTX2 was predominantly present in non-esterified form. Our study revealed a prolonged period of toxic contamination of shellfish in the absence of any causative organism, due to the continuing presence of DTX2 and, to a lesser extent, OA in mussel and oyster samples through the autumn and winter of 2015 in the Firth of Clyde. These results support the hypothesis proposed by Vale, 2006 [55], that esterified forms of OA and DTX2 in mussels and clams are eliminated more rapidly than free OA and DTX2 but that DTX2 is less esterified than OA in these species, leading to a build-up of free DTX2.

Johnson et al. [26] examined the OA group toxin profiles in 98 samples of mussels obtained from around Great Britain between 2011 and 2015 as part of the official control monitoring programme. They identified three different toxin profiles, the first (GB1 in Figure 8a) being dominated by OA in both free and ester form (about 86%), with a small amount of DTX1 (8%) and very little DTX2 (6%). The second profile (GB2) was also dominated by OA but with a higher proportion of OA in ester form, approximately 59% compared to 36% in GB1. The third profile (GB3) contained a much larger proportion of DTX2 (about 63%) present, mostly as free DTX2 (mean 58%). Pectenotoxins were absent in all the mussel samples tested. Similarly, in an analysis of toxin profiles from various shellfish species obtained around the coast of Scotland, England and Wales between 2011 and 2016, Dhanji-Rapkova et al. [16] identified three distinct profiles, with Profile 1 being dominated by OA (87%), Profile 2 more of a mix between OA (45%) and DTX2 (52%) and Profile 3 mostly composed of DTX2 (85%). A comparison between the toxin profiles in mussels determined from the Johnson et al. [26] investigation and the results obtained in the Firth of Clyde 2015 study (Figure 8) showed that the toxin profiles obtained for mussels in June and July were very similar to the profile for GB2. Okadaic acid contributed >80% to the total toxin content, with approximately twice as much OA in ester form compared with free OA. However, the September and October toxin profiles showed a much greater similarity with the profile for GB3 where DTX2 in both free and ester form contributed >63% to the total toxic potential.

Food business operators are required through regulation to ensure that unsafe products are not placed on the market and a number of relatively simple, rapid and inexpensive kits are commercially available that are used by the shellfish industry to test for the presence of DSTs in harvested shellfish. These use a variety of methods including quantitative enzyme linked immunosorbent assays, protein phosphatase inhibition assays and qualitative lateral flow immunoassays. The investigation by Johnson et al. [26] examined four of these rapid test kits to compare their performance with the results obtained by the official control method (LC-MS/MS) for a threshold of 80 μg OA eq./kg, which is half the MPL of OA group equivalent toxicity allowed in shellfish tissue. The authors found good agreement in the results for both toxin profiles GB1 and GB2, recorded as either positive or negative for the 0.5 MPL threshold but there was a larger proportion of false negatives for profile GB3 with the majority of the rapid test kits. Generally, the results from the rapid test kits gave a reliable indication of OA group toxin contamination in the mussels but performance was less accurate when there was a larger proportion of DTX2 present.

4. Conclusions

Our results confirm that the species diversity within *Dinophysis* populations in Scottish waters can vary interannually. *Dinophysis acuminata* is predominant in Scottish coastal waters and its presence is associated with contamination of shellfish with OA and DTX1, although occasional blooms of *D. acuta* can lead to prolonged contamination with DTX2. In some shellfish production areas, there is often a limited "window of opportunity" for harvesting between site closures due to spring/early summer contamination with paralytic shellfish toxins and those caused by diarrhetic shellfish toxins in mid/late summer. The decision to harvest may be based on a negative result returned by a rapid test kit if the tissue sample contains a high proportion of DTX2, although the regulatory LC-MS/MS test could return a positive result for a similar sample. This can result in expensive product recalls and the associated loss of consumer confidence for all shellfish products. Routine enumeration of *Dinophysis* to species level could provide early warning of potential contamination of shellfish with DTX2 and thus determine the choice of the most suitable kit for effective end-product testing. This would provide better protection to the health of consumers and reduce the potential impact to the shellfish aquaculture industry.

5. Materials and Methods

5.1. Study Areas

The two study sites are both located on the west coast of Scotland, an area characterised by islands and fjordic sea lochs that provide a sheltered location for much of Scotland's aquaculture industry. Loch Ewe is a fjordic sea loch on the Scottish west coast (Figure 1a), approximately 12 km long, with a mean depth of around 21 m and a maximum depth of 73 m [75]. It has only a slightly discernible sill at 33 m depth, resulting in it being associated with the more open waters of the North Minch [76,77]. Loch Ewe is part of the Scottish Coastal Observatory (SCObs) operated by Marine Science Scotland (MSS) where multiple physical, chemical and biological parameters are collected on a weekly basis [78]. Further south, the Firth of Clyde is a large fjordic basin with a number of associated sea lochs. It opens into the North Channel of the Irish Sea [79]. The regulatory monitoring points in this region were located on the southern end of the Kintyre peninsula, on the eastern side of the Firth of Clyde near Ayr and further north in Loch Striven and Loch Fyne (indicated by A-E in Figure 1b).

5.2. Phytoplankton Samples

Seawater samples were collected from classified shellfish production areas, the sampling method being either a PVC sampling tube or a bucket, depending on the depth of water at each site. The sampling tube allows for the collection of a depth-integrated water sample from 0–10 m. A well-mixed 500 mL (SAMS) or 1 L (MSS) sub-sample of this water was fixed on site, to obtain a final concentration of approximately 1% (SAMS) or 0.5% (MSS) acidic Lugol's iodine and then returned to the laboratory for analysis. The phytoplankton in a 50 mL sub-sample (detection limit 20 cells/L) was allowed to settle onto the base plate of a chamber for a minimum of 20 h before analysis, following the method described by Utermöhl, 1958 [80]. Cells belonging to the order Dinophysiales were identified and enumerated using inverted light microscopy and subsequent re-analysis of samples allowed assignation of cells to species level where this had not been recorded during the original routine analysis for the regulatory monitoring programme. Phytoplankton data collected through regulatory monitoring by both MSS (1996 to June 2005) and SAMS (September 2005 onwards) were examined to determine the prevalence and seasonality of *D. acuminata* and *D. acuta* in the Firth of Clyde and at the long-term MSS SCObs site in Loch Ewe.

Supplementary phytoplankton data were also available from a research cruise that was conducted between 8–9 September 2015 aboard RV Seòl Mara [24], with sampling taking place at stations around the Clyde Sea and in Loch Fyne (Figure 1b). Oxygen, temperature, salinity and fluorescence were recorded by CTD (SBE 19, Seabird Electronics) and water samples were collected by Niskin bottle into 500 mL opaque plastic bottles and preserved with acidic Lugol's iodine. Three depths were sampled at each station corresponding to surface, chlorophyll maximum and below the chlorophyll maximum, guided by CTD in-situ fluorescence data. Samples were analysed for the presence of phytoplankton following the Utermöhl method.

5.3. Shellfish Samples

Shellfish species collected from around the Firth of Clyde consisted of common mussels (*Mytilus edulis*), Pacific oysters (*Magallana gigas*) and razor clams (*Ensis* spp.) (Table 1). Samples were collected, packaged and transported to the Centre for Environment, Fisheries and Aquaculture Science (Cefas) within validated temperature-controlled containers, in accordance with Cefas guidance and protocols. Enough shellfish, with a minimum of ten organisms per sample, were taken to provide a sample characteristic of the Representative Monitoring Point (RMP) and a minimum weight of 100 g tissue once the shellfish were shucked.

Table 1. Number of phytoplankton and shellfish samples collected from around the Firth of Clyde between May and December 2015 and used in this study. The number of tissue samples containing total OA group equivalent toxicity exceeding the Maximum Permitted Level (MPL) of 160 μg OA eq./kg is also shown.

Site	Shellfish Species	Phytoplankton Samples	Tissue Samples	OA group Equiv. Toxicity > MPL
(A) Campbeltown Loch	Common mussels	16	28	15
(B) Loch Striven	Common mussels	6	22	9
(C) Loch Fyne: Ardkinglas	Common mussels	19	29	9
(D) Loch Fyne: Otter Ferry	Pacific oysters	19	31	0
(E) Barassie	Razor clams	19	20	0

Okadaic acid group toxins present in shellfish tissue were determined using a method validated at Cefas [81] based on that described by the EU Reference Method for lipophilic toxins, using liquid chromatography tandem mass spectrometry (LC-MS/MS). This method has been used for official control monitoring in the UK including Scotland since July 2011 [16]. Aliquots of 2.0 ± 0.01 g shellfish tissue from each sample were subjected to a double extraction each using 9 mL of methanol. Post-centrifugation, 0.2 μm filtered supernatants were subjected to both direct LC-MS/MS analysis and an alkaline hydrolysis step to liberate the esterified OA group toxins [82]. Two Waters, Acquity and Acquity *I*-class, (Waters Ltd., Manchester, UK) Ultra Performance Liquid Chromatographic (UPLC) systems were coupled to Waters Xevo TQ and Xevo TQ-S MS/MS systems respectively. A high pH LC method described by Gerssen et al. [14] was adopted with modifications [81]. Mobile phase A was prepared from 2 mM ammonium bicarbonate adjusted to pH 11 ± 0.2 with ammonium hydroxide. Mobile phase B was 2 mM ammonium bicarbonate in 90% acetonitrile, also adjusted to pH 11 ± 0.2 with ammonium hydroxide. On both systems, a Waters BEH C18 reverse phase UPLC column (2.1 × 50 mm, 1.7 μm) was used in series with a pre-column VanGuard cartridge. The mobile phase flow rate was held at 0.6 mL/min, with column temperatures, run times and injection volumes optimised for the two instruments independently. MS/MS parameters used were those given by Turner and Goya, 2015 [83].

Toxins in shellfish extracts were quantified against calibration solutions prepared from Certified Reference Material (CRM) standards obtained from the Institute of Biotoxin Metrology, National Research Council of Canada (NRCC). Chromatographic retention times together with two Selected Reaction Monitoring (SRM) transitions, optimised for each toxin, were utilised for qualitative identification of toxins, with the primary SRM used for quantitative purposes. Hydrolysed extracts were analysed alongside the unhydrolysed filtrates to enable the quantitation of both free OA group toxins (OA, DTX1 and DTX2) and OA group esters (DTX3s) [82]. Within the regulatory monitoring programme, results are reported as total μg OA equivalent/kg, with a Toxicity Equivalency Factor of 0.6 used for DTX2 [9]. Measurement uncertainty, determined for each shellfish species/toxin analogue combination, is then applied to each quantifiable toxin concentration and used to calculate an overall uncertainty for each total toxic potential estimation. As a precautionary measure, the higher value is used to determine whether the total OA equivalent/kg exceeds the MPL, although actual total OA equivalent/kg values are reported in this study. Okadaic acid group toxin values reported in excess of 400 μg OA eq./kg should be regarded as estimations, as such levels fall outside the operationally-defined linear working range of the instrument.

Additional MSS data on OA group toxins in common mussels were also available for Loch Ewe between 2001 and 2002 [13]. The concentrations of okadaic acid, DTX1 and DTX2 in 80% (*v*/*v*) aqueous methanol shellfish extracts were determined using an API 150EX single quadrupole mass spectrometer, equipped with a TurboIonspray source (Applied Biosystems, Warrington, UK). This was coupled to an Agilent 1100 series HPLC system (Agilent Technologies, West Lothian, UK) comprising of a de-gasser, quaternary pump and autosampler. A reversed-phase column was used for the analysis (Thermo Hypersil C_8 BDS, 50 × 2.1 mm, particle size 3 μm) with a 10 mm guard cartridge of the same stationary phase. The isocratic mobile phase consisted of 2 mM ammonium formate with 50 mM formic acid in 50% (*v*/*v*) acetonitrile. The flow rate and run time for both analyses were 0.25 mL/min and 10 min respectively. An aliquot of 5 μL was injected onto the analytical column. The mobile phase was directly infused into the mass spectrometer after 1.5 min and the initial mobile phase was put to waste using a switching valve.

Author Contributions: Conceptualization by S.C.S., A.D.T., K.D. and C.W.; S.C.S. and E.B. identified the *Dinophysis* from the regulatory monitoring samples and E.B. supplied information from the SCObs; Toxin data were collected by A.D.T. and E.B.; R.F.P. and S.M. conducted the Clyde field study and R.F.P., S.M. and E.M. performed sample and data analyses; The original draft was prepared by S.C.S., A.D.T., E.B., C.W., R.F.P. and K.D.; Review & editing was performed by S.C.S., A.D.T., E.B. and K.D.; S.C.S. prepared the figures and final version.

Funding: The laboratory analyses for biotoxins in shellfish were conducted by the Centre for Environment, Fisheries and Aquaculture Science (Cefas) Weymouth Laboratory, whilst the laboratory phytoplankton analyses were performed by the Scottish Association for Marine Science (SAMS) in Oban during 2015. The programmes were aimed at delivering the testing required for the statutory monitoring of biotoxins in shellfish and for identification and enumeration of potentially harmful algal species in selected shellfish harvesting areas, as described in EC Regulations 854/2004, 882/2004 and 2074/2005. They were funded by and delivered on behalf of, Food Standards Scotland (FSS), the national competent authority for food safety. Marine Science Scotland (MSS) phytoplankton data was collected as part of the SOAEFD and Food Standards Agency, UK Toxic Phytoplankton Monitoring Programme in Scotland and the Scottish Coastal Observatory (ST05a). Toxin analysis from 2001–2003 was performed under the Food Standards Agency, Scotland project B04008. The boat based field survey was funded by the BBSRC/NERC ShellEye project [grant reference NE/P011004/1]. R.F.P. was supported by a PhD studentship co-funded by FSS and SAMS, and K.D. was funded by BBSRC/NERC grant BB/M025934/1 and the NWE Europe Interreg project PRIMROSE.

Acknowledgments: All official control samples analysed and used to provide the data for this study were acquired and tested as part of the Food Standards Scotland funded regulatory marine biotoxin monitoring programme.

Conflicts of Interest: The authors declare no conflict of interest.

References and Notes

1. Davidson, K.; Bresnan, E. Shellfish toxicity in UK waters: A threat to human health? *Environ. Health* **2009**, *8*, S12. [CrossRef] [PubMed]
2. Reguera, B.; Riobó, P.; Rodríguez, F.; Díaz, P.A.; Pizarro, G.; Paz, B.; Franco, J.M.; Blanco, J. *Dinophysis* Toxins: Causative organisms, distribution and fate in shellfish. *Mar. Drugs* **2014**, *12*, 394–461. [CrossRef] [PubMed]
3. Smayda, T.J. Harmful Algal Bloom Communities in Scottish Coastal Waters: Relationship to Fish Farming and Regional Comparisons—A Review. 2006. Available online: http://www.gov.scot/Publications/2006/02/03095327/0 (accessed on 3 February 2006).
4. Trainer, V.L.; Moore, L.; Bill, B.D.; Adams, N.G.; Harrington, N.; Borchert, J.; da Silva, D.A.M.; Eberhart, B.-T.L. Diarrhetic shellfish toxins and other lipophilic toxins of human health concern in Washington State. *Mar. Drugs* **2013**, *11*, 1815–1835. [CrossRef] [PubMed]
5. Scoging, A.; Bahl, M. Diarrhetic shellfish poisoning in the UK. *Lancet* **1998**, *352*, 117. [CrossRef]
6. Whittle, K.; Gallacher, S. Marine toxins. *Br. Med. Bull.* **2000**, *56*, 236–253. [CrossRef] [PubMed]
7. Hinder, S.L.; Hays, G.C.; Brooks, C.J.; Davies, A.P.; Edwards, M.; Walne, A.W.; Gravenor, M.B. Toxic marine microalgae and shellfish poisoning in the British Isles: History, review of epidemiology and future implications. *Environ. Health* **2011**, *10*. [CrossRef] [PubMed]
8. McDougall, S.; Midgley, P. The Scottish live bivalve mollusc monitoring programme and Enforcement. Scottish food advisory committee report 2010. FSAS 11/08/01 19 pp.

9. European food safety Authority. Opinion of the Scientific Panel on Contaminants in the Food chain on a request from the European Commission on marine biotoxins in shellfish—Okadaic acid and analogues. *EFSA J.* **2008**, *589*, 1–62.
10. Whyte, C.; Swan, S.; Davidson, K. Changing wind patterns linked to unusually high *Dinophysis* blooms around the Shetland Islands, Scotland. *Harmful Algae* **2014**, *39*, 365–373. [CrossRef]
11. European Commission. Regulation (EC) No. 854/2004 of the European Parliament and of the Council of 29 April 2004 laying down specific rules for the organisation of official controls on products of animal origin intended for human consumption. *Off. J. Eur. Union* **2004**, Annex II, Chapter II, B, 1c and 4a.
12. Managing Shellfish Toxin Risks: Guidance For Harvesters and Processors. Available online: http://www.foodstandards.gov.scot/publications-and-research/managing-shellfish-toxin-risks-for-harvesters-and-processors (accessed on 30 May 2018).
13. Bresnan, E.; Fryer, R.; Hart, M.; Percy, L. Correlation between algal presence in water and toxin presence in shellfish. *Fish. Res. Serv. Contract Rep.* **2005**, *4*, 5–27.
14. Gerssen, A.; Mulder, P.P.J.; McElhinney, M.A.; de Boer, J. Liquid chromatography-tandem mass spectrometry for the detection of marine lipophilic toxins under alkaline conditions. *J. Chromatogr. A.* **2009**, *1216*, 1421–1430. [CrossRef] [PubMed]
15. Stobo, L.A.; Lacaze, J.-P.C.L.; Scott, A.C.; Petrie, J.; Turrell, E.A. Surveillance of algal toxins in shellfish from Scottish waters. *Toxicon* **2008**, *51*, 635–648. [CrossRef] [PubMed]
16. Dhanji-Rapkova, M.; O'Neill, A.; Maskrey, B.H.; Coates, L.; Teixeira Alves, M.; Kelly, R.J.; Hatfield, R.G.; Rowland-Pilgrim, S.J.; Lewis, A.M.; Algoet, M.; et al. Variability and profiles of lipophilic toxins in bivalves from Great Britain during five and a half years of monitoring: Okadaic acid, dinophysis toxins and pectenotoxins. *Harmful Algae* **2018**, *77*, 66–80. [CrossRef] [PubMed]
17. Edvardsen, B.; Shalchian-Tabrizi, K.; Jakobsen, K.S.; Medlin, L.K.; Dahl, E.; Brubak, S.; Paasche, E. Genetic variability and molecular phylogeny of *Dinophysis* species (Dinophyceae) from Norwegian waters inferred from single cell analysis of rDNA. *J. Phycol.* **2003**, *39*, 395–408. [CrossRef]
18. Stern, R.F.; Amorim, A.L.; Bresnan, E. Diversity and plastid types in *Dinophysis acuminata* complex (Dinophyceae) in Scottish waters. *Harmful Algae* **2014**, *39*, 223–231. [CrossRef]
19. Reguera, B.; Velo-Suárez, L.; Raine, R.; Park, M.G. Harmful *Dinophysis* species: A review. *Harmful Algae* **2012**, *14*, 87–106. [CrossRef]
20. Reguera, B.; González-Gil, S. Small cell and intermediate cell formation in species of *Dinophysis* (Dinophyceae, Dinophysiales). *J. Phycol.* **2001**, *37*, 318–333. [CrossRef]
21. Moita, M.T.; Sobrinho-Gonçalves, L.; Oliveira, P.B.; Palma, S.; Falcão, M. A bloom of *Dinophysis acuta* in a thin layer off North-West Portugal. *Afr. J. Mar. Sci.* **2006**, *28*, 265–269. [CrossRef]
22. González-Gil, S.; Pizarro, G.; Paz, B.; Velo-Suárez, L.; Reguera, B. Considerations on the toxigenic nature and prey sources of *Phalacroma rotundatum*. *Aquat. Microb. Ecol.* **2011**, *64*, 197–203. [CrossRef]
23. Foden, J.; Purdie, D.A.; Morris, S.; Nascimento, S. Epiphytic abundance and toxicity of *Prorocentrum lima* populations in the Fleet Lagoon, UK. *Harmful Algae* **2005**, *4*, 1063–1074. [CrossRef]
24. Paterson, R.F.; McNeill, S.; Mitchell, E.; Adams, T.; Swan, S.C.; Clarke, D.; Miller, P.I.; Bresnan, E.; Davidson, K. Environmental control of harmful dinoflagellates and diatoms in a fjordic system. *Harmful Algae* **2017**, *69*, 1–17. [CrossRef] [PubMed]
25. Morris, S.; Stubbs, B.; Brunet, C.; Davidson, K. Spatial distributions and temporal profiles of harmful phytoplankton and lipophilic toxins in Common mussels and Pacific oysters from four Scottish shellfish production areas (2009). Final project report to the Food Standards Agency in Scotland, 2010; p. 57.
26. Johnson, S.; Harrison, K.; Turner, A.D. Application of rapid test kits for the determination of *Diarrhetic Shellfish Poisoning* (DSP) toxins in bivalve molluscs from Great Britain. *Toxicon* **2016**, *111*, 121–129. [CrossRef] [PubMed]
27. Escalera, L.; Pazos, Y.; Doval, M.D.; Reguera, B. A comparison of integrated and discrete depth sampling for monitoring toxic species of *Dinophysis*. *Mar. Pollut. Bull.* **2012**, *64*, 106–113. [CrossRef] [PubMed]
28. Moita, M.T.; Pazos, Y.; Rocha, C.; Nolasco, R.; Oliveira, P.B. Toward predicting *Dinophysis blooms* off NW Iberia: A decade of events. *Harmful Algae* **2016**, *53*, 17–32. [CrossRef] [PubMed]
29. Díaz, P.A.; Reguera, B.; Ruiz-Villarreal, M.; Pazos, Y.; Velo-Suárez, L.; Berger, H.; Sourisseau, M. Climate variability and oceanographic settings associated with interannual variability in the initiation of *Dinophysis acuminata* blooms. *Mar. Drugs* **2013**, *11*, 2964–2981. [CrossRef] [PubMed]

30. Escalera, L.; Reguera, B.; Pazos, Y.; Moroño, A.; Cabanas, J.M. Are different species of *Dinophysis* selected by climatological conditions? *Afr. J. Mar. Sci.* **2006**, *28*, 283–288. [CrossRef]
31. Díaz, P.A.; Ruiz-Villarreal, M.; Pazos, Y.; Moita, T.; Reguera, B. Climate variability and *Dinophysis acuta* blooms in an upwelling system. *Harmful Algae* **2016**, *53*, 145–159. [CrossRef] [PubMed]
32. Jones, K.J.; Gowen, R.J. Influence of stratification and irradiance regime on summer phytoplankton composition in coastal and shelf seas of the British Isles. *Estuarine Coast. Shelf Sci.* **1990**, *30*, 557–567. [CrossRef]
33. Midgley, R.P.; Simpson, J.H.; Hyder, P.; Rippeth, T.P. Seasonal cycle of vertical structure and deep waters renewal in the Clyde Sea. *Estuarine Coast. Shelf Sci.* **2001**, *53*, 813–823. [CrossRef]
34. Edwards, M.; Johns, D.G.; Leterme, S.C.; Svendsen, E.; Richardson, A.J. Regional climate change and harmful algal blooms in the northeast Atlantic. *Limnol. Oceanogr.* **2006**, *51*, 820–829. [CrossRef]
35. Naustvoll, L.J.; Gustad, E.; Dahl, E. Monitoring of *Dinophysis* species and diarrhetic shellfish toxins in Flødevigen Bay, Norway: Inter-annual variability over a 25-year time-series. *Food Addit. Contam. Part A* **2012**, *29*, 1605–1615. [CrossRef] [PubMed]
36. Gobler, C.J.; Doherty, O.M.; Hattenrath-Lehmann, T.K.; Griffith, A.W.; Kang, Y.; Litaker, R.W. Ocean warming since 1982 has expanded the niche of toxic algal blooms in the North Atlantic and North Pacific oceans. *Proc. Natl. Acad. Sci. USA* **2017**, *114*, 4975–4980. [CrossRef] [PubMed]
37. Dees, P.; Bresnan, E.; Dale, A.C.; Edwards, M.; Johns, D.; Mouat, B.; Whyte, C.; Davidson, K. Harmful algal blooms in the Eastern North Atlantic ocean. *Proc. Natl. Acad. Sci. USA* **2017**, *114*, 124–126. [CrossRef] [PubMed]
38. Franks, P.J.S. Sink or swim: Accumulation of biomass at fronts. *Mar. Ecol. Prog. Ser.* **1992**, *82*, 1–12. [CrossRef]
39. Franks, P.J.S. Phytoplankton blooms at fronts: Patterns, scales and physical forcing. *Rev. Aquat. Sci.* **1992**, *6*, 121–137.
40. Raine, R. A review of the biophysical interactions relevant to the promotion of HABs in stratified systems: The case study of Ireland. *Deep Sea Res. Part II Top. Stud. Oceanogr.* **2014**, *101*, 21–31. [CrossRef]
41. Smayda, T.J.; Reynolds, C.S. Community Assembly in Marine Phytoplankton: Application of Recent Models to Harmful Dinoflagellate Blooms. *J. Plankton Res.* **2001**, *23*, 447–461. [CrossRef]
42. Raine, R.; Cosgrove, S.; Fennell, S.; Gregory, C.; Barnett, M.; Purdie, D.; Cave, R. Origins of *Dinophysis* blooms which impact Irish aquaculture. In *Marine and Freshwater Harmful Algae, Proceedings of the 17th International Conference on Harmful Algae, Florianópolis, Brazil, 9–14 October 2016*; Proença, L.A.O., Hallegraeff, G.M., Eds.; International Society for the Study of Harmful Algae: Paris, France, 2017; pp. 46–49.
43. Farrell, H.; Gentien, P.; Fernand, L.; Lunven, M.; Reguera, B.; González-Gil, S.; Raine, R. Scales characterising a high density thin layer of *Dinophysis acuta* Ehrenberg and its transport within a coastal jet. *Harmful Algae* **2012**, *15*, 36–46. [CrossRef]
44. Davidson, K.; Anderson, D.M.; Mateus, M.; Reguera, B.; Silke, J.; Sourisseau, M.; Maguire, J. Forecasting the risk of harmful algal blooms: Preface to the Asimuth special issue. *Harmful Algae* **2016**, *53*, 1–7. [CrossRef] [PubMed]
45. Svensson, S. Depuration of Okadaic acid (diarrhetic shellfish toxin) in mussels, *Mytilus edulis* (Linnaeus), feeding on different quantities of nontoxic algae. *Aquaculture* **2003**, *218*, 277–291. [CrossRef]
46. Bricelj, V.M.; Shumway, S.E. Paralytic shellfish toxins in bivalve molluscs: Occurrence, transfer kinetics and biotransformation. *Rev. Fish. Sci.* **1998**, *6*, 315–383. [CrossRef]
47. Sidari, L.; Nichetto, P.; Cok, S.; Sosa, S.; Tubaro, A.; Honsell, G.; Della Loggia, R. Phytoplankton selection by mussels and diarrhetic shellfish poisoning. *Mar. Biol.* **1998**, *131*, 103–111. [CrossRef]
48. Nielsen, L.T.; Hansen, P.J.; Krock, B.; Vismann, B. Accumulation, transformation and breakdown of DSP toxins from the toxic dinoflagellate *Dinophysis acuta* in blue mussels, *Mytilus edulis*. *Toxicon* **2016**, *117*, 84–93. [CrossRef] [PubMed]
49. Tong, M.; Smith, J.L.; Richlen, M.; Steidinger, K.A.; Kulis, D.M.; Fux, E.; Anderson, D.M. Characterization and comparison of toxin-producing isolates of *Dinophysis acuminata* from New England and Canada. *J. Phycol.* **2015**, *51*, 66–81. [CrossRef] [PubMed]
50. Hattenrath-Lehmann, T.K.; Marcoval, M.A.; Mittlesdorf, H.; Goleski, J.A.; Wang, Z.; Haynes, B.; Morton, S.L.; Gobler, C.J. Nitrogenous nutrients promote the growth and toxicity of *Dinophysis acuminata* during estuarine bloom events. *PLoS ONE* **2015**, *10*. [CrossRef] [PubMed]

51. Pizarro, G.; Escalera, L.; González-Gil, S.; Franco, J.M.; Reguera, B. Growth, behaviour and cell toxin quota of *Dinophysis acuta* during a daily cycle. *Mar. Ecol. Prog. Ser.* **2008**, *353*, 89–105. [CrossRef]
52. Pizarro, G.; Paz, B.; González-Gil, S.; Franco, J.M.; Reguera, B. Seasonal variability of lipophilic toxins during a *Dinophysis acuta* bloom in Western Iberia: Differences between picked cells and plankton concentrates. *Harmful Algae* **2009**, *8*, 926–937. [CrossRef]
53. Mafra, L.L.; Ribas, T.; Alves, T.P.; Proença, L.A.O.; Schramm, M.A.; Uchida, H.; Suzuki, T. Differential okadiac acid accumulation and detoxification by oysters and mussels during natural and simulated *Dinophysis* blooms. *Fish. Sci.* **2015**, *81*, 749–762. [CrossRef]
54. Vale, P. Differential dynamics of dinophysistoxins and pectenotoxins between blue mussel and common cockle: A phenomenon originating from the complex toxin profile of *Dinophysis acuta*. *Toxicon* **2004**, *44*, 123–134. [CrossRef] [PubMed]
55. Vale, P. Differential dynamics of dinophysistoxins and pectenotoxins, part II: Offshore bivalve species. *Toxicon* **2006**, *47*, 163–173. [CrossRef] [PubMed]
56. Lindegarth, S.; Torgersen, T.; Lundve, B.; Sandvik, M. Differential retention of okadaic acid (OA) group toxins and pectenotoxins (PTX) in the blue mussel, *Mytilus edulis* (L.) and European flat oyster, *Ostrea edulis* (L.). *J. Shellfish Res.* **2009**, *28*, 313–323. [CrossRef]
57. García-Altares, M.; Casanova, A.; Fernández-Tejedor, M.; Diogène, J.; de la Iglesia, P. Bloom of *Dinophysis* spp. dominated by *D. sacculus* and its related diarrhetic shellfish poisoning (DSP) outbreak in Alfacs Bay (Catalonia, NW Mediterranean Sea): Identification of DSP toxins in phytoplankton, shellfish and passive samplers. *Reg. Stud. Mar. Sci.* **2016**, *6*, 19–28. [CrossRef]
58. Hattenrath-Lehmann, T.K.; Lusty, M.W.; Wallace, R.B.; Haynes, B.; Wang, Z.; Broadwater, M.; Deeds, J.R.; Morton, S.L.; Hastback, W.; Porter, L.; et al. Evaluation of rapid, early warning approaches to track shellfish toxins associated with *Dinophysis* and *Alexandrium* blooms. *Mar. Drugs* **2018**, *16*. [CrossRef] [PubMed]
59. MacKenzie, L.; Beuzenberg, V.; Holland, P.; McNabb, P.; Suzuki, T.; Selwood, A. Pectenotoxin and okadaic acid-based toxin profiles in *Dinophysis acuta* and *Dinophysis acuminata* from New Zealand. *Harmful Algae* **2005**, *4*, 75–85. [CrossRef]
60. Suzuki, T.; Miyazono, A.; Baba, K.; Sugawara, R.; Kamiyama, T. LC-MS/MS analysis of okadaic acid analogues and other lipophilic toxins in single-cell isolates of several *Dinophysis* species collected in Hokkaido, Japan. *Harmful Algae* **2009**, *8*, 233–238. [CrossRef]
61. Kamiyama, T.; Suzuki, T. Production of dinophysistoxin-1 and pectenotoxin-2 by a culture of *Dinophysis acuminata* (Dinophyceae). *Harmful Algae* **2009**, *8*, 312–317. [CrossRef]
62. Blanco, J.; Álvarez, G.; Uribe, E. Identification of pectenotoxins in plankton, filter feeders and isolated cells of a *Dinophysis acuminata* with an atypical toxin profile from Chile. *Toxicon* **2007**, *49*, 710–716. [CrossRef] [PubMed]
63. Fux, E.; Smith, J.L.; Tong, M.; Guzmán, L.; Anderson, D.M. Toxin profiles of five geographical isolates of *Dinophysis* spp. from North and South America. *Toxicon* **2011**, *57*, 275–287. [CrossRef] [PubMed]
64. Fabro, E.; Almandoz, G.O.; Ferrario, M.; Tillmann, U.; Cembella, A.; Krock, B. Distribution of *Dinophysis* species and their association with lipophilic phycotoxins in plankton from the Argentine Sea. *Harmful Algae* **2016**, *59*, 31–41. [CrossRef] [PubMed]
65. Lindahl, O.; Lundve, B.; Johansen, M. Toxicity of *Dinophysis* spp. in relation to population density and environmental conditions on the Swedish west coast. *Harmful Algae* **2007**, *6*, 218–231. [CrossRef]
66. Jørgensen, K.; Andersen, P. Relation between the concentration of *Dinophysis acuminata* and diarrheic shellfish poisoning toxins in blue mussels (*Mytilus edulis*) during a toxic episode in the Limfjord (Denmark), 2006. *J. Shellfish Res.* **2007**, *26*, 1081–1087. [CrossRef]
67. Nielsen, L.T.; Krock, B.; Hansen, P.J. Effects of light and food availability on toxin production, growth and photosynthesis in *Dinophysis acuminata*. *Mar. Ecol. Prog. Ser.* **2012**, *471*, 37–50. [CrossRef]
68. Fernández, M.L.; Reguera, B.; Ramilo, I.; Martinez, A. Toxin content of *Dinophysis acuminata, D. acuta* and *D. caudata* from the Galician Rías Baixas. In Proceedings of the Ninth Conference on Harmful Algal Blooms, Hobart, Australia, 7–11 February 2000; Hallegraeff, G.M., Blackburn, S.I., Bolch, C.J., Lewis, R.J., Eds.; Intergovernmental Oceanographic Commission of UNESCO: Paris, France, 2001; pp. 360–363.
69. Vale, P.; de M Sampayo, M.A. Dinophysistoxin-2: A rare diarrhoeic toxin associated with *Dinophysis acuta*. *Toxicon* **2000**, *38*, 1599–1606. [CrossRef]

70. Marcaillou, C.; Gentien, P.; Lunven, M.; Le Grand, J.; Mondeguer, F.; Danilou, M.M.; Crassous, M.P.; Youenou, A. *Dinophysis acuminata* distribution and specific toxin content in relation to mussel contamination. In Proceedings of the Ninth Conference on Harmful Algal Blooms, Hobart, Australia, 7–11 February 2000; Hallegraeff, G.M., Blackburn, S.I., Bolch, C.J., Lewis, R.J., Eds.; Intergovernmental Oceanographic Commission of UNESCO: Paris, France, 2001; pp. 356–358.
71. James, K.J.; Bishop, A.G.; Healy, B.M.; Roden, C.; Sherlock, I.R.; Twohig, M.; Draisci, R.; Giannetti, L.; Lucentini, L. Efficient isolation of the rare diarrhoeic shellfish toxin, dinophysistoxin-2, from marine phytoplankton. *Toxicon* **1999**, *37*, 343–357. [CrossRef]
72. Puente, P.F.; Sáez, M.J.F.; Hamilton, B.; Furey, A.; James, K.J. Studies of polyether toxins in the marine phytoplankton, *Dinophysis acuta*, in Ireland using multiple tandem mass spectrometry. *Toxicon* **2004**, *44*, 919–926. [CrossRef] [PubMed]
73. Fux, E.; Gonzalez-Gil, S.; Lunven, M.; Gentien, P.; Hess, P. Production of diarrhetic shellfish poisoning toxins and pectenotoxins at depths within and below the euphotic zone. *Toxicon* **2010**, *56*, 1487–1496. [CrossRef] [PubMed]
74. Morris, S.; Stubbs, B.; Cook, A.; Milligan, S.; Quilliam, M.A. The First Report of the Co-Occurrence of Pectenotoxins, Okadaic Acid and Dinophysistoxin-2 in Shellfish from England. Cefas Publication. 2004. Available online: https://www.cefas.co.uk/publications/posters/30830web.pdf (accessed on 2 June 2018).
75. Edwards, A.; Sharples, F. Scottish sea lochs: A catalogue. Scottish Marine Biological Association. *Nat. Conserv. Counc.* **1986**, *110*, 250.
76. Bresnan, E.; Cook, K.B.; Hughes, S.L.; Hay, S.J.; Smith, K.; Walsham, P.; Webster, L. Seasonality of the plankton community at an east and west coast monitoring site in Scottish waters. *J. Sea Res.* **2015**, *105*, 16–29. [CrossRef]
77. O'Brien, T.D.; Wiebe, P.H.; Falkenhaug, T. ICES Cooperative Research Report. 2013. Available online: http://ices.dk/sites/pub/PublicationReports/CooperativeResearchReport(CRR)/crr318/CRR318Zooplankton.pdf (accessed on 12 June 2018).
78. Bresnan, E.; Cook, K.; Hindson, J.; Hughes, S.; Lacaze, J.-P.; Walsham, P.; Webster, L.; Turrell, W.R. The Scottish Coastal Observatory 1997–2013: Part 1—Executive Summary. Available online: https://www.gov.scot/Resource/0051/00513827.pdf (accessed on 26 September 2018).
79. Edwards, A.; Baxter, M.S.; Ellett, D.J.; Martin, J.H.A.; Meldrum, D.T.; Griffiths, C.R. Clyde Sea hydrography. *Proc. R. Soc. Edinburgh Sect. B Biol. Sci.* **1986**, *90*, 67–83.
80. Utermöhl, H. Zur Vervollkommnung der quantitativen Phytoplankton-Methodik. *Mitt. Int. Ver. Theor. Angew. Limnol.* **1958**, *9*, 1–3.
81. In-House Validation of an LC-MS/MS Method for the Determination of Lipophilic Toxins in Shellfish Species Typically Tested in the United Kingdom. Available online: https://www.food.gov.uk/sites/default/files/media/document/fs235004_0.pdf (accessed on 26 September 2018).
82. EU-Harmonised Standard Operating Procedure for Determination of Lipophilic Marine Biotoxins in Molluscs by LC-MS/MS. Available online: http://www.aecosan.msssi.gob.es/AECOSAN/docs/documentos/laboratorios/LNRBM/ARCHIVO2EU-Harmonised-SOP-LIPO-LCMSMS_Version5.pdf (accessed on 8 June 2018).
83. Turner, A.D.; Goya, A.B. Occurrence and profiles of lipophilic toxins in shellfish harvested from Argentina. *Toxicon* **2015**, *102*, 32–42. [CrossRef] [PubMed]

toxins

Article

Dinophysis Species and Diarrhetic Shellfish Toxins: 20 Years of Monitoring Program in Andalusia, South of Spain

Raúl Fernández *, Luz Mamán, David Jaén, Lourdes Fernández Fuentes, M. Asunción Ocaña and M. Mercedes Gordillo

Laboratory for the Quality Control of Fishery Resources, Agency for the Management of Agriculture and Fisheries of Andalusia, Ministry for Agriculture, Fisheries and Rural Development, Regional Government of Andalusia, 21459 Andalusia, Spain; luz.m.menendez@juntadeandalucia.es (L.M.); david.jaen@juntadeandalucia.es (D.J.); lourdes.fernandez.fuentes@juntadeandalucia.es (L.F.F.); mariaa.ocana@juntadeandalucia.es (M.A.O.); mariam.gordillo@juntadeandalucia.es (M.M.G.)

* Correspondence: raul.fernandez.lozano@juntadeandalucia.es; Tel.: +34-600-145-893

Received: 13 November 2018; Accepted: 26 March 2019; Published: 29 March 2019

Abstract: In Andalusia, the official monitoring program for toxic phytoplankton and marine biotoxins was launched in 1994 to comply with European legislation. Since then, there have been numerous episodes of DST (Diarrhetic shellfish toxins) associated with the proliferation of *Dinophysis* species. This article reviews two decades of time series data and assesses the effectiveness of the program established. The testing of lipophilic toxins and toxic phytoplankton is based on official methods harmonized and accredited since 2007 according to the standard UNE-EN-ISO 17025. The major species of *Dinophysis* identified were *D. acuminata* complex, *D. caudata*, *D. acuta* and *D. fortii*, with the main growth season being from early spring until the end of autumn. Both *D. acuminata* complex and *D. acuta* have been clearly associated with toxicity in molluscs. Despite the complexity of data obtained through monitoring programs, it is possible to provide early warning of potential health risks for most situations. This is the first report of *Dinophysis* species and their relation to DST events in a time series from Andalusia.

Keywords: *Dinophysis*; Diarrhetic shellfish toxins; marine biotoxins; blooms

Key Contribution: The analysis of the data has shown that not all the *Dinophysis* species identified in Andalusia with proven toxic potential have so far been associated with DST outbreaks in molluscs

1. Introduction

The implementation of monitoring programs for marine biotoxins in the wake of the findings of Yasumoto [1,2], at a scale dependent on the geographical scope of each competent administration, started in Andalusia in 1994. These findings demonstrated a relationship between outbreaks of diarrheal intoxication in humans, the ingestion of molluscs and the presence in the environment of *Dinophysis fortii* that was identified as the producer of toxins responsible for poisoning. This led to the monitoring programs to carry out both analysis of the mollusc toxin content and cell counts of the phytoplankton species whose toxicity was proven over time.

The European regulations applicable concerning food security [3,4] lay down the basic requirements and recommendations for the implementation of these programs. The program implemented in Andalusia has observed the guidelines established for the definition of areas and the frequency of monitoring. This study presents the data obtained from the start of monitoring and their analysis to answer the following question: Are the regulatory requirements for the analysis of toxic phytoplankton effective as an early-warning system for the risk of contamination in molluscs on the Andalusian coast?

The identification of some species of *Dinophysis* has led to much discussion and many scientific publications. The main issues have been reviewed by Reguera et al. [5]. Identification has been carried out based on morphometric characteristics mainly using light microscopy (LM), but the considerable intraspecific variability makes it difficult to clearly discriminate between some of the species. Nevertheless, LM is the method most used by monitoring programs. In any case, in Andalusia, the set of species given in the IOC Taxonomic Reference List of Toxic Microalgae [6] has been used as the basis for monitoring, and the region has acted according to the principle of maximum food security in situations of any doubt.

A group of new causative agents of shellfish poisoning, the Diarrhetic Shellfish Toxins (DST), was isolated and their structures determined in the 1980s [1,2]. In Andalusia, many cases of DST have been detected during the years of monitoring but not all the toxins in this group have been individually characterized.

Accumulation of the toxicity produced by microalgae in filter-feeders has also been the subject of study. However, important intra- and interspecific variability has been measured resulting from causes such as differences in filtration and clearance rates [7,8] or from selection mechanisms based on the quality and quantity of prey [9–11]. Such variability has become a parameter considered in the monitoring program.

For more than 20 years, species of the genus *Dinophysis* have been commonly found in almost all the sampling stations in Andalusia. The species clearly associated with toxicity phenomena in molluscs, have been *D. acuminata*/*D. ovum* and *D. acuta*. The accumulation of toxins above permitted levels triggers the activation of closure protocols for fisheries that can sometimes be prolonged for up to 6 months. All the species of the genus identified in the samples that at some time have formed part of the IOC list, are presented in this study along with toxicity levels of molluscs in each case when this has occurred.

2. Results

The distribution of areas in Andalusia (see Section 4.1) represents the complete set of mollusc habitats ranging in size between 12.6 ha and the 35,340.5 ha (average area 4842.4 ha). Smaller areas correspond to the perimeter of areas where aquaculture facilities are located.

All the information presented in this study comes from the sampling stations located in the above-mentioned areas. In each sampling, the choice of sampling points has been arbitrary within each area, except in areas where physico-chemical measurements of the water were already being made, at previously fixed points. Mollusc samples were usually selected at those points where there was high fishing activity.

2.1. Species of the Genus Dinophysis

Twenty *Dinophysis* species out of more than 100 that make up the genus [12] were identified on the Andalusian coast. Those *Dinophysis* cells considered gametes have been excluded from the reported counts. *Dinophysis* cells not identified to species level are reported as *Dinophysis* spp. Table 1 provides a species list along with the frequency of occurrence. The number of samples collected in the study period (20 years) was 34,329.

The difficulty in discriminating between *D. acuminata* and *D. ovum* has led us to follow the example of Lassus and Bardouil [13] or Bravo [14] who introduced the term "*Dinophysis acuminata* complex" that encompasses both, reflecting its great morphological variability.

Table 1. Species of the genus *Dinophysis* found in the samples. (34,329 samples).

Species	Frequency in Atlantic (%)	Frequency in Mediterranean (%)
Dinophysis acuminata Claparède & Lachmann, 1859	85.2	53.8
Dinophysis acuta Ehrenberg, 1839	19.4	9.6
Dinophysis argus (Phalacroma argus) F. Stein 1883	0.1	0.9
Dinophysis caudata Saville-Kent, 1881	54.7	55.3
Dinophysis amphora Balech 1971	<0.1	0
Dinophysis schroederi J. Pavillard 1909	0.2	0.9
Dinophysis cuneus (Phalacroma cuneus) F. Schütt 1895	0	0.1
Dinophysis doryphora (Phalacroma doryphorum) Stein 1883	0.2	0.9
Dinophysis fortii Pavillard, 1923	4.5	17.1
Dinophysis hastata F. Stein 1883	0.8	0.3
Dinophysis odiosa (Pavillard) Tai & Skogsberg 1934	3.3	0.5
Dinophysis pusilla Jörgensen 1923	<0.1	0.2
Dinophysis rapa (Phalacroma rapa) F. Stein 1883	0.2	6.8
Dinophysis sacculus Stein, 1883	2.5	2.7
Dinophysis schuettii G. Murray & Whitting 1899	4.7	5.6
Dinophysis similis Kofoid & Skogsberg 1928	<0.1	0.1
Dinophysis tripos Gourret, 1883	<0.1	2.1
Dinophysis mitra (Phalacroma mitra) F. Schütt, 1895	0.1	0.7
Phalacroma rotundatum (Dinophysis rotundata) (Claparéde & Lachmann) Kofoid & Michener, 1911	12.5	5.1
Dinophysis ovum [1] (F. Schütt) T.H. Abé	([1])	([1])
Dinophysis spp.	42.2	46.2

[1] Species identified from isolated specimens and kept in culture. Routinely, *Dinophysis ovum* are included in the *Dinophysis acuminata* complex.

The species with the highest frequency were *D. acuminata* complex, *D. caudata*, *D. acuta* and *D. fortii*.

Nearly all the species were detected in both the Atlantic and the Mediterranean areas, but some show marked differences in their repartition between the two areas. While *D. acuminata* complex, *D. acuta* and *D. rotundata* (*P. rotundatum)* are more frequent on the Atlantic coast, *D. fortii* and *D. rapa* (*P. rapa*) are more frequent in the Mediterranean Sea.

Taking into account that the sampling frequency was uniform all year long, it can be observed that *D. acuminata* complex is present almost all throughout the year, although it does not always trigger toxic outbreaks in molluscs (see Section 2.3).

The couple *D. acuminata* complex/*D. caudata* is frequent in the samples. In addition, it is accompanied at times by *D. acuta* and *D. fortii*. Similar associations have already been reported in temperate waters [5].

The set of species identified as *Dinophysis* spp. occurs very frequently in both sea areas. Although these species not known to be toxic, unusual high concentrations of some of them activated alert protocols.

2.2. Temporal Episodes of Dinophysis

The volume of data generated during the 20 years of monitoring subject to examination is very high, and data processing is needed to condense the redundancies into manageable form.

Figure 1 shows the choice of the appropriate number of clusters, to summarize the data, through the highest Simple Structure Index (SSI) [15]. It shows how the grouping of seven clusters best explains the variance in the data taking up 12 SSI clusters at maximum.

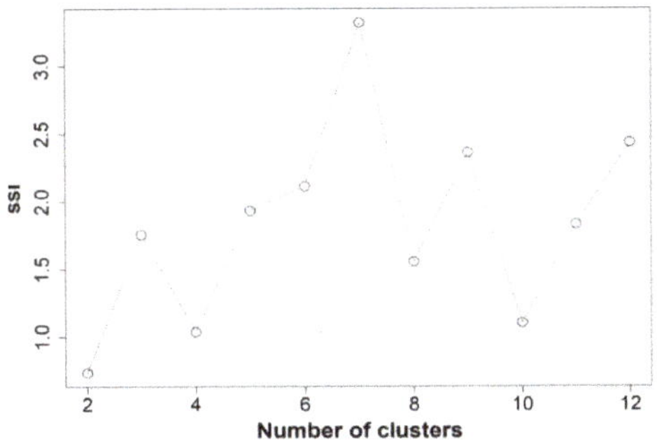

Figure 1. Optimizing the number of clusters through the SSI criterion. Number of samples analyzed 6659.

Figure 2 shows the distribution of the stations in the different groups. Appendix A (Figures A1–A7) and Appendix B (Figures A8–A11) shows a historical series of 20 years of their abundance values, along with toxin values in molluscs of a selected area of each cluster obtained.

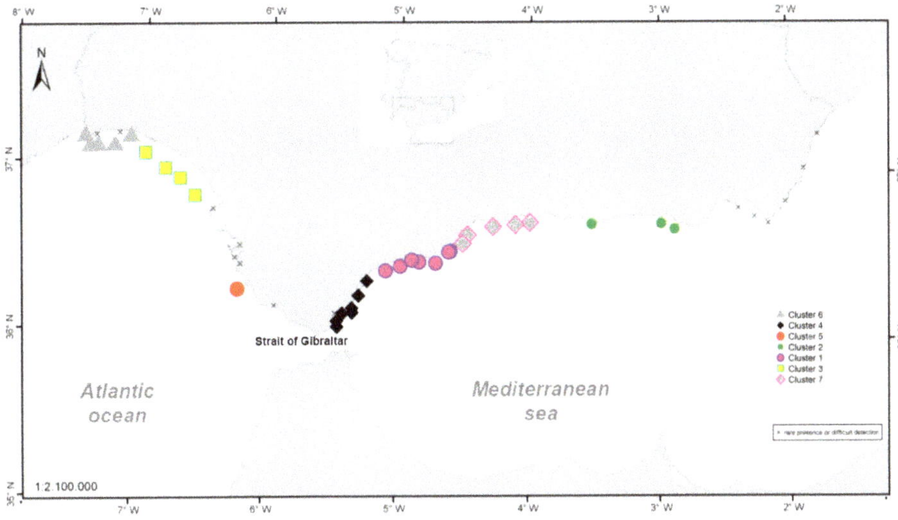

Figure 2. Result of the cluster analysis using the k-means non-hierarchical method. The areas excluded from the analysis (marqued with an "x") are those in which the presence of *Dinophysis* was detected with a very low frequency for various reasons: impossibility of quantifying samples due to organic matter or areas of low sampling frequency due to the absence of extractive activity.

As discussed in the previous section, the most frequent species in the coast of Andalusia are *D. acuminata* complex, *D. caudata*, *D. acuta* and *D. fortii*. Of these, *D. acuminata* complex and *D. acuta* are the only ones which have been partnered by co-occurrence with episodes of DST. Thus, the description of episodes presented in this work will be focused on both species.

Although *D. acuminata* complex is present almost all year round, the more substantial episodes are usually produced as a succession of between one and three pulses from the beginning of spring until the end of autumn. The period of growth of *D. acuta* is, however, more reduced, from summer to early autumn. Although the pattern mentioned for *D. acuminata* complex has been repeated in all the years of monitoring, *D. acuta* does not present such a recurrence, and they generally disappear for one or more years. The patterns found show similarity between different years of monitoring, while the abundance reached determines the degree of difference. Figure 3 shows the maximum levels of abundance where the difference can be seen.

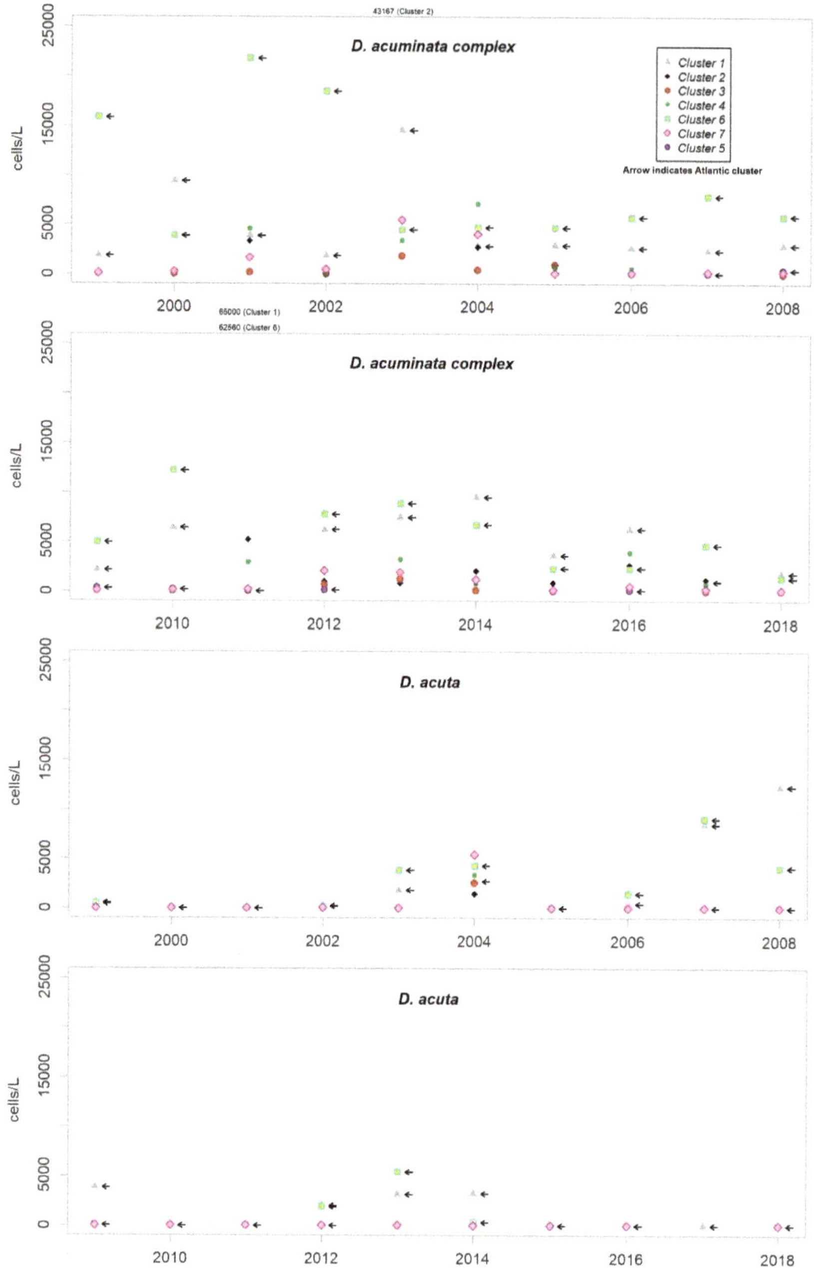

Figure 3. Annual maximum concentration (cells/L) of *Dinophysis acuminata* complex and *Dinophysis acuta* in each cluster throughout the monitoring period.

Although the presence of *D. acuminata* complex and *D. acuta* in the environment occurs during similar periods all along the coast of Andalusia, in general, there are notable differences in the intensity of the abundance between clusters 1 and 6 (Atlantic area) and the rest. Therefore, although there are frequent blooms of relatively high abundance in the Atlantic area, in the Mediterranean it is rare that either species exceeds 400 cells/l. However, cluster number 5 belongs to the Atlantic area and does not show the behaviour of the other neighbouring Atlantic clusters.

It sometimes happens, however, that a particular episode (characterized by a certain intensity) spreads to almost all the Andalusian coast in one direction or the other. Possible advection through the Strait of Gibraltar is suggested by the proximity of the dates of the growth pulses on both sides of the strait, but which also should be investigated using hydrodynamic models. In August 2001, August 2003, October 2004, July 2012, July 2013 and August 2014, episodes of *D. acuminata* complex were recorded with these features. *D. acuta* can be often detected along the entire coast, but not always; in August 2004, for example, a single case of unusually high intensity was recorded in all the areas monitored.

Episodes of special intensity of *D. acuta* occurred from the end of June to end of August 2007 and of *D. acuminata* complex from March to mid-April 2011, both in clusters 6 and 1. In the first episode, there were more than 2000 cells/L in 24.9% of the samples and more than 5000 cells/L in 4.7% (349 samples). A maximum value of 9080 cells/L occurred in cluster 6. In the second episode, a maximum of 65,000 cells/L (Cluster 1) was recorded, which was the highest concentration of *Dinophysis* species found during the years of monitoring. In this case, there were more than 2000 cells/L in 69.4% of the samples and more than 5000 cells/L in 47.9% (278 samples).

From 2014 on, a declining trend of abundance has been recorded for both species towards the western end (clusters 1 and 6). The *D. acuminata* complex had never shown this behavior (frequency of values above 2000 cells/L was drastically reduced) in the monitoring period.

The timing and abundance of other *Dinophysis* species is shown in Appendix B. None of them shows any obvious seasonal pattern or other type of temporary recurrence. The only condition found is spatial, so that while some species are detected in all areas sampled, others preferably appear in the Atlantic or the Mediterranean areas.

2.3. *Toxicity in Molluscs*

The criteria of the official monitoring programme aims to categorize some species of bivalve molluscs as indicators of each production area (administrative spatial unit). Therefore, in Andalusia, the species which have been monitored in areas of external waters where there have been major incidents with *Dinophysis*, have mainly been *Donax trunculus*, *Chamelea gallina*, *Mytilus galloprovincialis*, *Callista chione*, *Venus verrucosa* and *Cerastoderma edule*.

Levels of okadaic acid have been detected in all these areas when *D. acuminata* complex and/or *D. acuta* were present in the environment. There have also been cases, albeit few, in which samples showed toxicity but in which *Dinophysis* species or other organisms considered as DSP producers were not found; there were more cases in the period when the mouse bioassay method was used. Other substances that are part of the group of lipophilic toxins have been detected although on a smaller number of occasions. Levels of DTX-2 began to be measured at the beginning of June 2018 in *Donax trunculus* and *Mytilus galloprovincialis*. The episode has not finished yet. In the environment, the presence of mainly *Prorocentrum* cf. *texanum* has been accompanied by minor amounts of *D. acuminata* complex and *D. acuta*. Also, levels of yessotoxin were measured only in *Mytilus galloprovincialis* in the spring and summer of 2015 when in the water samples the presence mainly of *D. acuminata* complex was detected and, to a lesser extent, *D. acuta*, *D. fortii*, *D. caudata* and *P. rotundatum*.

The durations of the episodes usually correspond to the maintenance of the population of that or those phytoplankton species that generate them. There is thus good association between the detection of both parameters in qualitative terms. However, as it can be seen in Figure 4 which shows the pairs of cell concentration-toxicity values of parallel sampling, the levels of okadaic acid in molluscs do not correlate well with the concentration of the producer microalgae if the expected linear relationships are taken into account. Thus, it is not uncommon to find high values of okadaic acid with low values of phytoplankton and *vice versa*.

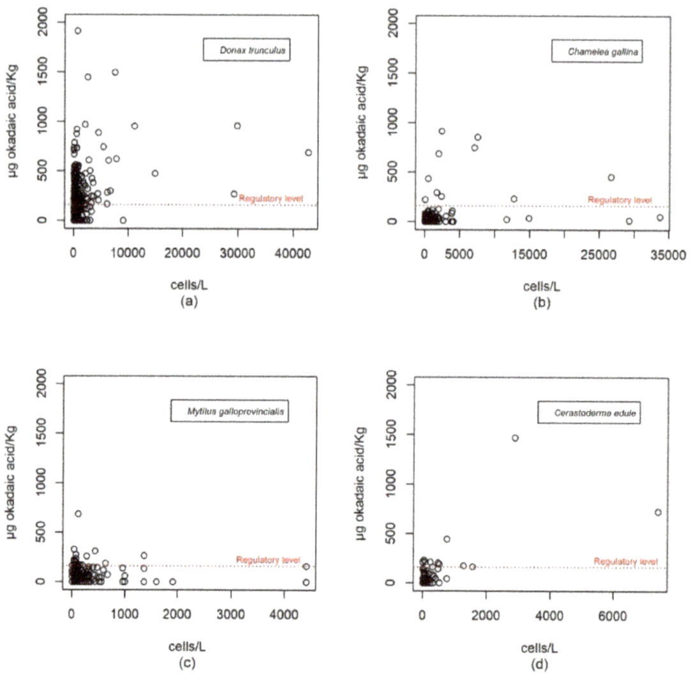

Figure 4. Toxicity in molluscs (µg okadaic acid/kg) versus concentration of *D. acuminata* complex + *D. acuta* (cells/L). The bivalve species with the highest toxic incidence have been selected. Data are not shown for mollusc species which, although they have a sufficient amount of data, have shown very little tendency to accumulate toxin. (**a**) *Donax trunculus;* (**b**) *Chamelea gallina;* (**c**) *Mytilus galloprovincialis;* (**d**) *Cerastoderma edule.*

Although there is not a good correlation between toxicity values in molluscs and the concentration of *Dinophysis* in parallel sampling, if each episode as a whole is considered, toxicity patterns in molluscs do correspond to the patterns of the producer phytoplankton species as might be expected. Thus, in general, there have been more incidents in the Atlantic area than in the Mediterranean area; episodes have occurred in warm seasons and there has been a trend toward a decrease in measured values over the last three years.

The time series of contamination episodes of bivalve molluscs, together with the abundance of DSP-producing microalgae is shown in Appendix A. It shows how smaller bivalve species (larger specimens rarely exceed 3–4 cm in their axis of maximum growth) are more prone to the accumulation of lipophilic toxins. In this way, maximum levels of toxicity (µg okadaic acid/kg) were 2665 in *D. trunculus*, 913 in *C. gallina* and 1468 in *C. edule*, whereas in larger species, there were 687 in *M. galloprovincialis*, 91 in *C. chione* and 28 in *V. verrucosa*. This difference has been verified for the pair *D. trunculus* and *C. gallina* (Figure 5) in 85 double samples taken, which has contributed to the selection of *Donax trunculus* as an indicator species for some harvesting areas.

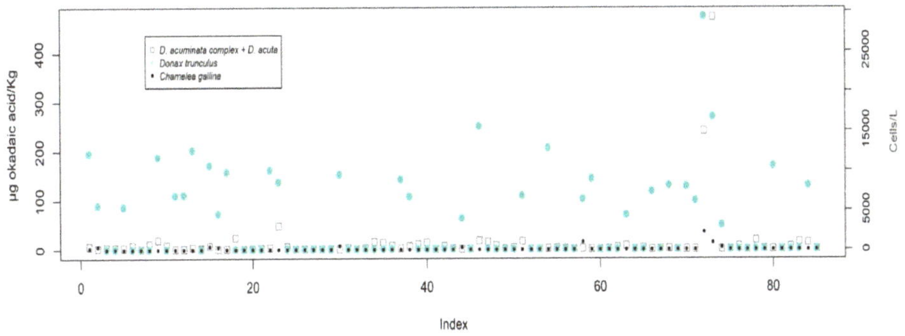

Figure 5. Toxicity in *D. trunculus* and *C. gallina* in simultaneous samples taken in the same area (x-axis: Sampling identification number). Accompanying the results is the concentration of *D. acuminata* complex being the majority *Dinophysis* species in the water sample taken at the same time.

In view of the results of the frequency distribution of accumulation and elimination daily rates (Figure 6), it is worth noting the symmetry and positive kurtosis. This means that, on the one hand, there are no appreciable differences between the speed of accumulation and elimination and, on the other hand, the values that are statistically considered as normal, do not exceed 25 µg okadaic acid/kg/day which, as has been said, are low values taking into account the extent of the range. This means that the occasions on which, starting from an absence of toxicity, the molluscs analyzed have the capacity to exceed the legal limit (160 µg okadaic acid/kg) for less than a week are statistically not significant (outliers; Figure 6).

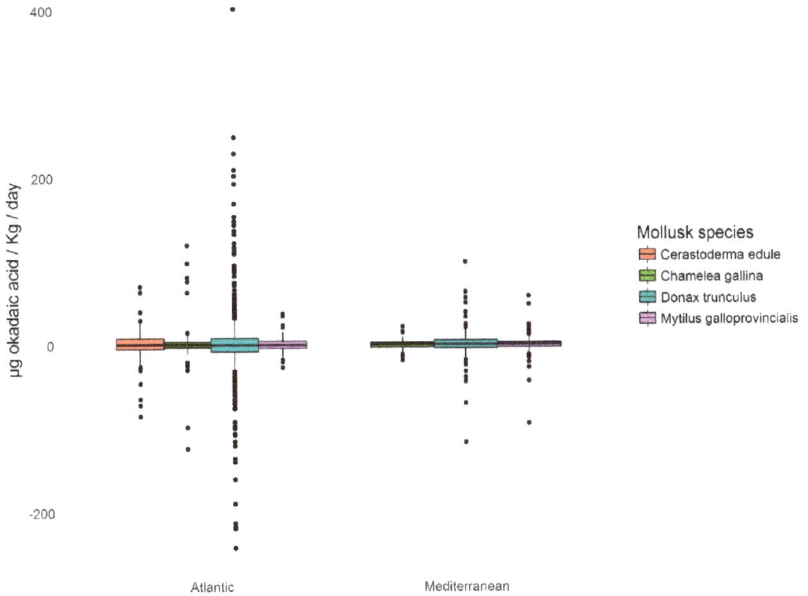

Figure 6. Box and whiskers of daily rate of accumulation / elimination of toxins (okadaic acid). In the same way that in Figure 4 the mollusc species with the highest toxic incidence have been selected, discarding those with a low tendency to accumulate.

The monitoring program of Andalusia establishes that once levels above the regulatory limit are detected in molluscs, temporary closures of fisheries must be triggered. They have been recorded in digital databases from 2007. The data presented (Tables 2 and 3) correspond to this period.

Table 2. Maximum annual closing period (days) of a fishery in an Atlantic area from 2007 to 2018.

Species [1]	2007	2008	2009	2010	2011	2012	2013	2014	2015	2016	2017	2018
Donax trunculus	161	63	51	99	45	112	55	126	125	47	46	-
Chamelea gallina	196	194	40	34	85	63	22	126	41	47	73	-
Mytilus galloprovincialis	0	0	0	54	13	147	63	4	27	34	0	-
Cerastoderma edule	0	0	0	0	34	14	34	43	30	32	0	0

[1] The mollusc species with the highest toxic incidence are shown, discarding those with a low tendency to accumulate. The latter are: *Ruditapes philippinarum, Scrobicularia plana, Polititapes rhomboides, Ruditapes decussatus, Dosinia* spp, *Polititapes aureus, Magallana gigas, Mimachlamys varia, Solen marginatus, Venus verrucosa, Acanthocardia tuberculata, Aequipecten opercularis and Pecten maximus.*

Table 3. Maximum annual closing period (days) of a fishery in a Mediterranean area from 2007 to 2018.

Species [1]	2007	2008	2009	2010	2011	2012	2013	2014	2015	2016	2017	2018
Donax trunculus	0	0	18	0	119	48	90	77	11	34	14	0
Chamelea gallina	0	0	18	0	126	51	113	77	71	34	14	0
Mytilus galloprovincialis	0	0	0	10	64	59	50	55	0	16	3	0
Callista chione	0	0	95	0	171	92	85	77	11	77	14	0
Venus verrucosa	0	0	0	0	98	32	113	59	0	34	14	0

[1] *The same as in Table 2.*

3. Discussion

Data from monitoring programs are usually complex in their processing. Regulatory changes lead to modifications in sampling plans in a way that they lose their regularity when frequency, spatial distribution or target species change. This study has taken into account such features when calculating parameters or obtaining general conclusions.

The polymorphic life cycle, feeding behaviour and phase of the cell cycle have been given by various authors as the causes of the wide morphological variation of certain species of *Dinophysis* [16,17]. This variation makes some species intermediate forms similar in shape, a fact that makes it often difficult to discriminate them as it is the case with the pairs: *D. acuminata/D. sacculus, D. acuminata/D. ovum, D. sacculus/D. pavilardii, D. caudata/D.tripos* mentioned by various authors according to the case [13,14,18,19]. For a monitoring program, this difficulty translates into the possibility of producing false positive or negative results in the risk assessment, taking into account possible differences in the toxic potential between species. An example of this was resolved in the Thermaikos Gulf, Greece [20] by considering *D. acuminata* and *D. ovum* as *D.* cf *acuminata*. A similar treatment has been decided in the monitoring program of Andalusia where *D. acuminata, D. ovum* and *D. sacculus* are treated as a whole as *D. acuminata* complex.

The species associated with DST outbreaks in Andalusia (*D. acuminata* complex and *D. acuta*) have also been considered as the main species responsible on the Galician coast in addition to *D. sacculus* [17,19,21]. Vale and Sampayo [22,23] consider *D. acuminata* and *D. acuta* as responsible for specific DST episodes along the Portuguese coast. These two species are considered again to be responsible for similar outbreaks in Sweden [24]. In the North Sea, around the island of Helgoland (Germany), *D. norvegica* joins *D. acuminata* as co-responsible for episodes of contamination in mussels. *D. acuminata* appears as the species of wider distribution concerning its association with toxic events. However, there are cases in which the responsibility of episodes of intoxication is attributed to less common species such as *D. fortii, D. rotundata, D. caudata, D. sacculus* and *D. tripos* in the east Adriatic [25]. In our program, although such species have been detected, there were two results:

toxicity was not observed in molluscs or the above-mentioned species of *Dinophysis* accompanied *D. acuminata* and/or *D. acuta* to a much lesser abundance.

It is important to mention the spatial coherence of the homogeneous areas obtained in the cluster analysis as there is no cluster covering non-neighbouring stations. It is also noteworthy that clusters mainly occupy coastal areas where the direction of the coast line is constant and that changes in that direction generate a different cluster. This feature seems to define a characteristic length of cluster dependent on such geomorphological characteristics that, in turn, could define hydrodynamic characteristics. This gives consistency to the conclusion derived from the analysis that the patterns and abundances of *D. acuminata* complex in the different stations of each cluster are similar.

The seasonal patterns of *Dinophysis* (growth pulses from the beginning of the spring until the end of autumn) in Andalusia do not differ from those found by the other authors in western Europe. It exceeds at the end points of the period mentioned by Smayda [26]: "the blooms of dinoflagellates occur in predominantly warm waters which are stratified from late spring to early autumn". Other authors have limited this same period as the one with the largest development of *Dinophysis* [27–31]. In general, although the most apparent growth peaks are given within this period, species such as *D. acuminata* complex are present throughout the rest of the year even though at very low concentrations. Nincevic-Gladan [25] revealed that of the 13 species detected in the east Adriatic coast, only *D. tripos* appeared in winter. Koukaras [20] noted that, at genus level, the episodes usually lasted between 3 and 4 months, and sporadically appeared throughout the rest of the year.

Many authors have reported and analysed the possible causes of the discrepancy between the values for toxicity in molluscs and the abundance of microalgae [24,32–34]. The causes mainly proposed are the presence of alternative food, environmental factors, the stratification of the water column that favours the development of thin layers of microalgae, or the variability in the toxin content per cell. In addition, other authors have studied the daily vertical migration of plankton [13,35–38], which translates into irregularity in daily food availability for molluscs. Discrepancy in the pairs of parallel sampling values (if a linear correlation is expected between cell numbers and toxicity) and the explanation of the inaccuracy of dinoflagellate abundance as an indicator of the true exposure suffered by molluscs throughout the previous week has been found in our data. This discrepancy may be a consequence of the factors above mentioned. In this way, the toxicity value in molluscs represents the result of a continuous exposure before the sample is taken, while the value of plankton concentration is representative of the moment of capture as molluscs have not yet responded.

The European regulations [3,4] says "production areas must be periodically monitored to check for the presence of toxin-producing plankton in production and relaying waters and biotoxins in live bivalve molluscs. The sampling frequency for toxin analysis in the molluscs is, as a general rule, to be weekly during the periods at which harvesting is allowed. This frequency may be reduced in specific areas, or for specific types of molluscs, if a risk assessment on toxins or phytoplankton occurrence suggests a very low risk of toxic episodes". On the other hand, it indicates that monitoring must be increased if there is evidence or suspicions of an increased risk. Such indications, in principle, leave no room for a lack of efficiency in the programs established at European level so, the answer to the initial question raised in this study, "Are the regulatory requirements for the analysis of toxic phytoplankton effective as an early-warning system of the risk of contamination of molluscs in the Andalusian coast?" would be "Yes". The problem lies in the risk assessment. In Andalusia, the check once a week of the concentration of phytoplankton, as discussed above, may have inaccuracies as indicators. An important number of cases in which molluscs had the capacity to exceed the legal limits in less than a week have been detected on our coast. Under these conditions, 11.6% of the cases were of *Donax trunculus*, 12.2% of *Cerastoderma edule*, 11.5% of *Mytilus galloprovincialis* and 11.4% of *Chamelea gallina*. Therefore, in order to prevent, to some extent, this risk from 2015 on, the uncertainty of the measure of toxicity needed to activate the intensification of sampling (48 h) was set in the criteria of the monitoring program as a factor to take into account. On the other hand, incidents with the toxicities of bivalve molluscs have been so important that there have been closures of fisheries for even half a year. A fact that shows the magnitude of the problem, bearing in mind that such fisheries represent a significant economic source at a local coastal scale. As has been mentioned, there have been numerous studies aimed at understanding the dynamics of the plankton's and molluscs' toxicities. Although there is increasing awareness of them, it remains necessary to expand knowledge which, with large sets of data of different nature, will shed light to the production of other indices or will suggest changes in sampling strategies to reduce the range of health risk.

4. Materials and Methods

All the data that underpin this article correspond to the information generated by the program for phytoplankton and biotoxins official monitoring established in Andalusia in 1994. The data generated were not recorded on a computer system until 1999. Therefore, this article refers to the period from then on. The information is available to the public and can be found at the web page http://www.cap.junta-andalucia.es/agriculturaypesca/moluzonasprodu/ of the Regional Ministry for Agriculture, Fisheries and Rural Development of Andalusia (Regional Government). That Ministry is conferred with the exclusive jurisdiction for fishing in inland waters, shellfish and aquaculture. The laboratory designated by the competent authority to perform the analyses corresponding to the official monitoring program is the *Laboratory for the Quality Control of Fishery Resources* which has developed its functions since 1996. The laboratory has been entitled to develop this monitoring since 2007, according to the UNE-EN-ISO 17025 standard.

4.1. Sampling Plan

The sampling stations in Figure 7 are represented by the centroid of the production area to which they belong. However, the point of capture of each sample can be placed in any position within the same area.

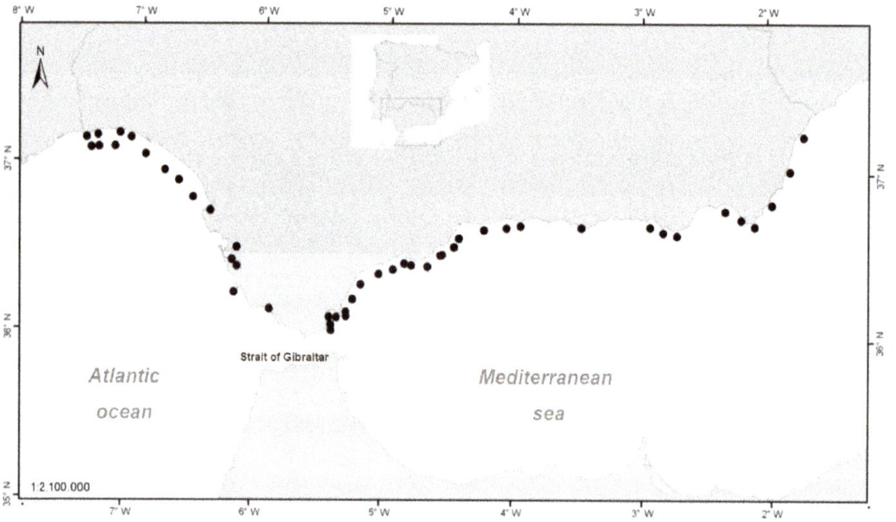

Figure 7. Centroids of the production areas declared by the Order of 15 July 1993 - BOJA (Spanish acronym for the Andalusian Official Gazette) No. 85 of 5 August 1993 [39]—which have been updated in successive orders.

Based on the operational capacity of the program, the sampling strategy has been adapted as far as possible to the European Regulations and their successive modifications. Thus, the sampling frequency was weekly at some stations from the beginning while others started on a fortnightly basis for water and quarterly for molluscs. However, this frequency has now been increased to include sampling all parameters in all production areas declared every week. The program has always allowed the possibility of increasing sampling if evidence of an increase of a toxicological risk is detected. The successive changes are detailed in Appendix C (Tables A1–A4).

4.2. Sampling Techniques

Water samples were collected using vertical hauls with bongo nets of mesh size 20 μm and a hose system [40]. Samples of molluscs from natural populations were collected using techniques traditionally used by the Andalusian shellfish sector. Samples were either taken at points of highest productive activity within each production area or provided by producers from their aquaculture facilities.

4.3. Analysis

Testing of lipophilic toxins and toxic phytoplankton are based on official methods harmonized and accredited since 2007 by ENAC (National Accreditation Entity-in Spanish) according to the standard UNE-EN-ISO 17025.

For the identification and enumeration of *Dinophysis* spp., the technique of Utermöhl [41] was used as recommended in European standard UNE-EN 15204 *Guidance standard on the enumeration of phytoplankton using inverted microscopy*.

Lipophilic toxin levels were determined according to the method described by Yasumoto et al. [42]. From 2011 on, the data presented correspond to analyses carried out using the European harmonized chemical technique (LC-MS/MS).

4.4. Data Processing

The processing and graphic presentations of the data are carried out using the free software for statistical analysis and graphics R in its 2013 version [15].

Given the huge volume of records (20 years), and for the submission of the time series, a cluster analysis was carried out on producing areas in order to reduce the datasets to be presented, excluding redundancy without losing relevant information. To do this, the K-means non-hierarchical cluster analysis (function in R: kmeans()) was used after developing the analysis of the optimal number of clusters (function in R: cascadeKM()) over a maximum of 12 clusters. (If more clusters were extracted, the purpose sought with the use of this technique would not be achieved). This is an unsupervised automatic method for pattern recognition, i.e., it is based on the response variable (concentration of *D. acuminata* complex) without seeking correlations with explanatory variables (e.g., environmental). For the response variable, the concentration of *Dinophysis acuminata* complex was chosen, as it provides more information because it has a high frequency in the samples. A total of 6659 samples were used after excluding very low incidence areas (see Figure 3) and extracting only quantifiable values. Thus, it is assumed that the homogeneous areas defined by *D. acuminata*, probably conditioned by the hydrodynamic characteristics, could be homogeneous also for the other species. In any case, the most relevant species in Andalusia is *D. acuminata* complex and the presentation of the information must adapt mainly to it. To obtain the optimal number of areas the "SSI" (Simple Structure Index) criterion has been used [43]. This is an index that combines three factors: (1) the greatest difference in the response variable between clusters, (2) the sizes of the most contrasting clusters and (3) the deviation of the variable in the cluster centers compared to its overall mean. It can be deduced that each factor separately indicates a more homogeneous selection of groups and thus, a higher SSI score implies a better partition.

The calculation of the daily rate of accumulation or elimination of toxins is carried out through the difference in toxicity measured between the samples from the same area in two successive samplings divided by the number of days, provided that between the two sampling there are not more than 11 days (maximum amplitude in samples obtained in working days of two consecutive weeks). This rate is a calculated value that indicates what would be the accumulation or elimination if every day between the two samples was kept constant. It represents, therefore, a theoretical daily value that must be taken with caution, understanding that there are probably days between the two samples with a higher and lower rate.

The information provided concerning the relative sensitivity among bivalve species identically exposed to microalgae of *Dinophysis* genus derives from parallel samples, if present, in which such species have been collected at the same time in the same area.

Author Contributions: Formal analysis, R.F.; investigation, R.F., L.M, D.J., L.F.F., M.A.O. and M.M.G.; writing—original draft preparation, R.F.; writing—review and editing, R.F., L.M.; supervision, L.M.

Funding: The editing of this article was funded by European funding programme INTERREG Atlantic Area with the proyect PRIMROSE, EAPA_182/2016.

Acknowledgments: Acknowledgments to Esther for her accurate translation into English. I would like to express my gratitude to all the staff of the Laboratory for the quality control of fishery resources and the sampling staff for their daily dedication to the hard task of extracting information from the sea.

Conflicts of Interest: The authors declare no conflict of interest.

Appendix A

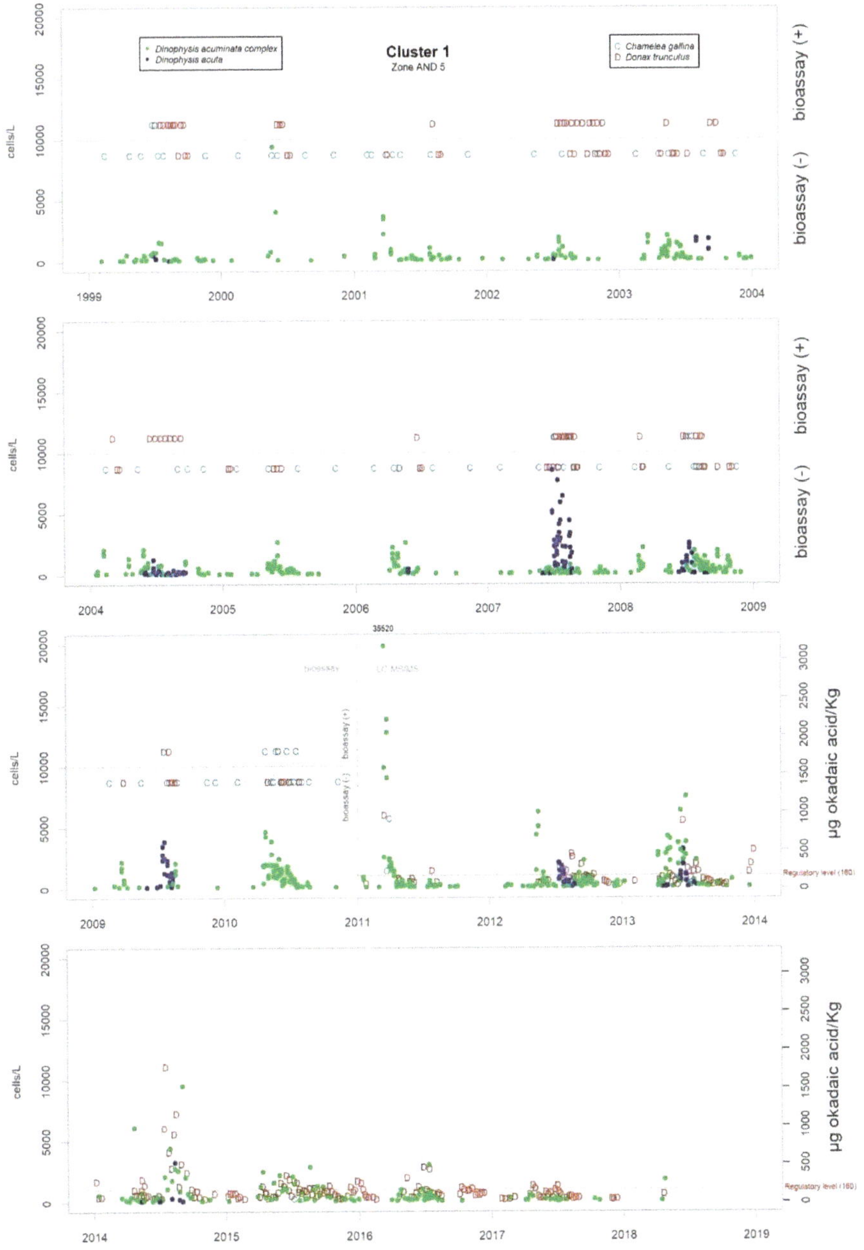

Figure A1. Temporal series of the abundance of *D. acuminata* and *D. acuta* and the concentration of okadaic acid in the species of mollusc monitored in each harvest area, in cluster 1. The order of the sequence of figures from Figure A1 to Figure A7 follows the geographic order of the clusters from west to east.

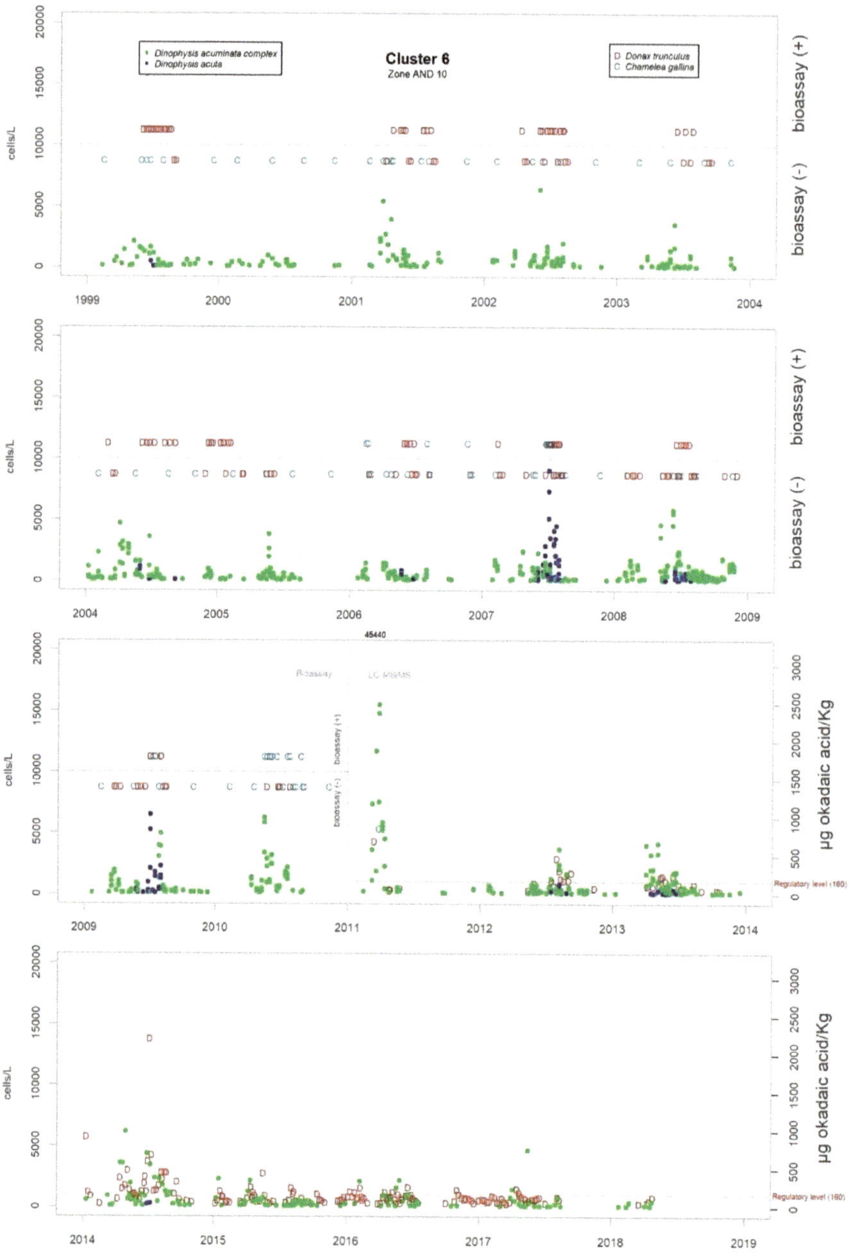

Figure A2. Temporal series of the abundance of *D. acuminata* and *D. acuta* and the concentration of okadaic acid in the species of mollusc monitored in each harvest area, in cluster 6. The order of the sequence of figures from Figure A1 to Figure A7 follows the geographic order of the clusters from west to east.

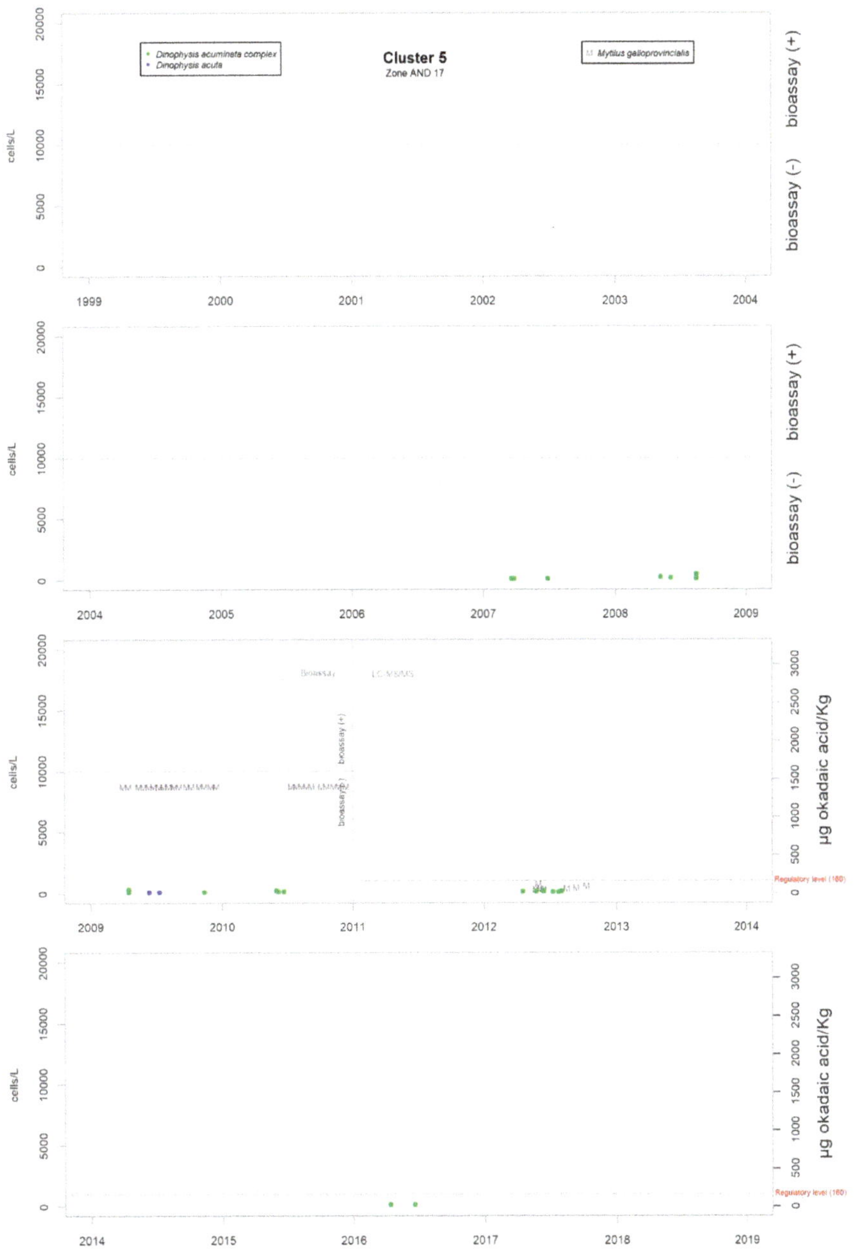

Figure A3. Temporal series of the abundance of *D. acuminata* and *D. acuta* and the concentration of okadaic acid in the species of mollusc monitored in each harvest area, in cluster 5. The order of the sequence of figures from Figure A1 to Figure A7 follows the geographic order of the clusters from west to east. The long periods of absence correspond to lack of sampling due to cessation of harvesting.

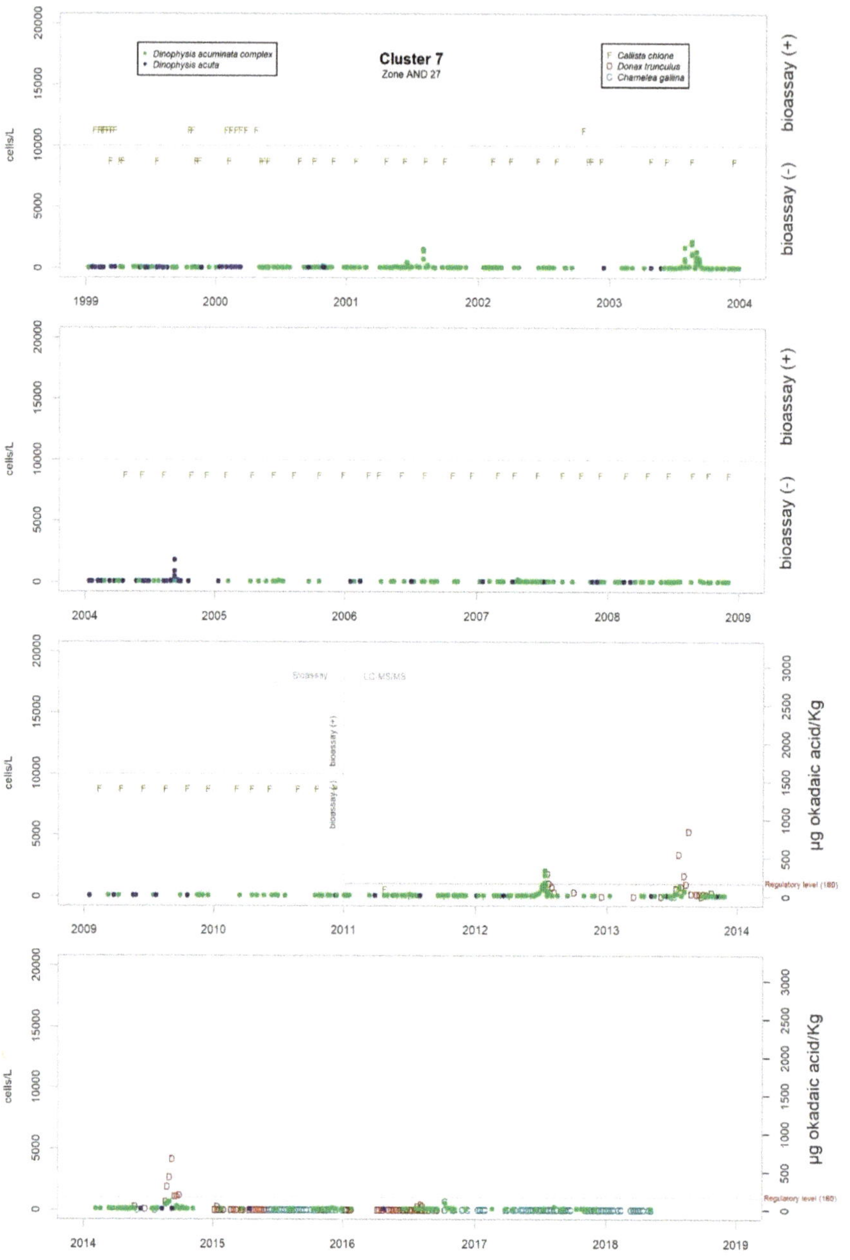

Figure A4. Temporal series of the abundance of *D. acuminata* and *D. acuta* and the concentration of okadaic acid in the species of mollusc monitored in each harvest area, in cluster 7. The order of the sequence of figures from Figure A1 to Figure A7 follows the geographic order of the clusters from west to east.

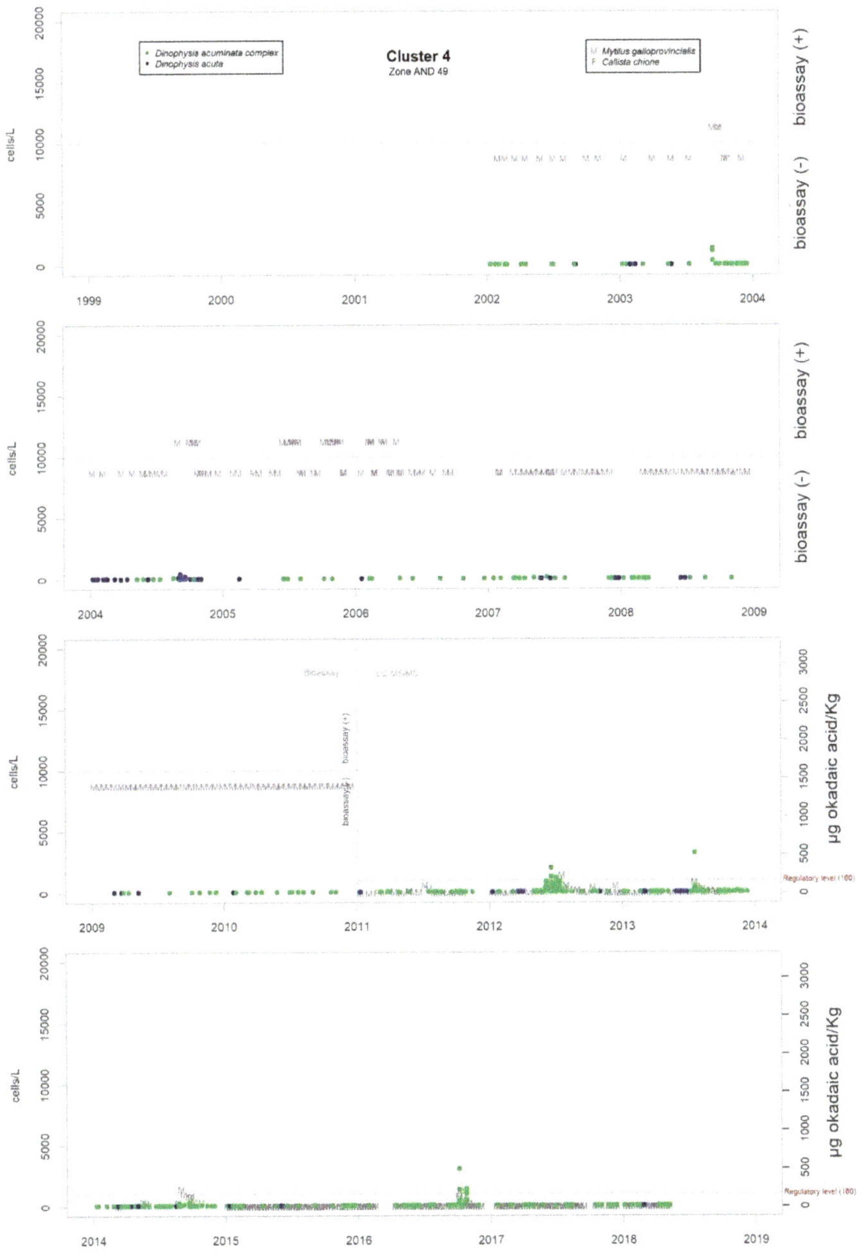

Figure A5. Temporal series of the abundance of *D. acuminata* and *D. acuta* and the concentration of okadaic acid in the species of mollusc monitored in each harvest area, in cluster 4. The order of the sequence of figures from Figure A1 to Figure A7 follows the geographic order of the clusters from west to east.

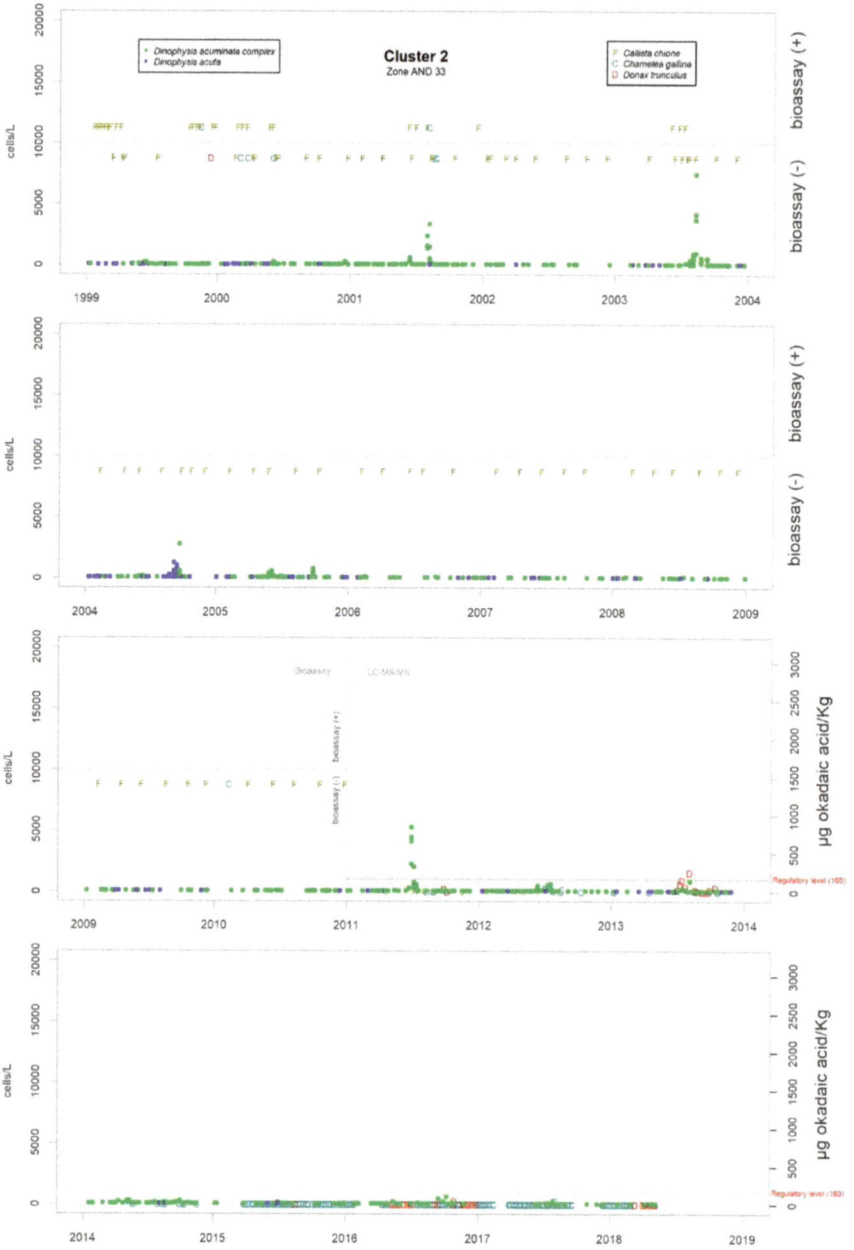

Figure A6. Temporal series of the abundance of *D. acuminata* and *D. acuta* and the concentration of okadaic acid in the species of mollusc monitored in each harvest area, in cluster 2. The order of the sequence of figures from Figure A1 to Figure A7 follows the geographic order of the clusters from west to east.

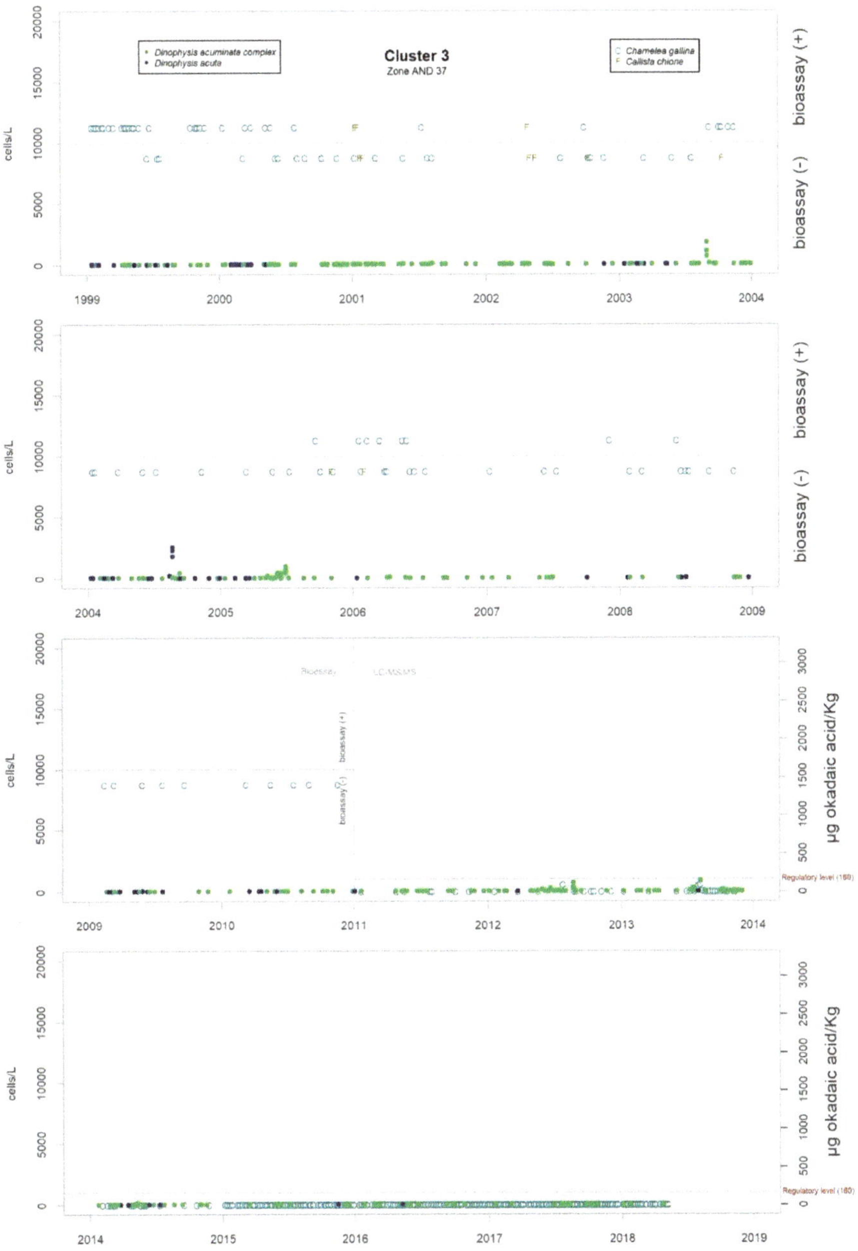

Figure A7. Temporal series of the abundance of *D. acuminata* and *D. acuta* and the concentration of okadaic acid in the species of mollusc monitored in each harvest area, in cluster 3. The order of the sequence of figures from Figure A1 to Figure A7 follows the geographic order of the clusters from west to east.

Appendix B

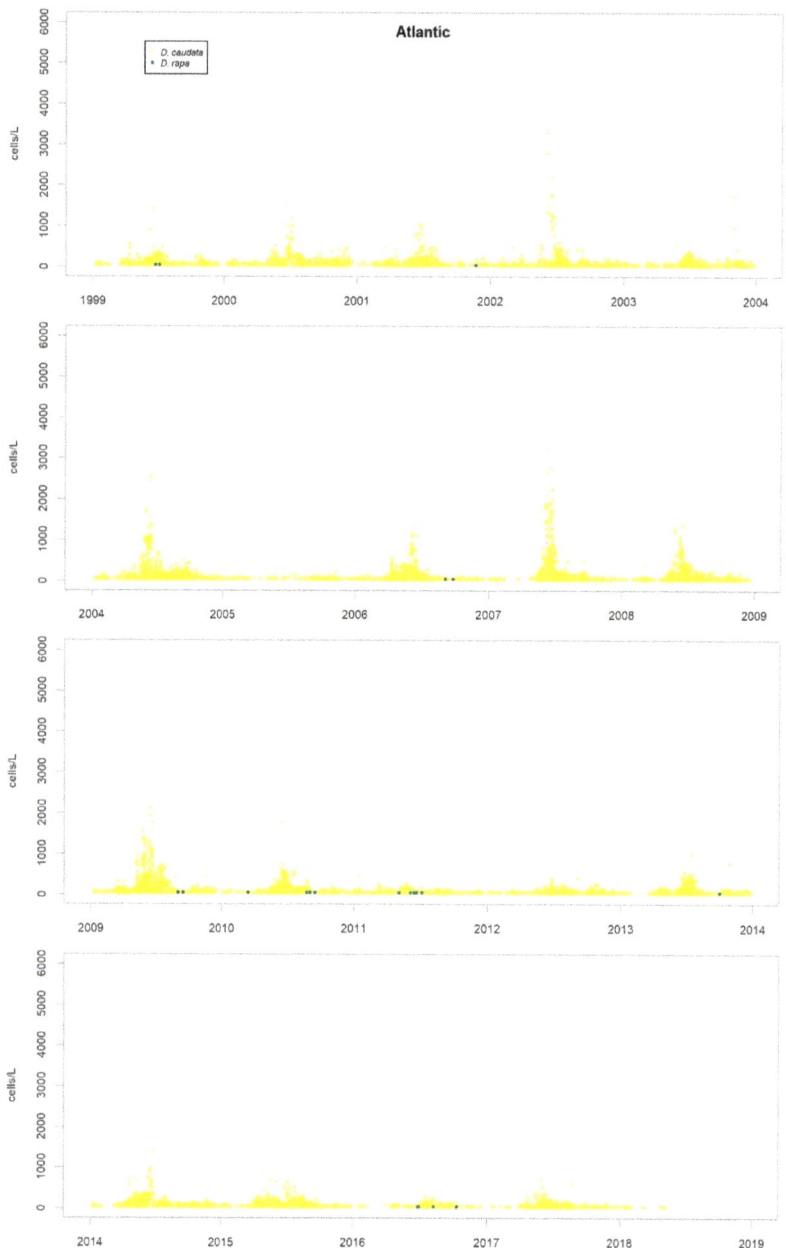

Figure A8. Temporal series of the abundance of *D. caudata* and *D. rapa* in the areas of the Atlantic Ocean.

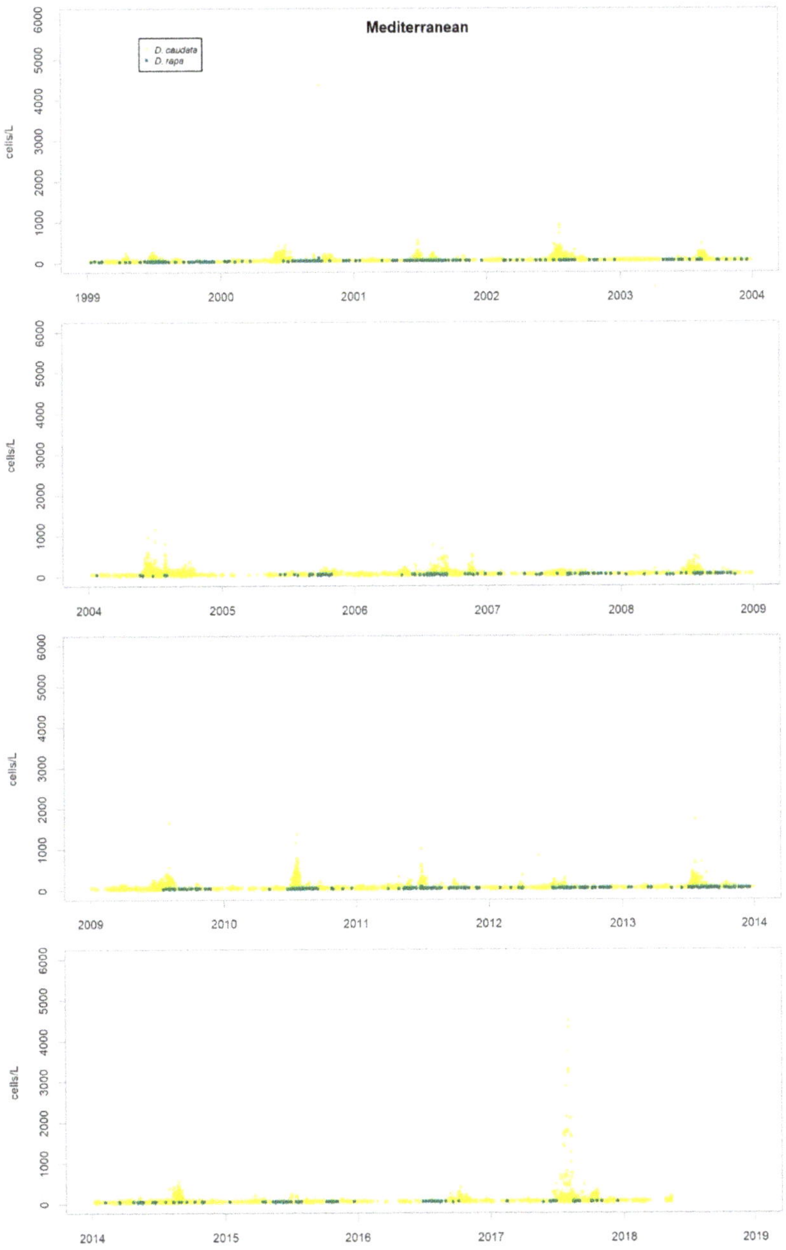

Figure A9. Temporal series of the abundance of *D. caudata* and *D. rapa* in the areas of the Mediterranean Sea.

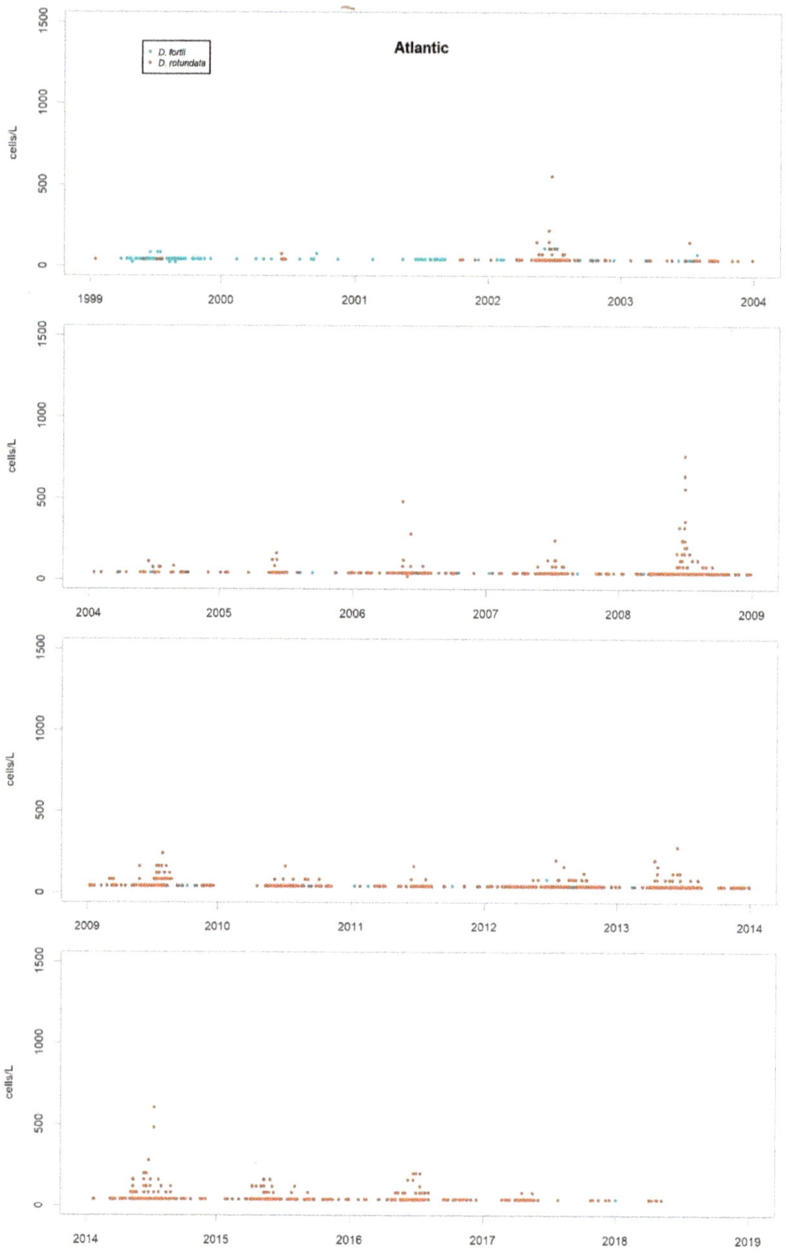

Figure A10. Temporal series of the abundance of *D. fortii and D. rotundata* in the areas of the Atlantic Ocean.

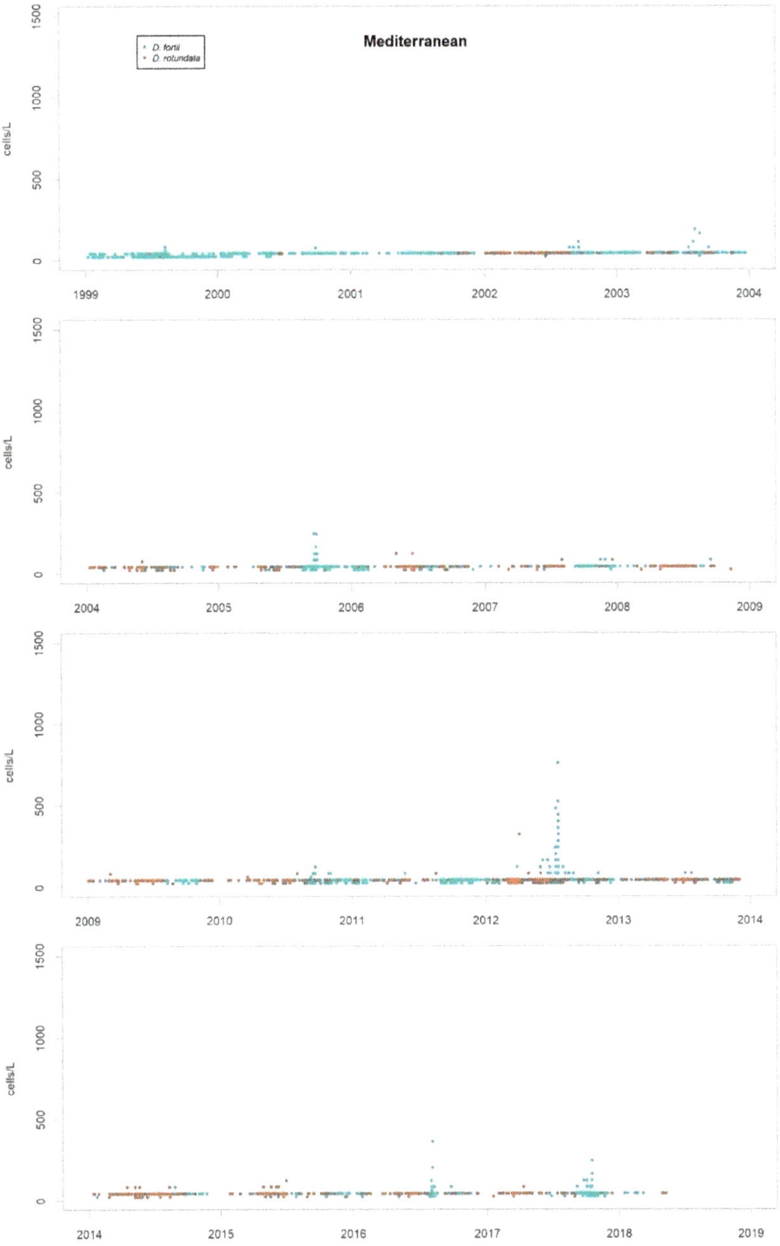

Figure A11. Temporal series of the abundance of *D. fortii and D. rotundata* in the areas of the Mediterranean Sea.

Appendix C

Table A1. Sampling frequencies in marine waters for the phytoplankton analysis from 1999 to 2008.

Frequency	1999	2000	2001	2002	2003	2004	2005	2006	2007	2008
Weekly	1–13, 21–24, 27–36 [1]	1–13, 21–24, 27–36	1–13, 21–24, 27–36	1–13, 21–24, 27–36	1–13, 21–24, 27–36	1–13, 21–24, 27–36	1–13, 21–24, 27–38, 40, 44	1–13, 21–24, 27–38, 40, 44	1–13, 21–24, 27–38, 40, 44	1–13, 21–24, 27–38, 40, 44
Biweekly	37–44	37–44	37–44	37–44	37–44	37–44	14–16, 18, 39, 41–43	14–16, 18, 39, 41–43	14–16, 18, 39, 41–43	14–16, 18, 39, 41–43
Monthly	14-20	14-20	14-20	14-20	14-20	14-20	17, 19, 20	17, 19, 20	17, 19, 20	17, 19, 20

[1] Data on the cells, identification number of the harvest area. To avoid clutter, the prefix AND- (through which they are officially known) has been omitted.

Table A2. Sampling frequencies in marine waters for phytoplankton analysis from 2009 to 2018.

Frequency	2009	2010	2011	2012	2013	2014	2015	2016	2017	2018
Weekly	1–13, 21–24, 27–38, 40, 44 [1]	1–13, 21–24, 27–38, 40, 44	1–13, 21–24, 27–38, 40, 44	1–13, 21–24, 27–38, 40, 44	All active zones	All active zones	All active zones	All active zones	All active zones	All active zones
Biweekly	14–16, 18, 39, 41–43	14–16, 18, 39, 41–43	14–16, 18, 39, 41–43	14–16, 18, 39, 41–43						
Monthly	17, 19, 20	17, 19, 20	17, 19, 20	17, 19, 20						

[1] Data on the cells, identification number of the harvest area. To avoid clutter, the prefix AND- (through which they are officially known) has been omitted.

Table A3. Sampling frequencies of molluscs for the analysis of lipophilic toxins from 1999 to 2008.

Frequency	1999	2000	2001	2002	2003	2004	2005	2006	2007	2008
Weekly										
Monthly	36 [1]	36	36	36	36	36	4, 7, 11, 24, 30	4, 7, 11, 24, 30	4, 7, 11, 24, 30	4, 7, 11, 24, 30
Bimonthly							24, 27–35, 37–44	24, 27–35, 37–44	24, 27–35, 37–44	24, 27–35, 37–44
Quarterly	1–35, 37–44	1–35, 37–44	1–35, 37–44	1–35, 37–44	1–35, 37–44	1–35, 37–44	1–3, 5, 6–10, 13–22	1–3, 5, 6–10, 13–22	1–3, 5, 6–10, 13–22	1–3, 5, 6–10, 13–22

[1] Data on the cells, identification number of the harvest area. To avoid clutter, the prefix AND- (through which they are officially known) has been omitted.

Table A4. Sampling frequencies of molluscs for the analysis of lipophilic toxins from 2009 to 2018.

Frequency	2009	2010	2011	2012	2013	2014	2015	2016	2017	2018
Weekly					All active zones [1]	All active zones [1]	All active zones [1]	All active zones [1]	All active zones [1]	All active zones [1]
Monthly	4, 7, 11, 24, 30	4, 7, 11, 24, 30	4, 7, 11, 24, 30	4, 7, 11, 24, 30						
Bimonthly	24, 27–35, 37–44	24, 27–35, 37–44	24, 27–35, 37–44	24, 27–35, 37–44						
Quarterly	1–3, 5, 6–10, 13–22	1–3, 5, 6–10, 13–22	1–3, 5, 6–10, 13–22	1–3, 5, 6–10, 13–22						

[1] Data on the cells, identification number of the harvest area. To avoid clutter, the prefix AND- (through which they are officially known) has been omitted. In areas of bivalve molluscs from aquaculture, monitoring was activated only during the production season.

References

1. Yasumoto, T.; Oshima, Y.; Yamaguchi, M. Occurrence of a new type of shellfish poisoning in the Tohoku district. *Bull. Jpn. Soc. Sci. Fish.* **1978**, *44*, 1249–1255. [CrossRef]
2. Yasumoto, T.; Oshima, Y.; Sugawara, W.; Fukuyo, Y.; Oguri, H.; Igarashi, T.; Fujita, N. Identification of Dinophysis fortii as the causative organism of diarrhetic shellfish poisoning in the Tohoku district. *Bull. Jpn. Soc. Sci. Fish.* **1980**, *46*, 1405–1411. [CrossRef]
3. Regulation (EC) No 853/2004 of the European Parliament and of the Council of 29 April 2004 Laying Down Specific Hygiene Rules for Food of Animal Origin. Available online: https://eur-lex.europa.eu/legal-content/EN/ALL/?uri=CELEX%3A32004R0853 (accessed on 27 March 2019).
4. Regulation (EC) No 854/2004 of the European Parliament and of the Council of 29 April 2004 laying Down Specific Rules for the Organisation of Official Controls on Products of Animal Origin Intended for Human Consumption. Available online: https://eur-lex.europa.eu/legal-content/EN/TXT/?uri=CELEX%3A32004R0854 (accessed on 27 March 2019).
5. Reguera, B.; Velo-Suarez, L.; Raine, R.; Gil Park, M. Harmful Dinophysis species: A review. *Harmful Algae* **2012**, *14*, 87–106. [CrossRef]
6. Zingone, A.; Larsen, J. (Eds.) *Dinophysiales*; IOC-UNESCO Taxonomic Reference List of Harmful Micro Algae. 2009. Available online: http://www.marinespecies.org/hab (accessed on 27 March 2019).
7. Gosling, E. *Bivalve Molluscs*; Blackwell Publishing: Oxford, UK, 2003.
8. Riisgård, H. On measurement of filtration rates in bivalves—The stony road to reliable data: Review and interpretation. *Mar. Ecol. Prog. Ser.* **2001**, *211*, 275–291. [CrossRef]
9. Kiørboe, T.; Mohlenberg, F. Particle selection in suspension-feeding bivalves. *Mar. Ecol. Prog.* **1981**, *5*, 291–296. [CrossRef]
10. Shumway, S.; Cucci, T.; Newell, R.; Clarice, M.Y. Particle selection, ingestion and absorption in filter-feeding bivalves. *J. Exp. Biol. Ecol.* **1985**, *91*, 77–92. [CrossRef]
11. Hégaret, H.; Wikfors, G.H.; Shumway, S.E. Diverse feeding responses of five species of bivalve mollusc when exposed to three species of harmful algae. *J. Shellfish Res.* **2007**, *26*, 549–559. [CrossRef]
12. Gómez, F. A list of free-living dinoflagellate species in the world's oceans. *Acta Bot. Croat.* **2005**, *64*, 129–212.
13. Lassus, P.; Bardouil, M. Le Complexe Dinophysis acuminata: Identification des espèces le long des côtes Françaises. *Cryptogam. Algol.* **1991**, *12*, 1–9.
14. Bravo, I.; Delgado, M.; Fraga, S.; Honsell, G.; Montresor, M.; Sampayo, M.A.M. The Dinophysis genus: Toxicity and species definition in Europe. In *Harmful Marine Algal Blooms*; Lassus, P., Arzul, G., Erard-Le Denn, E., Gentien, P., Marcaillou Le Baut, C., Eds.; Lavoisier: Paris, France, 1995; pp. 843–845.
15. R Core Team. R: A Language and Environment for Statistical Computing. R Foundation for Statistical Computing: Vienna, Austria. Available online: https://www.R-project.org/ (accessed on 27 March 2019).
16. Reguera, B.; González-Gil, S. Small cell and intermediate cell formation in species of Dinophysis (Dinophyceae, Dinophysiales). *J. Phycol.* **2001**, *37*, 318–333. [CrossRef]
17. Reguera, B.; Garcès, E.; Bravo, I.; Pazos, Y.; Ramilo, I. In situ division rates of several species of Dinophysis estimated by a postmitotic index. *Mar. Ecol. Prog. Ser.* **2003**, *249*, 117–131. [CrossRef]
18. Zingone, A.; Montresor, M.; Marino, D. Morphological variability of the potentially toxic dinoflagellate Dinophysis sacculus (Dinophyceae) and its taxonomic relationships with *D. pavillardii* and *D. acuminata*. *Eur. J. Phycol.* **1998**, *33*, 259–273. [CrossRef]
19. Reguera, B.; González-Gil, S.; Delgado, M. Dinophysis diegensis Kofoid is a life history stage of Dinophysis caudata Kent (Dinophyceae, Dinophysiales). *J. Phycol.* **2007**, *43*, 1083–1093. [CrossRef]
20. Koukaras, K.; Nikolaidis, G. Dinophysis blooms in Greek coastal waters (Thermaikos Gulf NW Aegean Sea). *J. Plankton Res.* **2004**, *26*, 445–457. [CrossRef]
21. Álvarez-Salgado, X.A.; Figueiras, F.G.; Fernández-Reiriz, M.J.; Labarta, U.; Peteiro, L.; Piedracoba, S. Control of lipophilic shellfish poisoning outbreaks by seasonal upwelling and continental runoff. *Harmful Algae* **2011**, *10*, 121–129. [CrossRef]
22. Vale, P.; Sampayo, M.A.M. Domoic acid in Portuguese shellfish and fish. *Toxicon* **2001**, *39*, 893–904. [CrossRef]
23. Vale, P.; Botelho, M.J.; Rodrigues, S.M.; Gomes, S.S.; Sampayo, M.A.M. Two decades of marine biotoxin monitoring in bivalves from Portugal (1986–2006): A review of exposure assessment. *Harmful Algae* **2008**, *7*, 11–25. [CrossRef]

24. Godhe, A.; Svensson, S.; Rehnstam-Holm, A.S. Oceanographic settings explain fluctuations in Dinophysis spp. and concentrations of diarrhetic shellfish toxin in the plankton community within a mussel farm area on the Swedish west coast. *Mar. Ecol. Prog. Ser.* **2002**, *240*, 71–83. [CrossRef]
25. Ninčević-Gladan, Ž.; Skejić, S.; Bužančić, M.; Marasović, I.; Arapov, J.; Ujević, I.; Bojanić, N.; Grbec, B.; Kušpilić, G.; Vidjak, O. Seasonal variability in Dinophysis spp. abundances and diarrhetic shellfish poisoning outbreaks along the eastern Adriatic coast. *Bot. Mar.* **2008**, *51*, 449–463. [CrossRef]
26. Smayda, T.; Reynolds, C.S. Community assemblage in marine phytoplankton: Application of recent models to harmful algae blooms. *J. Plankton Res.* **2001**, *23*, 447–461. [CrossRef]
27. Andersen, P.; Benedicte, H.; Emsholm, H. Toxicity of Dinophysis acuminata in Danish coastal waters. In *Harmful and Toxic Algal Blooms*; Yasumoto, T., Oshima, Y., Fukuyo, Y., Eds.; Intergovernmental Oceanographic Commission of UNESCO: Paris, France, 1996; pp. 281–284.
28. Palma, A.S.; Vilarinho, M.G.; Moita, M.T. Interannual trends in the longshore distribution of Dinophysis off the Portuguese coast. In *Harmful Algae*; Reguera, B., Blanco, J., Fernández, M.L., Wyatt, T., Eds.; Xunta de Galicia and Intergovernmental Oceanographic Commission of UNESCO Publishers: Paris, France, 1998; pp. 124–127.
29. Poletti, R.; Cettul, K.; Bovo, F.; Milandri, A.; Pompei, M.; Frate, R. Distribution of toxic dinoflagellates and their impact on shellfish along the northwest Adriatic coast. In *Harmful Algae*; Reguera, B., Blanco, J., Fernández, M.L., Wyatt, T., Eds.; Xunta de Galicia and Intergovernmental Oceanographic Commission of UNESCO: Paris, France, 1998; pp. 88–90.
30. Aubry, F.B.; Berton, A.; Bastianini, M.; Bertaggia, R.; Baroni, R.; Socal, G. Seasonal dynamics of Dinophysis in coastal waters of the NW Adriatic Sea (1990–1996). *Bot. Mar.* **2000**, *43*, 423–430. [CrossRef]
31. Vila, M.; Camp, J.; Garcès, E.; Masó, M.; Delgado, M. High resolution spatio-temporal detection of potentially harmful dinoflagellates in confined waters of the NW Mediterranean. *J. Plankton Res.* **2001**, *23*, 497–514. [CrossRef]
32. Dahl, E.; Johannessen, T. Relationship between occurrence of Dinophysis species and shellfish toxicity. *Phycologia* **2001**, *40*, 223–227. [CrossRef]
33. Van der Fels-Klerx, H.J.; Adamse, P.; Goedhart, P.W.; Poelman, M.; Pol-Hofstad, I.E.; van Egmond, H.; Gerssen, A. Monitoring phytoplankton and marine biotoxins in production waters of the Netherlands: Results after one decade. *Food Addit. Contam.* **2012**, *29*, 1616–1629. [CrossRef]
34. Bazzoni, A.M.; Mudadu, A.G.; Lorenzoni, G.; Soro, B.; Bardino, N.; Arras, I.; Sanna, G.; Vodret, B.; Bazzardi, R.; Marongiu, E.; Virgilio, S. Detection of Dinophysis species and associated okadaic acid in farmed shellfish: A two-year study from the western Mediterranean area. *J. Vet. Res.* **2018**, *62*, 137–144. [CrossRef] [PubMed]
35. Durant Clément, M.; Clément, J.C.; Moreau, A.; Jeanne, N.; Puiseux-Dao, S. New ecological and ultrastructural data on the dinoflagellate Dinophysis sp. from the French coast. *Mar. Biol.* **1988**, *97*, 37–44. [CrossRef]
36. MacKenzie, L. Does Dinophysis (Dinophyceae) have a sexual life cycle? *J. Phycol.* **1992**, *28*, 399–406. [CrossRef]
37. Villarino, M.L.; Figueiras, F.G.; Jones, K.J.; Álvarez-Salgado, X.A.; Richard, J.; Edwards, A. Evidence of in situ diel vertical migration of a red-tide microplankton species in Ría de Vigo (NW Spain). *Mar. Biol.* **1995**, *123*, 607–617. [CrossRef]
38. Delgado, M.; Garcès´, S.E.; Camp, J. Growth and behaviour of Dinophysis sacculus from NW Mediterranean Sea. In *Harmful and Toxic Algal Blooms*; Yasumoto, T., Oshima, Y., Fukuyo, Y., Eds.; Intergovernmental Oceanographic Commission of UNESCO: Sendai, Japan, 1996; pp. 261–264.
39. Order of 15 July 1993 (BOJA No. 85, of 5 August 1993), updated in the Order of 25 March 2003 (BOJA No. 65, of 4 April 2003), and again updated in the Order of 18 November 2008 (BOJA núm.18, of 5 December). Available online: https://juntadeandalucia.es/boja/1993/85/17 (accessed on 27 March 2019).
40. Lindahl, O. A dividable hose for phytoplankton sampling. In *Report of the Working Group on Exceptional Algal Blooms*; International Council for the Exploration of the Sea: Copenhagen, Denmark, 1986; Annex 3.
41. Utermöhl, H. Zur Vervollkommung der quantitativen Phytoplankton-Methodik. *Mitt Ver. Theor. Angew. Limnol.* **1958**, *9*, 1–38.

42. Yasumoto, T.; Murata, M.; Oshima, Y.; Matsumoto, K.; Clardy, J. Diarrhetic shellfish poisoning. In *Seafood Toxins*; Ragelis, E.P., Ed.; American Chemical Society: Washington, DC, USA, 1984; pp. 207–214.
43. Dimitriadou, E.; Dolnicar, S.; Weingessel, A. An Examination of indexes for determining the number of clusters in binary data sets. *Psychometrica* **2002**, *67*, 137–160. [CrossRef]

toxins

MDPI

Article

A Long-Term Time Series of *Dinophysis acuminata* Blooms and Associated Shellfish Toxin Contamination in Port Underwood, Marlborough Sounds, New Zealand

Lincoln A. Mackenzie

Cawthron Institute, 98 Halifax Street, Nelson 7010, New Zealand; lincoln.mackenzie@cawthron.org.nz; Tel.: +64-3-548-2319

Received: 5 December 2018; Accepted: 15 January 2019; Published: 1 February 2019

Abstract: Blooms of the dinoflagellate *Dinophysis acuminata* occur every year in an important mussel cultivation area in Port Underwood, Marlborough Sounds, New Zealand. Annual maximum cell numbers range from 1500–75,000 cells L^{-1} and over 25 years of weekly monitoring the *D. acuminata* bloom has never failed to exhibit peaks in abundance at some time between spring and autumn. During winter (June–August) the dinoflagellate is often undetectable, or at low levels ($\leq$100 cells L^{-1}), and the risk of diarrhetic shellfish poisoning (DSP)-toxin contamination over this period is negligible. Bloom occurrence may be coupled to the abundance of *D. acuminata* prey (*Mesodinium* sp.) but the mechanism by which it maintains its long-term residence in this hydrologically dynamic environment is unknown. The toxin profile of *D. acuminata* is dominated by pectenotoxin-2 (PTX-2) and dinophysistoxin-1 (DTX-1), but the cellular toxin content is low. It is rare that free DTX-1 is detected in mussels as this is invariably exclusively present as fatty acid-esters. In only five out of >2500 mussel samples over 16 years have the levels of total DTX-1 marginally exceeded the regulated level of 0.16 mg kg^{-1}. It is also rare that free PTX-2 is detected in mussels, as it is generally only present in its hydrolysed non-toxic PTX-2 seco acid form. The *D. acuminata* alert level of 1000 cells L^{-1} is often exceeded without DTX-1 residues increasing appreciably, and this level is considered too conservative.

Keywords: *Dinophysis acuminata*; dinophysistoxins; pectenotoxins; Port Underwood; New Zealand

Key Contribution: A unique perspective on the risk associated with blooms of *Dinophysis acuminata* is obtained by the examination of a long-term phytoplankton and shellfish toxin monitoring data set from New Zealand.

1. Introduction

Since the phenomenon was first identified [1,2], diarrhetic shellfish poisoning (DSP) caused by various species of planktonic dinoflagellate in the genus *Dinophysis* (and some benthic *Prorocentrum* spp.) has become a significant quality assurance issue for shellfish aquaculture worldwide. *Dinophysis* spp. produce a suite of lipophilic polyether secondary metabolites within the okadaic acid (OA, DTX-1, DTX-2) and pectenotoxin (PTX-1–PTX-11) families. These toxins are internationally regulated at a maximum permissible level of <0.16 mg kg^{-1} [3] and there is a high level of awareness in the New Zealand industry that the avoidance of the harvesting of shellfish contaminated with these toxin residues is essential.

Port Underwood is a 24 km^2 inlet on the north-east coast of the South Island, New Zealand (Figure 1), and is regarded as one of the most productive Greenshell™ mussel (*Perna canaliculus*) growing regions of the Marlborough Sounds. The high productivity of the inlet (approximately

8000 tonnes of mussels per annum) is attributed to the fertilising effects of local wind-induced upwelling and its proximity to the Wairau River out-welling plume. Since weekly toxic phytoplankton and marine biotoxin monitoring began in Port Underwood in the early 1990s, it has become apparent that the inlet has a resident population of *Dinophysis acuminata* that blooms for short periods every year between spring (September–October) and autumn (March–April).

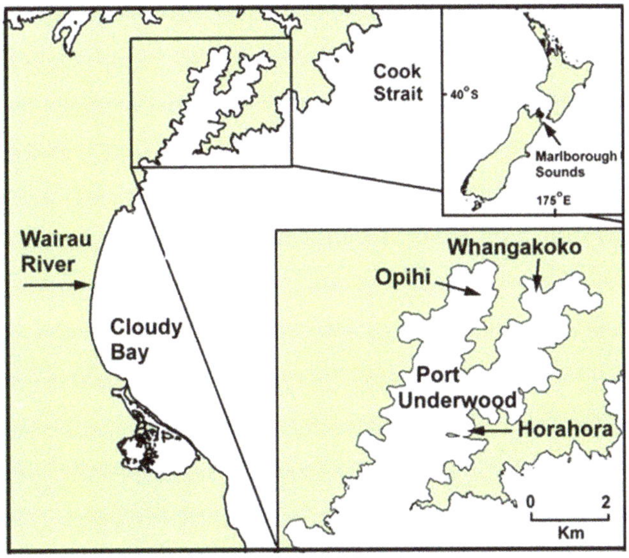

Figure 1. The geographic location of Port Underwood in the Marlborough Sounds region on the north-east coast of the South Island, New Zealand. The location of routine phytoplankton and shellfish monitoring sites (Opihi, Whangakoko, Horahora) in the inlet are indicated.

The cellular toxin content of the major pectenotoxin and okadaic acid group toxins in *Dinophysis acuta* and *Dinophysis acuminata* from various locations around the South Island coast of New Zealand has been described [4]. *D. acuminata* cells sampled from Port Underwood at various times showed low levels of okadaic acid (trace–0.4 pg/cell) and dinophysistoxin-1 (DTX-1) (0.1–0.5 pg $cell^{-1}$) but much higher levels of pectenotoxin-2 (PTX-2) (2.4–16.9 pg $cell^{-1}$). The cellular content of OA and its esters in *D. acuta* was 33 times higher and for PTX-2 and PTX-11, 8–42 times higher, respectively, than in *D. acuminata*. Only about 6% of total PTX-2 was present as the PTX-2 seco acid in *D. acuminata* cells. The toxin content of *D. acuminata* cells from Port Underwood was significantly lower than that of the same species from elsewhere in the South Island (Akaroa Harbour). DTX-1 was not detected in any *D. acuta* cells and DTX-2 was not detected in either species. A similarly low toxin content (0.01–1.8 pg OA + DTX-1 $cell^{-1}$) has been observed in *D. acuminata* cells from the north-western Atlantic [5].

Pectenotoxins are the predominant polyether macrolides found in the *Dinophysis* species throughout the world [6]. At least 11 PTX analogues have been described, with different degrees of toxicity as assayed by various methodologies [7]. Pectenotoxin 2 seco acid (PTX-2sa) was first isolated and described in mussels from the Marlborough Sounds, New Zealand and Ireland [8]. Subsequently, it was shown [9] that PTX-2sa was the product of the rapid enzymatic hydrolysis of PTX-2 within shellfish tissues and the esterase responsible for this conversion was isolated and characterised from the mussel hepatopancreas [10]. This enzymatic conversion severs the PTX-2 lactone ring essential for the biological activity of the molecule and thus, PTX-2sa loses its toxicity [7]. In the early 2000s, as the extent of PTX-2sa occurrence in New Zealand shellfish became apparent [11], an evaluation of the risk of this compound to consumers was undertaken [12]. This study concluded that available evidence suggested that PTX-2sa was harmless. The New Zealand shellfish regulatory authority (New Zealand Ministry for Primary Industries) sets a limit of 0.16 mg kg^{-1} okadaic acid equivalents that must not be exceeded in the edible portion of the shellfish. Okadaic acid group toxins (e.g., DTX-1) and pectenotoxins (e.g., PTX-2) are considered additive and, above this level, shellfish harvesting is prohibited. Pectenotoxin-seco acid analogues (e.g., PTX-2sa) are not considered a hazard and there is no non-permissible level.

The data presented here, accumulated over 25 years of weekly monitoring of phytoplankton and shellfish, provide a unique perspective on the magnitude of the DSP-toxin contamination problem in Port Underwood. Additional data from the occasional opportunistic sampling of the water column within the inlet illuminate some aspects of *D. acuminata* ecology and the environmental circumstances accompanying dinophysis-toxin contamination events.

2. Results and Discussion

2.1. Dinophysis acuminata *Morphology*

The vegetative cells of Port Underwood *D. acuminata* were on average (n = 10) 41.3 ± 2.7 μm (cell length) by 27.6 ± 1.6 μm (cell width) and, in terms of cell size and general morphology (Figure 2A), were consistent with descriptions of *D. acuminata* from elsewhere in the world [5]. A smaller morphotype (31 × 21 μm) was also commonly observed (Figure 2C), occasionally fusing with the larger morphotype. These fusing cells represent mating anisogamous gamete pairs and have been observed in several other *Dinophysis* species [13–15].

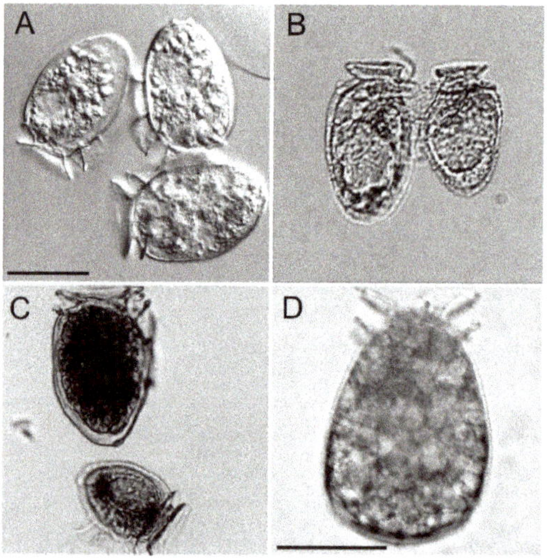

Figure 2. Specimens of *Dinophysis acuminata* from Port Underwood. (**A**) Live *D. acuminata* vegetative cells. (**B**) Conjugation of anisogamous gametes. (**C**) Large and small cell forms. (**D**) Dorsal view of a large, red, swollen cell. The scale bar (20 μm) in (**A**) also applies to (**B**,**C**). The scale bar in (**D**) is also 20 μm.

A third morphotype was comprised of large, swollen (50 × 33 μm), deeply red-pigmented cells that were most commonly observed during the early phases of bloom development (Figure 2D) It was believed these cells had recently fed on *Mesodinium* sp. prey [16] and that they played an important role in the subsequent rapid increase in cell numbers seen during subsequent blooms. Over the 25 years of monitoring in Port Underwood, larger cells of *D. acuta* have been observed on a few occasions. In October–November 2009, cell numbers of *D. acuta* briefly reached a maximum of 800 cells L^{-1} but no reportable associated toxicity in mussels occurred and this species has not played a significant role in DSP-toxin contamination events in this location to date.

2.2. *Frequency of* Dinophysis acuminata *Blooms*

Peaks in *D. acuminata* abundance occurred at some time between spring and autumn every year from 1994 to 2018 (Figures 3–5). Periods of relative abundance generally occurred at the same time at the three sampling sites and cell numbers were usually higher at the more inland sites (Whangakoko, Opihi) than at the Horahora site further towards the mouth of the inlet. The highest annual peak cell numbers usually occurred at the Whangakoko site and ranged from 2800–75,000 cells L^{-1}. Mid-winter (June–August) was the period when cells were most likely to be absent from the plankton (Figures 4 and 5), though even then there were a few occasions when cell numbers exceeded 1000 cell L^{-1}.

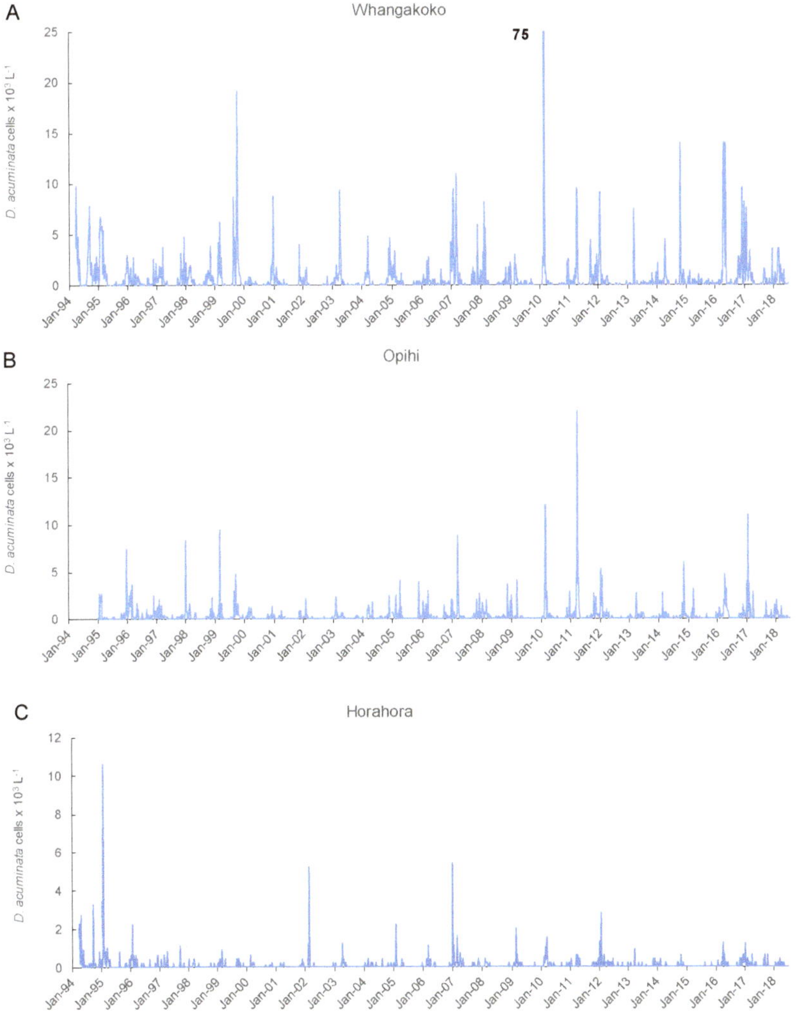

Figure 3. *Dinophysis acuminata* cells numbers ($\times 10^3$ L^{-1}) in 15 m water column tube samples collected weekly at three monitoring sites in Port Underwood 1994–2018. (**A**) Whangakoko Bay; (**B**) Opihi Bay; (**C**) Horahora Bay.

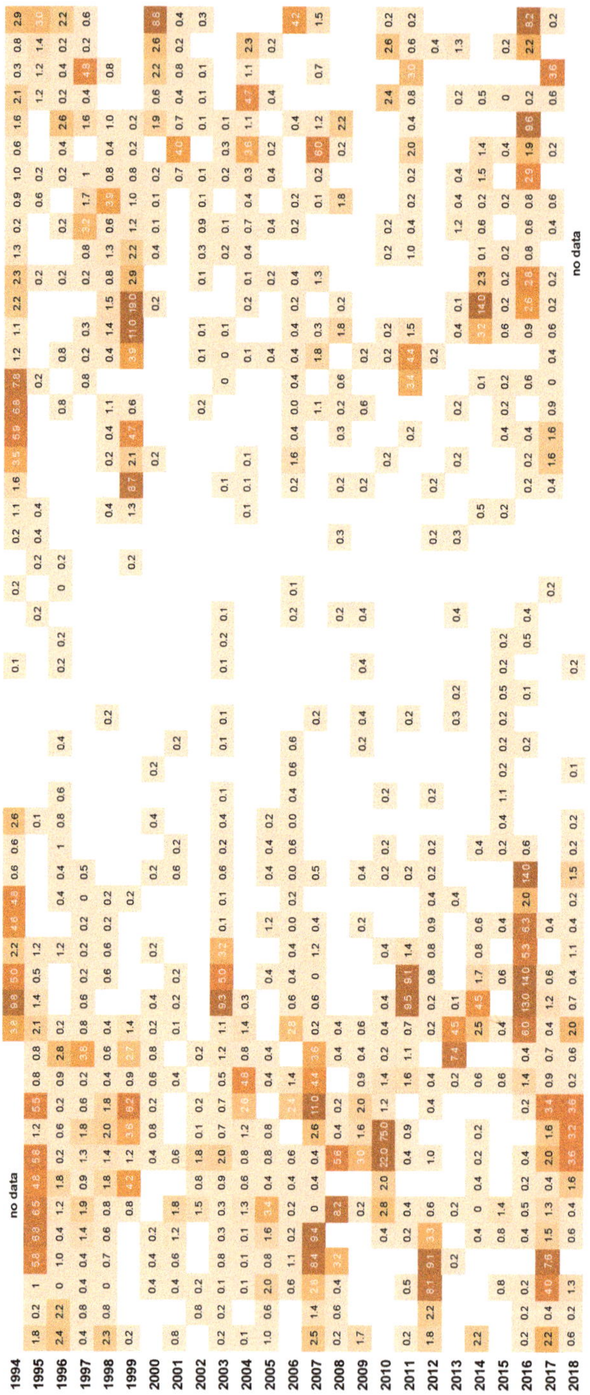

Figure 4. Cell counts (cells × 10^3 L^{-1}) of *Dinophysis. acuminata* in weekly 15 m tube samples from Whangakoko Bay, Port Underwood, March 1994–July 2018. Blank spaces indicate cell numbers $<10^2$ cells L^{-1}.

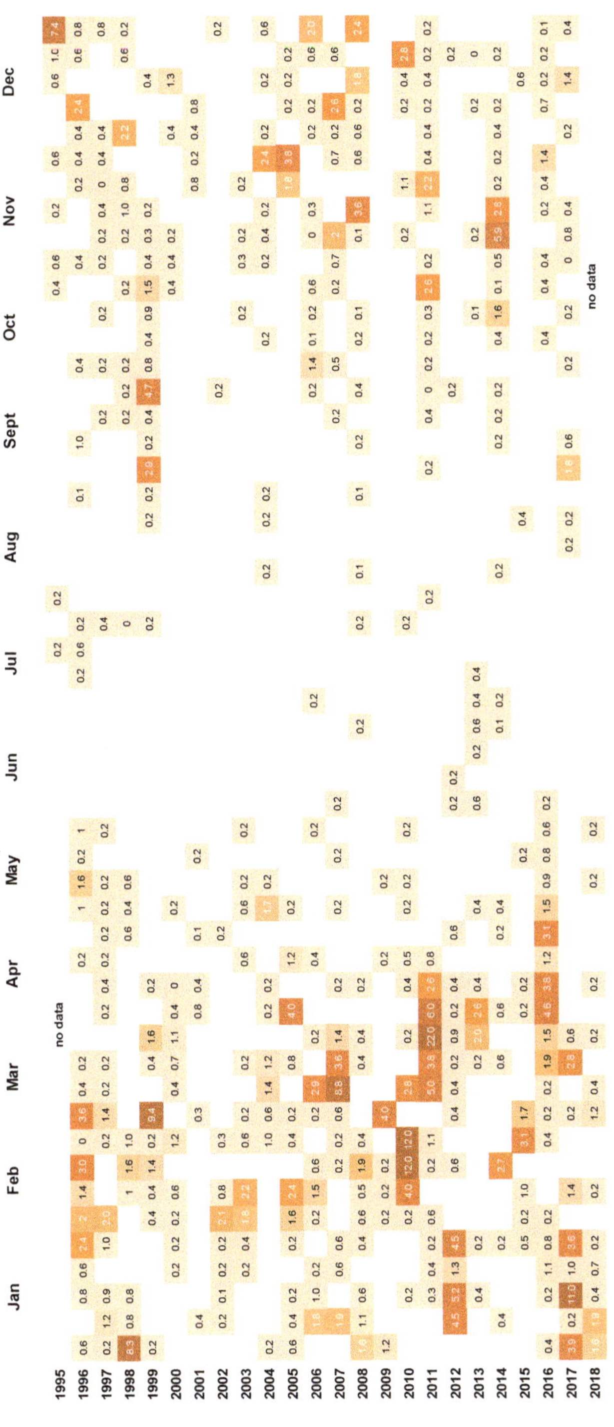

Figure 5. Cell counts (cells × 10^3 L^{-1}) of *Dinophysis acuminata* in weekly 15 m tube samples from Opihi Bay, Port Underwood, 1995–2018. Blank spaces indicate cell numbers <10^2 cells L^{-1}.

2.3. Spatial and Temporal Distribution of Blooms

D. acuminata blooms developed in the inland reaches of the two major arms of the inlet (Figures 6 and 7), becoming more widely dispersed (spatially and with depth) as the blooms matured (Figures 7 and 8). In early March 2004 (Figure 6), as the bloom was in its early stages, *D. acuminata* cell numbers were highest at 12–15 m depth, in association with a phytoplankton community dominated by diatoms (*Chaetoceros* spp.) and the phototrophic ciliate *Mesodinium* sp. A significant proportion of the *D. acuminata* populations at these depths (14% at 12 m and 23% at 15 m) were comprised of the large, swollen, red-pigmented cells described previously (Figure 2). These observations are consistent with a conceptual model of the *Dinophysis* spp. growth strategy [17,18] and it is believed that the appearance of these large cells signals the imminent rapid development of a bloom. In cultures of *D. acuminata* [16], cell division rates of up to 0.95 day^{-1} have been observed when light and *Mesodinium* sp. prey abundance were non-limiting.

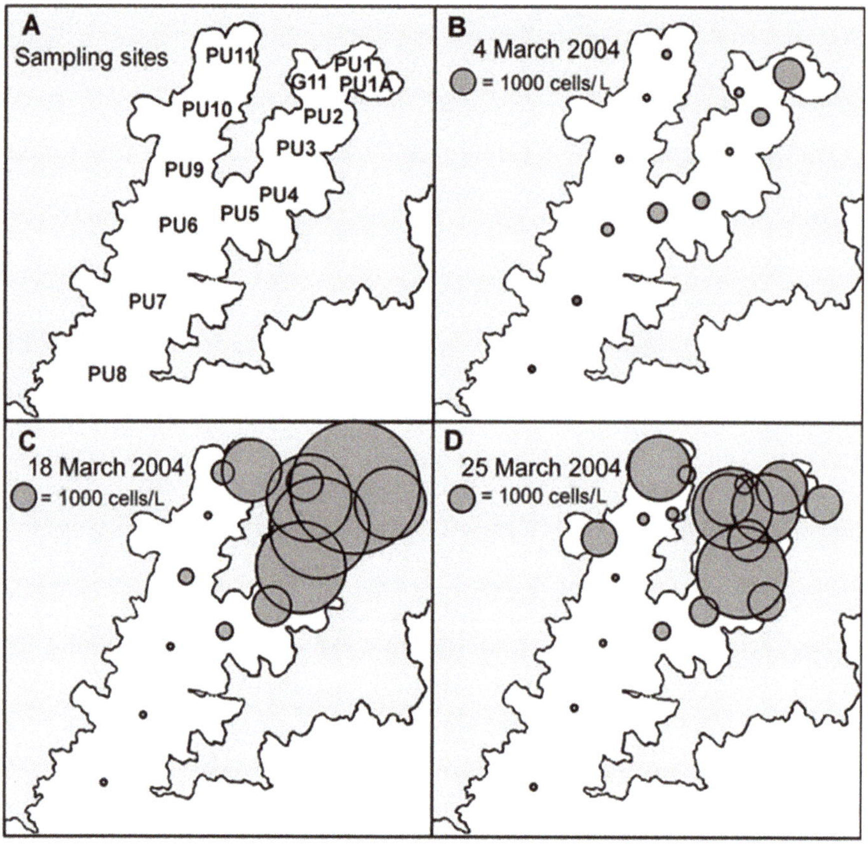

Figure 6. The distribution of cells in 15 m water column tube samples during a bloom of *Dinophysis acuminata* in Port Underwood, March 2004. (**A**) Sample site designations. (**B**) 4 March 2004; (**C**) 18 March 2004; (**D**) 25 March 2004.

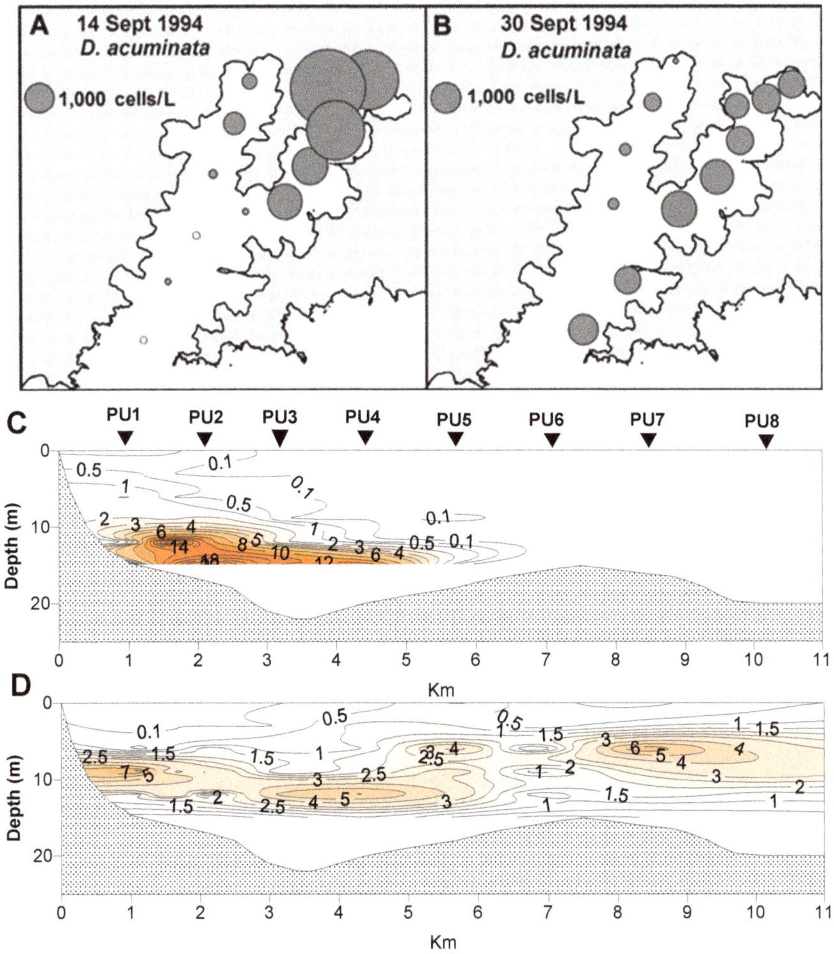

Figure 7. Spatial and vertical distribution of *Dinophysis acuminata* during a bloom between 14 Sept and 30 Sept 1994. (**A**,**B**) Spatial distribution of cells in 15 m tube samples. (**C**,**D**) The vertical distribution of cells along the Whangakoko Arm transect. The values are in cells × 10^3 L^{-1}. The site designations (PU1–PU8) are the same as shown in Figure 6.

D. acuminata blooms occurred at times when the water column was strongly stratified (due to salinity and temperature) but outside of the main phytoplankton bloom periods represented by high chlorophyll a concentrations (Figure 9). It has been observed elsewhere that *Dinophysis* populations tend to increase when the water column is thermally stratified [19,20].

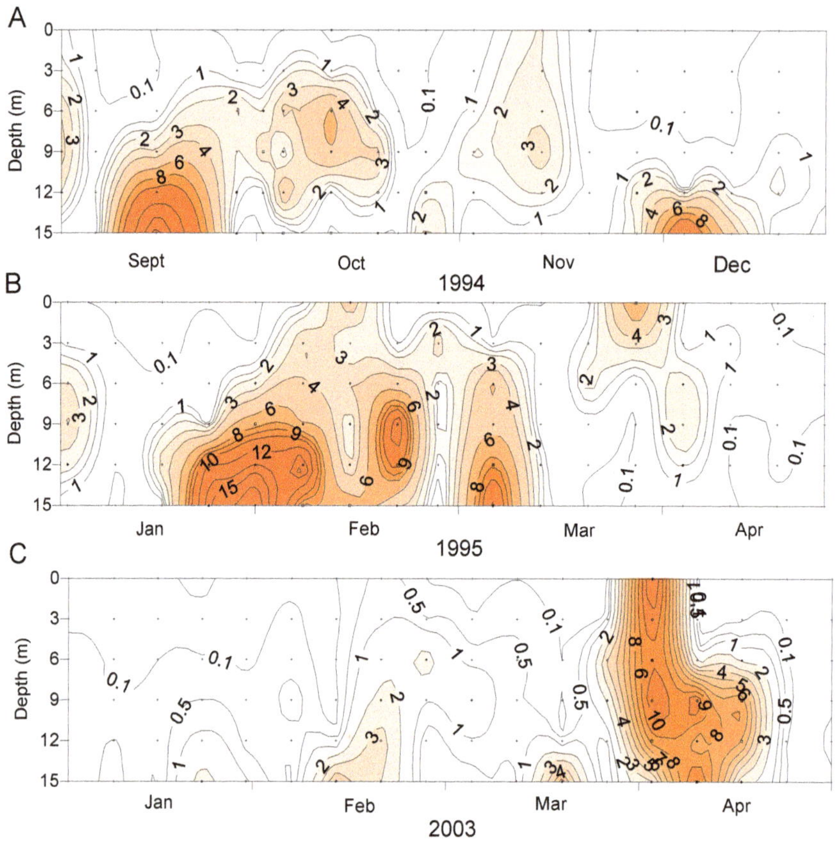

Figure 8. The vertical distribution of *Dinophysis acuminata* in the water column at Whangakoko, Port Underwood, at various times. (**A**) Sept–Dec 1995; (**B**) Jan–Apr 1995; (**C**) Jan–Apr 2003.

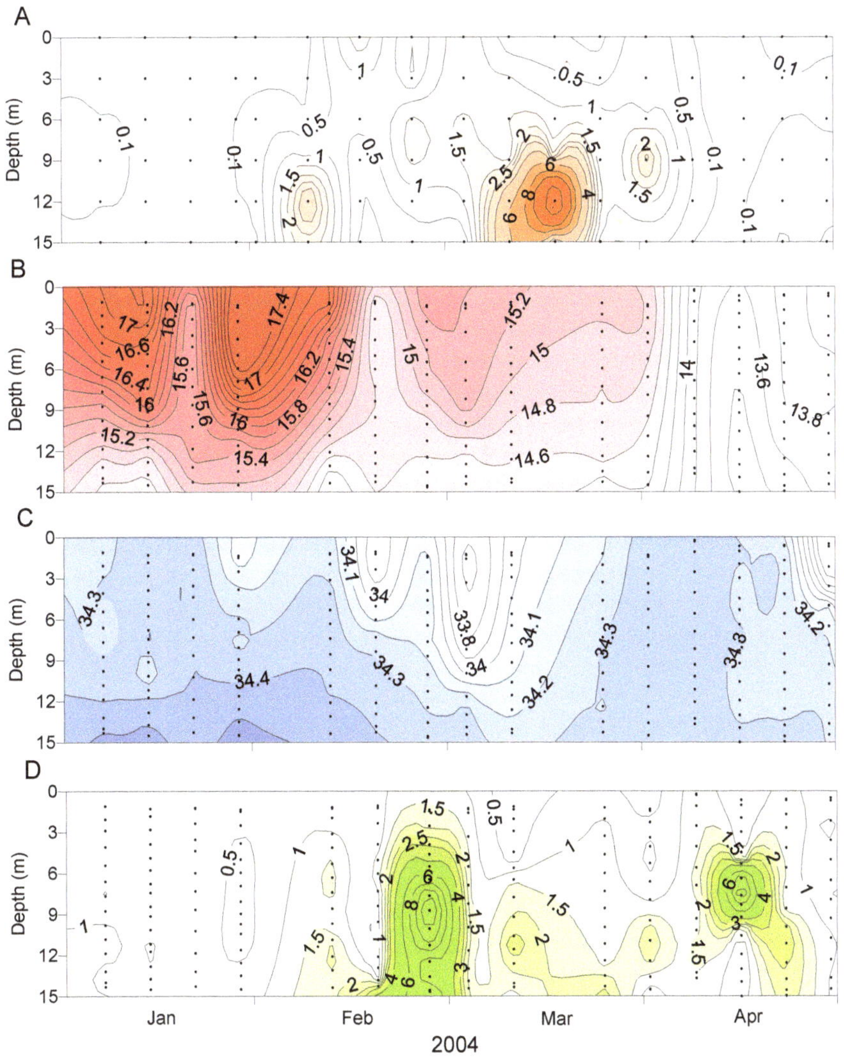

Figure 9. The progression of a *Dinophysis acuminata* bloom relative to the water column conditions at the Whangakoko site, January-April 2004. (**A**) *D. acuminata* cell numbers (cells × 10^3 L^{-1}). (**B**) Temperature (°C). (**C**) Salinity. (**D**) Chlorophyll a concentration (μg L^{-1}).

2.4. *Toxins Originating from* D. acuminata *in Cultivated Mussels (*Perna canaliculus*)*

Data from analyses using an LC-MS/MS multi-residue method for the determination of lipophilic algal toxins in shellfish [21,22] became available from early 2002.

On 14 occasions during *D. acuminata* blooms, the sampling of mussels at three depths on the vertical culture lines (near the surface, at 6 m, and at 12 m) was carried out (Figure 10). The distribution of the toxins in these shellfish (higher concentrations of PTX-2sa and total DTX-1 deeper in the water column) paralleled the depth distribution of *D. acuminata* cells (Figures 7–9).

A summary of the results of the weekly analysis of mussel tissues from the Whangakoko and Opihi monitoring sites (Figures 11 and 12) shows that PTX-2sa was present above the reporting level

(0.01 mg kg^{-1}) in the majority (70.6% and 54.5%, respectively) of samples analysed at both sites. At the Horahora site, 22.6% of samples had PTX-2sa above the reporting level. The maximum concentrations of PTX-2sa observed at Whangakoko, Opihi, and Horahora were 1.7 mg kg^{-1} (March 2013), 1.4 mg kg^{-1} (April 2005), and 0.24 mg kg^{-1} (October 2009), respectively. At Whangakoko, parent PTX-2 was only above the reporting level in 27 out of 860 samples analysed (3.1%), with a maximum concentration of 0.039 mg kg^{-1} in April 2016. At Opihi, only 1.1% of samples contained reportable levels of PTX-2, with a maximum concentration of 0.025 mg kg^{-1} (January 2012). At Horahora, free PTX-2 was not detected. It is likely that the concentrations of PTX-2sa were, in fact, significantly higher than those reported here, since PTX-2sa-esters were not included in these analyses. According to Torgeston et al. [23], >80% of PTX-2sa in mussels (*Mytilus edulis*) may be in the form of fatty acid esters, with 16:0 and 14:0 predominant. Likewise, Blanco et al. [24] found that the concentrations of PTX-2sa and the palmytol ester of PTX-2sa were approximately equivalent in the digestive gland of the surf clam *Mesodesma donacium*. They also found that PTX-2 and PTX-2sa were more rapidly eliminated from the digestive gland than PTX-2sa esters.

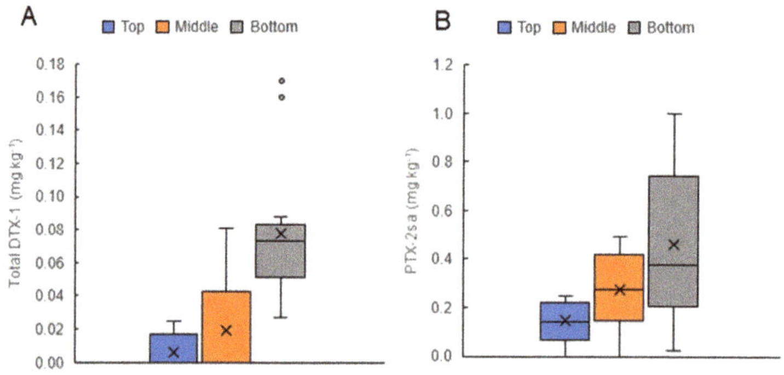

Figure 10. Summary of the depth distribution of total dinophysistoxin-1 (DTX-1) (**A**) and pectenotoxin-2sa (PTX-2sa) (**B**) Concentrations in Greenshell™ mussels on 14 occasions when samples were collected from the vertical mussel culture ropes, near the surface (Top), in the middle of the rope (approx. 6 m), and at the bottom of the rope (approx. 12 m). Error bars show the range of values. Horizontal lines are the medium values and crosses indicate the means. Dots show values considered outliers by this analysis (in this case, values at or above the regulatory level of 0.16 mg kg^{-1}).

Only a small proportion of samples between 2002 and 2018 had concentrations of total DTX-1 above the reporting level (Figures 10 and 11). DTX-1 was the only okadaic acid group toxin identified in Port Underwood mussels between 2002 and 2018 and was usually only detectable after the alkaline hydrolysis of fatty acid esters within the extracts. Free DTX-1 was only detected on a few occasions. At Whangakoko and Opihi, 8.5% and 4.2% of samples, respectively, had total DTX-1 above the reporting level (Figures 11 and 12). At Horahora, between February 2002 and July 2018 there was only one single report of DTX-1 in mussels (0.05 mg/kg) on 9 March 2010. The highest concentration of DTX-1 observed was 0.39 mg kg^{-1} at Whangakoko on 3 March 2010. Between October 2003 (when the alkaline hydrolysis procedure was introduced) and July 2018, 2307 samples were screened for the total DTX-1. Of these, only 11 samples (0.4%) had a total DTX-1 above 0.1 mg kg^{-1} and only 5 samples (0.2%) had concentrations at or above the regulatory level of 0.16 mg kg^{-1} (Figures 13 and 14). The cell numbers of *D. acuminata* on all of these occasions exceeded 5000 cells L^{-1} and were accompanied by peak concentrations of PTX-2sa (0.3–1.0 mg kg^{-1}). Abal et al. [25] have recently shown through the oral dosing of mice, that the toxicity equivalency factors (TEFs) between okadaic acid and dinophysistoxins −1 and 2 are ranked as OA = 1, DTX-1 = 1.5, and DTX-2 = 0.3. Applying a 1.5 factor to these, DTX-1 concentration data only slightly increased the number of samples exceeding 0.16 mg kg^{-1} from five to nine per 2307 samples analysed (0.2–0.3%).

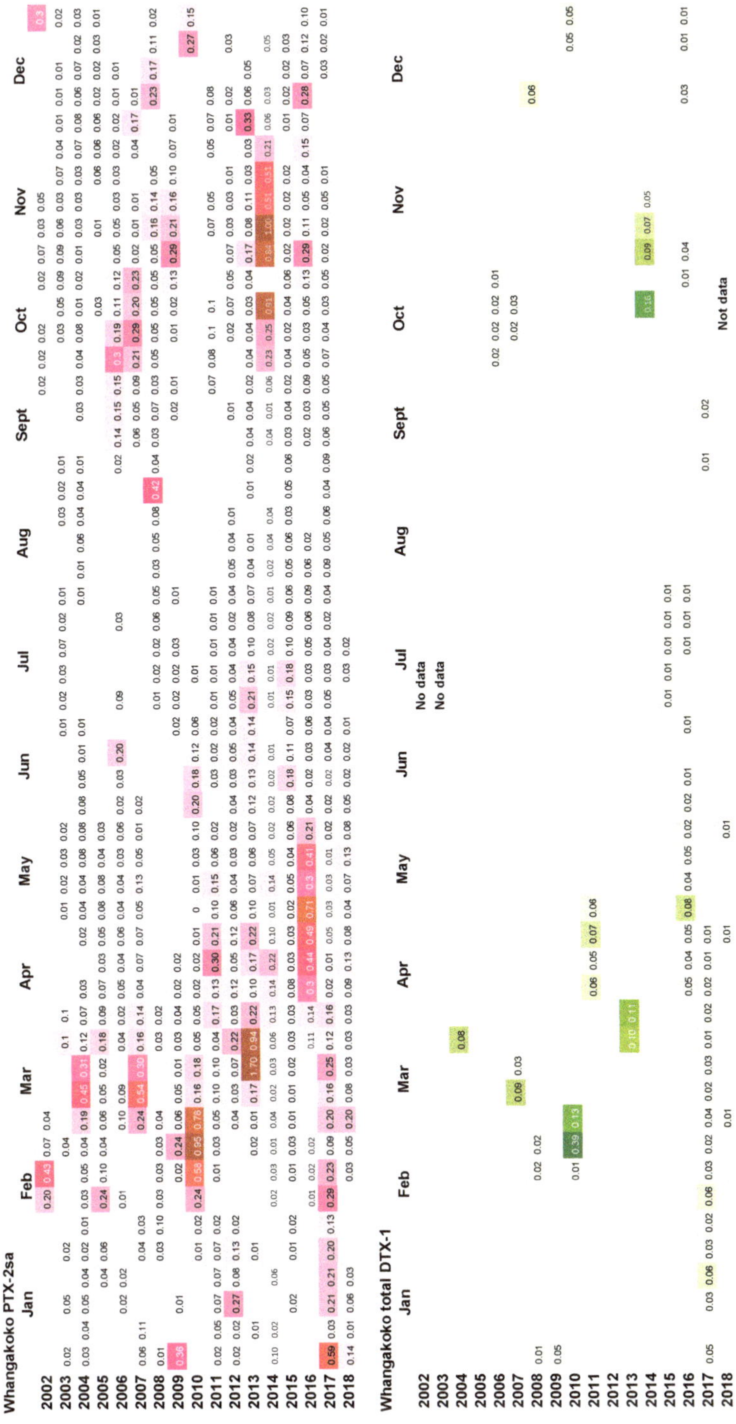

Figure 11. *Dinophysis acuminata* secondary metabolites (PTX-2sa and total DTX-1) in Greenshell™ mussels from Whangakoko, 2002–2018. Blank spaces indicate levels below the limit of reporting (<0.01 mg kg^{-1} of PTX-2sa and total DTX-1).

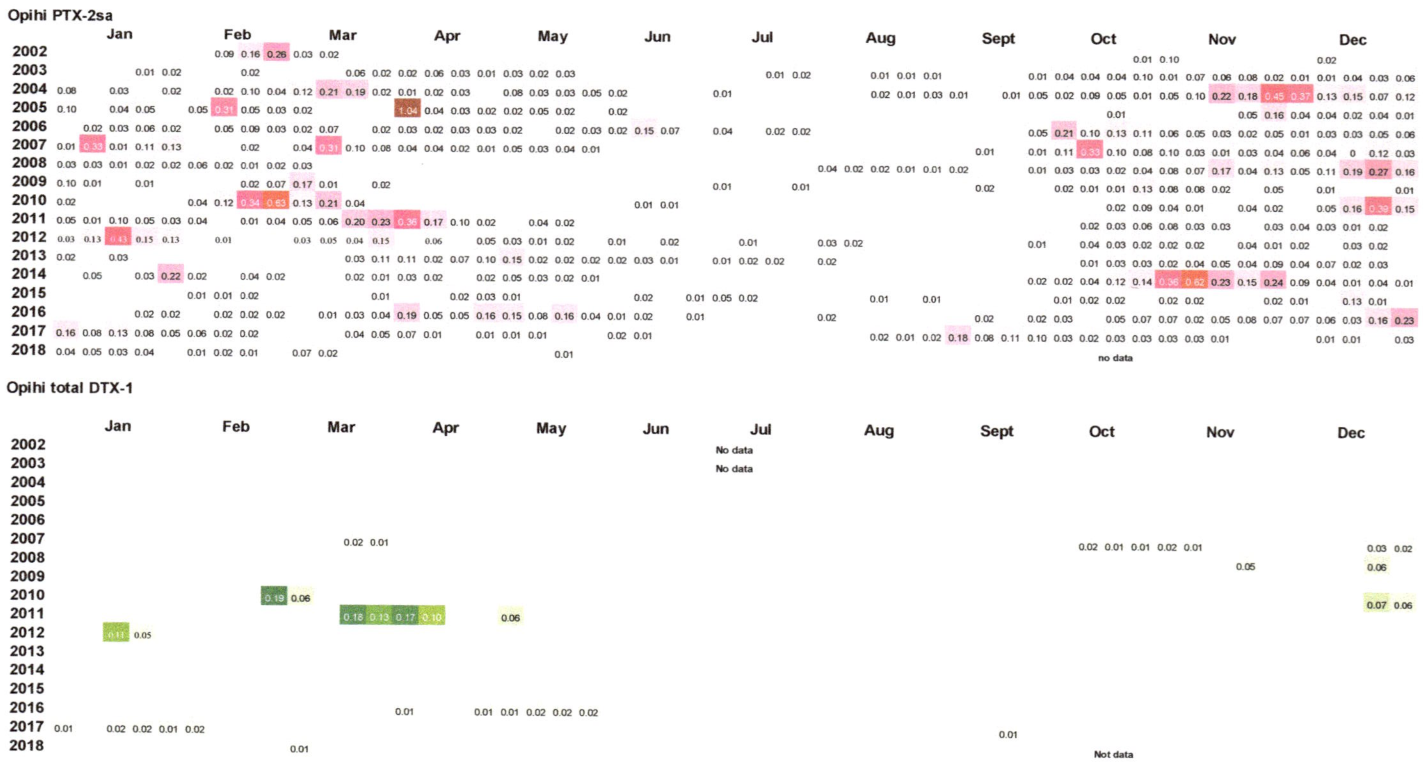

Figure 12. *Dinophysis acuminata* secondary metabolites (PTX-2sa and total DTX-1) in Greenshell^{TM} mussels from Opihi, 2002–2018. Blank spaces indicate levels below the limit of reporting (<0.01 mg kg^{-1} of PTX-2sa and total DTX-1).

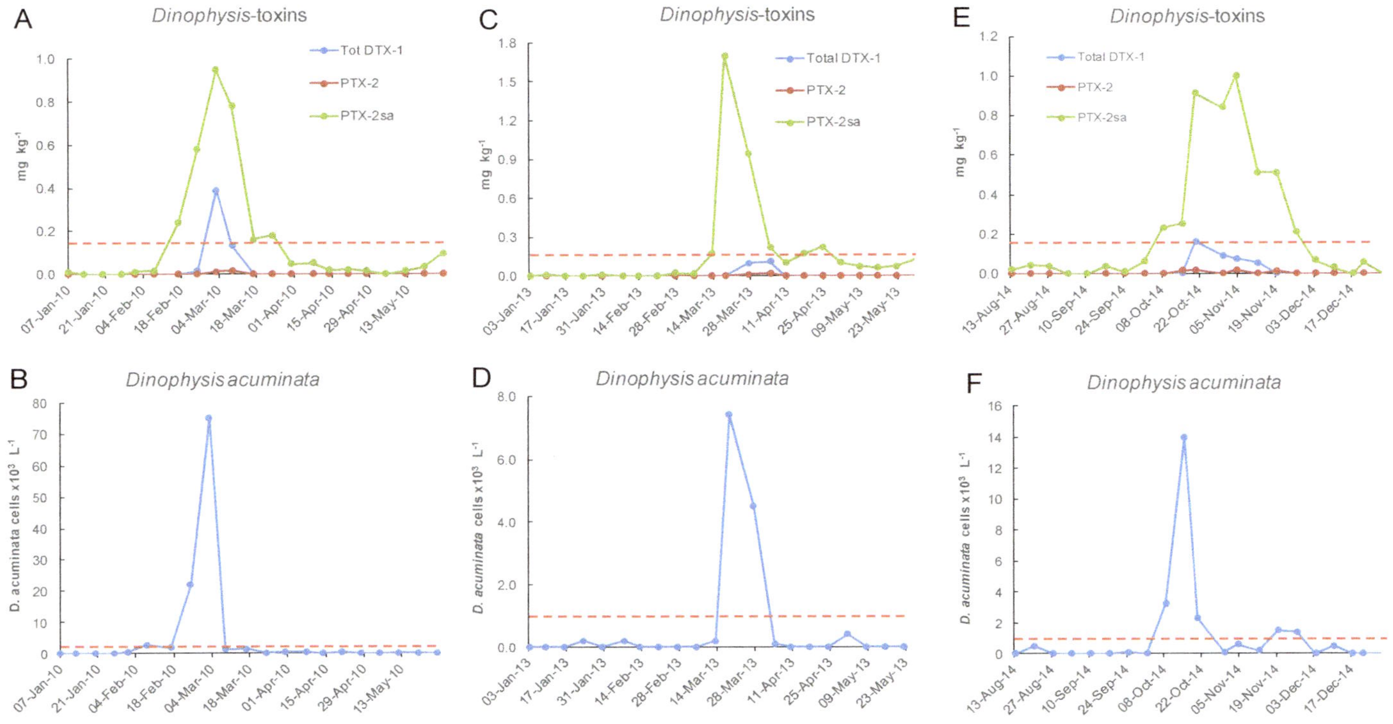

Figure 13. Three occasions between January 2002 and June 2018 at the Whangakoko sampling site when total DTX-1 approached or exceeded 0.1 mg kg^{-1}, in relation to the cell numbers of *Dinophysis acuminata* in the water column. (**A**,**B**) 7 Jan–26 May 2010; (**C**,**D**) 3 Jan–23 May 2013; (**E**,**F**) 17 Aug–28 Dec 2014. The dashed lines indicate the maximum permitted level of 0.16 mg kg^{-1} total DTX-1 in shellfish and the action level of 1×10^3 cells L^{-1} of *Dinophysis acuminata*.

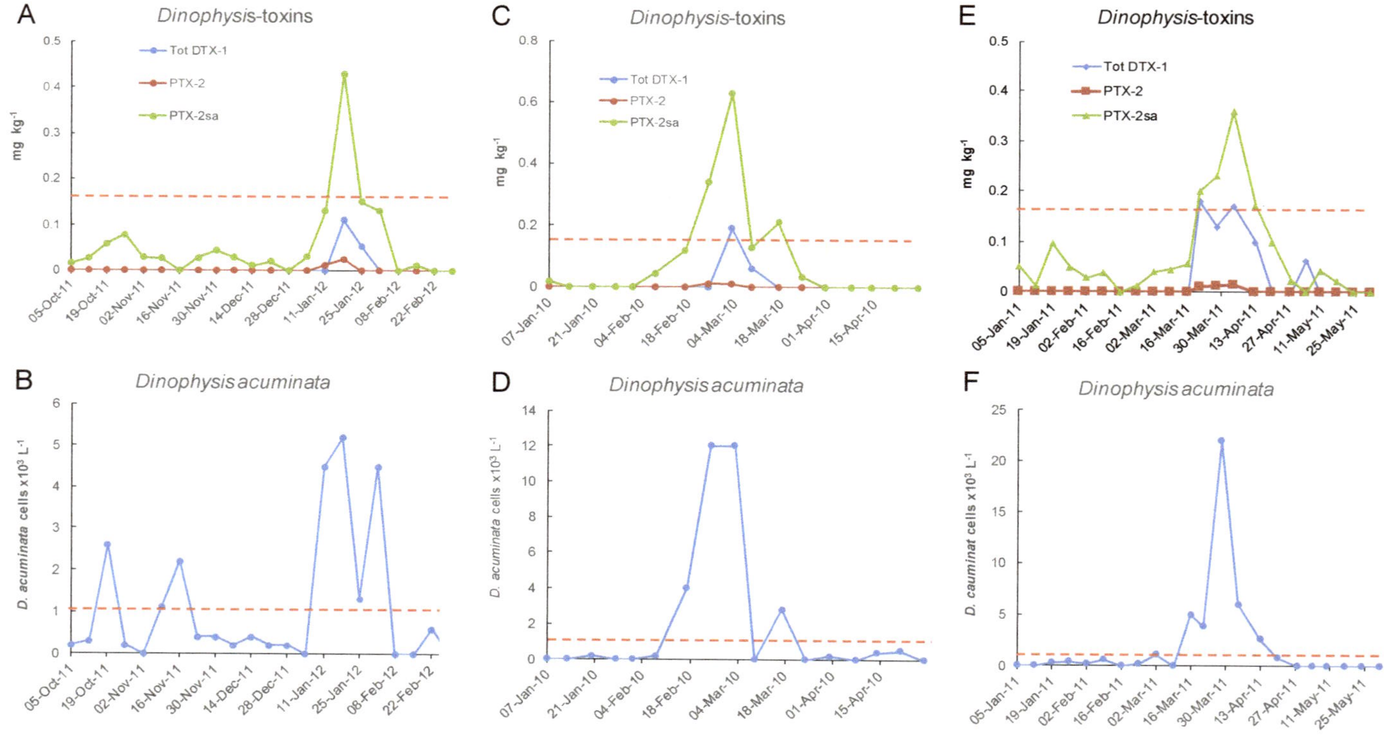

Figure 14. Three occasions between January 2007 and June 2018 at the Opihi sampling site when total DTX-1 approached or exceeded 0.1 mg/kg in relation to cell numbers of *Dinophysis acuminata* in the water column. (**A**,**B**) 8 Oct 2011 to 25 Feb 2012; (**C**,**D**) 7 Jan 2010 to 28 Apr 2010; (**E**,**F**) 5 Jan 2011 to 31 May 2011. The dashed lines indicate the maximum permitted level of 0.16 mg kg^{-1} total DTX-1 in shellfish and the action level of 1 × 10^{3} cells L^{-1} of *Dinophysis acuminata*.

3. Conclusions

Port Underwood has a resident population of *D. acuminata* that, over 24 years of continuous weekly monitoring, has never failed to bloom to some degree, at some time, from early spring to late autumn. Blooms developed in near-bottom waters in the most inland reaches of the inlet. It is believed that the abundance of *Mesodinium* sp. prey at depth may be an important precursor of the blooms. *Mesodinium* sp. is common in the inlet but cells are poorly preserved in Lugol's iodine and numbers were not recorded during routine monitoring, so no definitive data exists to demonstrate the relationship between populations of prey and predators. *D. acuminata* numbers rarely exceed 10,000 cells L^{-1} but low numbers of cells are present in the water column throughout much of the year. Cultivated mussels show evidence of this in the high proportion of samples that show low concentrations of (non-regulated) PTX-2sa in their flesh. The DTX-1 content of *D. acuminata* cells is low and only a small proportion of mussel samples show evidence of DTX-1 accumulation (primarily as DTX-1 fatty acid-esters) above the limit of reporting. Over 16 years of weekly LC-MS analysis, only a small proportion of mussel samples (0.2%) achieved or marginally exceeded the regulated level of 0.16 mg kg^{-1}. In every case when this level was reached, *D. acuminata* cell numbers exceeded 10,000 cells L^{-1}. Cell numbers of up to 5000 cells L^{-1} did not result in toxicity exceeding the regulatory limit, and the current action level of 1000 cells L^{-1} could be reviewed. It has been shown in cultured and natural populations of *Dinophysis* spp. [26,27] that the toxin quota can vary by an order of magnitude during the growing season, with the maximum cell content being exhibited during the stationary phase. It is possible that the toxin quota also varies temporally in the Port Underwood *D. acuminata* but the long-term data set presented here clearly shows that, given the inherent low toxicity of this population, any natural fluctuations in toxin quota are unlikely to be of any practical significance with respect to the toxin content of cultivated mussels. Increasing concentrations of PTX-2sa are a good indicator of the imminence of DTX-1 contamination and the addition of PTX-2sa ester quantification to the routine monitoring protocol would likely increase the sensitivity of this indicator.

4. Materials and Methods

Sea-water samples were collected weekly at three sites (Whangakoko, Opihi, and Horahora) in Port Underwood (Figure 1) with a tube sampler that provided a ≤15-metre depth-integrated sample of the water column. On some occasions, samples from selected depths were also collected with a van Dorn sampler. Surveys of water column properties (temperature, salinity, and chlorophyll a fluorescence) were carried out using a Chelsea Instruments "Aquapack" CTD instrument (West Molesly, Surrey, UK). Phytoplankton identification and counts were carried out on Lugol's iodine preserved samples, after the settling of 10 mL aliquots in Utermöhl chambers and examination under an inverted microscope.

Samples of Greenshell™ mussels (*Perna canaliculus*) were collected weekly from mussel culture long-lines at the same sites as the phytoplankton samples. Routinely, samples were collected from a depth of 6 m, although on some occasions during significant bloom events, additional samples were also collected from near the surface (top) and from a depth of 12 m (bottom). Phytoplankton and shellfish samples were couriered to the Cawthron phytoplankton and biotoxin laboratories and the results of the analyses were available within 24 hours of receipt of the samples.

Prior to 2002, diarrhetic shellfish poisoning (DSP) toxicity of shellfish samples was analysed using the standard mouse bioassay [2], after solvent extraction using the revised method of Hannah et al. [28]. However, because of the poor quantification and unreliability of the results of these tests, none of these data are included in this analysis.

From 2002, all mussel samples were analysed using the multi-residue LC-MS/MS method for lipophilic algal toxins developed and validated by McNabb et al. [21,22]. Shellfish tissue homogenates (from a minimum of 12 fresh specimens) were blended with 90% aqueous methanol and the centrifuged extract was cleaned-up with a hexane wash. LC-MS/MS was used for the quantitative analysis with reversed phase gradient elution (Luna C18 5μm 150 × 2mm column; acidic buffer), electrospray ionisation (positive and negative ion switching), and multiple reaction monitoring (MRM). The MRM channels were monitored in windows that covered the elution of the compounds of interest (precursor > daughter): okadaic acid −ve 803.5 > 255.0, +ve 827.5 > 723.4; DTX-1 −ve 817.5 > 255.2, +ve 841.5 > 723.4; PTX-2 +ve 876.6 > 823.2; PTX-2 seco acid +ve 894.5 > 823.5. Okadaic acid and PTX-2 were quantified with reference to certified reference materials (CRM-OA-d, CRM PTX2-b) from the National Research Council, Canada. DTX-1 and PTX-2 seco acid were also calibrated with reference to these standards after the application of relative response factors. Ester forms of dinophysistoxins (in this case, exclusively DTX-1 esters) were detected as the parent toxin following alkaline hydrolysis of the methanolic extract [29] and were reported as the total DTX-1.

Until 2016, the lower limits of reporting of PTX-2, PTX-2 seco acid, and total DTX-1, the only lipophilic toxin residues of any significance in these shellfish, were <0.01, <0.01, and <0.05 mg kg^{-1}, respectively. From 2016 onwards, the limit of reporting of the total DTX-1 was also reduced to <0.01 mg kg^{-1}.

Funding: This research was funded by the "Seafood Safety Platform" (New Zealand Ministry of Business Innovation and Employment Contract # CAWX 1801).

Acknowledgments: The author thanks the Marlborough Shellfish Quality Programme (MSQP) for permission to use their phytoplankton and shellfish biotoxin monitoring data in this presentation. Thanks also to Emillie Burger and Tony Bui at the Cawthron Institute for assistance in retrieving the data.

Conflicts of Interest: The author declares no conflicts of interest.

References

1. Yasumoto, T.; Oshima, Y.; Yamaguchi, M. Occurrence of a new type of shellfish poisoning in the Tohoku district. *Bull. Jpn. Soc. Sci. Fish.* **1978**, *44*, 1249–1255. [CrossRef]
2. Yasumoto, T.; Oshima, Y.; Sugawara, W.; Fukuyo, Y.; Oguri, H.; Igarashi, T.; Fujita, N. Identification of *Dinophysis fortii* as the causative organism of Diarrhetic Shellfish Poisoning. *Bull. Jpn. Soc. Sci. Fish.* **1980**, *46*, 1405–1411. [CrossRef]
3. European Parliament Council. Regulation (EC) 853 of April laying down specific hygiene rules for food of animal origin. *Off. J. Eur. Union* **2004**, *226*, 22–80.
4. MacKenzie, L.; Beuzenburg, V.; McNabb, P.; Holland, P.; Suzuki, T.; Neil, T.; Selwood, A. Pectenotoxin and okadaic acid based toxin profiles in *Dinophysis acuta* and *D. acuminata* from New Zealand. *Harmful Algae* **2004**, *4*, 75–85. [CrossRef]
5. Tong, M.; Smith, J.L.; Richlen, M.; Steidinger, K.A.; Kulis, D.M.; Fux, E.; Anderson, D.M. Characterization and comparison of toxin producing isolates s of *Diniophysis acuminata* from New England and Canada. *J. Phycol.* **2015**, *51*, 66–81. [CrossRef] [PubMed]
6. Draisci, R.; Lucentini, L.; Mascioni, A. Pectenotoxins and Yessotoxin: Chemistry, Toxicology, Pharmacology and Analysis. In *Seafood and Freshwater Toxins: Pharmacology Physiology, and Detection*; Botana, L.M., Ed.; Marcel Dekker Inc.: New York, NY, USA; Basel, Switzerland, 2000; pp. 289–324.
7. Munday, R. Toxicology of the pectenotoxins. In *Seafood and Freshwater Toxins: Pharmacology, Physiology and Detection*, 2nd ed.; Botana, L.M., Ed.; CRC Press: Boca Raton, FL, USA; London, UK; New York, NY, USA, 2008; pp. 371–380.
8. Daiguji, M.; Satake, M.; James, K.J.; Bishop, A.; Mackenzie, L.; Naoki, H.; Yasumoto, T. Structures of new Pectenotoxin analogs, Pectenotoxin-2 Seco acid and 7-epi-Pectenotoxin-2 seco acid, isolated from a dinoflagellate and Greenshell mussels. *Chem. Lett.* **1998**, *7*, 653–654. [CrossRef]
9. Suzuki, T.; Mackenzie, L.; Stirling, D.; Adamson, J. Pectenotoxin-2 Seco Acid: A toxin converted from Pectenotoxin-2 by the New Zealand Greenshell mussel *Perna canaliculus*. *Toxicon* **2001**, *39*, 507–514. [CrossRef]
10. MacKenzie, L.A.; Selwood, A.I.; Marshall, C. Isolation and characterization of an enzyme from the Greenshell™ mussel *Perna canaliculus* that hydrolyses pectenotoxins and esters of okadaic acid. *Toxicon* **2012**, *60*, 406–419. [CrossRef] [PubMed]

11. Mackenzie, L.; Holland, P.; McNabb, P.; Beuzenberg, V.; Selwood, A.; Suzuki, T. Complex toxin profiles in phytoplankton and Greenshell mussels (*Perna canaliculus*) revealed by LC-MS/MS analysis. *Toxicon* **2002**, *40*, 1321–1330. [CrossRef]
12. Mackenzie, L. *An Evaluation of the Risk to Consumers of Pectenotoxn-2 Seco Acid (PTX2-SA) Contamination of Greenshell^{TM} Mussels*; A Report for Marlborough Sounds Shellfish Quality Programme; Cawthron Report No. 750; Cawthron: Nelson, New Zealand, 2002; 50p.
13. MacKenzie, A.L. Does *Dinophysis* (Dinophyceae) have a sexual life cycle? *J. Phycol.* **1992**, *28*, 399–406. [CrossRef]
14. Reguera, B.; González-Gill, S. Small cell and intermediate cell formation in species of *Dinophysis* (Dinophyceae, Dinophysiales). *J. Phycol.* **2001**, *37*, 318–333. [CrossRef]
15. Koike, K.; Nishiyama, A.; Saitoh, K.; Imai, K.; Koike, K.; Kobiyama, A.; Ogata, T. Mechanism of gamete fusion in *Dinophysis fortii* (Dinophyceae, Dinophyta): Light microscopic and ultrastructural observations. *J. Phycol.* **2006**, *42*, 1247–1256. [CrossRef]
16. Park, M.G.; Kim, S.; Kim, H.S.; Myung, G.; Kang, Y.G.; Yih, W. First successful culture of the marine dinoflagellate *Dinophysis acuminata*. *Aquat. Microb. Ecol.* **2006**, *45*, 101–106. [CrossRef]
17. Reguera, B.; Velo-Suárez, L.; Raine, R.; Park, M.G. Harmful *Dinophysis* species: A review. *Harmful Algae* **2012**, *14*, 87–106. [CrossRef]
18. Velo-Suárez, L.; González-Gil, S.; Pazos, Y.; Reguera, B. The growth season of *Dinophysis acuminata* in an upwelling system embayment: A conceptual model based on in situ measurements. *Deep-Sea Res.* **2014**, *101*, 141–151. [CrossRef]
19. Maestrini, S.Y. Bloom dynamics and ecophysiology of *Dinophysis* spp. In *Physiological Ecology of Harmful Algal Blooms. NATO AI Series G. Ecological Science*; Anderson, D.M., Cembella, A.D., Hallegraeff, G.M., Eds.; Springer: Berlin/Heidelberg, Germany; New York, NY, USA, 1998; pp. 243–266.
20. Raine, R.; McDermott, G.; Silke, J.; Lyons, K.; Cusack, C. A simple short-range model for the prediction of harmful algal events in the bays of Southwest Ireland. *J. Mar. Syst.* **2010**, *83*, 150–157. [CrossRef]
21. McNabb, P.; Holland, P. Using LCMS to manage shellfish harvesting and protect public health. In *Molluscan Shellfish Safety*; Villalba, A., Reguera, B., Romalde, J., Beiras, R., Eds.; Xunta de Glaicia & IOC of UNESCO: Santiago de Compostela, Spain, 2003; pp. 179–186.
22. McNabb, P.; Selwood, A.I.; Holland, P.T. Multi-residue method for determination of algal toxins in shellfish: Single laboratory validation and inter-laboratory study. *J. AOAC Int.* **2005**, *88*, 761–772. [PubMed]
23. Torgersen, T.; Sanvik, M.; Lundve, B.; Lindegart, S. Profiles and levels of fatty acid esters of okadaic acid group toxins and pectenotoxins during toxin depuration. Part II: Blue mussels (*Mytilus edulis)* and flat oyster (*Ostrea edulis*). *Toxicon* **2008**, *52*, 418–427. [CrossRef]
24. Blanco, J.; Alvarez, G.; Rengel, J.; Diaz, R.; Marinao, C.; Martin, H.; Uribe, E. Accumulation and biotransformation of *Dinophysis* toxins by the surf clam *Mesodesma donacium*. *Toxins* **2018**, *10*, 314. [CrossRef] [PubMed]
25. Abal, P.; Louzao, M.C.; Suzuki, T.; Watanabe, R.; Vilarino, N.; Carrera, C.; Botana, A.M.; Vieytes, M.R.; Botana, L.M. Toxic action re-evaluation of Okadaic acid, Dinophysistoxin-1 and Dinophysistoxin-2: Toxicity equivalency factors based on the oral toxicity study. *Cell. Physiol. Biochem.* **2018**, *49*, 743–757. [CrossRef]
26. Kamiyama, T.; Nagai, S.; Miyamura, K. Effect of temperature on production of okadaic acid, dinophysistoxin-1 and pectenotoxin-2 by *Dinophysis acuminata* in culture experiments. *Aquat. Microb. Ecol.* **2010**, *60*, 193–202. [CrossRef]
27. Pizarro, G.; Paz, B.; González-Gil, S.; Franco, J.M.; Reguera, B. Seasonal variability of lipophilic toxins during a *Dinophysis acuta* bloom in Western Iberia: Differences between picked cells and plankton concentrates. *Harmful Algae* **2009**, *8*, 926–937. [CrossRef]
28. Hannah, D.J.; Till, D.G.; Deverall, T.; Jones, P.D.; Fry, J.M. Extraction of lipid-soluble marine biotoxins. *J. AOAC Int.* **1995**, *78*, 480–483.
29. Mountfort, D.O.; Suzuki, T.; Truman, P. Protein phosphatase inhibition assay adapted for determination of total DSP in contaminated mussels. *Toxicon* **2001**, *39*, 383–390. [CrossRef]

toxins

MDPI

Article

Diarrhetic Shellfish Toxin Monitoring in Commercial Wild Harvest Bivalve Shellfish in New South Wales, Australia

Hazel Farrell [1,*], Penelope Ajani [2], Shauna Murray [2], Phil Baker [1], Grant Webster [1], Steve Brett [3] and Anthony Zammit [1]

1. NSW Food Authority, 6 Avenue of the Americas, Newington, NSW 2127, Australia; phil.baker@dpi.nsw.gov.au (P.B.); grant.webster@dpi.nsw.gov.au (G.W.); anthony.zammit@dpi.nsw.gov.au (A.Z.)
2. Climate Change Cluster (C3), University of Technology Sydney, 15 Broadway, Ultimo, NSW 2007, Australia; penelope.ajani@uts.edu.au (P.A.); shauna.murray@uts.edu.au (S.M.)
3. Microalgal Services, 308 Tucker Rd, Ormond, VIC 3204, Australia; algae@bigpond.com

* Correspondence: hazel.farrell@dpi.nsw.gov.au; Tel.: +61-2-9741-4882

Received: 6 September 2018; Accepted: 23 October 2018; Published: 30 October 2018

Abstract: An end-product market survey on biotoxins in commercial wild harvest shellfish (*Plebidonax deltoides*, *Katelysia* spp., *Anadara granosa*, *Notocallista kingii*) during three harvest seasons (2015–2017) from the coast of New South Wales, Australia found 99.38% of samples were within regulatory limits. Diarrhetic shellfish toxins (DSTs) were present in 34.27% of 321 samples but only in pipis (*P. deltoides*), with two samples above the regulatory limit. Comparison of these market survey data to samples (phytoplankton in water and biotoxins in shellfish tissue) collected during the same period at wild harvest beaches demonstrated that, while elevated concentrations of *Dinophysis* were detected, a lag in detecting bloom events on two occasions meant that wild harvest shellfish with DSTs above the regulatory limit entered the marketplace. Concurrently, data (phytoplankton and biotoxin) from Sydney rock oyster (*Saccostrea glomerata*) harvest areas in estuaries adjacent to wild harvest beaches impacted by DSTs frequently showed elevated *Dinophysis* concentrations, but DSTs were not detected in oyster samples. These results highlighted a need for distinct management strategies for different shellfish species, particularly during *Dinophysis* bloom events. DSTs above the regulatory limit in pipis sampled from the marketplace suggested there is merit in looking at options to strengthen the current wild harvest biotoxin management strategies.

Keywords: diarrhetic shellfish toxins; *Dinophysis*; wild harvest; bivalve shellfish; pipis (*Plebidonax deltoides*); Sydney rock oyster (*Saccostrea glomerata*)

Key Contribution: Our findings demonstrated that *Dinophysis* spp. were the main source of DSTs on NSW wild harvest beaches. The detection of DST contaminated product above the regulatory limit within the marketplace suggested there is merit in looking at options to strengthen the current wild harvest management strategies.

1. Introduction

Bivalve shellfish are a major global commodity with current market analysis indicating a strong demand for limited available produce [1]. In a demanding market, consumer confidence is essential to support production increases. A major component of a bivalve shellfish safety program is the management and mitigation of the potential risks from biotoxins. Globally, the impact of algal toxins on shellfish aquaculture is variable. In some regions, there has been an apparent increase in the frequency and intensity of toxic events (e.g., recent paralytic shellfish toxins (PST) events in Tasmania [2,3]) but with effective monitoring and management, the risk of illness outbreaks can be minimised [4,5]. All biotoxin groups are of concern to shellfish safety managers, and more than one toxin group can occur concurrently. In the case of *Dinophysis* spp., certain species can produce diarrhetic shellfish toxins (Diarrhetic shellfish toxins (DSTs): okadaic acid (OA) and dinophysistoxins (DTX)) at very low cell densities (200 cells/L) [6–8]. OA, DTX 1, and DTX-3 are diarrheagenic and some OA/DTX analogues have been associated with tumor formation in laboratory studies on rodents [9–11]. Diarrhetic shellfish poisoning (DSP) was first described in the late 1970s following human illness outbreaks in Japan [12], yet early reports of gastrointestinal illness suspected as DSP date back to 1961 [7]. The acute symptoms of DSP are generally alleviated within a few days and no fatalities from acute cases of DSP have been recorded. Certain *Dinophysis* species can also produce pectenotoxins (PTX, previously part of the DST complex), although there is no known evidence that PTXs are toxic to humans [5]. Very high concentrations of *Dinophysis* can occur in thin layers and other micro and mesoscale oceanographic structures, which means that species of this genus can be difficult to detect [8,13–15]. These difficulties are compounded by the fact that *Dinophysis* species are generally mixotrophic, and the laboratory culture of species of this genus has only recently been achieved [16–23]. Until this development, verifying toxins produced by individual species and understanding the factors affecting toxin production have been challenging.

In New South Wales (NSW), Australia, bivalve shellfish aquaculture stretches along >2000 km of coastline with a farm gate value of more than $AUD 47 million per year [24]. The main cultivated species is the native Sydney rock oyster (*Saccostrea glomerata*). Other cultivated species include Pacific oyster (*Magallana gigas* formerly *Crassostrea gigas*), native oyster (*Ostrea angasi*), and blue mussel (*Mytilus edulis*). Seasonal (June–December) wild harvest shellfish collection from open beaches is focused on pipis ('clams', *Plebidonax deltoides*) at up to 16 beaches (Figure 1). Gathering of cockles (*Katelysia* spp., *Anadara granosa*) occurs within six oyster harvest areas, and a single operator collects clams (*Notocallista kingii*) through offshore dredging along the NSW south coast (~36°54.5′ S). Under the NSW Marine Biotoxin Management Plan [25], shellfish collected or grown for human consumption in NSW are subject to monitoring (phytoplankton in water adjacent to harvest areas and biotoxins in shellfish flesh) to ensure that the product is safe to eat.

Three types of biotoxins are currently known to occur in NSW (amnesic shellfish toxin (AST), diarrhetic shellfish toxins (DSTs) and paralytic shellfish toxins (PSTs)). In NSW, these toxin groups are routinely monitored (biotoxin testing of shellfish flesh and microscopic analysis of water samples for causative phytoplankton) in locations where shellfish are cultivated and harvested (or collected in terms of wild shellfish) for human consumption. Neurotoxic shellfish toxins (NSTs) and azaspiracid shellfish toxins (AZTs) have not been detected in NSW, or Australia, to date [3,26–29]. The permissible level of biotoxins in shellfish is regulated in Standard 1.4.1 clause 3 of the Australia New Zealand Food Standards Code [30] (The Code). The limits specified within The Code are similar to the European Union (EU) and the United States of America (USA) regulatory standards (Table 1).

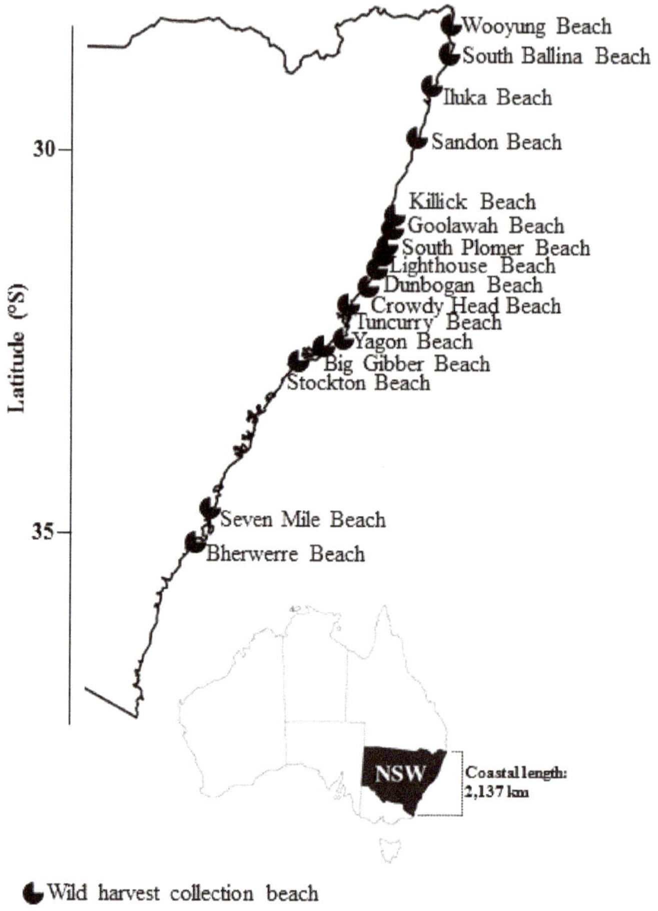

Figure 1. Location of wild harvest beaches in New South Wales (NSW), Australia from which pipis were harvested during the 2015–2017 harvest seasons.

Table 1. Regulatory limits for biotoxins in bivalve molluscs from the European Union (EU), United States of America (USA) and Australian legislation.

Toxin Group	EU [31]	USA [32]	Australia [30]
Amnesic shellfish toxin (AST, domoic acid equivalent)	20 mg/kg	20 mg/kg	20 mg/kg
Diarrhetic shellfish toxins (DSTs, okadaic acid equivalent)	0.16 mg/kg	0.16 mg/kg	0.20 mg/kg
Paralytic shellfish toxins (PSTs, saxitoxin equivalent)	0.80 mg/kg	0.80 mg/kg	0.80 mg/kg
Neurotoxic shellfish toxins (NSTs, brevetoxin-2 equivalent)	n/a [1]	0.8 ppm or 200 MU/kg	200 MU/kg
Azaspiracid shellfish toxins (AZTs)	0.16 mg/kg	0.16 mg/kg	n/a [2]

[1] not applicable, there are currently no EU regulatory limits for NSTs; [2] not applicable, AZTs have not been detected in Australia. If identified, international regulatory limits would apply.

Since the establishment of the current phytoplankton and biotoxin monitoring program by the NSW Food Authority in 2005, all three of the major toxin groups (AST, DSTs, PSTs) have been detected in shellfish tissue in NSW [29]. Biotoxin data from wild harvest beaches have shown detections of DSTs in pipis related to *Dinophysis* spp., with occasional reports of AST (NSW Food Authority 2018, unpublished data). While the NSW dataset did not report the presence of PSTs in pipis, PSTs, DSTs, and AST have been reported in shellfish species (cockles and clams) from similar intertidal or sandy-bottomed marine habitats (e.g., AST: razor clam (*Siliqua patula*) Washington State, USA [33–35], DSTs: littleneck clam (*Leukoma staminea*), varnish clam (*Nuttallia obscurata*), manila clam (*Ruditapes philippinarum* syn. *Venerupis philippinarum*) Washington State, USA [34] and PSTs: surf clam (tuatua, *Paphies subtriangulata*) Bay of Plenty, New Zealand [36]).

Historically, in NSW, most phytoplankton toxin-related illnesses have been linked to ciguatoxin in migratory and imported reef fish [37–39] rather than bivalve shellfish. To date, no illnesses linked to biotoxins from NSW oyster or mussel aquaculture areas have been reported (NSW Food Authority 2018, unpublished data). Before the establishment of routine monitoring on NSW wild harvest beaches, two illness outbreaks occurred following consumption of pipis. Both outbreaks were associated with DSTs in 1997 (north NSW coast; 102 cases including, 46 anecdotal) [40] and 1998 (mid-north NSW coast; >20 cases) [27,41]. In Australian waters, 36 species of *Dinophysis* have been documented [28,42,43], of which *Dinophysis acuminata* (Claparède and Lachmann), *Dinophysis acuta* (Ehrenberg), *Dinophysis caudata* (Saville-Kent), *Dinophysis fortii* (Pavillard), and *Dinophysis tripos* (Gourret) are known toxin producers, along with *Phalacroma mitra* (syn. *Dinophysis mitra*). Reports of *Dinophysis* and DST events elsewhere in Australia have been few, although the availability of long-term phytoplankton and biotoxin datasets across all Australian states is limited. A single case of DSP from pipis collected from a beach on North Stradbroke Island, Queensland was reported in 2000 [44]. DSTs above the regulatory limit have been reported in pipis from NSW (suspected *D. acuminata*) [45], in oysters from South Australia (*D. acuminata*) [46], and in mussels from Tasmania (*D. acuminata* and *D. fortii*) [47].

Given the frequent reports of DSTs both above and below the regulatory limit in wild harvest shellfish when compared to aquaculture shellfish in NSW [29,45], coupled with an increasing demand and value of pipis [48], further investigation into potential consumer risk from biotoxins was required. In the current study, an end-product survey was carried out over three wild harvest seasons (2015–2017) to evaluate the biotoxin management of wild shellfish harvest operations.

2. Results

2.1. Wild Harvest Shellfish End-Product Market Survey

Of the samples tested, 99.38% complied with regulatory limits. DSTs were detected only in pipi samples (40.59%, 110 of 271 samples). AST was detected in three pipi and two strawberry clam samples (maximum reported level = 3.50 mg/kg domoic acid (DA)). PSTs were not detected during the survey (Table 2). During the sampling period, two market survey samples exceeded the DST regulatory limit (0.20 mg/kg OA, Lighthouse Beach, Date of harvest (DOH) 19 December 2016, 0.23 mg/kg OA; Stockton Beach DOH 27 September 2017, 0.21 mg/kg OA).

Over the three wild harvest seasons, positive DST results in pipi samples were 82.35 (2015), 22.00 (2016), and 38.33 (2017) % across the state (Table 3). Okadaic acid was the single DST analogue identified during the survey. Examination of the spatial and temporal distribution of positive DST results (Table 4) indicated that positive detections at Stockton Beach (Figure 1) during the 2016 and 2017 wild harvest seasons occurred during weeks 33–39 (Table 4) earlier than beaches further north (weeks 45–52) (Table 4). This spatial pattern was not apparent during 2015 due to a shorter sampling window between November to December (Table 4). Data from 2015 to 2017 demonstrated that positive biotoxin results persisted throughout the wild harvest season once detected at most beaches (Table 4).

Table 2. All NSW wild harvest shellfish samples collected as part of the end-product market survey November 2015–December 2017. Each sample was a homogenate of the soft tissue of 15–20 individual shellfish.

Shellfish Type	*n* = 321	AST (No. Positive/Above Regulatory Limit)	DST (No. Positive/Above Regulatory Limit)	PST (No. Positive/Above Regulatory Limit)
Pipis (*Plebidonax deltoides*)	271	3/0	110/2	0/0
Cockles (*Katelysia* spp. *Anadara granosa*) [1]	47	0/0	0/0	0/0
Strawberry clam (cockle) (*Notocallista kingii*)	3	2/0	0/0	0/0

[1] Gymnodimine was detected in four samples (0.028, 0.041, 0.041, 0.072 mg/kg).

Table 3. All pipi samples (positive DST detections and total number of samples) from wild harvest beaches collected as part of the end-product market survey during the 2015, 2016, and 2017 wild harvest seasons. Each sample was a homogenate of the soft tissue of 15–20 individual shellfish.

Wild Harvest Beach (North–South)	2015 (Positive/Total)	2016 (Positive/Total)	2017 (Positive/Total)
South Ballina Beach	7/7	1/16	0/15
Iluka Beach	1/1	-	0/10
Killick Beach	-	1/5	3/12
Goolawah Beach	12/12	2/7	6/14
South Plomer Beach	-	0/1	-
Lighthouse Beach	13/13	5/11	2/3
Dunbogan Beach	-	3/6	6/7
Crowdy Head Beach	6/9	3/11	4/12
Tuncurry Beach	-	0/1	-
Yagon Beach	2/5	1/19	5/12
Big Gibber Beach	-	0/7	-
Stockton Beach	1/2	6/16	20/35
Unconfirmed [1]	0/2	-	-
Total	42/51	22/100	46/120

[1] Supplying co-op notified regarding labelling requirements.

2.2. Wild Shellfish Harvest Beaches Phytoplankton and Biotoxin Samples

During the 2015–2017 wild harvest seasons, 1097 phytoplankton samples were collected from sixteen wild harvest beaches (Table 5, Figure 1). The maximum concentration of *Dinophysis* spp. reported was 9330 cells/L from Stockton Beach (Table 5). Seventeen samples from six beaches contained concentrations of *Dinophysis* spp. above the phytoplankton action level (PAL) of 500 cells/L [25] (Table 5). Following the PAL exceedance and the subsequent biotoxin tests conducted, two shellfish (pipi) samples (2015 and 2017) exceeded the regulatory limit for DSTs (South Ballina 0.29 mg/kg OA, 0.03 mg/kg PTX2, October 2015 and Stockton Beach 0.46 mg/kg OA, October 2017) (Table 5, Figure 1). A pattern of elevated *Dinophysis* spp. concentrations detected at Stockton Beach (Figure 1) earlier than beaches further north was apparent (for example refer to Figure 2).

Table 4. Spatial and temporal distribution of okadaic acid (mg/kg OA) in pipi samples collected as part of an end-product wild harvest market survey (2015, 2016 and 2017 harvest seasons). The locations and week numbers listed correspond to the beach where the shellfish were collected and the harvest date, respectively. Where more than one sample was collected the range of results are provided, with the number of samples noted in brackets. For clarity of presentation, the okadaic results are round to two decimal places. The locations of wild harvest beaches listed each year in the order of north to south are shown in Figure 1.

	Week Number (2015)																											
Wild Harvest Beach	**25**	**26**	**27**	**28**	**29**	**30**	**31**	**32**	**33**	**34**	**35**	**36**	**37**	**38**	**39**	**40**	**41**	**42**	**43**	**44**	**45**	**46**	**47**	**48**	**49**	**50**	**51**	**52**
South Ballina Beach	No samping																									0.04-0.05 (5)	0.12	
Iluka Beach																							0.04					
Goolawah Beach																							0.03	0.03-0.07 (2)	0.05-0.09 (5)	0.05	0.17	0.16
Lighthouse Beach																							0.04	0.05-0.08 (4)	0.03-0.09 (5)		0.13	0.13
Crowdy Head Beach																							0.04	NEG (2)	0.03-0.04 (2)	NEG	0.03	
Yagon Beach																						NEG (2)			0.03 (2)			
Stockton Beach																						NEG					0.03	
	Week Number (2016)																											
Wild Harvest Beach	**25**	**26**	**27**	**28**	**29**	**30**	**31**	**32**	**33**	**34**	**35**	**36**	**37**	**38**	**39**	**40**	**41**	**42**	**43**	**44**	**45**	**46**	**47**	**48**	**49**	**50**	**51**	**52**
South Ballina Beach	NEG								NEG (2)				NEG (2)		NEG (2)	NEG	NEG	NEG	NEG (2)		NEG	NEG (2)	0.07					
Killick Beach	NEG														NEG			NEG			NEG			0.05				
Goolawah Beach				NEG							NEG				NEG		NEG				NEG		0.05	0.12				
South Plomer Beach	NEG																											
Lighthouse Beach				NEG							NEG				NEG (2)		NEG			NEG			0.06	0.12			0.03	0.16-0.23 (2)
Dunbogan Beach																		NEG		NEG	NEG			0.09			0.11	0.04
Crowdy Head Beach	NEG										0.056				NEG-0.03 (2)	NEG	NEG				NEG			NEG			NEG-0.03 (2)	NEG
Tuncurry Beach				NEG																								
Yagon Beach	NEG			NEG							NEG		0.061		NEG (2)	NEG	NEG	NEG (2)	NEG (2)	NEG	NEG (2)		NEG	NEG			NEG (2)	
Big Gibber Beach																	NEG			NEG	NEG (3)		NEG	NEG				
Stockton Beach	NEG			NEG					0.04-0.09 (2)		0.048		0.03-0.04 (2)		0.059	NEG	NEG	NEG	NEG	NEG	NEG		NEG					NEG
	Week Number (2017)																											
	25	**26**	**27**	**28**	**29**	**30**	**31**	**32**	**33**	**34**	**35**	**36**	**37**	**38**	**39**	**40**	**41**	**42**	**43**	**44**	**45**	**46**	**47**	**48**	**49**	**50**	**51**	**52**
South Ballina Beach													NEG	NEG (3)			NEG	NEG (3)				NEG (2)	NEG (3)		NEG (2)			
Iluka Beach									NEG						NEG	NEG		NEG (2)	NEG (2)			NEG			NEG	NEG		
Killick Beach					NEG											NEG (2)					NEG-0.03 (2)	NEG (2)	NEG-0.10 (2)			NEG-0.06 (3)		
Goolawah Beach																NEG (2)					NEG-0.03 (5)	0.03-0.04 (2)	0.03-0.04 (2)			NEG (3)		
Lighthouse Beach														NEG								0.06-0.09 (2)						
Dunbogan Beach					NEG																	0.08-0.12 (2)	0.11	0.06		0.05 (2)		
Crowdy Head Beach					NEG									NEG	0.03-0.04 (2)	NEG (5)						0.03	0.05					
Yagon Beach	NEG (2)				NEG				NEG					NEG-0.07 (3)	0.03	NEG-0.07 (2)	NEG						0.03					
Stockton Beach	NEG (2)				NEG				NEG (3)				NEG (2)	0.05-0.07 (2)	0.15-0.21 (3)							NEG-0.04 (3)	NEG-0.03 (4)	NEG-0.04 (3)	NEG-0.04 (3)	NEG-0.04 (5)	0.05-0.06 (4)	

NEG <0.025 mg/kg OA
< 0.2 mg/kg OA
> 0.2 mg/kg OA

Table 5. Summary of monitoring data (phytoplankton and biotoxin) from wild harvest beaches collected during the 2015, 2016, and 2017 wild harvest seasons.

Wild Harvest Monitoring Data	2015	2016	2017	All
No. of phytoplankton samples collected	310	411	376	1097
No. of phytoplankton samples >500 cells/L *Dinophysis* spp.	7	8	2	17
South Ballina Beach/Max cells/L *Dinophysis* spp.	2760	1760	-	-
Iluka Beach/Max cells/L *Dinophysis* spp.	520	-	-	-
Killick Beach/Max cells/L *Dinophysis* spp.	625	650	-	-
South Plomer/Max cells/L *Dinophysis* spp.	825	-	-	-
Stockton Beach/Max cells/L *Dinophysis* spp.	9330	-	530	-
Bherwerre Beach/Max cells/L *Dinophysis* spp.	-	-	500	-
No. of DST tests	10	10	6	26
No. of DST positive results	8 [1]	1 [2]	4	4
No. of DST results > 0.2 mg/kg OA	1	0	1	2

[1] Three positive test results were not quantified; [2] One positive test result was not quantified.

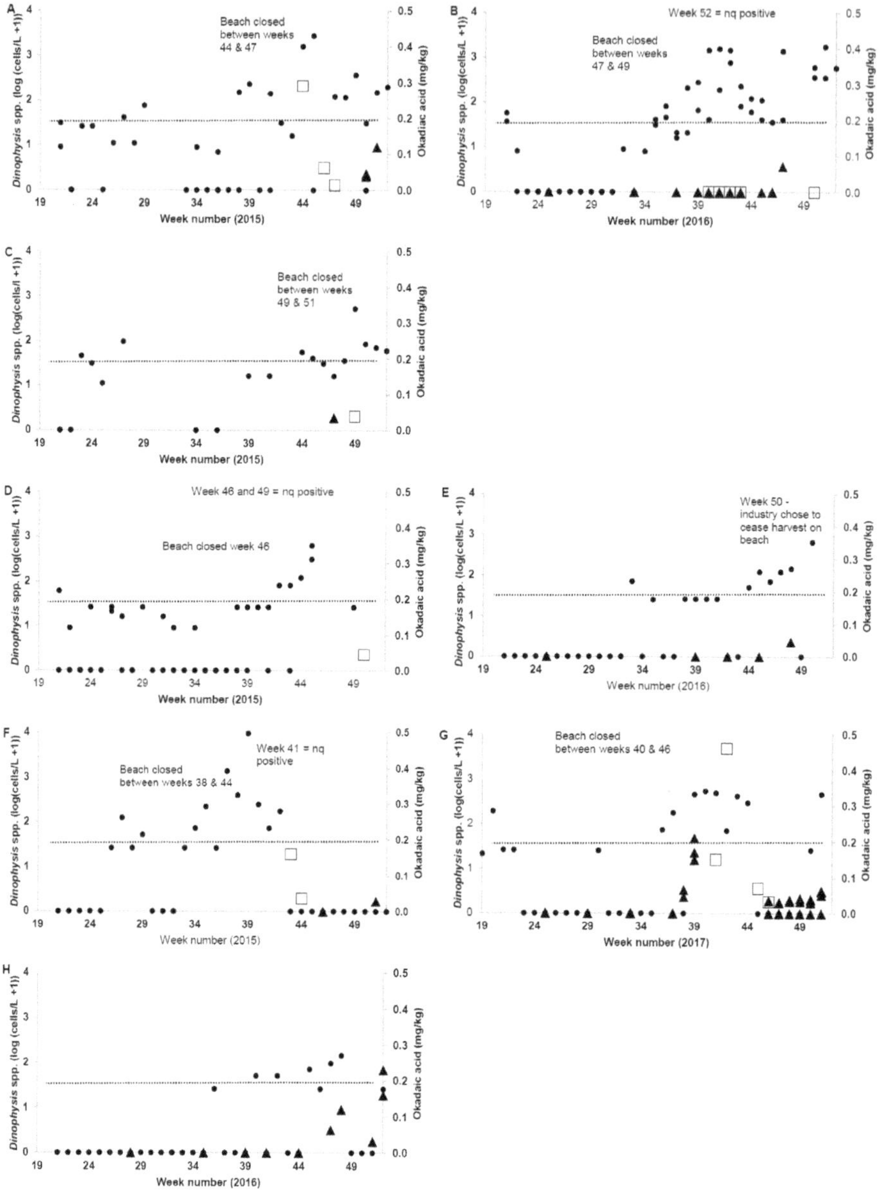

Figure 2. Temporal distribution of *Dinophysis* spp. (log (cells/L + 1), black circle) and okadaic acid (mg/kg) from market survey (black triangle) and routine monitoring (white square) biotoxin samples at South Ballina Beach 2015 (**A**) and 2016 (**B**); Iluka Beach 2015 (**C**); Killick Beach 2015 (**D**) and 2016 (**E**); Stockton Beach 2015 (**F**) and 2017 (**G**); and Lighthouse Beach 2016 (**H**). Note: a zero result is equivalent to <0.025 mg/kg OA, dashed line indicates regulatory limit of 0.2 mg/kg OA, nq = not quantified Wild harvest beaches are listed north to south and their locations are provided in Figure 1.

2.3. Comparison of Market Survey and Wild Shellfish Harvest Data

Market survey data were available for comparison to pipi wild harvest monitoring data for four (South Ballina Beach, Iluka Beach, Killick Beach and Stockton Beach) of the six locations where the PAL for *Dinophysis* spp. was exceeded (Table 5). For five of the six *Dinophysis* bloom events, biotoxin samples supported the existing biotoxin management plan, and all market survey results were below regulatory limits for DSTs (Figure 2A–F,H). On one occasion (Figure 2G), a biotoxin sample from pipis collected from Stockton Beach on 27 September 2017 (week 39) returned a positive result of 0.21 mg/kg OA. *Dinophysis* spp. concentrations were 448 cells/L in a seawater sample collected Stockton Beach during week 39 (24 September). Cell concentrations above the PAL (500 cells/L) for this group were not reported until week 40 (2 October). Biotoxin samples collected from the beach during weeks 41 (8 October) and 42 (15 October) returned positive results of 0.15 and 0.46 mg/kg OA, respectively (regulatory limit 0.2 mg/kg OA), while cell concentrations appeared to decline (480 and 69 cells/L for weeks 41 and 42, respectively).

At South Plomer Beach (2015) and Bherwerre Beach (2017), in lieu of biotoxin testing, the wild harvest industry chose to cease harvest when the PAL exceedances for *Dinophysis* spp. were reported (Table 5). No market survey samples were collected for either of these beaches.

An alternative comparison was the positive, above regulatory limit, biotoxin result of 0.23 mg/kg OA to phytoplankton results. The positive sample was from Lighthouse Beach (Figure 1) and pipis collected on 19 December 2016. The preceding phytoplankton samples from this beach did not indicate an increase in *Dinophysis* spp. (Figure 2H), with cell concentrations <150 cells/L.

2.4. Phytoplankton and Biotoxin Samples from Oyster and Mussel Harvest Areas

Up to ten species of *Dinophysis* were observed in water samples from shellfish aquaculture areas across the state (*D. acuminata*, *D. caudata*, *D. rotundata* (= *Phalacroma rotundatum*), *D. acuta*, *D. tripos*, *D. fortii*, *D. truncata*, *D. schroederi*, *D. mitra* (= *Phalacroma mitra*) and *D. hastata*) (refer Figure S1). *D. acuminata* was the most common species observed. *D. acuminata* was observed in all estuaries except for the Tweed River (Table 6). From the available data, *D. acuminata* was observed to be present in elevated (up to 3200 cells/L) concentrations on the north NSW coast between August and December (Table 6). The second most common species observed was *D. caudata* (Table 6). Maximum concentrations (up to 1500 cells/L) were reported between November and June, but the distribution of *D. caudata* between estuaries was more variable (Table 6). The other *Dinophysis* spp. observed did not exceed the 500 cells/L PAL and these species were generally observed south of 31°38′ S (data not shown). Biotoxin testing from shellfish aquaculture areas during this period did not detect DTX or OA positive results [29] (NSW Food Authority, unpublished data). Pectenotoxin-2 was detected at low concentrations (max 0.036 mg/kg) in two samples from Wonboyn Lake (37°17′ S) [29].

Table 6. Summary of *D. acuminata* and *D. caudata* reported from shellfish (oyster and mussel) producing estuaries north to south along the NSW coastline (November 2015–December 2017). Observations of cell concentrations above 500 cells/L are highlighted in bold, corresponding to the PAL for *Dinophysis* spp. applied to routine monitoring for wild shellfish harvest beaches.

Estuary (North–South)	Latitude (S)	No. of Sample Sites	Total Samples Per Site (November 2015–December 2017)	*D. acuminate* (No. of Observations/Max. Cells/L /Month of Max. Concentration)			*D. caudate* (No. of Observations/Max. Cells/L /Month of Max. Concentration)		
Tweed River	28°10′	1	45	-	-	-	3	**700**	December
Richmond River	28°53′	1	20	6	**650**	December	6	400	
Clarence River	29°25′	1	29	8	**850**	November	7	200	
Wooli River	29°53′	1	20	3	200		3	200	
Bellinger and Kalang Rivers	30°30′	2	29, 14	6	**2400**	November	8	200	
Nambucca River	30°39′	2	48, 43	10	**3200**	November	7	250	
Macleay River	30°52′	2	44, 20	3	50		2	50	
Hastings River	31°25′	3	45, 38, 23	27	**1100**	November	13	**1000**	December
Camden Haven River	31°38′	3	56, 34, 34	29	**650**	November	7	**900**	
Manning River	31°53′	3	53, 52, 41	39	**1700**	October	19	300	May
Wallis Lake	32°13′	3	58, 58, 59	54	**3700**	October	27	**550**	December
Port Stephens	32°42′	10	29, 34, 56, 56, 56, 57, 57, 56, 56, 56	44	**1000**	August	28	**850**	February
Brisbane Water	33°31′	4	55, 52, 37, 56	18	300		24	**1300**	April
Patonga River	33°32′	1	52	4	100		1	50	
Hawkesbury River	33°34′	3	61, 59, 20	14	300		25	350	
Georges River	34°01′	1	57	6	300		4	**500**	March
Shoalhaven and Crookhaven Rivers	34°53′	3	48, 48, 48	30	250		6	100	
Clyde River	35°42′	3	42, 56, 56	9	150		21	250	
Tuross Lake	36°04′	1	53	1	100		-	-	
Wagonga Inlet	36°13′	2	62, 62	27	350		36	**1500**	November
Bermagui River	36°26′	1	23	3	150		-	-	
Wapengo Lake	36°38′	2	57, 56	16	150		1	50	
Nelson Lagoon	36°41′	1	31	1	50		-	-	
Merimbula	36°54′	2	59, 59	15	400		25	**1300**	November
Pambula Lake	36°57′	1	60	11	250		2	100	
Twofold Bay	37°05′	3	48, 48, 48	42	**1400**	March	19	300	
Wonboyn River	37°17′	2	57, 57	18	250		41	**1000**	June

3. Discussion

Most wild shellfish harvest in NSW is focused on mid-north and north coast beaches and coincides with seasonal *Dinophysis* events during the Austral spring and summer months. Our study conducted over three consecutive wild harvest seasons in NSW highlighted DSTs as the main concern due to their presence in over one-third of the shellfish samples tested. On two occasions, DSTs were detected above the regulatory limit in the marketplace and suggested that the current wild harvest biotoxin management processes could be strengthened. In the first scenario, cell concentrations at Lighthouse Beach did not exceed the PAL for *Dinophysis* spp. This elevated DST result was reported following the annual closure of the harvest season, and further phytoplankton or biotoxin samples were not available to evaluate how or if the bloom progressed. During the second incident, *Dinophysis* concentrations at Stockton Beach did not exceed the PAL until a week after a DST result above the regulatory limit was detected. Both circumstances resulted in shellfish above the regulatory limit for DSTs entering the market. While no illnesses were reported related to these events, this study was an opportunity to consider improvements in the current wild harvest biotoxin management plans. While this study highlights the potential risk of DST contaminated product entering the marketplace, the emphasis on other biotoxin groups could be redirected if there was a shift in dominant harmful phytoplankton near existing beaches, or if the industry chose to relocate to a location where different biotoxins were present.

Dinophysis spp. cell densities reported from wild harvest beaches varied along the NSW coast. Without a full understanding of how pipis uptake and depurate DSTs it is difficult to elucidate the patterns involved. The dynamics of intertidal habitats are not readily comparable to studies of uptake and depuration of DSTs in mussels and oysters in planktonic environments (e.g., Pitcher et al. [49], Wallace 2011 [47]). As depuration of biotoxins from clams and pipis tends to be slower than oysters and mussels [5,36,50], this may result in prolonged periods where positive toxins are detected. As in other surf clams, pipis feed via a siphon. In the butter clam (*Saxidomus giganteus*) PSTs have been found to accumulate and be retained in the siphon [51], and we hypothesise that a similar mechanism could be occurring in pipis. Moreover, the uptake and depuration of toxins varies substantially between bivalve species. The northern quahog (*Mercenaria mercenaria*) can selectively feed during exposure to *Alexandrium* by retracting its siphon and closing its valve [52,53]. In contrast, selective feeding of *Dinophysis* spp. has been observed via examination of the gut of the Mediterranean mussel (*Mytilus galloprovincialis*) [54]. There is no information published on the uptake or depuration dynamics of DSTs by pipis specifically, and more investigation is required.

Other possible reasons for the disparities between the beach monitoring data and market survey data in this study could be attributed to the natural non-homogenous distribution of phytoplankton, toxin variability between individual cells or strains of *Dinophysis* spp., the current phytoplankton net sampling technique or a combination of these. In addition, knowledge of the bloom dynamics involved are limited by phytoplankton data reported to genus level only and lack of simultaneous environmental data (e.g., temperature, salinity, turbidity, current data). The current study demonstrated that weekly phytoplankton sampling alone was not sufficient to ensure that shellfish product with DSTs above the regulatory limit were not harvested. At Stockton Beach, the beach was closed to harvest following the report of the above DST regulatory limit market survey result. DST concentrations, both below and greater than twice the regulatory limit, were reported from shellfish (pipi) samples collected at Stockton Beach in the following weeks. The incorporation of routine biotoxin monitoring into the wild harvest monitoring program would improve understanding of variability in toxin concentrations over short time periods and unknown differences between toxic strains of *Dinophysis* in this region. Furthermore, and pending an appropriate risk analysis, a shift to a seasonal quota system for the NSW wild harvest shellfish industry could allow fishers to collect pipis during lower risk periods.

Concurrent phytoplankton data from shellfish aquaculture areas demonstrated that *D. acuminata* was the predominant *Dinophysis* species occurring in NSW estuaries, with greatest concentrations observed in estuaries north of 32°42′ S during the Austral spring and summer. Ajani et al. [55] have also reported peaks of *Dinophysis* cell concentrations during summer (January) offshore of

Sydney (Port Hacking). This information is comparable with other field studies of *Dinophysis* in Australia. Takahashi et al. [56] found that on North Stradbroke Island, Queensland, Australia that *Dinophysis* spp. were more common during warmer months, with *D. acuminata* only reported on open beaches between November and January. Reports on *Dinophysis* spp. in Australian waters have shown the genus to be "common but rarely abundant" [3,26–28,57]. A study on *Dinophysis* spp. within the upper reaches of the Hawkesbury river estuary demonstrated a similar seasonality to this study with *D. acuminata* and *D. caudata* having greatest abundances in spring and summer/autumn, respectively [57]. While phytoplankton sampling was by undertaken different methods in estuaries and beaches, data from the present study supports the view that *D. acuminata* was the main source of DSTs in pipis. More data are required to substantiate this extrapolation, but it is a likely explanation given that elevated concentrations of *Dinophysis* spp. and the presence of OA in wild harvest samples occurring within a similar season (early October onwards). Historical illnesses linked to DSTs in pipis from NSW were assumed to be caused by *D. caudata* and pectenotoxin-2 and pectenotoxin-2-seco acids [44]. It was later clarified that OA derivatives from *D. acuminata* had been the causative agents [58]. Additionally, *Prorocentrum* spp. were not considered to be a cause of DSTs in NSW [29]. While linked to toxin production historically elsewhere, *Prorocentrum* spp. have not been found to be toxin producing in NSW to date [29]. Negative DST results in estuarine shellfish harvest areas suggest that *Dinophysis acuminata* blooms in NSW originate offshore or along the coastline. Ajani et al. [26] also showed that *D. acuminata* was significantly more abundant at downstream sites when compared to upstream sites within NSW estuaries, thus, supporting the oceanic origin hypothesis. While further investigation is needed into if and how *Dinophysis* blooms are transported into NSW estuaries, similar along-shore transport has been observed for *Dinophysis* in other locations (e.g., Spain/Portugal [59], Ireland [14]).

More than twelve years of routine phytoplankton and biotoxin data from estuaries has demonstrated a low risk of DSTs and other phytoplankton toxin groups for NSW oyster consumers, and the current monitoring in estuaries is effective at minimising consumer risk [29]. Mussels generally accumulate DSTs more readily than oysters (e.g., Pitcher et al. [49]) and while during this study pipis were the main species affected by DSTs in NSW, oyster samples from South Australia have shown DSTs above the regulatory limit [46]. Worldwide, new cases and outbreaks of DST are still occurring (e.g., British Columbia [60], China [61], Brazil [62]). While the occurrence of DSTs has been variable in NSW [3,29,45], a DST event in Tasmania during 2016 was responsible for a recall of mussels from a location that was not previously known to be impacted by DSTs [63]. In a changing environment, where phytoplankton blooms are seemingly more frequent and intense [7,8,64,65], management strategies need to be adaptable to manage the potential risks for shellfish consumers. The use of sentinel species or passive samplers may be an option for risk management, but these techniques can have limitations depending on the harvest area conditions or targeted toxins (e.g., [66,67]). Historically, phytoplankton and biotoxin monitoring programs have been established following illness outbreaks (e.g., monitoring of wild harvest beaches in NSW following DSP events and Thermaikos Gulf in Thessaloniki, Greece [68]) but long-term data can help inform existing shellfish safety programs. For example, at the Coorong harvesting area in SA, routine biotoxin testing during the pipi harvest season occurs monthly at one location. This regime increases to a fortnightly sampling frequency for biotoxins at three sample locations during upwelling events, which can impact phytoplankton production (C. Wilkinson, *pers comm*).

In NSW, due to extended consecutive DST positive results during *Dinophysis* bloom events, pipi harvesters tend to relocate and operate in other open status beaches rather than continue testing at 'positive' beaches. Protection of consumers from biotoxin-related illnesses is critical in maintaining customer confidence in shellfish produce and to safeguard the growing wild harvest shellfish industry in NSW. More data are required to understand *Dinophysis* bloom dynamics and to substantiate that *D. acuminata* is the main source of DSTs in pipis in NSW. The notable occurrences of DST positives presented in this study suggest that there is merit in augmenting the current testing regime on wild harvest beaches by adopting a regime that includes frequent biotoxin monitoring. The development of more cost-effective, rapid and reliable test methods would improve risk management while maximising harvesting opportunities for industry.

4. Materials and Methods

4.1. End-Product Market Survey

4.1.1. End-Product Sample Collection (Shellfish)

End-product market survey shellfish sample collection focused on Sydney Fish Market, Sydney, Australia, as most wild harvest shellfish collected in NSW is consigned through the market for auction. Between November 2015 and December 2017, 323 wild harvest shellfish samples were collected (Table S1). Wild shellfish harvest is focused on mid-north and north coast beaches in NSW (Figure 1, Figure S2). Pipis were the predominant wild harvest shellfish available for sale at the time of sampling (Table 2). Sampling frequency was increased from monthly to weekly between September and December during each year (Table S1) in line with historical phytoplankton data and positive DST detections from wild harvest beaches in NSW [26,45]. Depending on the amount of wild harvest stock on sale, more than one sample from a wild harvest beach was collected, as often multiple licensed individuals collect shellfish on the same beach. In addition, on some beaches there were more than one wild harvest collection group operating (Table S2). Each shellfish sample was a homogenate of the soft tissue of 15–20 individual shellfish (min. 100 g of meat was collected). The samples were kept chilled and either delivered to a National Association of Testing Authorities (NATA) accredited biotoxin laboratory (Symbio Laboratories, Sydney) within 1 h of collection or frozen (−20 °C) for later analyses.

4.1.2. Biotoxin Testing of Shellfish Samples

All end-product market survey samples were screened for PSTs by high performance liquid chromatography (HPLC) [69]. Initial screening for PSTs included the analogues STX, GTX2,3, C1,2, GTX5, NEO, dcNEO, and GTX1,4. If a positive result was reported, pre-column oxidation was used to confirm concentrations of STX, GTX2,3, C1,2, GTX5, dcSTX, dcGTX2,3, NEO, dcNEO, GTX1,4, C3,4. AST (domoic acid (DA)), and DSTs (OA, dinophysistoxin 1 (DTX-1), dinophysistoxin 2 (DTX-2)), and pectenotoxin 2 (PTX-2) by liquid chromatography tandem mass spectrometry (LCMS/MS) [70–72]. The lipophilic toxins cylindrospermopsin, gymnodimine, spirolide 1, azaspiracid 1, azaspiracid 2, azaspiracid 3, and yessotoxin were also included as part of the LCMS/MS screen [71]. Positive toxin results were equivalent to $\geq$1.00 mg/kg DA (AST), $\geq$0.25 mg/kg OA equivalents (DSTs) and $\geq$0.10 mg/kg STX equivalents (PSTs).

4.2. Routine Monitoring at Shellfish Harvest or Collection Areas

4.2.1. Sample Collection for Phytoplankton Analyses (Water)

Phytoplankton and biotoxin data collected within the same timeframe as the market survey samples (November 2015–December 2017) from both wild harvest beaches and shellfish aquaculture areas were compared to the market survey data. The current NSW Food Authority monitoring program for phytoplankton and biotoxins in NSW distinguishes between aquaculture and wild shellfish harvest areas. The location of phytoplankton and biotoxin sample sites are designated as representative of the water filtered by shellfish in each location [25,73].

Routine phytoplankton samples for wild harvest shellfish and shellfish aquaculture areas are collected weekly and fortnightly during the open harvest status, respectively. Samples are collected by trained shellfish industry members. During each wild harvest season, a weekly phytoplankton sampling program was followed. Seawater samples (~50 L = 5 × 10 L buckets of seawater) were concentrated by a 20 µm mesh phytoplankton net (to ~500 mL) and preserved with Lugol's Iodine. When open for harvest, shellfish aquaculture areas were subject to the collection of fortnightly discrete sub surface (0.5 m) estuarine water samples (500–1000 mL), with a phytoplankton net surface drag sample collected at each sample site. Both samples were preserved with Lugol's Iodine for later analysis by microscope for potentially harmful species listed in Appendix 9 of the NSW Marine Biotoxin Management Plan [25]. Sub-samples (1 mL) of concentrated seawater samples from wild harvest beaches were analysed. Note that phytoplankton concentrations reported from wild harvest beach samples were identified to genus level only. Estuarine water samples from shellfish aquaculture areas were concentrated by gravity-assisted membrane filtration (5 μm) prior to analysis. Simultaneous phytoplankton net haul samples were utilised to assist with identification. As a cost saving measure, if a PAL is reported, industry may choose to delay sampling. For example, the wild harvest beaches can be closed for collection until subsequent phytoplankton and biotoxin testing demonstrates that any contamination has ceased (Figure 3).

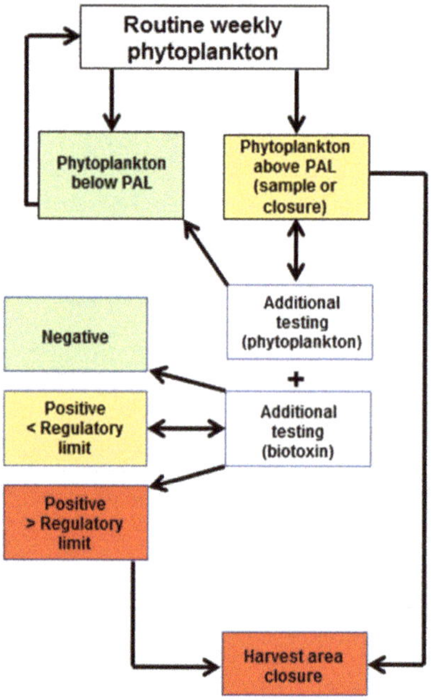

Figure 3. Phytoplankton and biotoxin monitoring program for wild harvest beaches in NSW [25].

4.2.2. Sample Collection for Biotoxin Testing (Shellfish)

On wild harvest beaches, biotoxin samples were collected when a PAL was exceeded (for example >500 cells/L *Dinophysis* spp.) [25]. Biotoxin sampling occurred weekly if a wild harvest beach was open and toxin levels were below regulatory limits. Shellfish aquaculture areas were also subject to routine monthly biotoxin sampling when the harvest areas were open for harvest. Shellfish tissue samples (12–14 individuals, min. 100 g flesh) were collected, shucked and frozen prior to dispatch for biotoxin analysis at a NATA accredited laboratory. Shellfish samples from aquaculture or wild harvest areas were analysed for biotoxins either by Jellett screening (Jellett Rapid Testing Ltd., Nova Scotia, Canada) or by the qualitative methods, as above.

Supplementary Materials: The following are available online at http://www.mdpi.com/2072-6651/10/11/446/s1, Table S1: Summary of frequency of wild harvest sample collection at Sydney Fish Market during the 2015, 2016 and 2017 wild harvest seasons, Table S2: All active wild harvest beaches along the New South Wales coast during the 2015, 2016 and 2017 wild harvest seasons. The number of wild harvest collection groups operating on each beach during each season is also provided, Figure S1: Images of *Dinophysis* spp. observed in NSW coastal waters under light (A–B and D–F) and calcofluor fluorescence (C,G) microscopy. A–C: *Dinophysis acuminata* D–E:

Dinophysis caudata, F–G: *Dinophysis tripos*. Images provided by Dr. S. Brett (Microalgal Services), Figure S2: Total weight (kg) of pipis sold each week from north (A) and south (B) coast NSW wild harvest beaches between 2012 and 2017 (data provided by Sydney Fish Market).

Author Contributions: Conceptualization, H.F., P.B., G.W. and A.Z.; Data curation, G.W. and S.B.; Formal analysis, H.F., P.A., S.M., P.B., G.W., S.B. and A.Z.; Investigation, H.F. and A.Z.; Methodology, H.F. and A.Z.; Project administration, H.F. and A.Z.; Supervision, A.Z.; Writing—original draft, H.F., P.A., S.M., P.B., G.W. and A.Z.; Writing—review & editing, H.F., P.A., S.M., P.B., G.W., S.B. and A.Z.

Funding: The wild harvest biotoxin market survey was carried out and funded by the NSW Food Authority. Wild harvest field data (phytoplankton and biotoxin testing) were funded by industry. Shellfish aquaculture area data were funded through the NSW Food Authority and industry.

Acknowledgments: Data for north and south coast pipi sales in NSW were provided by Sydney Fish Market. The authors greatly appreciate the assistance of QA staff at Sydney Fish Market. The authors wish to thank Alison Imlay and Lisa Szabo (NSW Food Authority) for their reviews of the manuscript. The authors also wish to thank the constructive input of the manuscript reviewers and editors.

Conflicts of Interest: The authors declare no conflict of interest.

References

1. Globefish. Globefish-Analysis and Information on World Fish Trade. Available online: http://www.fao.org/in-action/globefish/market-reports/resource-detail/en/c/1136590/ (accessed on 20 July 2018).
2. Campbell, A.; Hudson, D.; McLeod, C.; Nicholls, C.; Pointon, A. Tactical Research Fund: Review of the 2012 Paralytic Shellfish Toxin Event in Tasmania Associated with the Dinoflagellate Alga, *Alexandrium tamarense*. Fisheries Research and Development Corporation; FRDC Project 2012/060 2013; p. 94. Available online: http://www.safefish.com.au/Reports/Technical-Reports/Paralytic-Shellfish-Toxin-Event-2012-2013 (accessed on 20 July 2018).
3. Ajani, P.; Harwood, D.T.; Murray, S.A. Recent trends in marine phycotoxins from Australian coastal waters. *Mar. Drugs* **2017**, *15*, 33. [CrossRef] [PubMed]
4. Kiermeier, A.; McLeod, C.; Sumner, J. *Marinebiotoxins in Shellfish-Saxitoxin Group: Scientific Opinion of the Panel on Contamination in the Food Chain' by the European Food Safety Authority (EFSA)*; South Australian Research and Development Institute (SARDI): Adelaide, SA, Australia, 2009; p. 11.
5. Lawrence, J.; Loreal, H.; Toyofuku, H.; Hess, P.; Iddya, K.; Ababouch, L. Assessment and management of biotoxin risks in bivalve molluscs. *FAO Tech. Pap.* **2011**, *551*, 358. Available online: http://www.fao.org/docrep/015/i2356e/i2356e.pdf (accessed on 20 July 2018).
6. Taylor, F.J.R.; Fukuyo, Y.; Larsen, J.; Hallegraeff, G.M. Taxonomy of harmful dinoflagellates. In *Manual on Harmful Marine Microalgae*, 2nd ed.; Hallegraeff, G.M., Anderson, D.M., Cembella, A.D., Eds.; UNESCO: Paris, France, 2004; pp. 389–431.
7. Reguera, B.; Riobó, P.; Rodríguez, F.; Díaz, P.; Pizarro, G.; Paz, B.; Franco, J.; Blanco, J. *Dinophysis* toxins: Causative organisms, distribution and fate in shellfish. *Mar. Drugs* **2014**, *12*, 394–461. [CrossRef] [PubMed]
8. Reguera, B.; Velo-Suárez, L.; Raine, R.; Park, M.G. Harmful *Dinophysis* species: A review. *Harmful Algae* **2012**, *14*, 87–106. [CrossRef]
9. Suganuma, M.; Fujiki, H.; Suguri, H.; Yoshizawa, S.; Hirota, M.; Nakayasu, M.; Ojika, M.; Wakamatsu, K.; Yamada, K.; Sugimura, T. Okadaic acid: An additional non-phorbol-12-tetradecanoate-13-acetate-type tumor promoter. *Proc. Natl. Acad. Sci. USA* **1988**, *85*, 1768–1771. [CrossRef] [PubMed]
10. Suganuma, M.; Tatematsu, M.; Yatsunami, J.; Yoshizawa, S.; Okabe, S.; Uemura, D.; Fujiki, H. An alternative theory of tissue specificity by tumor promotion of okadaic acid in glandular stomach of sd rats. *Carcinogenesis* **1992**, *13*, 1841–1845. [CrossRef] [PubMed]
11. Fujiki, H.; Suganuma, M. Unique features of the okadaic acid activity class of tumor promoters. *J. Cancer Res. Clin. Oncol.* **1999**, *125*, 150–155. [CrossRef] [PubMed]
12. Murata, M.; Shimatani, M.; Sugitani, H.; Oshima, Y.; Yasumoto, T. Isolation and structural elucidation of the causative toxin of the diarrhetic shellfish poisoning. *Nippon Suisan Gakkaishi* **1982**, *48*, 549–552. [CrossRef]
13. Xie, H.; Lazure, P.; Gentien, P. Small scale retentive structures and *Dinophysis*. *J. Mar. Syst.* **2007**, *64*, 173–188. [CrossRef]

14. Farrell, H.; Gentien, P.; Fernand, L.; Lunven, M.; Reguera, B.; González-Gil, S.; Raine, R. Scales characterising a high density thin layer of *Dinophysis acuta* Ehrenberg and its transport within a coastal jet. *Harmful Algae* **2012**, *15*, 36–46. [CrossRef]
15. Velo-Suárez, L.; Reguera, B.; González-Gil, S.; Lunven, M.; Lazure, P.; Nézan, E.; Gentien, P. Application of a 3d lagrangian model to explain the decline of a *Dinophysis acuminata* bloom in the Bay of Biscay. *J. Mar. Syst.* **2010**, *83*, 242–252. [CrossRef]
16. Park, M.G.; Kim, S.; Kim, H.S.; Myung, G.; Kang, Y.; Yih, W. First successful culture of the marine dinoflagellate *Dinophysis acuminata*. *Aquat. Microb. Ecol.* **2006**, *45*, 101–106. [CrossRef]
17. Nishitani, G.; Nagai, S.; Sakiyama, S.; Kamiyama, T. Successful cultivation of the toxic dinoflagellate *Dinophysis caudata* (Dinophyceae). *Plankton Benthos Res.* **2008**, *3*, 78–85. [CrossRef]
18. Nagai, S.; Nitshitani, G.; Tomaru, Y.; Sakiyama, S.; Kamiyama, T. Predation by the toxic dinoflagellate *Dinophysis fortii* on the ciliate *Myrionecta rubra* and observation of sequestration of ciliate chloroplasts1. *J. Phycol.* **2008**, *44*, 909–922. [CrossRef] [PubMed]
19. Nishitani, G.; Nagai, S.; Takano, Y.; Sakiyama, S.; Baba, K.; Kamiyama, T. Growth characteristics and phylogenetic analysis of the marine dinoflagellate *Dinophysis infundibulus* (Dinophyceae). *Aquat. Microb. Ecol.* **2008**, *52*, 209–221. [CrossRef]
20. Rodríguez, F.; Escalera, L.; Reguera, B.; Rial, P.; Riobó, P.; de Jesús da Silva, T. Morphological variability, toxinology and genetics of the dinoflagellate *Dinophysis tripos* (Dinophysiaceae, Dinophysiales). *Harmful Algae* **2012**, *13*, 26–33. [CrossRef]
21. Nagai, S.; Suzuki, T.; Kamiyama, T. Successful cultivation of the toxic dinoflagellate *Dinophysis tripos* (Dinophyceae). *Plankton Benthos Res.* **2013**, *8*, 171–177. [CrossRef]
22. Basti, L.; Uchida, H.; Matsushima, R.; Watanabe, R.; Suzuki, T.; Yamatogi, T.; Nagai, S. Influence of temperature on growth and production of pectenotoxin-2 by a monoclonal culture of *Dinophysis caudata*. *Mar. Drugs* **2015**, *13*, 7124–7137. [CrossRef] [PubMed]
23. Jaén, D.; Mamán, L.; Domínguez, R.; Martín, E. First report of *Dinophysis acuta* in culture. *Harmful Algal News* **2009**, *39*, 1–2.
24. Jefferson, R. *Aquaculture Production Report 2016–2017*; NSW Department of Primary Industries: Taylors Beach, NSW, Australia, 2018; p. 12. Available online: https://www.dpi.nsw.gov.au/__data/assets/pdf_file/0009/750726/Aquaculture-Production-Report-2016-2017.pdf (accessed on 20 July 2018).
25. NSW FA. *Marine Biotoxin Management Plan*; NSW Food Authority: Newington, NSW, Australia, 2014; p. 36. Available online: http://www.foodauthority.nsw.gov.au/_Documents/industry/marine_biotoxin_management_plan.pdf (accessed on 20 July 2018).
26. Ajani, P.; Brett, S.; Krogh, M.; Scanes, P.; Webster, G.; Armand, L. The risk of harmful algal blooms (HABS) in the oyster-growing estuaries of New South Wales, Australia. *Environ. Monit. Assess.* **2013**, *185*, 5295–5316. [CrossRef] [PubMed]
27. Ajani, P.; Hallegraeff, G.M.; Pritchard, T. Historic overview of algal blooms in marine and estuarine waters of New South Wales, Australia. *Proc. Linn. Soc. NSW* **2001**, *123*, 1–22.
28. Ajani, P.; Ingleton, T.; Pritchard, T.; Armand, L. Microalgal blooms in the coastal waters of New South Wales, Australia. *Proc. Linn. Soc. NSW* **2011**, *133*, 15–31.
29. NSW FA. *Phytoplankton and Biotoxins in Nsw Shellfish Aquaculture Areas*; NSW Food Authority: Newington, NSW, Australia, 2017; p. 48. Available online: http://www.foodauthority.nsw.gov.au/_Documents/scienceandtechnical/phytoplankton_and_biotoxin_risk_assessment.pdf (accessed on 20 July 2018).
30. FSANZ. Australia New Zealand Food Standards Code. Food Standards Australia New Zealand, 2016. Available online: https://www.legislation.gov.au/Details/F2017C00305 (accessed on 20 July 2018).
31. EC-853. No 853/2004 of the European Parliament and of the Council of April 29, 2004. Laying down specific hygiene rules for food of animal origin. *Off. J. Eur. Union* **2004**, *139*, 55.
32. NSSP/US FDA. National shellfish sanitation program. In *Guide for the Control of Moluscan Shellfish: 2018 Revision*; 2018. Available online: https://www.fda.gov/food/guidanceregulation/federalstatefoodprograms/ucm2006754.htm (accessed on 20 July 2018).
33. Dyson, K.; Huppert, D.D. Regional economic impacts of razor clam beach closures due to harmful algal blooms (HABs) on the Pacific coast of Washington. *Harmful Algae* **2010**, *9*, 264–271. [CrossRef]

34. Trainer, V.L.; Moore, L.; Bill, B.D.; Adams, N.G.; Harrington, N.; Borchert, J.; Da Silva, D.A.M.; Eberhart, B.-T.L. Diarrhetic shellfish toxins and other lipophilic toxins of human health concern in Washington State. *Mar. Drugs* **2013**, *11*, 1815–1835. [CrossRef] [PubMed]
35. Anderson, D.M.; Hoagland, P.; Kaoru, Y.; White, A.W. Estimated Annual Economic Impacts from Harmful Algal Blooms (HABs) in the United States; DTIC Document: 2000. Available online: http://www.whoi.edu/cms/files/Economics_report_18564_23050.pdf (accessed on 20 July 2018).
36. MacKenzie, L.; White, D.; Adamson, J. Temporal variation and tissue localization of paralytic shellfish toxins in the New Zealand tuatua (surfclam), *Paphies subtriangulata*. *J. Shellfish Res.* **1996**, *15*, 735–740.
37. Farrell, H.; Murray, S.A.; Zammit, A.; Edwards, A.W. Management of ciguatoxin risk in eastern Australia. *Toxins* **2017**, *9*, 367. [CrossRef] [PubMed]
38. Farrell, H.; Zammit, A.; Harwood, D.T.; McNabb, P.; Shadboldt, C.; Manning, J.; Turahui, J.; van den Berg, D.; Szabo, L. Clinical diagnosis and chemical confirmation of ciguatera fish poisoning in New South Wales, Australia. *CDI* **2016**, *40*, E1–E6. [PubMed]
39. Farrell, H.; Zammit, A.; Harwood, D.T.; Murray, S. Is ciguatera moving south in Australia? *Harmful Algal News* **2016**, *54*, 5–6.
40. Quaine, J.; Kraa, E.; Holloway, J.; White, K.; McCarthy, R.; Delpech, V.; Trent, M.; McAnulty, J. Outbreak of gastroenteritis linked to eating pipis. *NSW Public Health Bull.* **1997**, *8*, 103–104.
41. MacKenzie, L.; Holland, P.; McNabb, P.; Beuzenberg, V.; Selwood, A.; Suzuki, T. Complex toxin profiles in phytoplankton and greenshell mussels (*Perna canaliculus*), revealed by LC-MS/MS analysis. *Toxicon* **2002**, *40*, 1321–1330. [CrossRef]
42. Hallegraeff, G.M.; Lucas, I.A.N. The marine dinoflagellate genus *Dinophysis* (Dinophyceae): Photosynthetic, neritic and non-photosynthetic, oceanic species. *Phycologia* **1988**, *27*, 25–42. [CrossRef]
43. McCarthy, P. Census of Australian Marine Dinoflagellates. 2018. Available online: http://www.anbg.gov.au/abrs/Dinoflagellates/index_Dino.html (accessed on 20 July 2018).
44. Burgess, V.; Shaw, G. Pectenotoxins—An issue for public health: A review of their comparative toxicology and metabolism. *Environ. Int.* **2001**, *27*, 275–283. [CrossRef]
45. Farrell, H.; Brett, S.; Webster, G.; Baker, P.; Zammit, A. A summary of harmful algal bloom monitoring and risk assessment in New South Wales, australia. In Proceedings of the 16th International Conference on Harmful Algae, Wellington, New Zealand, 27–31 October 2014; pp. 254–257.
46. Madigan, T.L.; Lee, K.G.; Padula, D.J.; McNabb, P.; Pointon, A.M. Diarrhetic shellfish poisoning (DSP) toxins in South Australian shellfish. *Harmful Algae* **2006**, *5*, 119–123. [CrossRef]
47. Wallace, G.M. Diarrhetic Shellfish Toxins in Tasmanian Coastal Waters: Causative Dinoflagellate Organisms, Dissolved Toxins and Shellfish Depuration. Ph.D. Thesis, University of Tasmania, Tasmania, Australia, 2011.
48. Sydney Fish Market. Annual Report 2017. 2017. Available online: https://www.sydneyfishmarket.com.au/our-company/annual-report (accessed on 20 July 2018).
49. Pitcher, G.C.; Krock, B.; Cembella, A.D. Accumulation of diarrhetic shellfish poisoning toxins in the oyster *Crassostrea gigas* and the mussel *Choromytilus meridionalis* in the southern benguela ecosystem. *Afr. J. Mar. Sci.* **2011**, *33*, 273–281. [CrossRef]
50. FAO Food and Nutrition Paper 80. In *UN Food and Agriculture Organization (FAO)*; FAO: Rome, Italy, 2004. Available online: http://www.fao.org/docrep/007/y5486e/y5486e00.htm (accessed on 20 July 2018).
51. Hégaret, H.; Wikfors, G.H.; Shumway, S.E. Biotoxin contamination and shellfish safety. In *Shellfish Safety and Quality*; Shumway, S.E., Rodrick, G.E., Eds.; Woodhead Publishing Limited: Cambridge, UK, 2009; pp. 43–82.
52. Mons, M.P.; Speijers, G.J.A. Paralytic Shellfish Poisoning: A Review. 1998. Available online: https://www.rivm.nl/bibliotheek/rapporten/388802005.html (accessed on 20 July 2018).
53. Fernández, M.L.; Shumway, S.E. Managment of shellfish resources. In *Manual on Harmful Marine Microalgae*; Hallegraeff, G.M., Anderson, D.M., Cembella, A.D., Eds.; UNESCO: Paris, France, 2004.
54. Sidari, L.; Nichetto, P.; Cok, S.; Sosa, S.; Tubaro, A.; Honsell, G.; Della Loggia, R. Phytoplankton selection by mussels, and diarrhetic shellfish poisoning. *Mar. Biol.* **1998**, *131*, 103–111. [CrossRef]
55. Ajani, P.; Lee, R.; Pritchard, T.; Krogh, M. Phytoplankton dynamics at a long-term coastal station off Sydney, Australia. *J. Coastal Res.* **2001**, 60–73.
56. Takahashi, E.; Yu, Q.; Eaglesham, G.; Connell, D.W.; McBroom, J.; Costanzo, S.; Shaw, G.R. Occurrence and seasonal variations of algal toxins in water, phytoplankton and shellfish from North Stradbroke Island, Queensland, Australia. *Mar. Environ. Res.* **2007**, *64*, 429–442. [CrossRef] [PubMed]

57. Ajani, P.; Larsson, M.E.; Rubio, A.; Bush, S.; Brett, S.; Farrell, H. Modelling bloom formation of the toxic dinoflagellates *Dinophysis acuminata* and *Dinophysis caudata* in a highly modified estuary, south eastern Australia. *Estuar. Coastal Shelf Sci.* **2016**, *183*, 95–106. [CrossRef]
58. Burgess, V.; Shaw, G. Investigations into the Toxicology of Pectenotoxin-2-Seco Acid and 7-Epi Pectenotoxin 2-Seco Acid to Aid in a Health Risk Assessment for the Consumption of Shellfish Contaminated with These Shellfish Toxins in Australia. Available online: http://www.frdc.com.au/Archived-Reports/FRDC%20Projects/2001-258-DLD.pdf (accessed on 20 July 2018).
59. Escalera, L.; Reguera, B.; Moita, T.; Pazos, Y.; Cerejo, M.; Cabanas, J.M.; Ruiz-Villarreal, M. Bloom dynamics of *Dinophysis acuta* in an upwelling system: In situ growth versus transport. *Harmful Algae* **2010**, *9*, 312–322. [CrossRef]
60. Taylor, M.; McIntyre, L.; Ritson, M.; Stone, J.; Bronson, R.; Bitzikos, O.; Rourke, W.; Galanis, E.; Outbreak Investigation, T. Outbreak of diarrhetic shellfish poisoning associated with mussels, British Columbia, Canada. *Mar. Drugs* **2013**, *11*, 1669–1676. [CrossRef] [PubMed]
61. Chen, T.; Xu, X.; Wei, J.; Chen, J.; Miu, R.; Huang, L.; Zhou, X.; Fu, Y.; Yan, R.; Wang, Z.; et al. Food-borne disease outbreak of diarrhetic shellfish poisoning due to toxic mussel consumption: The first recorded outbreak in China. *PLoS ONE* **2013**, *8*, e65049. [CrossRef] [PubMed]
62. Alves, T.; Mafra, L. Diel variations in cell abundance and trophic transfer of diarrheic toxins during a massive *Dinophysis* bloom in southern Brazil. *Toxins* **2018**, *10*, 232. [CrossRef] [PubMed]
63. O'Connor, T. Spring Bay mussels recalled in tasmania over algal toxin find. *ABC News*, 20 March 2016. Available online: https://www.abc.net.au/news/2016-03-19/spring-bay-mussels-recalled-in-tasmania-over-algal-toxin-find/7260250 (accessed on 20 July 2018).
64. Hallegraeff, G.M. Harmful algal blooms: A global overview. In *Manual on Harmful Marine Microalgae*; Hallegraeff, G.M., Anderson, D.M., Cembella, A.D., Eds.; UNESCO: Paris, France, 2003; pp. 24–49.
65. Hallegraeff, G.M. Ocean climate change, phytoplankton community responses, and harmful algal blooms: A formidable predictive challenge. *J. Phycol.* **2010**, *46*, 220–235. [CrossRef]
66. Pizarro, G.; Moroño, Á.; Paz, B.; Franco, J.; Pazos, Y.; Reguera, B. Evaluation of passive samplers as a monitoring tool for early warning of *Dinophysis* toxins in shellfish. *Mar. Drugs* **2013**, *11*, 3823. [CrossRef] [PubMed]
67. Hattenrath-Lehmann, T.K.; Lusty, M.W.; Wallace, R.B.; Haynes, B.; Wang, Z.; Broadwater, M.; Deeds, J.R.; Morton, S.L.; Hastback, W.; Porter, L.; et al. Evaluation of rapid, early warning approaches to track shellfish toxins associated with *Dinophysis* and *Alexandrium* blooms. *Mar. Drugs* **2018**, *16*, 28. [CrossRef] [PubMed]
68. Economou, V.; Papadopoulou, C.; Brett, M.; Kansouzidou, A.; Charalabopoulos, K.; Filioussis, G.; Seferiadis, K. Diarrheic shellfish poisoning due to toxic mussel consumption: The first recorded outbreak in Greece. *Food Addit. Contam.* **2007**, *24*, 297–305. [CrossRef] [PubMed]
69. Lawrence, J.F.; Niedzwiadek, B.; Menard, C. Quantitative determination of paralytic shellfish poisoning toxins in shellfish using prechromatographic oxidation and liquid chromatography with fluorescence detection: Collaborative study. *J. AOAC Int.* **2005**, *88*, 1714–1732. [PubMed]
70. van den Top, H.J.; Gerssen, A.; McCarron, P.; van Egmond, H.P. Quantitative determination of marine lipophilic toxins in mussels, oysters and cockles using liquid chromatography-mass spectrometry: Inter-laboratory validation study. *Food Addit. Contam.* **2011**, *28*, 1745–1757. [CrossRef] [PubMed]
71. Villar-Gonzalez, A.; Rodriguez-Velasco, M.L.; Gago-Martinez, A. Determination of lipophilic toxins by LC/MS/MS: Single-laboratory validation. *J. AOAC Int.* **2011**, *94*, 909–922. [PubMed]
72. AOAC. Domoic acid in mussels, liquid chromatographic method. *J. AOAC Int.* **2000**.
73. ASQAAC. *The Australian Shellfish Quality Assurance Program Operations Manual*; Australian Shellfish Quality Assurance Advisory Committee: Canberra, Australia, 2016; p. 46.

toxins

MDPI

Article

First Report of Okadaic Acid and Pectenotoxins in Individual Cells of *Dinophysis* and in Scallops *Argopecten purpuratus* from Perú

Alex Alcántara-Rubira *, Víctor Bárcena-Martínez *, Maribel Reyes-Paulino, Katherine Medina-Acaro, Lilibeth Valiente-Terrones, Angélica Rodríguez-Velásquez, Rolando Estrada-Jiménez * and Omar Flores-Salmón *

Organismo Nacional de Sanidad Pesquera (SANIPES), Av. Domingo Orué N° 165, Surquillo Lima 34, Perú; maribel.reyes@sanipes.gob.pe (M.R.-P.); katherine.medina@sanipes.gob.pe (K.M.-A.); locador203@sanipes.gob.pe (L.V.-T.); angelica.rodriguez@sanipes.gob.pe (A.R.-V.)

* Correspondence: alex.alcantara@sanipes.gob.pe (A.A.-R.); victor.barcena@sanipes.gob.pe (V.B.-M.); restradaj@gmail.com (R.E.-J.); omar.flores@sanipes.gob.pe (O.F.-S.); Tel.: +51-1-213-8570 (ext. 8020) (A.A.-R.); +51-1-213-8570 (ext. 8012) (V.B.-M.); +51-1-213-8570 (ext. 8018) (O.F.-S.)

Received: 25 September 2018; Accepted: 13 November 2018; Published: 23 November 2018

Abstract: Causative species of Harmful Algal Bloom (HAB) and toxins in commercially exploited molluscan shellfish species are monitored weekly from four classified shellfish production areas in Perú (three in the north and one in the south). Okadaic acid (OA) and pectenotoxins (PTXs) were detected in hand-picked cells of *Dinophysis* (*D. acuminata*-complex and *D. caudata*) and in scallops (*Argopecten purpuratus*), the most important commercial bivalve species in Perú. LC-MS analyses revealed two different toxin profiles associated with species of the *D. acuminata*-complex: (a) one with OA (0.3–8.0 pg cell^{-1}) and PTX2 (1.5–11.1 pg cell^{-1}) and (b) another with only PTX2 which included populations with different toxin cell quota (9.3–9.6 pg cell^{-1} and 5.8–9.2 pg cell^{-1}). Toxin results suggest the likely presence of two morphotypes of the *D. acuminata*-complex in the north, and only one of them in the south. Likewise, shellfish toxin analyses revealed the presence of PTX2 in all samples (10.3–34.8 μg kg^{-1}), but OA (7.7–15.2 μg kg^{-1}) only in the northern samples. Toxin levels were below the regulatory limits established for diarrhetic shellfish poisoning (DSP) and PTXs (160 μg OA kg^{-1}) in Perú, in all samples analyzed. This is the first report confirming the presence of OA and PTX in *Dinophysis* cells and in shellfish from Peruvian coastal waters.

Keywords: okadaic acid; pectenotoxins; *Dinophysis*; *D. acuminata*-complex; *D. caudata*; *Argopecten purpuratus*

Key Contribution: This study shows that the *D. acuminata*-complex in northern Peru produces OA and PTX2 and in the southern zone only PTX2. *D. caudata* only produces PTX2. No DTXs were detected in the analyzed cells. The same profile was observed in the scallop *Argopecten purpuratus*, suggesting that only these toxins are produced by the phytoplankton species analyzed in these areas.

---

1. Introduction

Diarrhetic shellfish poisoning (DSP) toxins cause a gastrointestinal human health syndrome with the main symptoms being nausea, diarrhea, vomiting, and gastrointestinal pain [1,2]. Okadaic acid (OA) and its congeners, dinophysistoxins (DTX1, DTX2), their high-polarity precursors (DTX4, DTX5), and their 7-*O*-acyl-derivatives ("DTX3") are liposoluble polyethers that have been designated as diarrhetic shellfish toxins [3–5]. Pectenotoxins are liposoluble, non-diarrheogenic, polyether lactones which may co-occur with DSP toxins and can be coeluted with them [6] using the usual extraction procedures. The two groups of toxins have been found in different species of *Dinophysis* (*D. acuminata*, *D. acuta*, *D. caudata*, *D. fortii*, *D. infundibula*, *D. miles*, *D. norvegica*, *D. ovum*, *D. sacculus*, *D. tripos*) and two species of *Phalacroma* (*P. mitra*, *P. rotundatum*) [5]. In addition, OA and its congeners have been found in several benthic species from the genus *Prorocentrum* (*P. concavum*, *P. texanum*, *P. arenarium*, *P. lima*) [5,7,8].

Filter-feeding bivalves accumulate algal toxins and are the main vectors transferring them to humans through the food web. DSP toxins and pectenotoxins (PTXs) pose a global threat to public health and aquaculture [9–12]. The analysis of DSP toxins for monitoring programmes in Perú have been carried out only by mouse bioassay [13], and there is no information on the toxin profiles of either the potentially toxic species of *Dinophysis* or of the contaminated molluscan shellfish. Nevertheless, *D. acuminata*, *D. caudata*, *D. tripos*, and *Phalacroma rotundatum* (=*Dinophysis rotundata*) have been reported in Peruvian coastal waters [14], and their toxins associated with positive results for lipophilic toxins in mouse bioassays [13]. There have also been reports on the occurrence of the benthic dinoflagellate *Prorocentrum lima* [13], but to date this species has not been associated with DSP events in Perú.

During 2017 and 2018, seawater and shellfish samples were collected from classified shellfish production areas (Figure 1), in the framework of the Molluscan Shellfish Safety Programme (PCMB) of the National Fisheries Health Organization of Perú (SANIPES), to establish the relationship between the toxic profiles detected in shellfish and the occurrence of potentially toxic dinoflagellates.

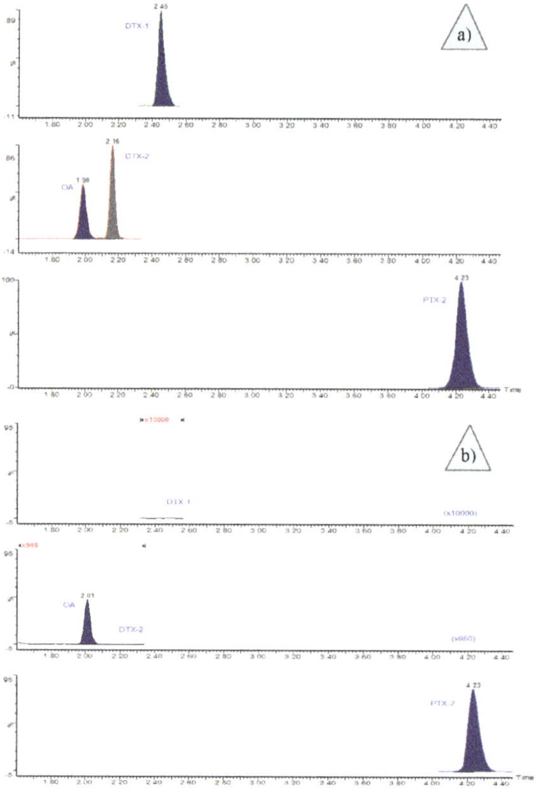

Figure 1. Selective ion chromatograms from the LC-MS/MS analyses of isolated cells of *Dinophysis acuminata*-complex in: (**a**) multitoxin standard, 3 ng mL^{-1}; and (**b**) chromatogram of the sample from Bahía de Sechura-Vichayo, where the absence of DTX1 (increase ×10,000) and DTX2 (increase ×950) was observed.

2. Results

Chromatograms from the LC-MS/MS analyses of hand-picked cells showed that the toxin profile of *Dinophysis acuminata*-complex cells from the northernmost production area (Sechura Bay) included OA and PTX2 (Figure 1b).

Other toxins, such as DTX1 and DTX2, were not found (LOD = 0.16 ng mL^{-1}). In contrast, only PTX2 was detected in the analyses of picked cells of *Dinophysis* cf. *acuminata* and *D. caudate* from the other three areas (i.e., Independencia Bay, Samanco Bay, and Salinas), with an average toxin content of 9.3 pg PTX2 $cell^{-1}$ (Table 1).

Table 1. Toxin content in isolated cells of *Dinophysis*.

Date (d/m/y)	Location	Sampling Depth (m)	Species	Picked Cells (No.)	OA (pg $Cell^{-1}$)	PTX2 (pg $Cell^{-1}$)
27/01/2017	Independencia Bay	0–8	*D. acuminata*-complex	150	<LOD *	9.6
09/02/2017	Samanco Bay	0–15	*D. caudata*	92	<LOD *	9.2
10/04/2017	Salinas	0–15	*D. acuminata*-complex	204	<LOD *	9.3
24/03/2018	Sechura Bay (Vichayo)	0–15	*D. acuminata*-complex	440	0.8	11.1
24/03/2018	Sechura Bay (Puerto Rico)	0–15	*D. acuminata*-complex	400	0.3	1.5
14/04/2018	Sechura Bay (Parachique)	0–15	*D. caudata*	400	<LOD *	5.8

* LOD: 0.16 ng mL^{-1}. OA: okadaic acid; PTX: pectenotoxin.

The same profile of toxins present in the cells was detected in the shellfish *Argopecten purpuratus* from the same production areas (Table 2).

Table 2. Toxin content in *Argopecten purpuratus* (whole flesh).

Date d/m/y	Place	OA µg kg^{-1} Post-Hydrolysis	PTX2 µg kg^{-1}
27/01/2017	Independencia Bay-El Queso	<LOD *	22.2
09/02/2017	Samanco Bay	<LOD *	20.3
10/04/2017	Salinas	<LOD *	10.3
14/04/2018	Sechura Bay-Puerto Rico	10.4	34.8
14/04/2018	Sechura Bay-Barrancos	8.6	20.8
14/04/2018	Sechura Bay-San Pedro	15.2	27.6
05/05/2018	Sechura Bay-Las Delicias	7.7	10.7

* LOD: 1.6 µg kg^{-1}.

3. Discussion

Okadaic acid and PTX2 were detected in both *Dinophysis* cells and scallops. In some cases, both toxins were present but in others only PTX2 was detected. There are previous reports on *Dinophysis* species with a toxin profile constituted by only PTX2. That was the case with *D. acuminata* cells isolated from Inglesa Bay [15] and from Reloncaví estuary [4], both from Chile, as well as with *D. caudata* from the Galician Rías Bajas, northwest Spain [16] and *D. acuminata* from Danish waters [17]. Likewise, our analyses of shellfish meat from the same areas in Perú were in agreement with the toxin profiles of the dinoflagellates, that is, just PTX-2 (10.3–22.2 µg PTX2 kg^{-1} meat) and no traces of OA in the areas where *Dinophysis* species had the same profile.

The Peruvian strains of *Dinophysis* seemed to contain much lower amounts of toxin per cell than those reported from Galicia, Spain (*D. caudata*: 100.0–127.4 pg PTX2 $cell^{-1}$) [16] and from Chile (*D. acuminata*: 180 pg PTX2 $cell^{-1}$), which had a toxin content one order of magnitude higher than the Peruvian strains (Table 2).

Cells of *Dinophysis acuminata*-complex around Sechura Bay showed a higher variability in their PTX2 content, with values ranging from 1.5 to 11.1 pg cell^{-1} and to a lesser extent in their OA cell quota (from 0.3 to 0.8 pg cell^{-1}). We do not know if this variability is due to the co-occurrence of different species of the *D.* cf. *acuminata* in the same area. Nevertheless, previous laboratory experiments and field data have shown a large variability of toxin content per cell of *Dinophysis* associated with different phases of the population growth and their interaction with environmental conditions [18]. More studies, including physiological and genetic factors affecting toxin profiles and content, are needed to clarify these questions. The presence of OA and PTX2 has been also reported in *D. acuminata* from Lake Orbetello, Italy [19] and in New Zealand [20], USA [4], and Japan [21], where other toxins (e.g., DTX1 and some PTX analogues) were also reported.

D. caudata from the same bay had 5.8 pg PTX2 cell^{-1}. Therefore, there was a co-occurrence of two toxic *Dinophysis* species in this area. Scallop samples ("concha de abanico") during the occurrence of these species reached toxin levels ranging from 7.7 to 15.2 μg OA kg^{-1} and from 10.7 to 34.8 μg PTX2 kg^{-1} (Table 2).

The low toxin content found in *Dinophysis* cells in Perú suggests a low risk of DSP toxins accumulation in shellfish above the regulatory levels. That was the case during the 2 years (maximum levels in Independencia Bay: <LOD OA and 22.2 μg kg^{-1} PTX2; Samanco Bay: <LODOA and 16.4 μg kg^{-1} PTX2; Salinas: <LOD OA and 12.2 μg kg^{-1} PTX2; Sechura Bay-Puerto Rico: 10.4 μg kg^{-1} OA and 48.2 μg kg^{-1} PTX2; Sechura Bay-Barrancos: 8.6 μg kg^{-1} OA and 21.0 μg kg^{-1}; Sechura Bay-San Pedro: 15.2 μg kg^{-1} OA and 43.7 μg kg^{-1} PTX2; and Sechura Bay-Las Delicias: 7.7 μg kg^{-1} OA y 19.6 μg kg^{-1}, June 2016–May 2018) of toxin monitoring of scallops, *A. purpuratus*, by LC-MS/MS. During this period, toxin levels never reached regulatory limits, although *Dinophysis* densities above 10^4·cells L^{-1} were recorded. *Dinophysis* densities of around 10^3 cells L^{-1} are considered a bloom, and have often been related to toxic outbreaks in other parts of the world [5].

4. Conclusions

The toxin profiles, including OA and PTX2, of several species of *Dinophysis* and of scallops (*Argopecten purpuratus*) from shellfish production areas in Perú were characterized. Different species included in the *Dinophysis acuminata*-complex and *D. caudata*, producers of toxins regulated by the EU, co-occur in northern Perú. The toxic species of *Dinophysis* from Sechura Bay, Samanco Bay, Salinas, and Independencia Bay showed low cell-toxin content (pg cell^{-1}) in comparison with those reported for the same species in other parts of the world, although more studies, including physiological and genetic factors affecting toxin profiles and content, are needed. *Dinophysis acuminata*-complex and *D. caudate* are most likely the main species concerning molluscan shellfish safety in Perú.

5. Materials and Methods

5.1. Field Sampling

Seawater and shellfish samples for the analyses of potentially toxic phytoplankton and shellfish toxins were collected weekly in the framework of the National Molluscan Shellfish Safety Programme (PCMB) of the National Fisheries Health Organization of Perú (SANIPES), which is the national competent authority for the control of seafood safety. Samples from classified shellfish production areas were analyzed at the SANIPES official laboratory. During 2017 and the first half of 2018, seawater and scallops (*Argopecten purpuratus* "concha de abanico") samples were collected at the fixed monitoring stations in Sechura Bay, Samanco Bay, Salinas, and Independencia Bay (Figure 2) for analyses. The objective was to determine the toxin profiles in the plankton and shellfish at the time of detection of lipophilic shellfish toxins. Two kinds of water samples were collected at each station for phytoplankton analyses: (i) vertical net-hauls (10 μm mesh size), with no fixatives added, for the identification of the species in vivo and for single cell isolations; (ii) depth-integrated hose-samples (hose length 15 m), which were immediately fixed with acid Lugol's solution, for quantitative analyses by the standard Utermöhl method [22].

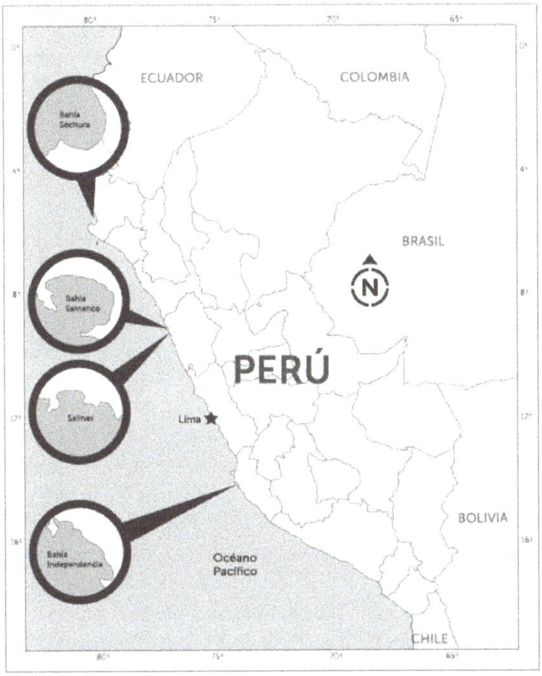

Figure 2. Location of sampling stations.

5.2. Single Cell Isolations

Cells of *Dinophysis caudata* and *D. acuminata*-complex (two different morphotypes *D.* cf. *acuminata* and *D.* cf. *ovum*) (Figure 3) were isolated one by one from the plankton net-haul concentrates with a microcapillary pipette under an inverted microscope Olympus IX71, at 200× magnification. Each picked cell was transferred three times through drops of sterile seawater and finally placed (with as little seawater as possible) in a 1.5 mL Eppendorf tube with 500 μL methanol, and kept at −20 °C until analysis.

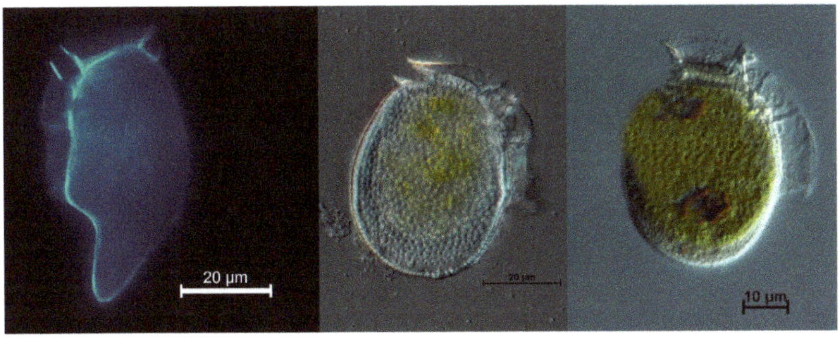

Figure 3. *Dinophysis* cells isolated from Samanco Bay, Perú. (**Left**) Epifluorescence of *Dinophysis caudata;* (**middle**) and (**right**) DIC micrographs of cells of the *Dinophysis acuminata*-complex.

5.3. Standards and Reagents

LC-MS grade methanol (MeOH) and acetonitrile (CH_3CN) were used for the extraction and analyses of toxins by liquid chromatography coupled to mass spectrometry (LC-MS). Analytical-grade ammonium hydroxide, sodium hydroxide (NaOH), and hydrochloric acid (HCl) were used for the mobile phase and hydrolysis. Ultrapure water was obtained with a Sartorius (Arium Pro) purification system. Certified reference solutions for okadaic acid CRM-OA-d (batch #20141119), dinophysistoxin-2 CRM-DTX2-b (batch #20150819), dinophysistoxin-1 CRM-DTX1-b (batch #20151209), and pectenotoxin-2 CRM-PTX2-b (batch #20120516) were obtained from NRC-CNRC.

5.4. Toxins Extraction

5.4.1. From Isolated Cells of *Dinophysis*

To prepare for LC/MS analysis, samples kept frozen in Eppendorf tubes were transferred to a 2-mL microtube, the remains in the Eppendorf tube were washed twice with 200 µL of methanol, incorporated to the microtube, and mixed in a vortex prior to being dried at 40 °C under a flow of nitrogen gas. The dried toxin extract was re-suspended in 500 µL of methanol, mixed in a vortex, and filtered through 0.2 µm pore size nylon filters (Sterlitech, 13 mm) as described in [23].

5.4.2. From Shellfish Meat

Whole flesh samples of 12–15 scallops, *Argopecten purpuratus*, were homogenized and a 2 ± 0.05 g subsample, weighed on an analytical scale (Precisa, LX 220A), was placed in a 50 mL centrifuge tube and extracted twice with 9 mL methanol, stirred with a vortex (Thermo, maxi mix II) for 3 min, and centrifuged at 2000× *g* (Thermo, Sorvall ST 16R) for 10 min at a temperature of 20 °C. The supernatants were transferred and mixed in a volumetric flask and made up to 20 mL with methanol. To explore the presence of esterified derivatives of OA and DTXs, an aliquot of the methanolic extract was taken for alkaline hydrolysis.

The alkaline hydrolysis was carried out by adding 125 µL of 2.5 N NaOH to 1 mL of the methanolic extract, vortexing the mixture for 0.5 min, heating it for 40 min at 76 °C, and finally neutralizing the added NaOH with an equivalent amount of 2.5 N HCl.

Finally, all extracts (raw and hydrolyzed) were filtered through a 0.2 µm pore size nylon filter (Chromafil®Xtra, 25 mm) following the recommended protocols from the European Union Reference Laboratory for Marine Biotoxins [24].

5.5. LC-MS/MS Analyses

For LC-MS/MS analysis of the lipophilic toxins, a Waters Acquity I Class chromatograph coupled to a triple quadrupole mass spectrometer Waters XEVO-TQS by means of an electrospray interface (ESI) was used. Analytical separation was performed following a modification of the method developed by Gerssen et al. [25], with an Acquity UPLC® BEH C18 (1.7 µm, 2.1 × 100 mm) column kept at 40 °C. A binary gradient elution was used, with phase A consisting of H_2O and phase B of 90% CH_3CN, both containing ammonium hydroxide 6.7 mM (approximate pH of 11). The gradient started with 30% B, that proportion was kept for 1 min and then linearly increased to 90% B in 4 min. It was maintained at that proportion for 1 min, returned to the initial proportion in 0.1 min, and maintained for equilibration during 1.5 min before the next injection. The flow rate was 0.4 mL min^{-1} and the injection volume was 2 µL. The mass spectrometer was operated in both ESI positive and negative modes, the cone voltage was 3.0 kV, desolvation gas temperature was 500 °C with an N_2 flow of 1000 L h^{-1} and a source temperature of 150 °C. Voltage parameters of the cone and collision energy were optimized during the tuning phase by direct infusion in alkaline medium. Product ions used for the quantification of each toxin in microalgae and shellfish and the MS/MS conditions for the multiple reaction monitoring (MRM) for each molecule are shown in Table 3.

Table 3. Multiple reaction monitoring (MRM) and MS/MS of each toxin from the shellfish analysis.

Toxins	ESI Mode	Ion		Cone Voltage (V)	Collision Energy (CE) (eV)	Dwell (s)
		Precursor (*m*/*z*)	Product (*m*/*z*)			
OA	ESI^-	803.5	255.1 * 113.0	30	50 60	0.05
DTX1	ESI^-	817.5	255.1 * 113.0	30	50 60	0.05
DTX2	ESI^-	803.5	255.1 * 113.0	30	50 60	0.05
PTX1	ESI^+	892.5	821.5 * 213.3	30	30 40	0.02
PTX2	ESI^+	876.6	823.5 * 213.1	30	20 40	0.20

* Transitions used for the phytoplankton analyses. ESI: electrospray ionization.

Author Contributions: Conceptualization, A.A.-R., V.B.-M. and O.F.-S.; Investigation, A.A.-R., V.B.-M., M.R.-P., K.M.-A., A.R.-V. and L.V.-T.; Project administration, A.A.-R.; Visualization, A.A.-R., V.B.-M. and O.F.-S.; Writing—original draft, A.A.-R., V.B.-M. and O.F.-S.; Writing—review & editing, A.A.-R., V.B.-M., O.F.-S. and R.E.-J.

Funding: This work was funded by the National Programme of Bivalve Molluscs of the National Fisheries Health Organization of Perú, an autonomous entity attached to the Ministry of Production.

Acknowledgments: The authors acknowledge the Shellfish Monitoring Program of Bivalve Molluscs of the National Fisheries Health Organization of Perú for supplying shellfish and seawater samples for this study. We also thank Beatriz Reguera (Spanish Institute of Oceanography (IEO), Oceanographic Centre of Vigo) and Juan Blanco (Marine Research Centre—CIMA, Pontevedra 36620, Spain) for reviewing and translating this work.

Conflicts of Interest: The authors declare that there are no conflicts of interest.

References

1. Yasumoto, T.; Murata, M.; Oshima, Y.; Sano, M.; Matsumoto, G.K.; Clardy, J. Diarrhetic shellfish toxins. *Tetrahedron* **1985**, *41*, 1019–1025. [CrossRef]
2. Yasumoto, T.; Oshima, Y.; Yamaguchi, M. Occurrence of a new type of shellfish poisoning in the Tohoku district. *NIPPON SUISAN GAKKAISHI* **1978**, *44*, 1249–1255. [CrossRef]
3. Yasumoto, T.; Murata, M. Polyether Toxins Involved in Seafood Poisoning. In *Marine Toxins*; Hall, S., Strichartz, G., Eds.; American Chemical Society: Washington, DC, USA, 1990; Volume 418, pp. 120–132.
4. Fux, E.; Smith, J.L.; Tong, M.; Guzmán, L.; Anderson, D.M. Toxin profiles of five geographical isolates of *Dinophysis* spp. from North and South America. *Toxicon* **2011**, *57*, 275–287. [CrossRef] [PubMed]
5. Reguera, B.; Riobó, P.; Rodríguez, F.; Díaz, P.; Pizarro, G.; Paz, B.; Franco, J.; Blanco, J. Dinophysis Toxins: Causative Organisms, Distribution and Fate in Shellfish. *Mar. Drugs* **2014**, *12*, 394–461. [CrossRef] [PubMed]
6. Blanco, J.; Moroño, Á.; Fernández, M.L. Toxic episodes in shellfish, produced by lipophilic phycotoxins: An overview. *Galician J. Mar. Resour.* **2005**, *1*, 1–70.
7. Van Dolah, F.M. Marine Algal Toxins: Origins, Health Effects, and Their Increased Occurrence. *Environ. Health Perspect.* **2000**, *108*, 9. [CrossRef] [PubMed]
8. Reguera, B. *Biología, Autoecología y Toxinología de las Principales Especies del Género Dinophysis Asociadas a Episodios de Intoxicación Diarreogénica por Bivalvos (DSP)*; Universidad de Barcelona: Barcelona, España, 2003.
9. Jørgensen, K.; Andersen, P. Relation between the concentration of *Dinophysis acuminata* and diarrheic shellfish poisoning toxins in blue mussels (*Mytilus edulis*) during a toxic episode in the Limfjord (DENMARK), 2006. *J. Shellfish Res.* **2007**, *26*, 1081–1087. [CrossRef]
10. Nincevic-Gladan, Z.; Skejic, S.; Arapov, J.; Buzancic, M.; Bojanic, N.; Ujevic, I.; Kuspilic, G.; Grbec, B.; Vidjack, O. Seasonal variability in *Dinophysis* spp. abundances and diarrhetic shellfish poisoning outbreaks along the eastern Adriatic coast. *Botanica Mar.* **2008**, *51*, 449–463. [CrossRef]
11. Hossen, V.; Jourdan-da Silva, N.; Guillois-Bécel, Y.; Marchal, J.; Krys, S. Food poisoning outbreaks linked to mussels contaminated with okadaic acid and ester dinophysistoxin-3 in France, June 2009. *Eurosurveillance* **2011**, 16. [CrossRef]

12. Reguera, B.; Velo-Suárez, L.; Raine, R.; Park, M.G. Harmful Dinophysis species: A review. *Harmful Algae* **2012**, *14*, 87–106. [CrossRef]
13. Sanchez, S.; Bernales, A.; Delgado, E.; Carmen Chang, F.D.; Jacobo, N.; Quispe, J. Variability and Biogeographical Distribution of Harmful Algal Blooms in Bays of High Productivity Off Peruvian Coast (2012–2015). *J. Environ. Anal.Toxicol.* **2017**, *7*. [CrossRef]
14. Ochoa, N.; Gómez, O.; Sánchez, S.; Delgado, E. Diversidad de Diatomeas y Dinoflagelados Marinos del Perú. *Bol. Inst. Mar. Perú* **1999**, *18*, 1–14.
15. Blanco, J.; Álvarez, G.; Uribe, E. Identification of pectenotoxins in plankton, filter feeders, and isolated cells of a *Dinophysis acuminata* with an atypical toxin profile, from Chile. *Toxicon* **2007**, *49*, 710–716. [CrossRef] [PubMed]
16. Fernández, M.L.; Reguera, B.; González-Gil, S.; Míguez, A. Pectenotoxin-2 in single-cell isolates of *Dinophysis caudata* and *Dinophysis acuta* from the Galician Rías (NW Spain). *Toxicon* **2006**, *48*, 477–490. [CrossRef] [PubMed]
17. Nielsen, L.T.; Krock, B.; Hansen, P.J. Production and excretion of okadaic acid, pectenotoxin-2 and a novel dinophysistoxin from the DSP-causing marine dinoflagellate *Dinophysis acuta*—Effects of light, food availability and growth phase. *Harmful Algae* **2013**, *23*, 34–45. [CrossRef]
18. Pizarro, G.; Paz, B.; Gonzalez-Gil, S.; Franco, J.M.; Reguera, B. Seasonal variability of lipophilic toxins during a *Dinophysis acuta* bloom in Western Iberia: Differences between picked cells and plankton concentrates. *Harmful Algae* **2009**, *8*, 926–937. [CrossRef]
19. Pigozzi, S.; Ceredi, A.; Milandri, A.; Pompei, M.; Buzzichelli, S.; Macori, G.; Susini, F.; Forletta, R. Pectenotoxin and okadaic acid-based toxin profiles in phytoplankton and shellfish from Orbetello Lagoon, Italy. In Proceedings of the 7th International Conference on Molluscan Shellfish Safety, Nantes, France, 14–19 June 2009; Available online: https://www.researchgate.net/profile/Guerrino_Macori2/publication/304776353_Pectenotoxin_and_okadaic_acid-based_toxin_profiles_in_phytoplankton_and_shellfish_from_Orbetello_Lagoon_Italy/links/577a35e608ae355e74f05c29/Pectenotoxin-and-okadaic-acid-based-toxin-profiles-in-phytoplankton-and-shellfish-from-Orbetello-Lagoon-Italy.pdf (accessed on 17 November 2018). [CrossRef]
20. MacKenzie, L.; Beuzenberg, V.; Holland, P.; McNabb, P.; Suzuki, T.; Selwood, A. Pectenotoxin and okadaic acid-based toxin profiles in *Dinophysis acuta* and *Dinophysis acuminata* from New Zealand. *Harmful Algae* **2005**, *4*, 75–85. [CrossRef]
21. Nagai, S.; Suzuki, T.; Nishikawa, T.; Kamiyama, T. Differences in the production and excretion kinetics of okadaic acid, dinophysistoxin-1, and pectenotoxin-2 between cultures of *Dinophysis acuminata* and *Dinophysis fortii* isolated from western Japan. *J.Phycol.* **2011**, *47*, 1326–1337. [CrossRef] [PubMed]
22. Utermöhl, H. Zur Vervollkommung der quantitativen phytoplankton-methodik. *Mitt Int. Ver Limnol.* **1958**, *9*, 38.
23. Raho, N.; Pizarro, G.; Escalera, L.; Reguera, B.; Marín, I. Morphology, toxin composition and molecular analysis of *Dinophysis ovum* Schütt, a dinoflagellate of the "*Dinophysis acuminata* complex". *Harmful Algae* **2008**, *7*, 839–848. [CrossRef]
24. European Union Reference Laboratory for Marine Biotoxins. EU-Harmonised Standard Operating Procedure for Determination of Lipophilic Marine Biotoxins in Molluscs by LC-MS/MS, V.5. Available online: http://aesan.msssi.gob.es/en/CRLMB/web/home.shtml (accessed on 15 March 2017).
25. Gerssen, A.; Mulder, P.P.J.; McElhinney, M.A.; de Boer, J. Liquid chromatography–tandem mass spectrometry method for the detection of marine lipophilic toxins under alkaline conditions. *J. Chromatogr. A* **2009**, *1216*, 1421–1430. [CrossRef] [PubMed]

toxins

MDPI

Article

Interannual Variability of *Dinophysis acuminata* and *Protoceratium reticulatum* in a Chilean Fjord: Insights from the Realized Niche Analysis

Catharina Alves-de-Souza [1,*], José Luis Iriarte [2,3] and Jorge I. Mardones [4]

1 Algal Resources Collection, MARBIONC, University of North Carolina Wilmington, 5600 Marvin Moss K. Lane, Wilmington, NC 29409, USA

2 Instituto de Acuicultura and Centro de Investigación Dinámica de Ecosistemas Marinos de Altas Latitudes—IDEAL, Universidad Austral de Chile, Puerto Montt 5480000, Chile; jiriarte@uach.cl

3 COPAS-Sur Austral, Centro de Investigación Oceanográfica en el Pacífico Sur-Oriental (COPAS), Universidad de Concepción, Concepción 4030000, Chile

4 Instituto de Fomento Pesquero (IFOP), Centro de Estudios de Algas Nocivas (CREAN), Padre Harter 574, Puerto Montt 5501679, Chile; jorge.mardones@ifop.cl

* Correspondence: cathsouza@gmail.com; Tel.: +1-910-962-2409

Received: 1 December 2018; Accepted: 31 December 2018; Published: 5 January 2019

Abstract: Here, we present the interannual distribution of *Dinophysis acuminata* and *Protoceratium reticulatum* over a 10-year period in the Reloncaví Fjord, a highly stratified fjord in southern Chile. A realized subniche approach based on the Within Outlying Mean Index (WitOMI) was used to decompose the species' realized niche into realized subniches (found within subsets of environmental conditions). The interannual distribution of both *D. acuminata* and *P. reticulatum* summer blooms was strongly influenced by climatological regional events, i.e., El Niño Southern Oscillation (ENSO) and the Southern Annual Mode (SAM). The two species showed distinct niche preferences, with blooms of *D. acuminata* occurring under La Niña conditions (cold years) and low river streamflow whereas *P. reticulatum* blooms were observed in years of El Niño conditions and positive SAM phase. The biological constraint exerted on the species was further estimated based on the difference between the existing fundamental subniche and the realized subniche. The observed patterns suggested that *D. acuminata* was subject to strong biological constraint during the studied period, probably as a result of low cell densities of its putative prey (the mixotrophic ciliate *Mesodinium* cf. *rubrum*) usually observed in the studied area.

Keywords: *Dinophysis acuminata*; *Protoceratium reticulatum*; Reloncaví Fjord; OMI analysis; WitOMI analysis; *Mesodinium* cf. *rubrum*; El Niño Southern Oscillation; Southern Annual Mode

Key Contribution: First description of the interannual variability of *D. acuminata* and *P. reticulatum* in the Reloncaví Fjord showed blooms of these species strongly linked to climatological events of regional scale (i.e., ENSO and SAM): Blooms of *D. acuminata* were observed in cold years (La Niña conditions) and low streamflow whereas blooms of *P. reticulatum* were observed in warm years (El Niño conditions) and positive SAM phase. *D. acuminata* suffered strong biological constraint, presumably due to low concentration of its putative prey *M.* cf. *rubrum*.

1. Introduction

Diarrhetic Shellfish Poisoning (DSP) is a gastrointestinal syndrome caused by the consumption of shellfish contaminated with okadaic acid (OA) and dinophysistoxins (DTXs) produced by certain dinoflagellates of the genus *Dinophysis* and, to a lesser extent, by benthic *Prorocentrum* species [1]. DSP outbreaks caused by *Dinophysis* spp. have been mainly reported from temperate areas with well-developed aquaculture activities, mostly in Europe, Japan, and Chile [2]. Although only OA and DTXs have been linked to DSP [3], other lipophilic toxins (LSTs) such as pectenotoxins (PTXs) and yessotoxins (YTXs) are also included in seafood safety regulations because they are toxic to mice following intraperitoneal injection of lipophilic shellfish extracts, and, in the case of PTXs, have been shown to promote tumor formation in mammals [4]. PTXs production have been linked only to *Dinophysis* species while YTXs are known to be produced by the dinoflagellates *Protoceratium reticulatum*, *Lingulodinium polyedrum*, *Gonyaulax spinifera* and *G. taylorii* [4–6]. Azaspiracids (AZAs), produced by dinoflagellates of the genus *Azadinium* [7], have diarrheagenic effect on humans and are included in the European Union (EU) seafood safety regulations [4].

D. acuta and *D. acuminata* are the most frequent and abundant *Dinophysis* species in southern Chile's fjords (53–41° S) [8–13]. DSP have been of special concern in this geographical area since the 1970s, when intoxications by diarrhetic toxins were first reported following the consumption of contaminated shellfish extracted from the Reloncaví Sound [14]. DTX-1 and DTX-3 are the predominant DSP toxins in southern Chile [15–17]. The chronicle occurrence of these toxins in bivalves from this area during spring–summer is usually associated with *D. acuta* [18] and less frequently with *D. acuminata* [9,19]. DTX-1 has been detected in plankton samples from this region [20,21], although the causative organism remains to be identified. More recently, DTX-2 has been detected in the plankton associated with the presence of *D. acuta* [13]. PTXs presence in southern Chile have been detected in filter feeders [22], plankton assemblages [13,20], and Diaion® resin passive samplers [23], with the production of PTX-2 by *D. acuminata* confirmed in isolates from this area [24]. Finally, YTXs have been recorded in southern Chile both in bivalves and plankton samples containing *P. reticulatum* [12,21,25,26], whereas AZAs have been detected only in bivalves [27].

Despite the evident impact of DSP events in southern Chile, few field studies have focused on the ecological characterization of *Dinophysis* spp. in this area [8,10,21,28]. The available evidence from seasonal surveys points to the importance of persistent saline stratification and increased temperature to high cell densities of *D. acuminata* during spring–summer in the inner portion of fjords [28], where they have been observed forming thin layers associated with the pycnocline [21]. However, these findings were based on seasonal studies carried out over only 1–2 years without considering inter-annual environmental variability. On the other hand, information on *P. reticulatum* is especially scarce and restricted to an apparent preference of this species by high temperatures due to its occurrence during summer in southern Chilean fjords [21]. Although YTXs are not linked to DSP intoxications, moderate levels of these toxins under the EU regulation (1 mg K^{-1}; [5]) have been linked to false positives in DSP mouse bioassays in southern Chile [21] which can lead to the unnecessary closure of areas to shellfish extraction. Thus, *P. reticulatum* distribution should also be determined when assessing the environmental conditions promoting the development of *Dinophysis* spp. and the conditions leading to high DSP toxicity in bivalves in southern Chile.

Here, we present the interannual distribution of *Dinophysis* spp. and *P. reticulatum* from May 2006 to February 2017 in a highly stratified estuarine system in southern Chile, the Reloncaví Fjord (~41.6° S). Our main goal was to obtain insight on the environmental conditions accounting for differences between years where *D. acuminata* and *P. reticulatum* blooms were observed and the ones without blooms of these species. For that, environmental conditions affecting spatio-temporal distribution of the two species over the 10-year time series were determined following a niche approach based on the Outlying Mean Index (OMI) [29]. Then, the Within Outlying Mean Index (WitOMI) [30,31] was used to decompose the species' realized niche into realized subniches (found within subsets of environmental conditions) to estimate the impact of biological constraints on *D. acuminata* and *P. reticulatum* populations. Further WitOMI analyses for *D. acuminata* considering a complementary dataset (spring–summer 2008/2009) were performed, for which additional data on nutrient data and density of the ciliate *Mesodinium* cf. *rubrum* (the putative *Dinophysis* prey, [32]) were available.

2. Results

2.1. Physical and Meteorological Conditions

The 10-year time series (May 2006 to February 2017) was obtained as part of a harmful algae monitoring program carried out by the Chilean Fishing Promotion Institute (IFOP; "Instituto de Fomento Pesquero") at nine sampling stations (Figure 1): three in the Reloncaví Sound near to the mouth of the fjord (stations 1 to 3), four in the middle (stations 4 to 7) and two at the head (stations 8 to 9) of the fjord. The Reloncaví Fjord was characterized by strong spatio-temporal environmental heterogeneity regarding water temperature and salinity. Average maximal and minimal subsurface (depth ~ 1 m) water temperatures were 19 ± 2.2 °C and 8.2 ± 2.3 °C, respectively, with similar values observed among the different sampling stations in each season of the year (Figure 2A and Figure S1A). Maximal subsurface water temperatures were observed in January 2008 (22 °C) and January 2017 (22.6 °C) (Southern Hemisphere summer) while the lowest absolute value was observed in May 2006 (6.2 ± 2.2 °C). Subsurface salinity showed extreme oscillations (0.77–32.54 PSU) in all sampling stations throughout the study period (Figure 2B). Although no consistent seasonal pattern was observed regarding subsurface salinity values (Figure S1B), a clear spatial gradient was observed for this variable with lower values (<15 PSU) mostly observed in the inner part of the fjord (sampling stations 4 to 9).

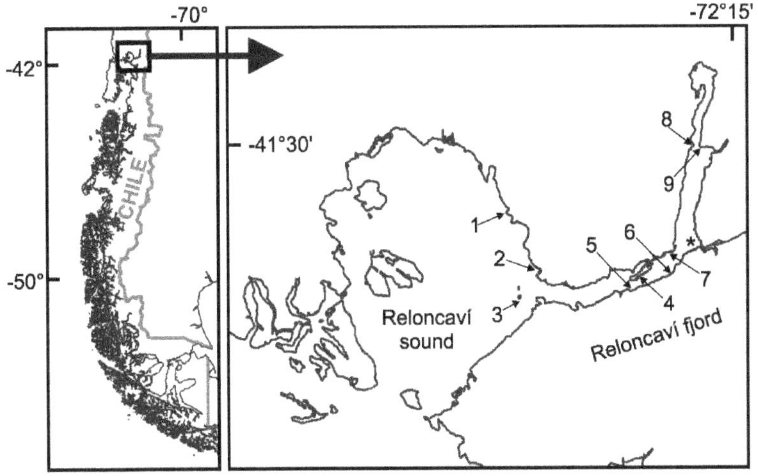

Figure 1. Location of the nine sampling stations in the Reloncaví Fjord. The asterisk indicates the position of the Puelo River's inflow in the fjord.

Salinity was strongly stratified in the upper surface layer for the majority of the studied period. This vertical structure was due to significant differences in salinity between fresher near-surface waters (<15 PSU) and saltier subsurface marine waters (>30 PSU) (Figure S2). Less pronounced stratification was rarely observed and only during winter months, when higher salinities were occasionally observed in the upper layer. The Brunt–Väisälä buoyancy frequency (N_{BV}), a proxy of the water column stratification [33], oscillated between 0.001 s^{-1} (homogeneous water column) to 0.15 s^{-1} (stratification with a sharp pycnocline), although stratification with a more gradual pycnocline was more frequently observed (N_{BV} ~ 0.025 s^{-1}) (Figure S1C,I). The pycnocline depth oscillated between 2 and 9 m (Figure S1D). Besides temperature, seasonal variability was also related to precipitation with this variable strongly correlated to streamflow from the Puelo River (R = 0.58; $p < 0.05$). Higher values for both variables were mostly observed during winter months, although a second precipitation peak was observed during spring for some years (Figure 2C and Figure S1E,F). Interannual variability was related to oscillation in the El Niño Southern Oscillation (ENSO) (here accessed through the Niño 3.4 index) and the Southern Annual Mode (SAM) (Figure 2D,E and Figure S1G,H).

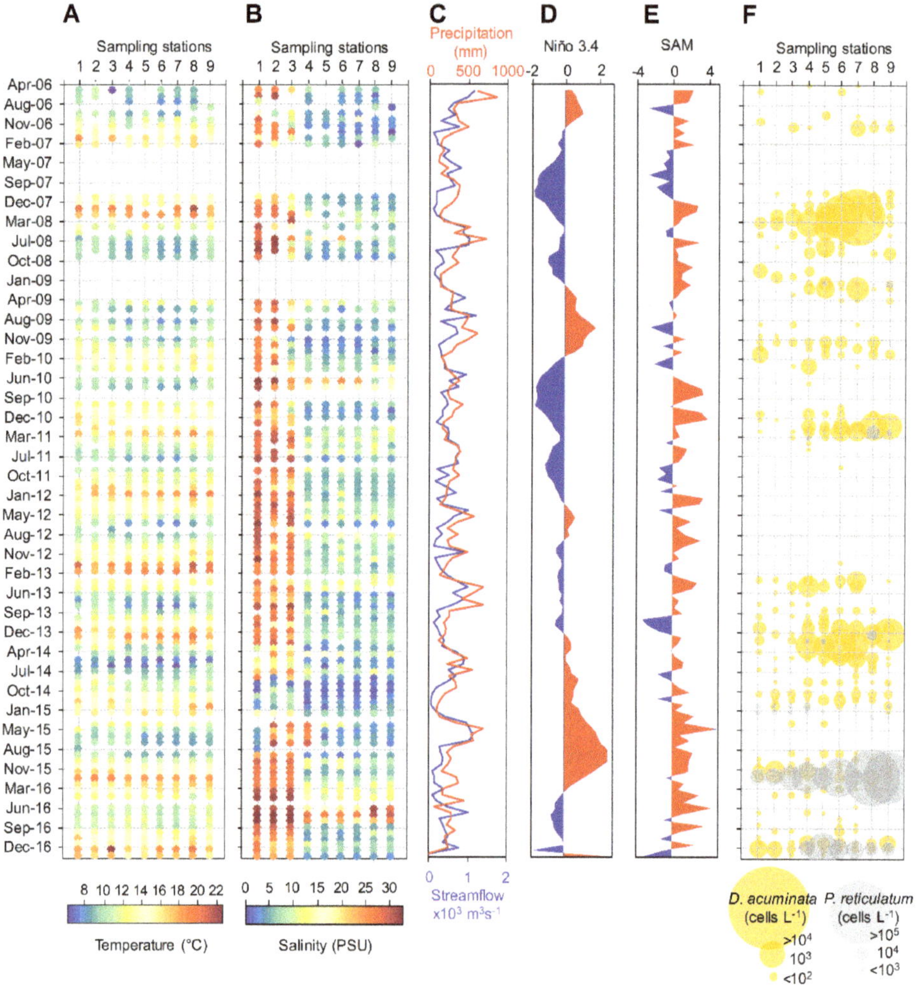

Figure 2. Spatio-temporal variability of physical conditions of the water column, meteorological conditions and potentially toxic dinoflagellate species in the Reloncaví Fjord for the 10-year time series. (**A**) subsurface water temperature, (**B**) subsurface salinity, (**C**) precipitation and streamflow from the Puelo River, (**D**) Niño 3.4 index, (**E**) Marshall Southern Annular Mode index (SAM), (**F**) cell density of *Dinophysis acuminata* and *Protoceratium reticulatum*.

2.2. Spatio-Temporal Distribution of *Dinophysis* spp. and *P. reticulatum*

Five *Dinophysis* species were identified in the Reloncaví Fjord during the 10-year time series. *D. acuminata* was the most frequent species (present in 26% of the samples), followed by *D. punctata* (2% of the samples). *D. acuta*, *D. caudata* and *D. tripos* were less frequently observed (<1% of the samples). Other unidentified species were also observed and jointly quantified as *Dinophysis* spp. (present in only 5% of the samples). During the study period, *D. acuminata* was the only *Dinophysis* species with cell densities higher than the considered as bloom level for species of this genus (i.e., cell densities > 1000 cells L^{-1} [34]) Although *D. acuminata* was observed in all sampling stations, high cell densities of this species (>1000 cells L^{-1}) were usually present in the inner portion of the fjord during the spring–summer months (October to March). Blooms of *D. acuminata* were observed in the years 2008 (11,300 cells L^{-1}), 2011 (2800 cells L^{-1}) and 2014 (4200 cells L^{-1}), mostly during summer months (Figure 2F and Figure S3A). An exception was observed in the spring of 2008 when a bloom of this species was observed in the head of the fjord (2500 cells L^{-1}). High cell densities (>1000 cells L^{-1}) were also occasionally observed for this species during autumn and winter months. Although moderate densities of *P. reticulatum* (>1000 cells L^{-1}) were occasionally observed throughout the study, blooms of this species were observed in 2016 (175,700 cells L^{-1}) and 2017 (62,600 cells L^{-1}), always during the summer (Figure 2F and Figure S3B).

2.3. Niche Analysis

The Outlying Mean Index (OMI) was used to determine the combination of environmental variables that maximized average species marginality (i.e., the Euclidean distance between the mean habitat condition used by the species and the mean habitat condition of the sampling space [29]). A preliminary analysis using all samples (n = 839; not shown) indicated a strong spatial gradient due to differences in subsurface salinity observed between stations located in the exterior and the inner part of the fjord (Figure 2B). To remove the effect due to the spatial variability, only data for sampling stations 4 to 9 were included in a posterior analysis (n = 564). The OMI analysis considering only the samples from the inner part of the fjord depicted environmental gradients related to both seasonal and interannual temporal scales (Figure 3A). Together, the first two OMI axes explained 95% of the total explained variability. The OMI axis 1 accounted for the seasonal variability with the spring–summer period positively related to subsurface water temperature and negatively related to both precipitation and streamflow from the Puelo River, whereas the OMI axis 2 accounted for the interannual variability related mainly to the SAM and Niño 3.4 indexes as well as subsurface salinity. The *envfit* test [35] pointed out temperature, streamflow, SAM index as the variables accounting for most of total explained variability (R^2 = 0.88, 0.55 and 0.33, respectively; $p < 0.01$).

The OMI (i.e., species marginality) depends on the deviation from a theoretical ubiquitous, uniformly distributed species that would occur under all available habitat conditions (i.e., observed in all samples) (OMI = 0) and is inversely related to the tolerance index (an estimate of niche breath) [29]. Species with low OMI occur in typical (or common) habitats of the sampling region. They usually show high tolerance and are associated with a wide range of environmental conditions (i.e., generalists). On the contrary, species with high OMI occur in atypical habitats and are expected to have low tolerance associated with a distribution across a limited range of environmental conditions (i.e., specialists). From the six species included in the analysis, *D. acuminata*, *D. caudata*, *D. tripos*, and *P. reticulatum* showed significant OMIs ($p < 0.05$). The most uniformly distributed species was *D. acuminata* (OMI = 0.6) (used typical habitat), whereas *D. caudata* was the most specialized species followed by *D. tripos* and *P. reticulatum* (OMI = 18.80, 5.84 and 5.75, respectively) (using more atypical habitat) (Table S1).

In the OMI multivariate space, the polygon formed by all samples corresponded to the "realized environmental space" whereas the polygon formed only by the samples where a given species is present correspond do the "realized niche" of the species [36]. Both *D. acuminata* and *P. reticulatum* occupied large portions of the realized environmental space (Figure 3A,B), with the later showing a comparatively narrower realized niche (tolerance = 3.26 and 1.07, respectively). *D. acuminata* and *P. reticulatum* showed high residual tolerance when compared to the other species (8.77 and 8.38, respectively) and for both species this niche parameter accounted for more than 50% of their variability (which indicates that most variability in the niche of the two species was not explained by the environmental variables included in the analysis).

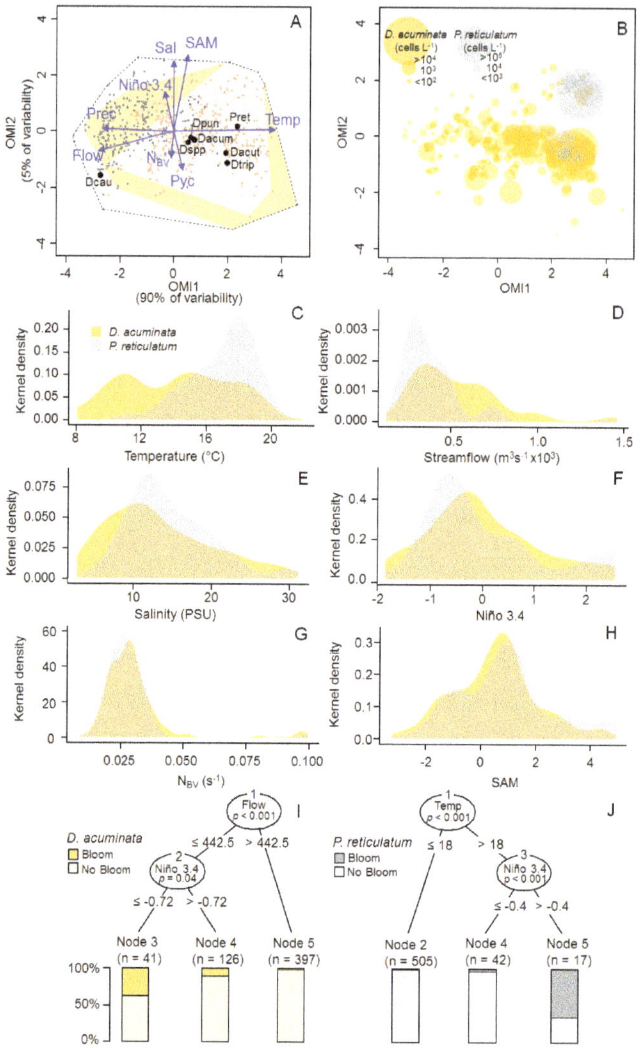

Figure 3. (**A**) Outlying Mean Index (OMI) analysis of the five *Dinophysis* species and *P. reticulatum* for the entire sampling period in the inner portion of the fjord (sampling stations 4 to 9). Blue vectors show relationship with the physical and meteorological variables. Samples from the spring–summer and autumn–winter periods are depicted in orange and grey, respectively. The dashed line delimitates the realized environmental space (i.e., sampling domain) whereas the yellow and grey polygons represent the realized niches of *D. acuminata* and *P. reticulatum*, respectively. The black dots represent the mean habitat condition used by the different species (i.e., species' niche positions). Dacum = *D. acuminata*, Dacut = *D. acuta*, Dcau = *D. caudata*, Dpun = *D. puncata*, Dtrip = *D. tripos*, Pret = *P. reticulatum*; Flow = Puelo River's Streamflow, Niño 3.4 = Niño 3.4 index, N_{BV} = Brunt–Väisälä buoyancy frequency, Pyc = depth of the pycnocline, Prec = precipitation, Sal = subsurface salinity, Temp = subsurface water temperature, SAM = Marshall Southern Annular Mode index. (**B**) Distribution of cell densities of *D. acuminata* and *P. reticulatum* in the OMI multivariate space. (**C**–**H**) Kernel density estimation (KDE) plots showing the frequency of occurrence (presence/absence) of *D. acuminata* and *P. reticulatum* related to different environmental variables. (**I**,**J**) Conditional inference trees showing main variables associated with blooms of *D. acuminata* (**I**) and *P. reticulatum* (**J**).

Kernel density estimation (KDE) plots obtained separately for each variable (Figure 3C–H) revealed some patterns regarding the presence/absence of these two species and environmental conditions. Based on that, *D. acuminata* were more frequently observed in conditions with salinities lower than 15 PSU, whereas *P. reticulatum* showed preference for temperatures between 16 and 18 °C and salinity between 10 and 15 PSU. Both species were related to Puelo River's streamflow lower than 1000 $m^3 s^{-1}$, negative to slightly positive values of the Niño 3.4 index, slightly positive values of the SAM index and N_{BV} values of ~0.025 s^{-1} (which was indicative of stratified conditions with a gradual pycnocline). Conditional inference trees indicated streamflow lower than 500 $m^3 s^{-1}$ associated with negative values of the Niño 3.4 index (<−0.4) as the conditions leading to *D. acuminata* blooms (Figure 3I). On the other hand, blooms of *P. reticulatum* occurred under temperatures higher than 18 °C and values of the Niño 3.4 index higher than −0.7 (Figure 3J).

2.4. Subniche Analysis

The Within Outlying Mean Index (WitOMI) [30] was used to decompose the ecological niche of the different species into subniches (i.e., subset of habitat conditions used by a species) taking into account interannual subsets of samples. This analysis is a refinement of the OMI analysis and provides estimations of niche shifts under different subsets of habitat conditions [31]. Considering that temperature was the main factor determining the distribution of the species in the OMI analysis when taking into account all samples and that dinoflagellate blooms were observed mostly during summer months, we decide to perform the subniche analysis considering only the samples for this season of the year (n = 167) to remove the effect of seasonal variability. As we aimed to detect the main conditions leading to the formation of blooms, only moderate to high cell densities for these two species were considered (≥1000 and ≥10,000 cells L^{-1} for *D. acuminata* and *P. reticulatum*, respectively).

2.4.1. Subsets

Summer samples from a given year were classified according to the occurrence/absence of blooms of different dinoflagellate species in the Reloncaví Fjord. Although the dinoflagellate *Prorocentrum micans* was not considered in this study, a massive bloom of this species was observed in March 2009 [37]. Thus, summer samples of this year were considered as a separate subset. According to this criterion, four subsets were recognized: (1) summer samples of years with *D. acuminata* blooms (2008, 2011, and 2014), (2) summer samples of year 2009 for which the massive *P. micans* bloom was observed, (3) summer samples of years where *P. reticulatum* blooms were observed (2015, 2016 and 2017), and (4) summer samples of years where no dinoflagellate bloom was observed.

The first two axes of the OMI analysis considering only samples from the summer period explained 89% of the total variability (Figure 4A). The OMI axis 1 accounted for the environmental temporal variability within the summer period and it was positively related to subsurface water temperature, subsurface salinity and SAM index and negatively related to precipitation and N_{BV}. The OMI axis 2 accounted for the interannual variability and was positively related to the Niño 3.4 index and streamflow. The *envfit* test indicated the Niño 3.4 index, streamflow and the SAM index as the main variables accounting for the total explained variability (R^2 = 0.62, 0.43 and 0.36, respectively; $p < 0.01$).

The four recognized subsets were distributed along the OMI axis 2 (Figure 4A). The function *subkrandtest* (implemented in the package 'subniche' in R) indicated that the main differences among the four subsets were given by the Niño 3.4 index, Puelo River's streamflow, depth of the pycnocline and subsurface salinity whereas no significant differences were observed regarding subsurface temperature, N_{BV} and the SAM index (Figure 4B–G; $p > 0.001$). Subset 1 (summers from years where *D. acuminata* blooms were observed) was characterized by low streamflow and negative values of the Niño 3.4 index. These conditions were also observed for subset 2 (summer months from the year where the massive bloom of *P. micans* was observed; [37]). Subset 3 (summer samples from years where *P. reticulatum* blooms were observed) was characterized by high Puelo River's streamflow, positive values of the Niño 3.4 index associated with slightly higher subsurface salinities and more superficial pycnocline when compared to the other subsets. Subset 4 (summers of years with no dinoflagellate blooms) was characterized by lower salinity and neutral values of the Niño 3.4 index. Although no significant difference was observed for the SAM index, this index showed a broader range in subsets 3 and 4, when compared to subsets 1 and 2.

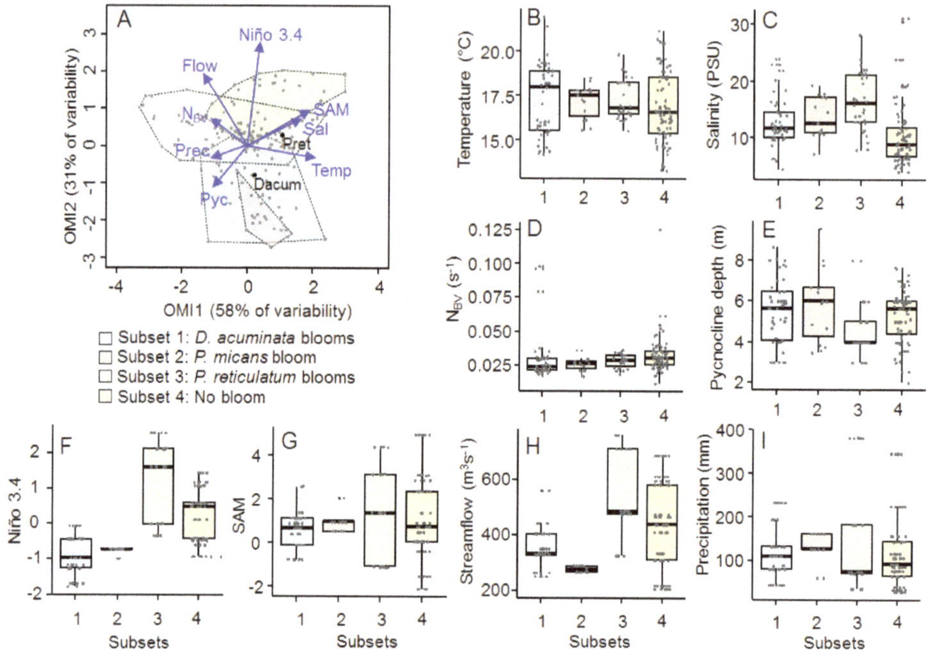

Figure 4. (**A**) Distribution of the four subsets in the OMI multivariate space considering only the summer period in the inner portion of the Reloncaví Fjord (sampling stations 4 to 9) and their relationship with environmental variables (blue vectors; see Figure 3 for meaning of labels). (**B–I**) Boxplots showing differences in the four subsets regarding subsurface water temperature (**B**), subsurface salinity (**C**), N_{BV} (Brunt–Väisälä buoyancy frequency) (**D**), pycnocline depth (**E**), Niño 3.4 index (F), SAM index (**G**), Puelo River's streamflow (**H**) and precipitation (**I**). Horizontal lines indicate the median for the different variables.

A clear separation between *D. acuminata* and *P. reticulatum* was shown by plotting their cell densities in the OMI multivariate ordination space of the summer period (Figure 5). As expected, the two species were related to the same conditions previously described as typical for the subsets where their blooms were observed (subsets 1 and 3, respectively) (Figure 5A,G). Additional conditional inference tree analysis, taking into account only the samples from the summer period, indicated that blooms of *D. acuminata* were mainly related to low streamflow whereas blooms of *P. reticulatum* were related to positive values of the Niño 3.4 and SAM indexes (not shown).

2.4.2. Subniches

The WitOMI analysis allowed the calculation of two additional marginalities: the WitOMIG (i.e., Euclidean distance between the mean habitat condition used by the species in the subset and the mean habitat condition of the sampling domain) and the WitOMIG$_k$ (i.e., Euclidean distance between the mean habitat condition used by the species in the subset and the mean habitat condition of the subset). In ecological terms, the WitOMIG allows the detection of shifts in the mean habitat conditions used by the species in each subniche whereas the WitOMIG$_k$ represents the marginality of the species within the subset (i.e., if the species uses typical or atypical habitat in the subset) [30].

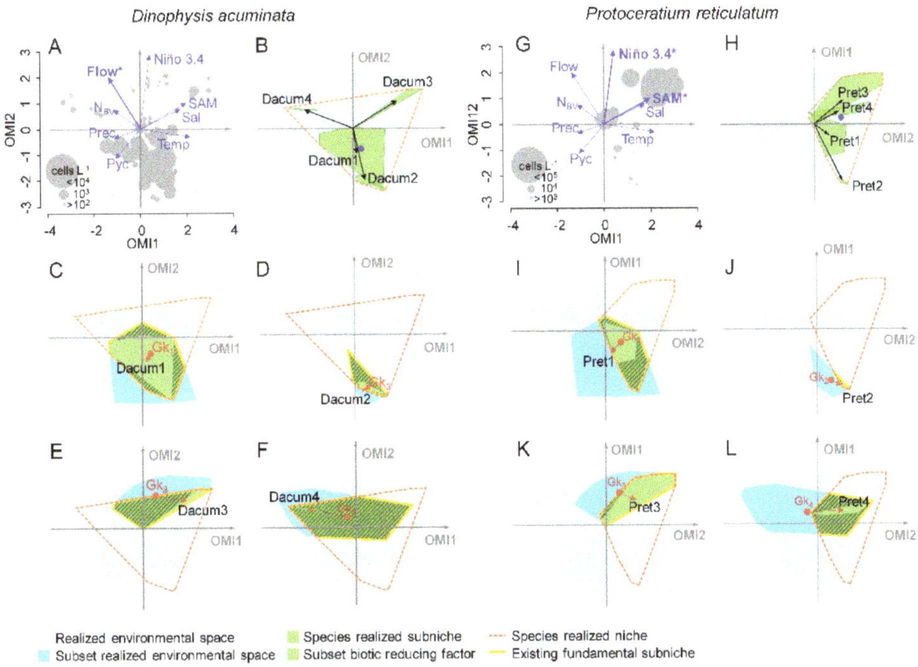

Figure 5. (**A–F**) *Dinophysis acuminata* and (**G–L**) *Protoceratium reticulatum* subniches' dynamics considering only the summer period in the inner portion of the Reloncaví Fjord (sampling stations 4 to 9) and their relationship with the physical and meteorological variables (blue vectors; see Figure 3 for meaning of labels). Main variables associated with bloom conditions for both species (detected by conditional inference tree analyses) are indicated with asterisks. The blue dots represent the mean habitat condition used by the species in the entire sampling domain (i.e., species' niche position) whereas the black labels represent the mean habitat condition used by the species in the subset (i.e., species' subniche position). The black and red vectors represent species marginalities (i.e., WitOMIG and WitOMIG$_k$, respectively). The red dots represent the mean habitat condition in each subset (G_k). The light blue polygon represents the realized environmental space (i.e., sampling domain). For each species, the existing fundamental subniches (polygons delimited by yellow lines) are given by the overlap between the subsets (dark blue polygons) and the species' realized niche (polygon delimited by dashed orange line). The difference between the existing fundamental subniche and the species subniche (light green polygons) is the "subset biotic reducing factor" (green area highlighted by diagonal lines), which correspond to the biological constraint exerted on the species that can be caused either by negative biological interactions or species dispersal limitations.

Based on this approach, we detected significant shifts in the subniche position of *D. acuminata* and *P. reticulatum* in the different subsets (Figure 5B,H). Although *D. acuminata* was distributed over the entire summer period, its used habitat was more marginal in the subsets 2, 3 and 4 (WitOMIG = 13.54, 6.40 and 10.54, respectively) than in subset 1 (WitOMIG = 1.74) (Table S2). This suggest that *D. acuminata* had a preference for the environmental habitat conditions in the subset 1. Furthermore, this species was significantly less marginal in subset 1 (WitOMIG$_k$ = 0.16; Figure 5C) when compared to subsets 2, 3 and 4 (WitOMIG$_k$ = 1.66, 2.66 and 5.56, respectively; Figure 5D–F). On the other hand, *P. reticulatum* used more common habitat in subset 1 and 3 (WitOMIG = 3.14 and 3.12, respectively) when compared to subsets 2 and 4 (WitOMIG = 12.34 and 5.44, respectively) (Table S2). Although, *P. reticulatum* showed similar marginality in the first two subsets, its realized subniche was comparatively broader in subset 3 than in subset 1 (tolerance = 1.08 and 0.24, respectively).

In the OMI multivariate space, the overlap between the polygon formed by samples of a subset and the polygon formed by the realized niche of a given species generates a third polygon that constitutes the "fundamental subniche" of this species. The area delimited by the difference between the fundamental subniche and the realized subniche correspond to the "subset biotic reducing factor", i.e., biological constraint (S_B) exerted on the species subniche that can be caused either by negative biological interactions or species dispersal limitations [30]. Both *D. acuminata* and *P. reticulatum* occupied a large position of their fundamental subniches in the subsets where their blooms were observed (subset 1 and 3, respectively) (Figure 5C,L).

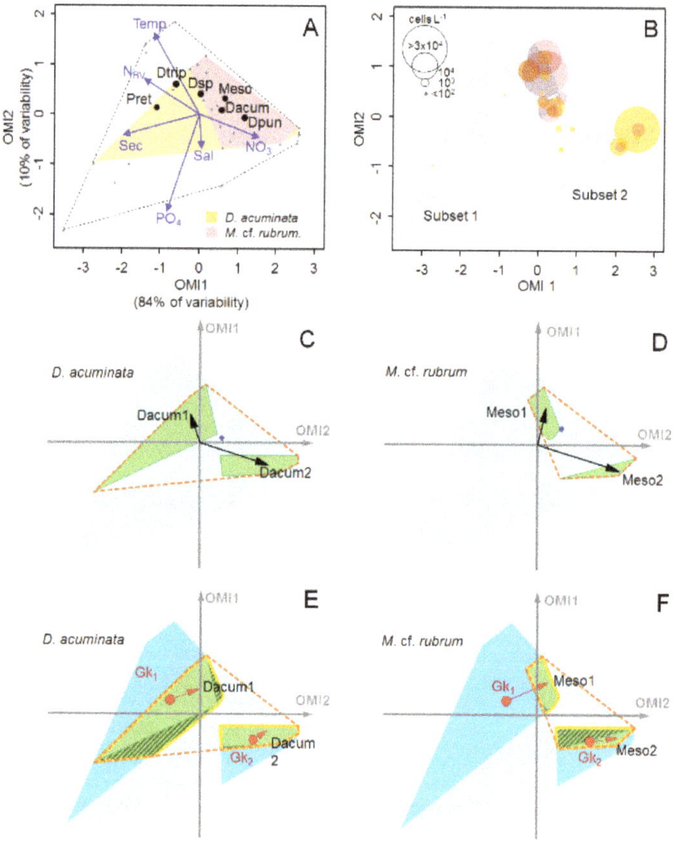

Figure 6. (**A**) OMI analysis for the summer–spring period 2008/2009 in the sampling station 8. The blue vectors show relationship with the physical and meteorological variables (see Figure 3 for meaning of labels). The black dashed line delimitates the realized environmental space (i.e., sampling domain) whereas the yellow and pink polygons represent the realize niches of *D. acuminata* and *M.* cf. *rubrum*, respectively. The black dots represent the mean habitat condition used by the different species (i.e., species' niche positions). Dacum = *D. acuminata*, Dpun = *D. puncata*, Dtrip = *D. tripos*, Dsp = *Dinophysis* sp., Meso = *Mesodinium* cf. *rubrum*, Pret = *P. reticulatum*. (**B**) Distribution of cell densities of *D. acuminata* and *M.* cf. *rubrum* in the OMI multivariate space. Blue polygons represent the two subsets. (**C, E**) *D. acuminata* and (**D, F**) *M.* cf. *rubrum* subniches' dynamics (see Figure 5 for meaning of dots, arrows and polygons).

To further assess the relative importance of biotic interactions on the subniche dynamics of *D. acuminata*, we performed an additional WitOMI analysis using a complementary dataset (previously published by Alves-de-Souza et al. [21]) that includes information on nutrient concentrations and the ciliate *M.* cf. *rubrum*. This sub-dataset was based on samples obtained every 2–3 weeks between October 2008 and March 2009 (spring–summer) from sampling station 8 (See Alves-de-Souza et al. [21] for a description of the environmental conditions during this period). The first two axes of the OMI analysis for this sub-dataset explained 94% of the variability. *D. acuminata* occupied common habitat (OMI = 0.35, tolerance = 1.69) when compared to *M.* cf. *rubrum* that was more marginal and showed a narrower realized niche (OMI = 0.52, tolerance = 0.45) (Figure 6A). Two subsets were stablished by k-mean cluster analysis of the OMI sample scores (see Methods). The OMI axis, positively related to the subset 2 (where *D. acuminata* bloom occurred), was mostly explained by NO_3^- and Secchi disk (proxy of water transparency), whereas the OMI axis 2 was related to the subset 1 (higher *M.* cf. *rubrum* cell densities) and explained mainly by temperature and PO_4^{3-} (Figure 6A,B). Although PO_4^{3-} was the variable that accounted for most of the explained variability (*envfit*; $R^2 = 0.84$), the species distribution along the OMI axis 1 seems to have been more related to Secchi disk, temperature and NO_3^- ($R^2 = 0.79, 0.77, 0.50$, respectively). Both *D. acuminata* and *M.* cf. *rubrum*. showed shifts in the subniche position and marginality (Figure 6C,D), with a stronger biotic constraint on *D. acuminata* in the realized subniche of the subset 1 (in samples where *M.* cf. *rubrum* was absent) (Figure 6E). Similarly, a strong biotic constraint on *M.* cf. *rubrum* was observed in the subset 2, concomitantly with *D. acuminata* blooms (Figure 6F).

3. Discussion

3.1. Seasonal and Interannual Variability

D. acuminata and *P. reticulatum* are widespread HAB species observed in temperate areas worldwide [34,38]. High densities of these two species have been previously reported during summer months in southern Chilean fjords [9,21,28,39]. Although they are frequently observed in low densities (<100 cells L^{-1}) [11,40,41], their blooms have being mostly regarded as episodic events of erratic occurrence. Here, we present for the first time evidence indicating that, far from having a random occurrence, blooms of both *D. acuminata* and *P. reticulatum* in the Reloncaví Fjord (and probably other fjord systems in southern Chile) are seasonal periodic events related to climatic and hydrological events of regional scale (i.e., ENSO, SAM). Moreover, our results showed that both species have different niche preferences that explain their seasonal and interannual distribution.

Results from the niche analysis considering the entire sampling period indicated that temperature and streamflow from the Puelo River were the main environmental factors associated with the seasonal variability in the Reloncaví Fjord (*envfit*; R^2 = 0.88 and 0.55, respectively) (Figure 3A). The reduced freshwater streamflow values during summer months were in agreement with the historical trend reported for this fjord, characterized by a streamflow bimodal regime with two main peaks in winter and spring related to precipitation and snowmelt, respectively [42,43]. Although blooms of both *D. acuminata* and *P. reticulatum* were associated with low streamflow (Figure 3D), the restricted occurrence of *P. reticulatum* during summer months seemed to be primarily determined by a preference of this species for surface water temperatures between 16 °C and 18 °C (Figure 3C), as previously reported for this species in culture experiments [44,45]. However, despite the fact that optimal temperatures were observed every summer, blooms of the species were only observed in years with values of the Niño 3.4 index higher than −0.4 (Figure 3J). *D. acuminata* presence was associated with a wide range of temperatures (Figure 3C) as usually observed for this species in other parts of the world [34]. These results were in disagreement with those previously reported for the Pitipalena Fjord (38°47′ S; 72°56′ W), where high temperature was suggested as a triggering factor for blooms of this species [28]. Instead, reduced streamflow from the Puelo River was found to be the main variable explaining high cell densities of *D. acuminata* in the Reloncaví Fjord during summer months, although blooms of this species were only observed in years with values of the Niño 3.4 index lower than −0.72 (Figure 3I).

The conditional inference trees suggest a hierarchical relevance of variables acting at different temporal scales in the formation of *D. acuminata* and *P. reticulatum* blooms. For both species, the first nodes of the trees were related to environmental conditions that were more relevant at the seasonal scale (i.e., low streamflow for *D. acuminata* and high temperature for *P. reticulatum*), whereas the second node depicted the main variable acting at the interannual scale (Niño 3.4 for both species) (Figure 3I,J). Shifts in the relative importance of environmental conditions according to the considered temporal scale have been previously reported for other microbial communities [46–48], with the interplay between factors acting at both seasonal and interannual scales determining the time-window of species occurrence [49]. In the specific case of the Reloncaví Fjord, our results indicate that although the time window for occurrence of *D. acuminata* and *P. reticulatum* are determined by variables acting at the seasonal scale, the formation of their blooms are ultimately defined by hydrological and climatological conditions acting at an interannual scale.

3.2. Summer Subsets

The niche and subniche analyses considering only the summer dataset allowed us to obtain a better understanding of the factors behind the interannual variability in blooms of *D. acuminata* and *P. reticulatum* during the 10-year time series (Figures 4 and 5). These analyses indicated that the interannual distribution of the two species was also related to the SAM index in addition to the effect of streamflow and Niño 3.4 index (*envfit*; R^2 = 0.36, 0.62 and 0.43, respectively; $p < 0.01$). Although reduced Puelo River's streamflow is generally observed in summer months, when compared to winter and spring [42,43], summers with *D. acuminata* blooms (subset 1) were characterized by even lower values of streamflow than the typically observed for this season of the year (Figures 4H and 5A) in association with the most negative values of the Niño 3.4 index (la Niña conditions) for the studied period (Figure 3F) (*subkrandtest*; $p < 0.001$ for both streamflow and Niño 3.4 indexes). On the other hand, summers with *P. reticulatum* blooms (subset 3) were characterized by positive values of the Niño 3.4 index (El Niño conditions) (*subkrandtest*; $p < 0.001$). This subset was further differentiated by higher variability in the SAM index, with a median value that was slightly more positive than the observed median values for the other subsets (Figure 4G). Although these differences were not significant (*subkrandtest*; $p = 0.128$), higher *P. reticulatum* cell densities were positively related to the SAM index (Figure 5G). This was further confirmed by a conditional inference tree considering only the summer dataset, which indicated positive values for both Niño 3.4 and SAM indexes as the main conditions associated with blooms of this species. These conditions were associated with higher salinities and shallower pycnoclines in the subset 3 (Figure 4C,E) (*subkrandtest*; $p = 0.128$).

ENSO is a coupled ocean-atmosphere phenomenon over the equatorial Pacific, characterized by irregular fluctuations between warm (El Niño) and cold (La Niña) conditions in the sea surface temperature, whereas SAM is an atmospheric mode of circulation that appears to modulate the air temperature over the southern tip of South America caused by pressure anomalies between the Antarctic and the 40–50° S circumpolar band [50]. The El Niño conditions are related to increase in the sea surface pressure (SLP) and weakening of westerlies in the southern extreme of the continent that may result in lower precipitation in western Patagonia when compared to average conditions [51]. At the same time, positive SAM levels lead to the intensification of the westerlies around the Antarctic periphery and weakening around 40° S, causing lower precipitation and increased air temperature over western Patagonia [43,52].

The relevance of the ENSO/SAM interplay for the occurrence of harmful algal blooms (HABs) in southern Chilean fjords has been demonstrate in a previous study, where it explained the formation of the most impressive HAB observed to date in southern Chile caused by the phytoflagellate *Pseudochatonella verruculosa* (Dictyochophyceae) in February–March 2016 [43]. As this bloom was observed just after the *P. reticulatum* bloom in January 2016 (the denser bloom of this species in the entire 10-year time series), both events were likely affected in a similar way by the existing climatological conditions. At this opportunity, Leon-Muñoz et al. [43] proposed that the combination between the strong El Niño event and the positive phase of SAM led to very dry conditions (both in terms of low precipitation and reduced freshwater input) associated with high radiation and reduced westerly wind, which in turn resulted in weakening of vertical stratification and the consequent advection of more saline and nutrient rich waters that ultimately determined the formation of the *P. verruculosa* bloom. Our data does not entirely support this hypothesis as (1) no significant difference among the different summer subsets was detected regarding either precipitation or the Brunt–Väisälä frequency (proxy of vertical stratification) and (2) the Puelo River's streamflow levels for subset 3 (that includes the summer 2016) were actually higher when compared to the other summer subsets (*subkrandtest*; $p > 0.001$). This discrepancy could be explained by the differential treatment of the data as well as the considered time-window in both studies: while Leon-Muñoz et al. [43] detected a decreasing trend for both precipitation and river streamflow based on accumulated annual values of these variables in the last five decades, we based our conclusions on the comparison of monthly values only in the last decade. Similarly, analyses reinforcing our conclusions were based on hundreds of CTD profiles collected during throughout the study period. Although it is clear that a trend does exist regarding the decrease in precipitation and Puelo River's streamflow in the Reloncaví Fjord [42,43], our results indicate that it was not the factor explaining the *P. verruculosa* and *P. reticulatum* blooms during the summer 2016. Instead, blooms of both species were explained by an increase in salinity (as suggested by Leon-Muñoz et al. [43]) likely caused by the shallowing of the pycnocline that facilitated the advection of more saline and (supposedly) nutrient rich water to the surface.

Of special notice was the occurrence of the massive bloom of the dinoflagellate *P. micans* in the summer 2009 (~10^5 cells L^{-1}; [37]), despite the fact that environmental and climatological conditions (low Puelo River's streamflow and La Niña conditions) seemed to be favorable for *D. acuminata* blooms. This was interesting, as both species seem to have an overlap on their realized subniches. The reason for this discrepancy could be potentially related to variables that were not considered in the present study (e.g., dissolved inorganic nutrient concentrations). While both species are mixotrophic, they show very distinctive nutritional strategies: *P. micans* seems to be mostly facultative mixotroph, whereas *D. acuminata* relies on both photosynthesis and feeding on the ciliate *M.* cf. *rubrum* [34]. While *D. acuminata* shows high affinity by regenerate nitrogen sources (i.e., ammonia and urea) [53,54], a positive relationship between blooms of *M.* cf. *rubrum* and nitrate concentrations have been observed [55]. Available nutrient information for the head of the Reloncaví Fjord indicated that both nitrate and silicic acid concentrations were significantly lower in summer 2009 when compared to summer 2008 [21], which could have potentially favored the *P. micans* bloom formation.

The reduced river streamflow in the subsets 1 and 2 associated with negative values of Niño 3.4 index is intriguing, since higher precipitations could be expected during La Niña conditions [50]. The absence of significant differences in precipitation among the subsets could be explained by the lack of a clear signal in El Niño/La Niña conditions in the southern extreme of South America regarding precipitation [50]. While precipitation and streamflow were correlated ($R = 0.58$; $p > 0.01$) [42], no significant differences among the four subsets were detected regarding the former variable. This suggests that river streamflow levels during the study period depended mostly on snowmelt that could be expected to be less important in colder years (La Niña conditions). Another interesting aspect is the counter intuitive lack of correlation between streamflow levels and the depth of the pycnocline, with subsets 1 and 3 (with lower streamflow) showing deeper pycnoclines when compared to subset 3 (with higher streamflow). The explanation for this remains elusive, but could be related to microscale oceanographic aspects, such as internal waves or seiches [56].

3.3. Subniches and Reducing Biotic Factors

Several aspects revealed by the subniche analysis (Figure 5) further confirmed the preference of *D. acuminata* and *P. reticulatum* for the environmental conditions observed in the subsets where their blooms occurred (subsets 1 and 3, respectively). First, the broader realized subniches of the two species in their respective subsets (indicated by larger tolerances in Table S2) indicated a better efficiency in using the available resources [30]. This is also evidenced by a larger occupied portion of their fundamental subniches in these subsets (i.e., fundamental and realized niches have similar areas) (Figure 5C,L). The unfavorable conditions for *D. acuminata* and *P. reticulatum* in the years without dinoflagellate blooms (subset 4) are reflected in larger values of WitOMIG for both species in this subset (indicated by the length of the red arrows in Figure 5F,M).

One of the advantages of the WitOMI analysis is that it allows the estimation of the biological constraints (S_B) exerted on the species, which is proportional to the space unoccupied by the species in its fundamental subniche (indicated by the green area highlighted by diagonal lines in Figure 5) [30]. This absence is interpreted as caused by biological constraint and can be due either to negative biotic interactions (e.g., parasitism, predation) or dispersal limitation of the species itself [57]. Interestingly, both *D. acuminata* and *P. reticulatum* showed a smaller unoccupied portion of their fundamental niches (attributed to biological constraint) in the subsets where their blooms were observed (Figure 6C,L, respectively). In the case of *D. acuminata*, the magnitude of biological constraint was even more impressive in the subset 4 (years without dinoflagellate blooms) (Figure 5F).

Although these results need to be interpreted with caution, the observed pattern shown in Figure 5C–F suggest that *D. acuminata* occurrence in the Reloncaví Fjord during the studied period was mostly modulated by biological constraints. Among the biotic factors affecting *Dinophysis* spp. dynamics, the availability of its prey (the ciliate *M.* cf. *rubrum*) is by far the most relevant [58]. Species of this genus are obligate mixotrophs that require both feeding on *M.* cf. *rubrum* and light for sustained growth [32,58–60]. In addition, M. cf. *rubrum* also depends on the ingestion of live prey to sustain growth (i.e., cryptophytes of the genera *Teleaulax* and *Geminigera*) [61]. In field populations, *Dinophysis* species may be under prey limitation for long periods, with maximal cell densities being preceded or co-occurring with high densities of *M.* cf. *rubrum* ciliates, resulting in predator–prey encounters and interactions [62–64], suggesting that the presence of the *Dinophysis-Mesodinium*-cryptophytes food chain may be used as a good indicator of upcoming *Dinophysis* spp. blooms [64].

D. acuminata blooms in co-occurrence with *M.* cf. *rubrum* was previously reported in the Reloncaví Fjord in a study using a sampling frequency of 2–3 weeks [21]. In this study, we revisited this dataset using the WitOMI approach to estimate the degree of biological constraint on both species during their period of co-occurrence. As the S_B estimation is based on the absence of the species in sampling units where it should be present (as they are encompassed into the species fundamental niche), this approach can be extremely useful to obtain insights on biotic interactions involving time-lags (such as predator–prey interactions) even when short-frequency data are not available. Indeed, the clear mismatch between maximal cell densities of *D. acuminata* and *M.* cf. *rubrum* (Figure 6B) was congruent with the time-lagged correlation observed in other studies [62–64], whereas the strongest biological constraint on *D. acuminata* was observed in periods where *M.* cf. *rubrum* was absent (Figure 6E). Similarly, a strong biotic constraint on the ciliate was observed concomitantly to highest *D. acuminata* cell densities (Figure 6F).

3.4. Additional Aspects Affecting D. acuminata

Although *D. acuminata* is observed under a broad range of environmental conditions, blooms of this species are consistently associated with increased stratification [65]. Similarly, physical driving forces (e.g., wind and/or currents) causing accumulation/dispersion of *D. acuminata* cells have been pointed out as an important factor [66–69]. DSP events in bays used for shellfish production are frequently observed after the transport of *D. acuminata* cells from the near continental shelf [70–72], where they are frequently found in dense populations (>10^4 cells L^{-1}) occurring in thin layers [73,74].

Formation of *D. acuminata* blooms within coastal areas is better understood in upwelling influenced systems, more specifically the Galician rías [34]. In these systems, *D. acuminata* blooms are mostly initiated after the advection of cells from offshore ("pelagic seed banks") with upwelled waters [62], although blooms can also be originated from persistence of autochthonous winter populations [75]. In both cases, accumulation of cells in the pycnocline and encounter with the mixotrophic ciliate *M.* cf. *rubrum* lead to cell proliferation [62,63].

By comparison, little is known about the environmental conditions leading to the development of *D. acuminata* blooms in fjords. The information from Swedish fjords points out to the formation of *D. acuminata* thin layers associated with strong stratification caused by freshwater input from land run-off, e.g., [76,77], whereas the interannual variability of this species seems to be related to climatic events of regional scale (i.e., the North Atlantic Oscillation; NAO) [78] favoring the entrainment and advection of cells from offshore [79]. Although we also established a link between the climate conditions and *D. acuminata* interannual variability, it is not clear how the reduction in river streamflow during La Niña conditions ultimately leads to high *D. acuminata* cell densities. Similarly to the observed blooms from their Swedish counterparts, blooms of *D. acuminata* in southern Chile fjords are more frequently reported from permanent salinity-driven stratified systems [39,40], where they show heterogeneous vertical distribution associated with the pycnocline [21,28]. Results from an intertidal experiment in the Patipalena Fjord [28] indicate that the vertical distribution of *D. acuminata* cells is affected by the vertical movement of the pycnocline caused by shear instabilities. Thus, a possibility to be explored is if changes in the streamflow levels affect the microscale circulation features patterns in southern Chilean fjords that could favor the accumulation of cells in the pycnocline.

Another important aspect to be clarified is the origin of the *D. acuminata* populations occurring inside the Reloncaví Fjord. The spatial patterns observed during the 10-year time series (Figure 1F) indicate that the highest cell densities of *D. acuminata* are first observed in areas close to the head of the fjords and posteriorly in the middle portion. Although this suggest that blooms originated in the interior of the fjord and posteriorly transported to the external locations through the surface outflow [80], it is not clear if they are originated from persistent winter populations or advected cells that could enter the fjord through the inflow layer. High *D. acuminata* cell densities correspondent to what is widely considered as bloom level for this species (>1000 cells L^{-1}) are occasionally observed during winter conditions (likely remnants from summer blooms). As *Dinophysis* species can survive without prey for months [32,81], these winter cells could constitute suitable inoculum for the next spring–summer populations [34]. Finally, the viability of putative *D. acuminata* overwintering cells (i.e., cells with reddish pigmentation observed at the end of growth season) observed in bottom layers of Reloncaví Fjord [34] should be determined.

The final major question to be answered is if the interannual variability observed in this study was due to factors affecting *D. acuminata* per se or the effect of the environmental conditions on its putative prey. While blooms of *M.* cf. *rubrum* ciliates are a common occurrence in the upwelling areas off Central-Northern Chile [82], the limited quantitative information on the occurrence of *M.* cf. *rubrum* ciliates in southern Chilean fjords and adjacent seas indicates that they are present in low cell densities throughout the year with maximal cell concentrations (and episodic blooms) observed during summer–spring months [21,82,83]. This suggests that the environmental conditions for their development are not usually suitable for mass proliferation within the zone of fjords and channels further south. Of note is the fact that the denser blooms of *M.* cf. *rubrum* ciliates in southern Chile were reported under La Niña conditions, in the years 1975 [84] and 1978 [85] for the Straits of Magellan (54°01′ S; 71°46′ W) and Aysén Fjord (45°22′ S; 73°04′ W), respectively. Thus, one hypothesis to be assessed is if oceanographic conditions during La Niña would facilitate the advection and development of offshore populations in the zone of fjords and channels which would posteriorly result in *Dinophysis* blooms.

3.5. Concluding Remarks

The interannual variability in *D. acuminata* and *P. reticulatum* in the Reloncaví Fjord was strongly linked to climatological events of regional scale (i.e., ENSO and SAM), with cold years (La Niña condition) associated with low Puelo River's streamflow being more favorable to the development of *D. acuminata* blooms, whereas strong El Niño events coupled to the positive phase of the SAM index lead to *P. reticulatum* blooms. These outcomes become more relevant as anthropogenic climate changes has been reported to cause a tendency in SAM toward its positive phase [52], which could change the current scenario characterizing dinoflagellate blooms in southern Chilean fjords.

4. Materials and Methods

4.1. Study Area and Datasets

The Reloncaví Fjord (~41.6° S), located in the uppermost region of the Chilean fjord zone, is the site of one of the largest mytilid Chilean production areas (Figure 1). The fjord is 60-km long, has a surface of 170 km^2, a maximum depth of 460 m and constitutes a representative model for other fjords in the region. The fjord has an annual average streamflow of 650 $m^3\ s^{-1}$ and a pluvio-nival regime. Its circulation is mostly regulated by freshwater input from the Puelo River, which drains a trans-Andean watershed and empties into the middle of Reloncaví Fjord and reaches its maximum streamflow in winter (rainfall) and spring (snowmelt) [43]. Streamflow of the Puelo River is significantly correlated with the streamflow of other rivers that drain into the middle and head of the Reloncaví Fjord as well as with the other main tributary rivers of the coastal systems in western Patagonia [86].

Phytoplankton samples were collected from integrated hose-samplers (0–10 m) and immediately fixed with 1% Lugol's solution. Potentially toxic algae were quantified using an inverted microscope (Olympus CKX41) using sedimentation chambers (20 mL) at 400×, according to Utermöhl [87]. Water temperature (°C), salinity (PSU) and density (σt) profiles were obtained using a Seabird 19 CTD. The Brunt–Väisälä buoyancy frequency (N_{BV}, s^{-1}) was estimated based on changes of water density over depth [33]. The N_{BV} was estimated for every 1-m interval and the largest value was used as representative of the water column stratification. Monthly accumulated values for streamflow and precipitation data for the hydrological stations Carrera Basilio (41°36′16″ S, 72°12′23″ W) and Puelo (41°39′4″ S, 72°18′42″ W) were obtained from the Climate Explorer [88]. Monthly values for the Niño 3.4 index and the Marshall Southern Annular Mode (SAM) index were obtained from the U.S. National Oceanic and Atmospheric Administration (NOAA) [89]. As the IFOP data series misses information on nutrient concentrations, a complementary analysis was performed using an additional dataset obtained from samples collected every 2–3 weeks from October 2008 and March 2009 from sampling station 8 (published by Alves-de-Souza et al. [21]). CTD (Sea Bird 19-plus) casts were used to obtain real time vertical profiles of salinity, temperature and fluorescence. Guided by the profile reading, five depths were selected: subsurface (1), above (2) and below (3) the pycnocline, the fluorescence maximum (4) and 16 m (5). Besides the variables above mentioned, this dataset includes concentration of NO_3^-, PO_4^{3-} and $Si(OH)_4$, water transparency (Secchi disc), as well as the cell densities of the ciliate *M.* cf. *rubrum*. For a detailed description on the sample collection and analyses regarding this dataset, see Alves-de-Souza et al. [21].

4.2. Statistical Analysis

Before the analysis, the 10-year dataset (n = 1170) was inspected in order to exclude the sampling dates for which abiotic measurements were not available. Cell densities were previously transformed [ln(x+1)] to reduce the effect of dominant species whereas environmental variables were standardized to values between 0 and 1, based on the minimum and maximum values of each variable [48]. All the statistical analyses described as follows were performed in R software (R Core Team, 2013) using packages freely available on the CRAN repository [90].

4.2.1. Niche Analysis

Data were arranged in one matrix containing the algal cell densities (*Dinophysis* species and *P. reticulatum*) and a second matrix containing the environmental variables (i.e., subsurface water temperature, subsurface salinity, Brunt–Väisälä frequency, Niño 3.4 index and SAM index). The OMI analysis [29] was performed using the function *niche* in the 'ade4' package [91]. The reasoning behind the OMI analysis was described in detail by Dolédec et al. [29]. Briefly, a PCA was first performed using the environmental matrix to determine the position of the sampling units (SUs) in the multivariate space, with the origin of the PCA axes corresponding to the center of gravity (*G*) of the SUs (i.e., represents the average mean habitat of the sampling domain). Based on the distribution of the species in the different SUs, a center of gravity was calculated for each species considering only the samples where the species occurred. This center of gravity represents the mean habitat condition used by the species. The OMIs for the different species were then estimated by the Euclidean distance between the species center of gravity and *G*. The total inertia is proportional to the average marginality of species and represents a quantification of the influence of the environmental variables on the niche separation of the species [29]. The statistical significance of the calculated marginalities (i.e., OMIs) were tested using Monte Carlo permutations included in the packages 'ade4' (10,000 permutations).

4.2.2. Subniche analysis

The WitOMI calculation was performed using the package 'subniche' [36] considering the same species and environmental variables mentioned previously for the OMI analysis. The WitOMI is based on parameters similar to the ones calculated in the OMI analysis, but instead of using the entire sampling domain, it considers one subset at time [30]. For the 10-year data series, the subsets were defined a priori (as explained in the Results section), whereas for the complementary WitOMI analysis using the dataset previously published by Alves-de-Souza et al. [21], the subsets were defined by a k-mean cluster analysis of the OMI scores of the SUs using the function *fact* of the package 'knitr' [92], with the optimal number of clusters previously determined using the function *fviz_nbclust* of the package 'factoextra' [93]. In both cases, the center of gravity of the SUs (G_k) (i.e., mean habitat condition in the subset), and the center of gravity of the different species in the subset (i.e., mean habitat condition used for the species in the subset) were calculated. Based on these parameters, the two additional marginalities (WitOMI*G* and WitOMIG_k) were calculated. For a detailed explanation on the WitOMI analysis, see Karasiewicz et al. [30].

The function *subkrandtest* in the package 'subniche' was used to check for differences in the physical and meteorological conditions among the four subsets. The null hypothesis in this test being that "G_k is not different from the overall habitat condition represented by *G*" [94]. The statistical significances of the calculated marginalities (WitOMI*G* and WitOMIG_k) were tested using the function *subnikrandtest* in the 'subniche' package. In the case of the WitOMI*G*, the null hypothesis is that "each species within a subset is uninfluenced by its overall average condition" whereas for the WitOMI*Gk* the null hypothesis states that "each species within a subset is uninfluenced by its subset average condition" [94]. Both functions are based on Monte Carlo permutation test (10,000 permutations). A tutorial for the WitOMI analysis is available at [94].

4.2.3. Relevance of Environmental Variables

Correlation among variables was checked by Pearson analysis. The function *envfit* from the package 'vegan' [35] was used to fit the environmental variables to the OMI scores. To visualize the frequency of occurrence (based on presence/absence) of *D. acuminata* and *P. reticulatum* related to the different environmental variables, Kernel density estimation (KDE) plots were obtained using the function *geom-density* of the package 'ggplot2' [95]. Finally, the relative importance of the different environmental variables to *D. acuminata* and *P. reticulatum* blooms was accessed by conditional inference tree analysis using the function *ctree* in the package 'party' [96]. For that, the density of the two species was converted to a categorical variable with two levels: "bloom" and "no bloom". Bloom levels were stablished as higher than 1000 and 10,000 cells L^{-1} for *D. acuminata* [34] and *P. reticulatum* [97], respectively. Although the conditional inference tree analyses for both species considered all the environmental variables (i.e., water temperature, salinity, Brunt–Väisälä frequency, Niño 3.4 index and SAM index) only the significant variables ($p < 0.05$) associated with blooms were depicted in the trees.

Supplementary Materials: The following are available online at http://www.mdpi.com/2072-6651/11/1/19/s1. Figure S1: (A–H) Box-plots showing seasonal median values for the physical and meteorological variables in the different years. (I) Examples of salinity vertical profiles related to the different values of the Brunt–Väisälä buoyancy frequency. Figure S2: Salinity vertical profiles. Figure S3: Box-plots showing seasonal median values for *Dinophysis acuminata* (A) and *Protoceratium reticulatum* (B) in the different years. Table S1: Niche parameters estimated through the OMI analysis for the five *Dinophysis* species and *Protoceratium reticulatum* in the Reloncaví Fjord during the 10-year time series. Table S2: Subniche parameters estimated through the WitOMI analysis of *Dinophysis acuminata* (Dacum) and *Protoceratium reticulatum* (Pret) in the Reloncaví Fjord for the summer months during the 10-year time series.

Author Contributions: Conceptualization, C.A.-d.-S. and J.I.M.; Data curation, C.A.-d.-S. and J.I.M.; Formal analysis, C.A.-d.-S.; Funding acquisition, C.A.-d.-S. and J.I.M.; Investigation, C.A.-d.-S., J.L.I. and J.I.M. Methodology, C.A.-d.-S.; Project administration, C.A.-d.-S. and J.I.M.; Supervision, C.A.-d.-S. and J.I.M.; Visualization, C.A.-d.-S.; Writing—original draft, C.A.-d.-S.; Writing—review and editing, C.A.-d.-S., J.L.I. and J.I.M.

Funding: C.A.S. was supported by the UNCW's Marine Biotechnology Program (MARBIONC) funded by the State of North Carolina (U.S.A.).

Acknowledgments: We are grateful to the Chilean Fishing Promotion Institute (IFOP; "Instituto de Fomento Pesquero") for allowing us access to the data used in this work. We are also appreciative of Aaron Cooke and Thomas Williamson for the English review of the manuscript and Emma Cascales for her help in the processing of CTD data. The general view of "Harmful Bloom Algae" perspective for sub-antarctic Patagonian fjords is in the framework of the FONDAP—IDEAL Center (Program 15150003).

Conflicts of Interest: The authors declare no conflict of interest.

References

1. van Dolah, F. Marine algal toxins: Origins, health effects, and their increased occurrence. *Environ. Health Perspect.* **2000**, *108*, 133–141. [CrossRef] [PubMed]
2. Reguera, B.; Riobó, P.; Rodríguez, F.; Díaz, P.A.; Pizarro, G.; Paz, B.; Franco, J.M.; Blanco, J. *Dinophysis* toxins: Causative organisms, distribution and fate in shellfish. *Mar. Drugs* **2014**, *12*, 394–461. [CrossRef] [PubMed]
3. Hamano, Y.; Kinoshita, Y.; Yasumoto, T. Enteropathogenicity of diarrhetic shellfish toxins in intestinal models. *J. Food Hyg. Soc. Jpn.* **1986**, *27*, 375–379. [CrossRef]
4. Blanco, J.; Moroño, A.; Fernández, M.L. Toxic episodes in shellfish, produced by lipophilic phycotoxins: An overview. *Rev. Gal. Rec. Mar. (Monog.)* **2005**, *1*, 1–70.
5. Tubaro, A.; Dell'Ovo, V.; Sosa, S.; Florio, C. Yessotoxins: A toxicological overview. *Toxicon* **2010**, *56*, 163–172. [CrossRef] [PubMed]
6. Álvarez, G.; Uribe, E.; Regueiro, J.; Blanco, J.; Fraga, S. *Gonyaulax taylorii*, a new yessotoxins-producer dinoflagellate species from Chilean waters. *Harmful Algae* **2016**, *58*, 8–15. [CrossRef]
7. Tillmann, U.; Elbrächter, M.; Krock, B.; John, U.; Cembella, A. *Azadinium spinosum* gen. et sp. nov. (Dinophyceae) identified as a primary producer of azaspiracid toxins. *Eur. J. Phycol.* **2009**, *44*, 63–79. [CrossRef]
8. Muñoz, F.; Avaria, S.; Sieveiï, H.; Prado, R. Presencia de dinoflagelados toxicos del genero *Dinophysis* en el seno Aysén, Chile. *Rev. Biol. Mar.* **1992**, *27*, 187–212.
9. Uribe, J.C.; García, C.; Rivas, M.; Lagos, N. First report of diarrhetic shellfish toxins in Magellanic Fjords, southern Chile. *J. Shellfish Res.* **2001**, *20*, 69–74.
10. Cassis, D.; Muñoz, P.; Avaria, S. Variación temporal del fitoplancton entre 1993 y 1998 en una estación fija del seno Aysén, Chile (45°26′S 73°00′W). *Rev. Biol. Mar. Oceanogr.* **2002**, *37*, 43–65. [CrossRef]
11. Seguel, M.; Tocornal, M.A.; Sfeir, A. Floraciones algales nocivas en los canales y fiordos del sur de Chile. *Cienc. Tecnol. Mar.* **2005**, *28*, 5–13.

12. Pizarro, G.; Paz, B.; Alarcón, C.; Toro, C.; Frangópulos, M.; Salgado, P.; Olave, C.; Zamora, C.; Pacheco, H.; Guzmán, L. Winter distribution of toxic, potentially toxic phytoplankton, and shellfish toxins in fjords and channels of the Aysén region, Chile. *Lat. Am. J. Aquat. Res.* **2018**, *46*, 120–139. [CrossRef]
13. Moreno-Pino, M.; Krock, B.; De la Iglesia, R.; Echenique-Subiabre, I.; Pizarro, G.; Vásquez, M.; Trefault, N. Next Generation Sequencing and mass spectrometry reveal high taxonomic diversity and complex phytoplankton-phycotoxins patterns in Southeastern Pacific fjords. *Toxicon* **2018**. [CrossRef] [PubMed]
14. Guzmán, L.; Campodónico, E. Mareas rojas en Chile. *Interciencia* **1978**, *3*, 144–149.
15. Zhao, J.; Lembeye, G.; Cenci, G.; Wall, B.; Yasumoto, T. Determination of okadaic acid and dinophysistoxin-1 in mussels from Chile, Italy and Ireland. In *Toxic Phytoplankton Blooms in the Sea*; Smayda, T.J., Shimizu, Y., Eds.; Elsevier: Amsterdam, The Netherlands, 1993; pp. 587–592.
16. García, C.; González, V.; Cornejo, C.; Palma-Fleming, H.; Lagos, N. First evidence of dinophisistoxin-1 and carcinogenic polycyclic aromatic hydrocarbons in smoked bivalves collected in the patagonic fjords. *Toxicon* **2004**, *43*, 121–131. [CrossRef]
17. García, C.; Pruzzo, N.; Rodríguez-Unda, N.; Contreras, C.; Lagos, N. First evidence of Okadaic acid acyl-derivative and dinophysistoxin-3 in mussel samples collected in Chiloe Island, southern Chile. *J. Toxicol. Sci.* **2010**, *35*, 335–344. [CrossRef] [PubMed]
18. Lembeye, G.; Yasumoto, T.; Zhao, J.; Fernández, R. DSP outbreak in Chilean Fjords. In *Toxic Phytoplankton Blooms in the Sea*; Smayda, T.J., Shimizu, Y., Eds.; Elsevier: Amsterdam, The Netherlands, 1993; pp. 525–529.
19. Garcia, C.; Rodriguez-Unda, N.; Contreras, C.; Barriga, A.; Lagos, N. Lipophilic toxin profiles detected in farmed and benthic mussels populations from the most relevant production zones in southern Chile. *Food Addit. Contam. A* **2012**, *29*, 1011–1020. [CrossRef] [PubMed]
20. Trefault, N.; Krock, B.; Delherbe, N.; Cembella, A.; Vásquez, M. Latitudinal transects in the southeastern Pacific Ocean reveal a diverse but patchy distribution of phycotoxins. *Toxicon* **2011**, *58*, 389–397. [CrossRef] [PubMed]
21. Alves-de-Souza, C.; Varela, D.; Contreras, C.; de La Iglesia, P.; Fernández, P.; Hipp, B.; Hernández, C.; Riobó, P.; Reguera, B.; Franco, J.M. Seasonal variability of *Dinophysis* spp. and *Protoceratium reticulatum* associated to lipophilic shellfish toxins in a strongly stratified Chilean fjord. *Deep Sea Res. II Top. Stud. Oceanogr.* **2014**, *101*, 152–162. [CrossRef]
22. Goto, H.; Igarashi, T.; Watai, M.; Yasumoto, T.; Gomez, O.V.; Valdivia, G.L.; Noren, E.; Gisselson, L.A.; Graneli, E. Worldwide occurrence of pectenotoxins and yessotoxins in shellfish and phytoplankton. In *Harmful Algal Blooms 2000, Proceedings of the IX International Conference on Harmful Alga Blooms, Hobart, Australia, 7–11 February 2000*; Hallegraeff, G., Blackburn, S.I., Bolch, C.J., Lewis, R.J., Eds.; Intergovernmental Oceanographic Commission of UNESCO: Paris, France, 2001; p. 49.
23. Pizarro, G.; Alarcón, C.; Franco, J.M.; Escalera, L.; Reguera, B.; Vidal, G.; Palma, M.; Guzmán, L. Distribución espacial de *Dinophysis* spp. y detección de toxinas DSP en el agua mediante resinas DIAION (verano 2006, X región de Chile). *Cienc. Tecnol. Mar.* **2011**, *34*, 31–48.
24. Fux, E.; Smith, J.L.; Tong, M.; Guzmán, L.; Anderson, D.M. Toxin profiles of five geographical isolates of *Dinophysis* spp. from North and South America. *Toxicon* **2011**, *57*, 275–287. [CrossRef] [PubMed]
25. Villarroel, O. Detección de toxina paralizante, diarreica y amnésica en mariscos de la XI región por cromatografía de alta resolución (HPLC) y bioensayo de ratón. *Cienc. Tecnol. Mar.* **2004**, *27*, 33–42.
26. Yasumoto, T.; Takizawa, A. Fluorometric measurement of yessotoxins in shellfish by highpressure liquid chromatography. *Biosci. Biotechnol. Biochem.* **1997**, *61*, 1775–1777. [CrossRef] [PubMed]
27. López-Rivera, A.; O'callaghan, K.; Moriarty, M.; O'driscoll, D.; Hamilton, B.; Lehane, M.; James, K.; Furey, A. First evidence of azaspiracids (AZAs): A family of lipophilic polyether marine toxins in scallops (*Argopecten purpuratus*) and mussels (*Mytilus chilensis*) collected in two regions of Chile. *Toxicon* **2010**, *55*, 692–701. [CrossRef] [PubMed]
28. Díaz, P.; Molinet, C.; Caceres, M.A.; Valle-Levinson, A. Seasonal and intratidal distribution of *Dinophysis* spp. in a Chilean fjord. *Harmful Algae* **2011**, *10*, 155–164. [CrossRef]
29. Dolédec, S.; Chessel, D.; Gimaret-Carpentier, C. Niche separation in community analysis: A new method. *Ecology* **2000**, *81*, 2914–2927. [CrossRef]

30. Karasiewicz, S.; Dolédec, S.; Lefebvre, S. Within outlying mean indexes: Refining the OMI analysis for the realized niche decomposition. *PeerJ* **2017**, *5*, e3364. [CrossRef] [PubMed]
31. Karasiewicz, S.; Breton, E.; Lefebvre, A.; Fariñas, T.H.; Lefebvre, S. Realized niche analysis of phytoplankton communities involving HAB: *Phaeocystis* spp. as a case study. *Harmful Algae* **2018**, *72*, 1–13. [CrossRef] [PubMed]
32. Park, M.G.; Kim, S.; Kim, H.S.; Myung, G.; Kang, Y.G.; Yih, W. First successful culture of the marine dinoflagellate *Dinophysis acuminata*. *Aquat. Microb. Ecol.* **2006**, *45*, 101–106. [CrossRef]
33. Jennings, E.; Jones, S.; Arvola, L.; Staehr, P.A.; Gaiser, E.; Jones, I.D.; Weathers, K.; Weyhenmeyer, G.A.; Chiu, C.-Y.; de Eyto, E. Effects of weather-related episodic events in lakes: An analysis based on high frequency data. *Freshw. Biol.* **2012**, *57*, 589–601. [CrossRef]
34. Reguera, B.; Velo-Suárez, L.; Raine, R.; Park, M.G. Harmful *Dinophysis* species: A review. *Harmful Algae* **2012**, *14*, 87–106. [CrossRef]
35. Oksanen, J.; Kindt, R.; Legendre, P.; O'Hara, B.; Henry, M.; Stevens, H. The vegan package. *Commun. Ecol. Package* **2007**, *10*, 631–637.
36. Karasiewicz, S. Within Outlying Mean Indexes: Refining the OMI Analysis. R Package Version 0.9.7. Available online: https://cran.r-project.org/web/packages/subniche/subniche.pdf (accessed on 2 January 2018).
37. Alves-de-Souza, C.; Varela, D.; Iriarte, J.L.; González, H.E.; Guillou, L. Infection dynamics of Amoebophryidae parasitoids on harmful dinoflagellates in a southern Chilean fjord dominated by diatoms. *Aquat. Microb. Ecol.* **2012**, *66*, 183–187. [CrossRef]
38. Rodríguez, J.J.G.; Miron, A.S.; García, M.d.C.C.; Belarbi, E.H.; Camacho, F.G.; Chisti, Y.; Grima, E.M. Macronutrients requirements of the dinoflagellate *Protoceratium reticulatum*. *Harmful Algae* **2009**, *8*, 239–246. [CrossRef]
39. Clément, A.; Lembeye, G.; Lassus, P.; Le Baut, C. Bloom superficial no tóxico de *Dinophysis* cf. *acuminata* en el fiordo Reloncaví. XIV Jornadas de Ciencias del Mar y I Jornada chilena de Salmonicultura. In Proceedings of the XIV Jornadas de Ciencias del Mar & I Jornada Chilena de Salmonicultura, Puerto Montt, Chile, 23–25 May 1994; p. 83.
40. Lembeye, G.; Molinet, C.; Marcos, N.; Sfeir, A.; Clément, A.; Rojas, X. *Seguimiento de la Toxicidad en Recursos Pesqueros de Importancia Comercial en la X y XI Región (Proyecto FIP-IT/97-49)*; Universidad Austral de Chile: Puerto Montt, Chile, 1997; p. 86.
41. Uribe, J.C.; Guzmán, L.; Jara, S. *Monitoreo Mensual de la Marea Roja en la XI y XII Regiones (Proyecto FIP-IT/93-16)*; Universidad de Magallanes: Punta Arenas, Chile, 1995; p. 282.
42. Castillo, M.I.; Cifuentes, U.; Pizarro, O.; Djurfeldt, L.; Caceres, M. Seasonal hydrography and surface outflow in a fjord with a deep sill: The Reloncaví Fjord, Chile. *Ocean Sci.* **2016**, *12*, 533–544. [CrossRef]
43. León-Muñoz, J.; Marcé, R.; Iriarte, J. Influence of hydrological regime of an Andean river on salinity, temperature and oxygen in a Patagonia fjord, Chile. *N. Z. J. Mar. Freshw.* **2013**, *47*, 515–528. [CrossRef]
44. Paz, B.; Vázquez, J.A.; Riobó, P.; Franco, J.M. Study of the effect of temperature, irradiance and salinity on growth and yessotoxin production by the dinoflagellate *Protoceratium reticulatum* in culture by using a kinetic and factorial approach. *Mar. Environ. Res.* **2006**, *62*, 286–300. [CrossRef] [PubMed]
45. Röder, K.; Hantzsche, F.M.; Gebühr, C.; Miene, C.; Helbig, T.; Krock, B.; Hoppenrath, M.; Luckas, B.; Gerdts, G. Effects of salinity, temperature and nutrients on growth, cellular characteristics and yessotoxin production of *Protoceratium reticulatum*. *Harmful Algae* **2012**, *15*, 59–70. [CrossRef]
46. Hatosy, S.M.; Martiny, J.B.; Sachdeva, R.; Steele, J.; Fuhrman, J.A.; Martiny, A.C. Beta diversity of marine bacteria depends on temporal scale. *Ecology* **2013**, *94*, 1898–1904. [CrossRef] [PubMed]
47. Reynolds, C. Temporal scales of variability in pelagic environments and the response of phytoplankton. *Freshw. Biol.* **1990**, *23*, 25–53. [CrossRef]
48. Alves-de-Souza, C.; Benevides, T.S.; Santos, J.B.; Von Dassow, P.; Guillou, L.; Menezes, M. Does environmental heterogeneity explain temporal β diversity of small eukaryotic phytoplankton? Example from a tropical eutrophic coastal lagoon. *J. Plankton Res.* **2017**, *39*, 698–714. [CrossRef]
49. Alves-de-Souza, C.; Benevides, T.; Menezes, M.; Jeanthon, C.; Guillou, L. First report of vampyrellid predator-prey dynamics in a marine system. *ISME J.* **2019**, in press. [CrossRef] [PubMed]

50. Garreaud, R. The Andes climate and weather. *Adv. Geosci.* **2009**, *22*, 3–11. [CrossRef]
51. Montecinos, A.; Aceituno, P. Seasonality of the ENSO-related rainfall variability in central Chile and associated circulation anomalies. *J. Clim.* **2003**, *16*, 281–296. [CrossRef]
52. Garreaud, R. Record-breaking climate anomalies lead to severe drought and environmental disruption in western Patagonia in 2016. *Clim. Res.* **2018**, *74*, 217–229. [CrossRef]
53. Seeyave, S.; Probyn, T.; Pitcher, G.; Lucas, M.; Purdie, D. Nitrogen nutrition in assemblages dominated by *Pseudo-nitzschia* spp., *Alexandrium catenella* and *Dinophysis acuminata* off the west coast of South Africa. *Mar. Ecol. Prog. Ser.* **2009**, *379*, 91–107. [CrossRef]
54. Hernández-Urcera, J.; Rial, P.; García-Portela, M.; Lourés, P.; Kilcoyne, J.; Rodríguez, F.; Fernández-Villamarín, A.; Reguera, B. Notes on the cultivation of two mixotrophic *Dinophysis* species and their ciliate prey *Mesodinium rubrum*. *Toxins* **2018**, *10*, 505. [CrossRef]
55. Crawford, D.W. *Mesodinium rubrum*: The phytoplankter that wasn't. *Mar. Ecol. Prog. Ser.* **1989**, *58*, 161–174. [CrossRef]
56. Valle-Levinson, A.; Sarkar, N.; Sanay, R.; Soto, D.; León, J. Spatial structure of hydrography and flow in a Chilean fjord, Estuario Reloncaví. *Estuar. Coasts* **2007**, *30*, 113–126. [CrossRef]
57. Peterson, A.T. Ecological niche conservatism: A time-structured review of evidence. *J. Biogeogr.* **2011**, *38*, 817–827. [CrossRef]
58. Riisgaard, K.; Hansen, P.J. Role of food uptake for photosynthesis, growth and survival of the mixotrophic dinoflagellate *Dinophysis acuminata*. *Mar. Ecol. Prog. Ser.* **2009**, *381*, 51–62. [CrossRef]
59. Hansen, P.J.; Nielsen, L.T.; Johnson, M.; Berge, T.; Flynn, K.J. Acquired phototrophy in *Mesodinium* and *Dinophysis*—A review of cellular organization, prey selectivity, nutrient uptake and bioenergetics. *Harmful Algae* **2013**, *28*, 126–139. [CrossRef]
60. Jiang, H.; Kulis, D.M.; Brosnahan, M.L.; Anderson, D.M. Behavioral and mechanistic characteristics of the predator-prey interaction between the dinoflagellate *Dinophysis acuminata* and the ciliate *Mesodinium rubrum*. *Harmful Algae* **2018**, *77*, 43–54. [CrossRef] [PubMed]
61. Gustafson Jr, D.E.; Stoecker, D.K.; Johnson, M.D.; Van Heukelem, W.F.; Sneider, K. Cryptophyte algae are robbed of their organelles by the marine ciliate *Mesodinium rubrum*. *Nature* **2000**, *405*, 1049. [CrossRef]
62. Velo-Suárez, L.; González-Gil, S.; Pazos, Y.; Reguera, B. The growth season of *Dinophysis acuminata* in an upwelling system embayment: A conceptual model based on in situ measurements. *Deep Sea Res. II Top. Stud. Oceanogr.* **2014**, *101*, 141–151. [CrossRef]
63. Moita, M.T.; Pazos, Y.; Rocha, C.; Nolasco, R.; Oliveira, P.B. Toward predicting *Dinophysis* blooms off NW Iberia: A decade of events. *Harmful Algae* **2016**, *53*, 17–32. [CrossRef] [PubMed]
64. Harred, L.B.; Campbell, L. Predicting harmful algal blooms: A case study with *Dinophysis ovum* in the Gulf of Mexico. *J. Plankton Res.* **2014**, *36*, 1434–1445. [CrossRef]
65. Maestrini, S.Y. Bloom dynamics and ecophysiology of *Dinophysis* spp. In *Physiological Ecology of Harmful Algal Blooms*; Anderson, D., Cembella, A., Hallegraeff, G., Eds.; Springer-Verlag: Berlin/Heidelberg, Germany; New York, NY, USA, 1998; pp. 243–266.
66. Xie, H.; Lazure, P.; Gentien, P. Small scale retentive structures and *Dinophysis*. *J. Mar. Syst.* **2007**, *64*, 173–188. [CrossRef]
67. Soudant, D.; Beliaeff, B.; Thomas, G. Explaining *Dinophysis* cf. *acuminata* abundance in Antifer (Normandy, France) using dynamic linear regression. *Mar. Ecol. Prog. Ser.* **1997**, *156*, 67–74. [CrossRef]
68. Koukaras, K.; Nikolaidis, G. *Dinophysis* blooms in Greek coastal waters (Thermaikos Gulf, NW Aegean Sea). *J. Plankton Res.* **2004**, *26*, 445–457. [CrossRef]
69. Velo-Suárez, L.; Reguera, B.; González-Gil, S.; Lunven, M.; Lazure, P.; Nézan, E.; Gentien, P. Application of a 3D Lagrangian model to explain the decline of a *Dinophysis acuminata* bloom in the Bay of Biscay. *J. Mar. Syst.* **2010**, *83*, 242–252. [CrossRef]
70. Delmas, D.; Herbland, A.; Maestrini, S.Y. Do *Dinophysis* spp. come from the open sea along the French Atlantic coast? In *Toxic Phytoplankton Blooms in the Sea*; Smayda, T.J., Shimizu, Y., Eds.; Elsevier: Amsterdam, The Netherlands, 1993; pp. 489–494.

71. Batifoulier, F.; Lazure, P.; Velo-Suarez, L.; Maurer, D.; Bonneton, P.; Charria, G.; Dupuy, C.; Gentien, P. Distribution of *Dinophysis* species in the Bay of Biscay and possible transport pathways to Arcachon Bay. *J. Mar. Syst.* **2013**, *109*, S273–S283. [CrossRef]
72. Raine, R. A review of the biophysical interactions relevant to the promotion of HABs in stratified systems: The case study of Ireland. *Deep Sea Res. II Top. Stud. Oceanogr.* **2014**, *101*, 21–31. [CrossRef]
73. Raine, R.; Farrell, H.; Gentien, P.; Fernand, L.; Lunven, M.; Reguera, B.; Gill, S.G. Transport of toxin producing dinoflagellate populations along the coast of Ireland within a seasonal coastal jet. ICES CM2010/N:05. Available online: http://www.ices.dk/sites/pub/CM%20Doccuments/CM-2010/N/N0510.pdf (accessed on 27 November 2018).
74. Velo-Suarez, L.; Gonzalez-Gil, S.; Gentien, P.; Lunven, M.; Bechemin, C.; Fernand, L.; Raine, R.; Reguera, B. Thin layers of *Pseudo-nitzschia* spp. and the fate of *Dinophysis acuminata* during an upwelling-downwelling cycle in a Galician Ria. *Limnol. Oceanogr.* **2008**, *53*, 1816. [CrossRef]
75. Díaz, P.A.; Reguera, B.; Ruiz-Villarreal, M.; Pazos, Y.; Velo-Suárez, L.; Berger, H.; Sourisseau, M. Climate variability and oceanographic settings associated with interannual variability in the initiation of *Dinophysis acuminata* blooms. *Mar. Drugs* **2013**, *11*, 2964–2981. [CrossRef] [PubMed]
76. Lindahl, O.; Lundve, B.; Johansen, M. Toxicity of *Dinophysis* spp. in relation to population density and environmental conditions on the Swedish west coast. *Harmful Algae* **2007**, *6*, 218–231. [CrossRef]
77. Berdalet, E.; McManus, M.; Ross, O.; Burchard, H.; Chavez, F.; Jaffe, J.; Jenkinson, I.; Kudela, R.; Lips, I.; Lips, U. Understanding harmful algae in stratified systems: Review of progress and future directions. *Deep Sea Res. II Top. Stud. Oceanogr.* **2014**, *101*, 4–20. [CrossRef]
78. Belgrano, A.; Lindahl, O.; Hernroth, B. North Atlantic Oscillation primary productivity and toxic phytoplankton in the Gullmar Fjord, Sweden (1985–1996). *Proc. R. Soc. Lond. B Biol. Sci.* **1999**, *266*, 425–430. [CrossRef]
79. Lindahl, O. Hydrodynamical processes: A trigger and source for flagellate blooms along the Skagerrak coasts? In *Ecology of Fjords and Coastal Waters*; Smayda, T.J., Shimizu, Y., Eds.; Elsevier Science Publishers BV: Amsterdam, The Netherlands, 1993; pp. 105–112.
80. Meire, L.; Mortensen, J.; Rysgaard, S.; Bendtsen, J.; Boone, W.; Meire, P.; Meysman, F.J. Spring bloom dynamics in a subarctic fjord influenced by tidewater outlet glaciers (Godthåbsfjord, SW Greenland). *J. Geophys. Res. Biogeosci.* **2016**, *121*, 1581–1592. [CrossRef]
81. Nishitani, G.; Nagai, S.; Takano, Y.; Sakiyama, S.; Baba, K.; Kamiyama, T. Growth characteristics and phylogenetic analysis of the marine dinoflagellate *Dinophysis infundibulus* (Dinophyceae). *Aquat. Microb. Ecol.* **2008**, *52*, 209–221. [CrossRef]
82. Rodríguez, L. Revisión del fenómeno de Marea Roja en Chile. *Rev. Biol. Mar.* **1985**, *21*, 173–197.
83. Toro, J.E.; Paredes, P.I.; Villagra, D.J.; Senn, C.M. Seasonal variation in the phytoplanktonic community, seston and environmental variables during a 2-year period and oyster growth at two mariculture sites, southern Chile. *Mar. Ecol.* **1999**, *20*, 63–89. [CrossRef]
84. Campodónico, I.; Guzmán, L.; Lembeye, G. Una discoloración causada por el ciliado *Mesodinium rubrum* (Lohmann) en Ensenada Wilson, Magallanes. *Ans. Inst. Pat.* **1975**, *6*, 225–239.
85. Jara, S. Observations on a red tide caused by *Mesodinium rubrum* (Lohmann) in the Aysén Fjord (Chile). *Cienc. Tecnol. Mar.* **1985**, *9*, 53–63.
86. Lara, A.; Villalba, R.; Urrutia, R. A 400-year tree-ring record of the Puelo River summer-fall streamflow in the Valdivian Rainforest eco-region, Chile. *Clim. Chang.* **2008**, *86*, 331–356. [CrossRef]
87. Utermöhl, H. Zur vendlhommung der quantitativen Phytoplankton-Methodik. *Mitt. Int. Ver. Theor. Angew. Limnol.* **1958**, *9*, 1–38.
88. Climate Explorer. Available online: http://explorador.cr2.cl (accessed on 24 May 2018).
89. NOAA: Global Climate Observing System (GCOS) Working Group on Surface Pressure (WG-SP). Available online: https://www.esrl.noaa.gov/psd/gcos_wgsp/Timeseries (accessed on 25 May 2018).
90. CRAN: The Comprehensive R Archive Network. Available online: https://cran.r-project.org/ (accessed on 25 May 2018).

91. Dray, S.; Dufour, A.-B. The ade4 package: Implementing the duality diagram for ecologists. *J. Stat. Softw.* **2007**, *22*, 1–20. [CrossRef]
92. Xie, Y. A General-Purpose Package for Dynamic Report Generation in R. R Package Version 1.21. Available online: https://cran.r-project.org/web/packages/knitr/knitr.pdf (accessed on 14 April 2018).
93. Kassambara, A.; Mundt, F. Extract and Visualize the Results of Multivariate Data Analyses. R Package Version 1.0.5. Available online: https://cran.r-project.org/web/packages/factoextra/factoextra.pdf (accessed on 2 January 2018).
94. Karasiewicz, S. Subniche Documentation for the Within Outlying Mean Indexes calculations (WitOMI). Available online: https://github.com/KarasiewiczStephane/WitOMI (accessed on 2 January 2018).
95. Wickham, H. ggplot2—Elegant graphics for data analysis. *J. Stat. Softw.* **2010**, *35*, 65–88.
96. Hothorn, T.; Zeileis, A. partykit: A modular toolkit for recursive partitioning in R. *J. Mach. Learn. Res.* **2015**, *16*, 3905–3909.
97. Álvarez, G.; Uribe, E.; Díaz, R.; Braun, M.; Mariño, C.; Blanco, J. Bloom of the Yessotoxin producing dinoflagellate Protoceratium reticulatum (Dinophyceae) in Northern Chile. *J. Sea Res.* **2011**, *65*, 427–434. [CrossRef]

toxins

MDPI

Article

Mesoscale Dynamics and Niche Segregation of Two *Dinophysis* Species in Galician-Portuguese Coastal Waters

Patricio A. Díaz [1,2,*], Beatriz Reguera [1], Teresa Moita [3,4], Isabel Bravo [1], Manuel Ruiz-Villarreal [5] and Santiago Fraga [1]

1 Instituto Español de Oceanografía (IEO), Centro Oceanográfico de Vigo, Subida a Radio Faro 50, 36390 Vigo, Spain; beatriz.reguera@ieo.es (B.R.); isabel.bravo@ieo.es (I.B.); santi.fraga.ieo.vigo@gmail.com (S.F.)
2 Centro i~mar & CeBiB, Universidad de Los Lagos, 557 Puerto Montt, Chile
3 Instituto Português do Mar e da Atmosfera (IPMA), Av. Brasília, 1449-006 Lisboa, Portugal; tmoitagarnel@gmail.com
4 CCMAR, Universidade do Algarve, Campus de Gambelas, 8005-339 Faro, Portugal
5 Instituto Español de Oceanografía (IEO), Centro Oceanográfico de A Coruña, Muelle das Ánimas s/n, 15001 A Coruña, Spain; manuel.ruiz@ieo.es
* Correspondence: patricio.diaz@ulagos.cl; Tel.: +56-65-2322423

Received: 1 December 2018; Accepted: 31 December 2018; Published: 14 January 2019

Abstract: Blooms of *Dinophysis acuminata* occur every year in Galicia (northwest Spain), between spring and autumn. These blooms contaminate shellfish with lipophilic toxins and cause lengthy harvesting bans. They are often followed by short-lived blooms of *Dinophysis acuta*, associated with northward longshore transport, at the end of the upwelling season. During the summers of 1989 and 1990, dense blooms of *D. acuta* developed in situ, initially co-occurring with *D. acuminata* and later with the paralytic shellfish toxin-producer *Gymnodinium catenatum*. Unexplored data from three cruises carried out before, during, and following autumn blooms (13–14, 27–28 September and 11–12 October) in 1990 showed *D. acuta* distribution in shelf waters within the 50 m and 130 m isobaths, delimited by the upwelling front. A joint review of monitoring data from Galicia and Portugal provided a mesoscale view of anomalies in SST and other hydroclimatic factors associated with a northward displacement of the center of gravity of *D. acuta* populations. At the microscale, re-examination of the vertical segregation of cell maxima in the light of current knowledge, improved our understanding of niche differentiation between the two species of *Dinophysis*. Results here improve local transport models and forecast of *Dinophysis* events, the main cause of shellfish harvesting bans in the most important mussel production area in Europe.

Keywords: *Dinophysis acuta*; *Dinophysis acuminata*; DSP; physical–biological interactions; niche partitioning; climatic anomaly

Key Contribution: Large positive SST anomalies combined with moderate upwelling and persistent thermal stratification were associated with the early decline of *D. acuminata* and its replacement by *Dinophysis acuta* in northwestern Iberian coastal waters and a poleward shift of the species distribution. The co-occurrence of *D. acuminata* with *D. acuta* from July to August showed a niche partitioning of the two toxic species; concentration of okadaic acid in raft mussels was a useful indicator of the vertical distribution of the species.

1. Introduction

Potentially toxic dinoflagellate species of the genus *Dinophysis* are distributed worldwide. To date, around twelve species of *Dinophysis* have been found to produce two kinds of lipophilic toxins:

diarrhetic shellfish poisoning (DSP) toxins and/or pectenotoxins (PTXs) [1]. These toxins are retained by filter feeding bivalves and are the main cause of shellfish harvesting bans in western Europe [2]. These bans are enforced when shellfish contamination with DSP toxins and PTXs exceeds the Regulatory Levels (RL) established by European Union directives [3] (herein referred to as "DSP event"). DSP events may occur with moderate cell densities, i.e., a few hundred cells per liter, and blooms of *Dinophysis* (densities > 10^3 cell L^{-1}) are defined as "low biomass blooms of toxin producing microalgae which are transferred through the food web" [1].

Negative impacts of *Dinophysis* blooms, namely of *D. acuminata* and *D. acuta*, are particularly severe in the Galician Rías Baixas and northern Portugal, northwestern Iberia, where harvesting bans may last more than nine months in the most affected shellfish production areas [1,4,5]. This region, located on the northern limit of the Canary Current upwelling system (Figure 1A,B), is subject to a seasonal upwelling regime due to latitudinal shifts of the Azores high- and the Iceland low-pressure systems [6]. Predominant northerly winds from April to September provoke upwelling, and southerly winds from October to March lead to downwelling. In early spring and summer, northerly winds create jets of cold upwelled water on the shelf, and a southward flow of offshore surface waters, the Portuguese Coastal Current (PCC) [7,8] (Figure 1). A poleward countercurrent, the Portuguese Coastal Undercurrent (PCUC), also known as the Poleward Surface Slope Current, or the Iberian Poleward Current (IPC), transports warmer and saltier subtropical water to the north [9,10]. In addition, during the autumn transition from the upwelling to downwelling season, a relatively narrow poleward warm flow has been described on the inner shelf, the "inner shelf countercurrent", inshore of a southward moving tongue of previously upwelled water [11,12].

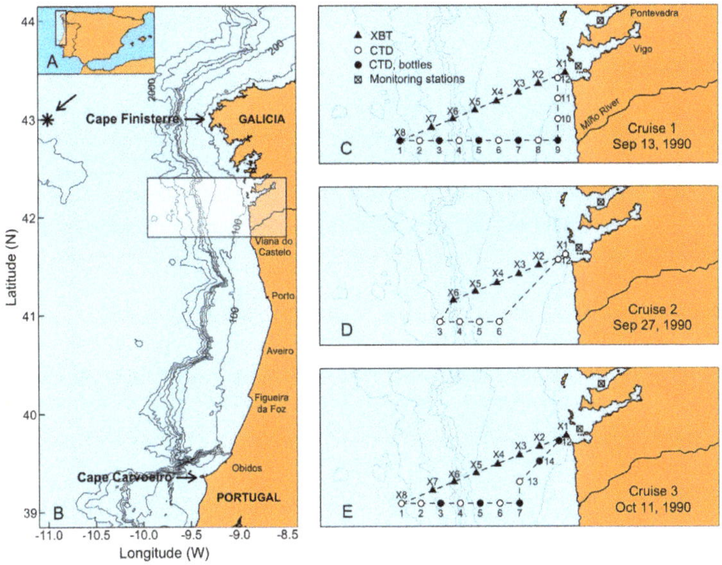

Figure 1. Map of the study area showing (**A**) Iberian Peninsula, (**B**) Northwest Iberia and location of the sampling station (asterisk) for upwelling index estimates, and (**C–E**) location of the sampling stations during the three cruises and of the two monitoring stations in Ría de Vigo and Ría de Pontevedra.

Upwelling has been identified as the main physical factor controlling phytoplankton dominance in the Galician Rías [13–15] and changes in upwelling patterns related to changes in phytoplankton community composition and in the frequency of toxic algae events [13,14,16]. On a seasonal scale, initiation or intensification of PSP (*Gymnodinium catenatum*) and DSP (*Dinophysis*) events have been associated with upwelling relaxation at the end of the upwelling season. The inner shelf countercurrent has been related with a northward transport of harmful dinoflagellates from northern Portuguese waters towards the Galician Rías Baixas [11,17]. On a smaller spatiotemporal scale, the highest risk of toxic events occurs during relaxation/downwelling between upwelling pulses (transport), or with calm weather and a stratified water column following upwelling (in situ growth) [18–20].

Previous studies in the region have shown that *D. acuminata* and *D. acuta* exhibit marked differences in their phenology [21–24] and occur associated with different microplankton assemblages throughout the annual succession [25]. Thus, the initiation of the *D. acuminata* growth season has been shown to be tightly coupled to the beginning of the upwelling season (March to September) and establishment of a shallow early spring pycnocline [26]. Earlier (March) DSP events caused by this species have been related to anomalous wind patterns the preceding winter [27]. In contrast, *D. acuta*, a mid-to-late summer species in northern Portugal, thrives under thermal stratification combined with moderate upwelling (Figure 1B) [28,29]. High densities of *D. acuta* in the Rías Baixas are usually found only at the end of the upwelling season (autumn transition) associated with upwelling relaxation and longshore transport [21,30,31]. But during exceptionally hot and dry summers combined with moderate upwelling pulses, *D. acuta* was found to grow in the Rías Baixas at the same time as and later replacing *D. acuminata* [23]. In addition, toxic blooms of the chain former *Gymnodinium catenatum*, producer of paralytic shellfish poisoning (PSP) toxins, occurs in some years in the autumn [11,32]. Blooms of *G. catenatum* have been also related to longshore transport at the end of the upwelling season, but a time lag of approximately seven days (two consecutive samplings) was usually observed in the Galician HAB monitoring between the sudden peaks of this species from 1986 to 1990 and the preceding maxima of *D. acuta* (unpubl. data). This time lag suggests different locations of the source populations for each species' blooms.

In 1990, exceptional summer blooms of *D. acuta*, in terms of cell density and time of co-occurrence with *D. acuminata*, developed in situ in the Galician Rías Baixas [18,33]. Later, during the autumn transition, there were simultaneous blooms of *D. acuta* and *G. catenatum*. Three research cruises were carried out on the Galician shelf to measure physical properties of the sea surface and water column, nutrients and HAB species distribution before, during and after the intense autumn blooms, in addition to the routine monitoring in shellfish production areas. The objective of these cruises was to identify the origin of the inoculum populations of *G. catenatum* [34] and no information was provided about the accompanying populations of *Dinophysis*. Here, unexplored results from these cruises, in addition to monitoring data from the rías of Pontevedra and Vigo and from the northern Portuguese coast are re-examined in the light of current knowledge with a focus on the co-occurring *Dinophysis* species. Results obtained here contribute to parameterize mesoscale environmental conditions associated with exceptional blooms of *D. acuta* developed that year and most important, the niche partitioning between *D. acuta* and *D. acuminata* explaining their spatiotemporal segregation. This information is used to refine local transport models and improve capabilities to forecast toxic events in the Galician Rías Baixas.

2. Results

2.1. Meteorological and Hydrographic Conditions

Summer 1990 in northwest Spain was extremely hot and dry. Positive air temperature anomalies were +2.6 °C (maximum of 36.6 °C on 20 July) in July and +2.0 °C in August compared with the 47-y (1967–2013) mean. Total rainfall from June to September in 1990 (118 mm) was less than half the mean value (263 mm) for the same period in the last 47-y (Figure 2A). In contrast, a significant positive anomaly was observed in autumn rainfall, with more than double the monthly mean (210 mm) during October (428 mm) (Figure 2A).

Estimates of the Cumulative Upwelling Index (CUI) showed that in 1990, the start of the upwelling season or "spring transition", on 21 March, was within the normal time-window observed in the climatological mean (1967–2013), but the autumn transition, on 24 September, was two weeks earlier

(Figure 2B). Thus, the second cruise was three days after the end of the upwelling season. The Total Upwelling Magnitude Index (TUMI), 81,280 m^3 s^{-1} km^{-1}, from 12 March to 30 September, was slightly above the 47-y mean (69,650 m^3 s^{-1} km^{-1}). At the event scale (7–10 days), the year 1990 was a "normal" year, presenting average patterns in its sequence of upwelling-relaxation cycles during spring and summer (Figure 2C).

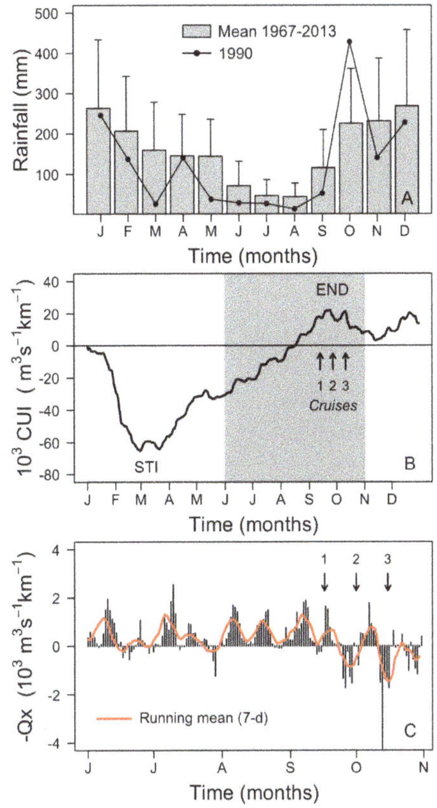

Figure 2. (**A**) Monthly rainfall (mm) in 1990 and the 30-y (1961–1990) monthly mean at Vigo airport. Whiskers indicate standard deviation. (**B**) Cumulative upwelling index (CUI) observed at 43° N in the Canary Current upwelling system in 1990. Upwelling and downwelling transitions are indicated. (**C**) Daily Ekman transport (m^3 s^{-1} km^{-1}) estimated at 43° N, from June to October 1990. Arrows indicate the initiation day of the three shelf water cruises.

From mid-June to early August the top 10 m of the water column were thermally stratified (Figure 3A). Stratification and sea surface temperature (SST) (22 °C) reached record values for the area in late July [18,33]. During August, there was evidence of a strong (1700–2200 m^3 s^{-1} km^{-1}) upwelling pulse (SST 15 °C, 10 µM nitrates at 15 m) after the first week followed by intermittent intrusions of colder water and increments of nitrate levels alternated with periods of rewarming and increased stratification that were not as marked as in July (Figure 3B). These intermittent upwelling pulses were followed by significant increases of chl *a* concentrations with a maximum value of ~8 µg chl *a* L^{-1} at the surface on 8 August (Figure 3C). During the last third of September, nitrate levels declined to almost undetectable levels, bottom temperatures increased, and progressive mixing took place in response to a few days of upwelling relaxation before downwelling. These conditions are common in the area at the end of the upwelling season, which in 1990 occurred two weeks earlier than the 47-y mean.

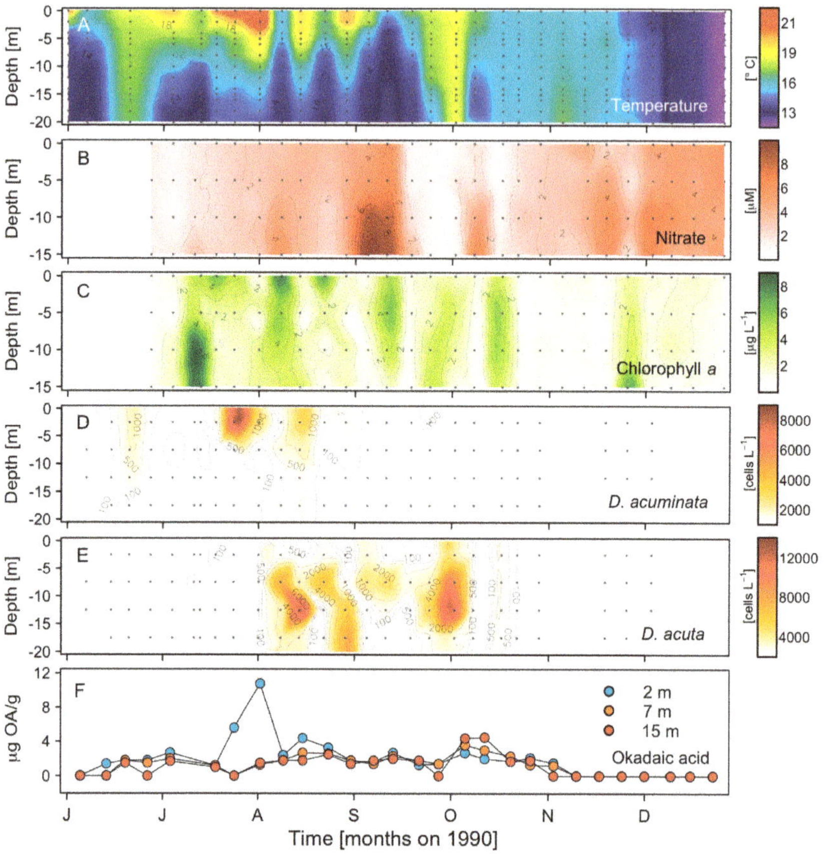

Figure 3. Time series of (**A**) temperature (°C), (**B**) nitrate (μM), (**C**) chlorophyll *a* (μg L^{-1}), (**D**) *D. acuminata*, and (**E**) *D. acuta* cell densities (cells L^{-1}); (**F**) Okadaic acid in mussels (3 depths) digestive glands (μg g^{-1} HP), from June to December 1990 at a monitoring station (P2) in Ría de Pontevedra. Isotherms are drawn at intervals of 1 °C. Gray dots indicate depth and time of measurements. *Dinophysis* contour plots were made with cell density estimates from integrated (0–5 m, 5–10 m, and 10–15 m) tube samples plotted at 2.5, 7.5, and 12.5 m.

2.2. *Seasonal Variability of* Dinophysis *Species and Microphytoplankton in Ría de Pontevedra*

During June and the first half of July, moderate (10^2–10^3 cells L^{-1}) densities of *D. acuminata* were observed in the warmer top 0–5 m layer (Figure 3D). Maximal densities were found on 23 July (8.3×10^3 cell L^{-1}) in the same layer, followed by almost undetectable levels after the strong upwelling pulse (2200 m^3 s^{-1} km^{-1}) in early August. A second surface maximum developed by mid-August (2.2×10^3 cell L^{-1}). A new decline followed, very low numbers were detected in September, and cells of *D. acuminata* were no longer detected either in the hose or in net samples in October. *Dinophysis acuta*, first detected on 10 July, exhibited low densities (max. 160 cell L^{-1}) that month. Rapid growth took place in early August, with a maximum of 14×10^3 cell L^{-1} found at 10–15 m on 13 August (Figure 3E), co-occurring with the second peak of *D. acuminata* at the surface. The depths of *D. acuta* maxima followed the vertical excursions of the isotherms. A second peak of 13.8×10^3 cells L^{-1}

occurred at 10–15 m on 2 October following downwelling and the species was no longer detected after 22 October (Figure 3E).

During June, small centric colony-forming diatoms (*Leptocylindrus minimus*, *Leptocylindrus danicus*, *Guinardia delicatula*, and *Dactyliosolen fragilissimus*) represented over 90% of the microphytoplankton accompanied by nanoplanktonic flagellates. In early July, *Pseudo-nitzschia seriata*-group species constituted >87%, and *Tripos fusus* was the most abundant dinoflagellate. In the second half of July, during maximal stratification, red patches of the ciliate *Mesodinium* cf *rubrum* were observed on the surface at noon, and *Proboscia alata*, and to a lesser extent *Pseudo-nizschia* spp., *Leptocylindrus* spp., and *T. fusus* were the most abundant species in the samples. Diatoms, in particular *P. alata*, *Rhizosolenia shrubsolei*, *L. danicus*, and *L. minimus*, were still dominant (>95%) at the three depth intervals all through August. The last two diatoms were dominant in the top 10 m in September, while *Gymnodinium* spp. were the most abundant in the 10–15 m layer at the end of that month. Thus, from June to September, when nutrients were high (Figure 3B), diatoms and small flagellates predominated and *Dinophysis* species (*D. acuminata* + *D. acuta*) represented a small proportion (1–5%) of the microphytoplankton community. The situation changed abruptly on 2 October, following some days of upwelling relaxation, when a sudden peak of *G. catenatum*, co-occurring with *D. acuta*, became the main component of a dinoflagellate (*T. fusus*, *Protoperidinium divergens*, and *Prorocentrum triestinum*)-dominated microplankton community with no diatoms. There was a lag of approximately five days between the cell maxima of *D. acuta* and *G. catenatum* at the monitoring station in the mouth of Ría de Vigo (Figure 4). After 8 October, diatoms reoccurred and together with small flagellates were the main component of a very sparse phytoplankton population.

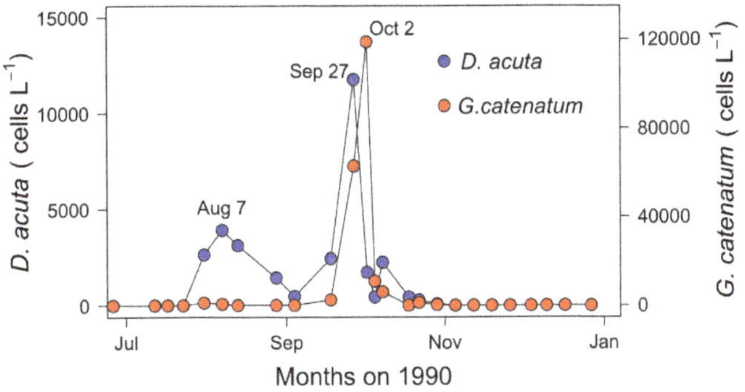

Figure 4. Distribution of *D. acuta* and *G. catenatum* cell maxima in the vertically integrated (0–5, 5–10, and 10–15 m) samples from a monitoring station at the mouth of Ría de Vigo (Figure 1).

2.3. Distribution of OA with Depth in Raft Mussels

Results from the monitoring of okadaic acid (OA) at three depths of the mussel ropes showed low levels of OA (1.4 $\mu g\ g^{-1}$ HP) in mussels from 7 and 15 m in early June, and a moderate progressive increase (up to 3 $\mu g\ g^{-1}$ HP) during June until mid-July. Between 17 and 31 July, OA levels at 2 m increased, coinciding with the surface maximum of *D. acuminata*, to the highest value of the season (10.8 $\mu g\ g^{-1}$ HP). In August (1.9–3.0 $\mu g\ g^{-1}$ HP) and September (1.5–1.8 $\mu g\ g^{-1}$ HP), there was an even distribution of the toxin with depth, with the exception of a small peak (4.4 $\mu g\ g^{-1}$ HP) at 2 m coinciding with the second maximum of *D. acuminata* before the population declined. A new increase with a maximum at 15 m (4.7 $\mu g\ g^{-1}$ HP) was detected at the same time and depth as the peak of *D. acuta*. From 8 October onward, OA levels gradually decreased, becoming undetectable by the end of the month at 15 m and on 5 November at 2 and 7 m.

Assuming for *Mytilus galloprovincialis* an average whole flesh:digestive gland weight ratio of 11:1 [35] and that approximately 80% of the toxins are accumulated in the digestive gland, the maximum level of OA observed in late July would be equivalent to approximately 1230 μg OA 100 g^{-1} meat, i.e., 7.7-fold higher than the RL.

2.4. Hydrodynamic Conditions on Shelf Before, During, and after the Autumn DSP and PSP Events

Cruise 1 (13–14 September). During the first cruise, there was offshore Ekman transport and upwelling associated with the onset of northerly winds the preceding days (Figure 2). The cruise coincided with an intense intrusion of cold water in bottom layers into the rías and with the export of surface ría waters to the shelf (Figure 5A). The upwelling pulse in the shelf–rías system was characterized by a marked upwelling front about 19 nm off the coast (~150 m isobath) with a gradient of 2.3 °C in 1.6 nm (Figure 5 A,B). The phytoplankton community on the inshore side of the front was dominated by the same diatoms than inside the rías, i.e., *L. danicus*, *L. minimus*, and by species of *Pseudo-nizschia seriata*-group spp. Seaward of the front there was a sharp decline in chlorophyll *a* fluorescence, and a dominance of small flagellates; values of salinity (>35.9) and temperature (>18 °C) corresponded to those typical of the Iberian Poleward Current (IPC) [9]. *D. acuta* cells were only observed at stations on the inshore side of the upwelling front. Maximum cell densities (9×10^3 cell L^{-1}) were observed at the base of the pycnocline (20 m) on a shelf station (50 m isobaths) close to the mouth of the Miño River (station 9) (Figures 5B and 6A).

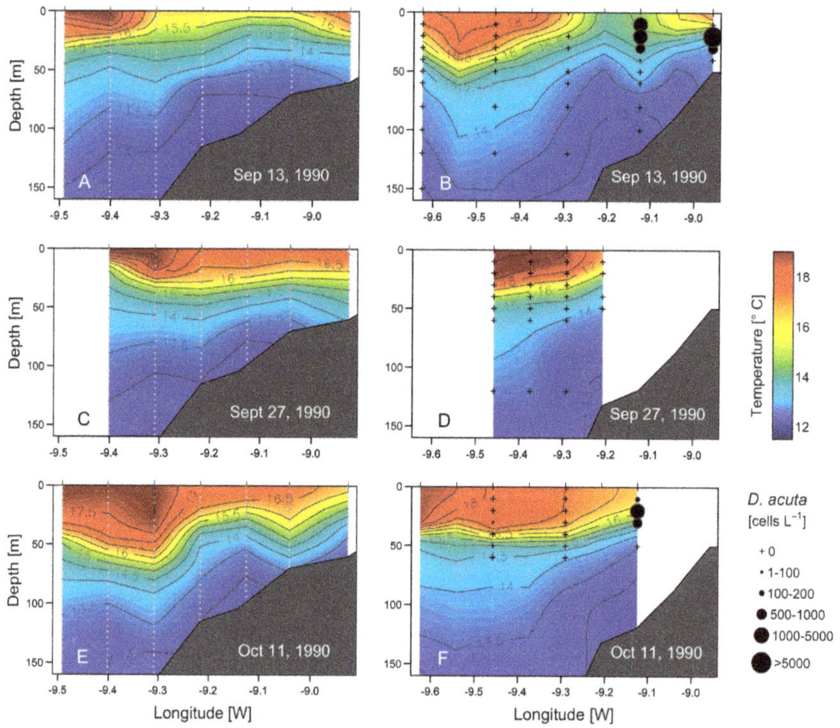

Figure 5. Vertical distribution of (**A**,**C**,**E**) temperature (°C), measured with XBT, in transects diagonal to the coast (left) and (**B**,**D**,**F**) temperature (CTD casts) and *D. acuta* cells density (bottle samples) in transects perpendicular to the coast (right) sampled during the three cruises on the Galician shelf (see Figure 1).

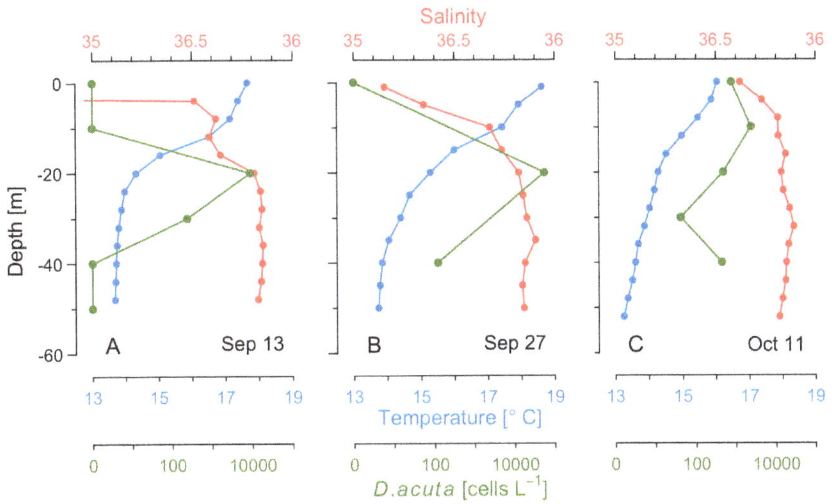

Figure 6. Vertical profiles of temperature (blue), salinity (red), and *D. acuta* cell densities (green), on the adjacent shelf during three cruises on (**A**) 13–14 September, (**B**) 27–28 September, and (**C**) 11–12 October.

Cruise 2 (27–28 September). Following some days of downwelling relaxation, a low pressure system off the western Iberian peninsula caused a shift from northerly to southerly winds on 25 September (Figure 2) resulting in onshore transport of the warmer (19 °C), more saline water located seaward of the front in the previous cruise, and lowering of the pycnocline over the whole shelf to the outer reaches of Ría de Vigo (Figure 5C). Maximal densities of *D. acuta* (5.4×10^4 cells L^{-1}) associated with marked vertical gradients (3.3 °C/20 m) were found at the base of the pycnocline at 20 m on a shelf station (station 12, 100 m isobath) close to the southern mouth of Ría de Vigo (Figure 6B). *G. catenatum*, below detection levels in the previous cruise, reached a maximum of 6.2×10^4 cells L^{-1} at 10 m at the monitoring station in the mouth of Ría de Vigo.

Cruise 3 (11–12 October) Renewed northerly winds at the beginning of October, after an intense upwelling event, led to positive Ekman transport (maximum value, 2000 m^3 s^{-1} km^{-1} on 7 October) and inflow of cold nutrient rich waters into the rías from below with surface outflow of warmer, less saline water from the rías. This re-established a strong thermal stratification and coastward shoaling of the 13.5–16.5 °C isotherms that reached the surface at the mouth of Ría de Vigo (Figure 5E). A new upwelling front developed, much closer to the coast than the one observed during the first cruise (Figure 5E,F). These conditions coincided with the decline of *G. catenatum*. Maximum values of 1–5 $\times$ 10^2 cells L^{-1} of this species were detected in the mouth of Ría de Vigo and adjacent shelf stations. Bloom levels (>10^3 cells L^{-1}) of *D. acuta* persisted at all stations sampled, with cell maxima at 10 m, below the warmer and saltier surface layer (Figure 6C).

2.5. Thermohaline Conditions Associated with Dinophysis *and* G. catenatum *Shelf Maxima*

Cell densities of toxigenic species (*D. acuminata*, *D. acuta*, and *G. catenatum*) plotted over TS diagrams during the three cruises showed that cell maxima of the three species were located in the mixed surface layer (< 30 m). This water layer is delimited by a seasonal thermocline (Figure 7). *D. acuminata* was detected in low densities (max. 120 cells L^{-1}) during the first and second cruises which showed salinities <35.5 and temperatures of 16 to 18 °C (Figure 7A). Plots of *D. acuta* cell densities on TS diagrams showed that it was most abundant in a salinity range of 35.4 to 35.9 and a temperature of 14 to 18 °C (Figure 7B). The cell maximum (5.4×10^4 cells L^{-1}) observed during the second cruise was associated with the 26.5 σt isopycnal (Figure 7B). In the case of *G. catenatum*, highest cell densities were associated with a temperature of 14 to 18 °C and salinity 35.4 (Figure 7C). This water mass, although similar in temperature to the warm offshore water, had a lower salinity.

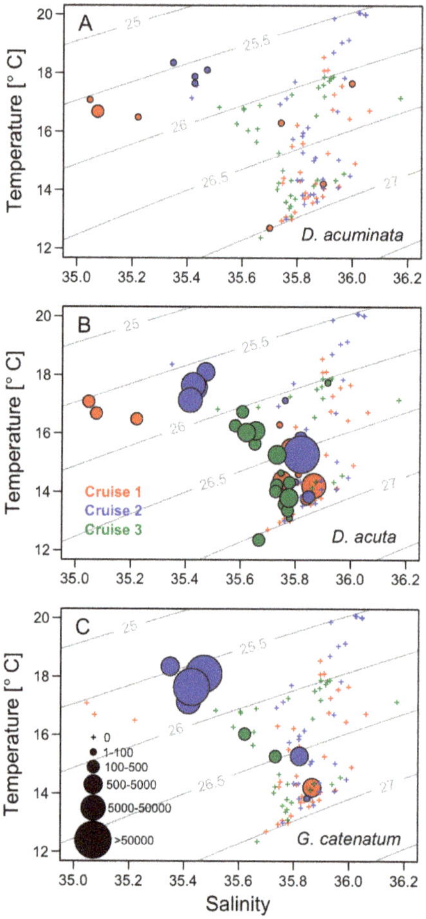

Figure 7. Cell densities (cells L^{-1}) of (**A**) *D. acuminata*, (**B**) *D. acuta*, and (**C**) *G. catenatum* plotted over TS diagrams from the three shelf cruises from September to October 1990. Contour lines (gray) represent isopycnals spaced at intervals of 0.5 σ.

Images from the AVHRR sensors, corresponding to the day pass of the satellite over the study area on 10 October revealed a surface poleward flow characterized by SST values >18 °C (Figure 8), which correspond to the signature of the Iberian Poleward Current, IPC. These agree with the surface salinity (>35.9) and temperature (>18 °C) values observed at the offshore stations (stations 1 and 2) on 11 October during the third cruise.

2.6. Mesoscale Dynamics of D. acuta *in Galician-Portuguese Coastal Waters*

Mesoscale dynamics of *D. acuta* cell density distribution estimated from weekly monitoring sampling at different sites along northwestern Iberian coastal waters, from Cape Carvoeiro, Portugal to Cape Finisterre, Spain between July and October 1990, were compared with the distribution in the same area observed in 2005 (Figure 9). In July 1990, low to moderate density (10^2–10^3 cells L^{-1}) populations of *D. acuta* were detected throughout Galician-northern Portuguese coastal waters.

Densities progressively increased reaching a maximum off Aveiro (2.9×10^4 cells L^{-1}) on 30 July and off Ría de Vigo (3.5×10^4 cells L^{-1}) on 13 August.

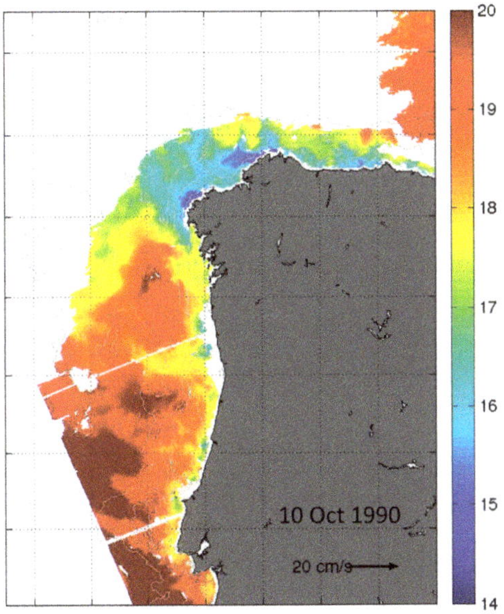

Figure 8. Sea Surface Temperature (SST) from AVHRR (2-km) satellite data on 10 October 1990. White patches represent clouds.

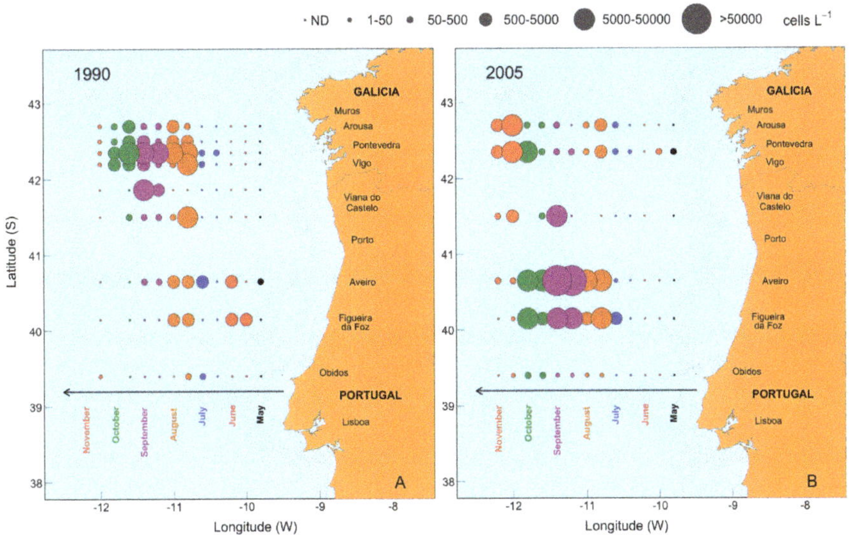

Figure 9. Seasonal variability, from June to November, of *D. acuta* cell maxima at monitoring sites in Galicia and northern Portugal in 1990 (**A**) and 2005 (**B**). Isobaths are shown in gray. The 2005 map is modified from Escalera et al. [30].

From mid-August onwards, the Galician Rías became the center of gravity (the region of highest population density) of the late summer *D. acuta* population distributed from Óbidos, Portugal to the Galician Rías. This population showed a seasonal bimodal distribution in the Galician Rías, with a second maximum of 2×10^4 cells L^{-1} observed in Ría de Pontevedra in early autumn (24 September) (Figure 9A). At the same time, cell densities 1–2 orders of magnitude lower (<1×10^3 cells L^{-1}) were detected off Aveiro. From 8 October onwards, cell densities declined, and they were below detection levels at most stations by the end of the month. Thus, in 1990 the growth season of *D. acuta* started and finished earlier in northern Portugal and showed a bimodal pattern with an unusual summer growth on the Galician coast, where the center of gravity of the population was located throughout August and September. The situation was quite different in 2005, a year which exhibited the most typical seasonal pattern of *D. acuta* populations in northwestern Iberia. In 2005, *D. acuta* populations developed in Portuguese coastal waters in summer, reaching record values off Aveiro in late August, and declined in late October. On the Galician coast, *D. acuta* densities were extremely low in summer. High densities were detected in late October associated with northward longshore transport by the end of the upwelling season [30] (Figure 9B). Therefore, during 2005, the center of gravity of the summer distribution of *D. acuta* population was off Aveiro, which is the common situation for the seasonal distribution of this species [28,29].

3. Discussion

HAB species respond to changes in local hydrodynamics that may be driven by large-scale atmospheric processes. Nevertheless, knowledge about the time scales over which preceding conditions shape communities and their biomass is scarce [36]. In 1990, the seasonal spatial variability of *D. acuta* on the Galician northern Portuguese shelf showed a northward drift and was characterized by unusually early dense (>10^4 cells L^{-1}) summer blooms. These blooms were associated with exceptional hydroclimatic conditions in summer, including positive anomalies of SST (over 2 °C) on the Galician shelf and in the Rías. These anomalies were a large scale phenomenon which also affected plankton communities in the North Sea and other northeast Atlantic coastal regions [37,38]. A second "normal" bloom occurred at the end of the upwelling season co-occurring with a PSP event of *G. catenatum*. Although both *D. acuta* events (late summer and early autumn) during 1990 reached similar population densities (2–3×10^4 cells L^{-1}), they developed under distinct meteorological and oceanographic conditions. The hydroclimatic process implicated in the onset, development, and decline of these exceptional events is discussed here with the overall objective of "identification of key past events which will be re-analyzed and used for training the modelling system".

3.1. *Initiation of* D. acuta *Summer Bloom and the Replacement of* D. acuminata

HABs may be triggered by different mechanisms promoted by physical, chemical and biological conditions optimal for bloom development [39]. In 1990, the exceptional *D. acuta* summer bloom coincided with extreme climate anomalies, characterized by very hot and dry summer conditions. These local weather conditions were accompanied by an upper-level high-pressure anomaly in late July and early August (data not shown). Likewise, Cloern et al. [36] reported extreme climate anomalies associated with an exceptional bloom of the red tide forming dinoflagellate *Akashiwo sanguinea* in San Francisco Bay during summer 2004. Nevertheless, similar summer blooms have not been observed in the Galician Rías since then, despite new records of high summer temperatures.

Recently, Díaz, et al. [33], based on a 29-y time series (1985–2013) analysis of monitoring data from the Galician Rías, suggested that a long period of stable, thermally-driven stratification is necessary for in situ development of summer populations of *D. acuta*. These authors suggested that exceptional in situ development of these populations (mainly July–August) appeared related to an optimal combination of SST (>17 °C), water column stability (>6 weeks) and values of upwelling close to the historic mean. These conditions would keep stability in the stratified top layer down to a favorable depth for *D. acuta*. In summer 1990, as well as in 1989, these "optimal environmental conditions" were observed. Recent laboratory studies have shown that *Dinophysis* species, including *D. acuta*, are obligate mixotrophs which require live ciliate prey (e.g., *Mesodinium* spp.) and light for sustained growth, but they are also able to survive for long periods of time (up to two months) without prey [40,41]. Nevertheless, predator and prey have different environmental requirements, their populations only coincide occasionally [42], and *Dinophysis* populations may often be prey-limited [43]. Monitoring data reported a dominance of *Mesodinium* cf *rubrum* within the microplankton community during the second half of July. Thus, the exceptional summer bloom of *D. acuta* in 1990 may be understood as a local response to an optimal coupling of physical (persistent thermal stratification) and biological conditions (prey availability) promoting in situ growth on the Galician shelf.

The sequential development of *D. acuminata* and *D. acuta* populations, the former with a much longer growth season than the second, is observed in all the geographic areas where these two HAB species commonly occur [44]. This is the case in northwestern Iberia, where a wider continental shelf enhances stratification and the development of dense populations of *D. acuta* in summer with a center of gravity off Aveiro [28]. But in the Galician Rías, in situ growth in summer is very weak (if it is present at all) and DSP outbreaks associated with this species are in the autumn, at the end of the upwelling season and due to longshore transport and accumulation [30]. During the exceptional years (1989 and 1990) described above, *D. acuta* exhibited a seasonal bimodal distribution characterized by two annual peaks. The first maximum, in late summer, associated with in situ growth and the second maximum in the autumn transition linked to physical transport [30].

A detailed understanding of the species-specific processes involved in the replacement of *D. acuminata* by *D. acuta* in late summer during exceptional summer conditions has not so far been achieved. A plausible explanation was given by Escalera et al. [23], who suggested that in the Galician Rías Baixas this replacement appeared to be associated with the establishment of deeper thermoclines. These authors described the 2003 scenario, with a high temperature (~20 °C) in the top layer (1–5 m) during a very hot summer. *Dinophysis acuta* was present and replaced *D. acuminata*, but at very low cell densities. The year 2003 was also characterized by having extremely weak upwelling pulses. This situation was recently reinterpreted in the light of new knowledge on *Dinophysis* feeding-behavior [33]. The low intensity upwelling pulses and subsequent low nutrient levels in the euphotic layer in 2003 would have prevented the development of high densities of *Mesodinium*, and its cryptophyte prey, both part of the food chain required to promote *Dinophysis* growth.

3.2. Niche Partitioning and Specific Requirements of *D. acuminata* and *D. acuta*

Species can differentiate their niche in many ways, such as by consuming different foods, or using different parts of the environment. The spatial and temporal complexity of upwelling dynamics can create a variety of niche opportunities for phytoplankton populations, including HAB species. In these systems, phytoplankton populations are much more dependent of turbulence (physical control) and nutrient availability [45]. Further, the large species diversity observed indicate that the adaptations and behavioral strategies are varied [46]. Recently, Smayda [47] suggested that different morphological traits allow dinoflagellates exploit the complex niche structure of upwelling systems without the need for special adaptations.

In this work we studied the population dynamics of two dinoflagellate species of *Dinophysis*—*D. acuminata*, and *D. acuta*—which are both kleptoplastic mixotrophs, i.e., they perform photosynthesis with "stolen" plastids from their prey. The two species have identical partial (23 S rDNA) sequences of their plastid *psbA* gene and both are successfully cultivated in the laboratory with the phototrophic ciliate *Mesodinium rubrum* [48]. Therefore, if the two species share the same prey, they would not be able to co-occur unless they occupied different positions in the water column. Results here show that when *D. acuminata* and *D. acuta* coincided in time (August 1990), their maxima occupied different water masses, suggesting a "niche partitioning" with depth. This vertical segregation may be associated with the species-specific response to environmental factors, such as light (quality and intensity) and turbulence.

Recent laboratory experiments with the two species have shown that *Dinophysis acuta* is more susceptible to photodamage, under high light intensities (370–650 µmol photons m^{-2} s^{-1}) than *D. acuminata*, but survives better with low light (10 µmol photons m^{-2} s^{-1}) and endures longer periods (28 d) in the dark [49]. *D. acuta* is better adapted to low light intensities and photosynthesizes better with blue light, the only wavelength reaching the lower limit of the euphotic zone, and its swimming capacity [46] enables it to succeed in deeper pycnoclines than *D. acuminata*. These features might explain its vertical distribution in summer in the Galician Rías, close to or associated with the pycnocline, whereas *D. acuminata* cell maxima aggregate nearer the surface. The vertical distribution of OA on the raft mussel ropes, with a marked peak at 2 m, provided evidence of the aggregation of *D. acuminata* near the surface in late July. From mid-August onwards, when *D. acuta* became the dominant *Dinophysis* species in the rías, the similar levels of OA in mussels from the three depths sampled suggests this species performed a daily vertical migration.

Morphologically, *D. acuminata* and *D. acuta* are also quite distinct. *D. acuta*, with a biovolume 3 times larger than *D. acuminata*, is much more dorsoventrally compressed than *D. acuminata*, which is rounded. These differences enable *D. acuminata* to endure higher values of turbulence near the surface. In contrast, *D. acuta* moves in layers, close to the pycnocline, with decreased rates of kinetic energy dissipation (ε). Experimental work with cultures of the two species subject to three different levels of turbulence confirmed that *D. acuta* was more sensitive to high levels of turbulence than *D. acuminata* [50]. All these differences in morphology and adaptations to distinct environmental conditions would define the realized niche of each species of *Dinophysis* and justify their co-occurrence in time but at different levels in the water column, even considering their competition for the same prey.

3.3. *Inoculum Source for Bloom Development*

Results from northern Portugal shelf waters have shown that the highest cell densities of *D. acuta* always occurred at the inner-shelf margin. [51]. The best documented example was reported by Moita et al. [29] who described an intense bloom of *D. acuta* (5×10^4 cells L^{-1}) restricted to a subsurface thin layer (between 18 and 20 m depth) within the pycnocline extending 30 km offshore.

The three cruises discussed here were originally planned in 1990 to investigate the origin of the inoculum population leading to abrupt increments of *G. catenatum* in the Galician Rías during relaxation at the end of the upwelling season [32]. One hypothesis was that the inoculum for *G. catenatum* blooms was transported by the Iberian Poleward Current. Results here showed that the phytoplankton in the IPC was mainly composed of small flagellates and that *D. acuta* and *G. catenatum* were always found at shelf stations close to the coast, but not at offshore stations. Early suspicions of longshore transport of *G. catenatum* came after observations on the mesoscale dynamics of blooms of this species in 1985 and 1994. Populations of *G. catenatum* were detected in retention areas formed on the lee side of upwelling plumes off Capes Roca and Carvoeiro during summer before blooming in northwestern Iberia in the autumn [52]. These autumn blooms were very sudden, during upwelling relaxation, and were interpreted as a result of advection from shelf populations into the Galician Rías [32]. Twenty years later, improved knowledge on the hydrodynamics and the development of predictive transport models in northwestern Iberia have provided a clearer picture of the mesoscale circulation at the end of the upwelling season and the identification of a poleward inner coastal current [17,53]. This inner poleward current has been associated with the northward transport of *D. acuminata* and *G. catenatum* populations [11], a view supported by observations from Escalera et al. [30] during the intense 2005 bloom of *D. acuta* in the Galician Rías. Estimates of in situ division rates of *D. acuta* throughout its seasonal occurrence that year showed that during the autumn bloom, cells were not dividing at all, so the rapid increase in net growth had to be the result of transport rather than in situ growth. Running of a local hydrodynamic model with data from the autumns of 2005 and 2013 confirmed a northwards advection in an inner shelf current as a plausible mechanism of northwards transport of *D. acuta* from Portugal to Galicia [53]. Surveys in the Celtic Sea, southwestern Ireland, provided evidence of the direct transport of a high-density patch of *D. acuta*, forming a subsurface thin layer within a coastal jet along the south coast of Ireland; the 5-m thick thin layer was centered at 20 m depth and did not coincide with the deeper (30 m) chlorophyll maximum [54]. The main unresolved issue with *Dinophysis* blooms and their contamination of shellfish with DSP toxins in Ireland was the identification of their source. Recent surveys have given evidence for extensive *D. acuta* bloom development in summer in the productive region close to the Celtic Sea Front, a tidal front extending from southeast Ireland to Britain [55]. Therefore, the source population of *D. acuta* would be about 300 km away from the aquaculture sites in Bantry Bay where their impact is maximal, i.e., a similar distance than that from the Aveiro "center of gravity" of *D. acuta* distribution in northwestern Iberia to the intensive mussel aquaculture sites in the Galician Rías Baixas. Likewise, the formation of a tidal front in the warm season has been pointed to as an essential requirement for the development of *D. acuta* blooms in the Firth of Clyde in western Scotland [56]. In the case of the Iberian blooms, the upwelling front at the time the cruises took place established the borders between oceanic water populations dominated by small flagellates, and those in the nutrient-rich shelf waters dominated by microplanktonic dinoflagellates and diatoms. The toxic dinoflagellate populations of concern were distributed on the inner shelf waters, far from the front. A much earlier cruise would have been needed, before bloom initiation, to explore the origin of the inoculum. Nevertheless, results on the distribution of scattered cells of *D. acuta* during the *Morena* cruise in May 1993 confirmed the prebloom distribution of the "pelagic seed banks", sensu Smayda [57] of this species were restricted to the northern half of the Portuguese shelf [58].

3.4. OA Distribution with Depth in Raft Mussels. Implications for Shellfish Exploitation

The sequence of *D. acuminata* (June-early August) and *D. acuta* (August–October) events observed in the Galician Rías in 1990 caused mussel harvesting bans from 9 July to 17 November, with significant economic losses [59]. Based on the vertical distribution of OA and *Dinophysis* species presented here (Figure 4E), it was concluded that *D. acuminata* blooms were associated with mussel toxicity from June to early August, and those of *D. acuta* with the late summer to autumn toxicity. It was also suggested that the smaller-sized *D. acuminata* had a stronger toxic potential than the larger *D. acuta*. We draw special attention to the fact that only OA was measured in the HPLC analyses performed in the 1990s, and that according to the analyses of picked cells from the region [60], it was assumed that OA was the only toxin present in *D. acuta* strains from Galicia. Dinophysistoxin 2 (DTX2) was not described until 1992 [61] and the widespread presence of PTX2 in Galician shellfish during blooms of *D. acuta*, *D. caudata*, and *D. tripos*, until 2002 [62]. *Dinophysis acuta* has a complex toxin profile including OA, DTX2, and PTX2 in addition to small amounts of OA diol-esters and PTX11. It is also known that different years may bring strains with different toxin profiles [63]. In any case, it is certain that the toxin content in mussels exposed to the *D. acuta* bloom in the Galician Rías Baixas in 1990 was much higher than the estimates given at the time.

A remarkable difference was observed in the vertical distribution of OA during the cell maxima of *D. acuminata* and *D. acuta*. The overwhelmingly higher values of toxin content in surface (2 m) mussels in late July and the second peak in early August suggest that *D. acuminata* kept aggregated in the top water layer. This suggestion agrees with observations in recent years on the vertical distribution of this species during cell cycle studies and a couple of 2-week spring cruises in the Galician Rías and adjacent shelf [42,64]. In contrast, the even vertical distribution of toxin content when the bloom was dominated by *D. acuta* (from mid-August to November), suggests a daily vertical migration of the species within the depth range of the mussel ropes (2–12 m).

Recently, Díaz et al. [33] proposed a conceptual model based on a 29-year (1985–2013) time series of weekly observations, to explain the seasonal variability of *D. acuminata* and *D. acuta* in the Galician Rías Baixas. According to this model, years with exceptional summer blooms of *D. acuta* (such as 1989 and 1990), or even worse, with very intense autumn blooms, following spring-summer blooms of *D. acuminata*, have more severe socioeconomic impacts. This is explained by the extended duration of the *Dinophysis* bloom season, which causes a longer period of harvesting bans. The latter scenario is worsened when the autumn blooms of *D. acuta* end very late in the year, when phytoplankton is scarce and mussels take much longer time to eliminate the toxins. That was the case in 2005, when lipophilic toxins accumulated until mid-November did not clear until March 2006 [30]. In addition, toxin analyses at the monitoring center are more complex when mussels are exposed to *D. acuta* than to *D. acuminata*, and DTX2 takes longer than OA to be eliminated.

In summary, the development of *D. acuta* blooms, following those of *D. acuminata*, may represent the worst scenario for the shellfish producers in terms of duration of harvesting bans and the complexity added to the regulation LC-MS analyses of lipophilic toxins. Vertical heterogeneities in toxin distribution stress the importance of appropriate sampling strategies including sample collection at different depth of the mussel ropes.

4. Conclusions

The unusual persistence of thermal stratification for 2 months, combined with moderate upwelling during the summer of 1990 and presumably the abundance of prey in the Galician-Portuguese shelf (northwest Iberia), was associated with a northwards shift in the mesoscale distribution of *D. acuta*. Cell maxima of this species, restricted to a 20 km-wide band, on the shelf, between the 50 and −130 m isobaths, and vertically segregated from the co-occurring *G. catenatum*, were observed at the depth of maximal thermal gradient. Conditions associated with the overlap of summer populations of *D. acuminata* and *D. acuta* in 1990 in the Galician Rías Baixas provided new insights into the niche-partitioning of two mixotrophs sharing the same ciliate prey and where the concentrations of okadaic acid in raft mussels can be used as an indicator of the vertical distribution of both *Dinophysis* species.

5. Materials and Methods

5.1. Study Area

The study area, northwest Iberia (~39.5°–42.5° N; 09° W), is comprised by the Galician Rías Baixas, the northern half of the Portuguese coast and the adjacent shelf. The Galician Rías Baixas are four flooded estuaries, site of intensive raft cultivation of Mediterranean mussel (*Mytilus galloprovincialis*) with production exceeding 250×10^3 t per year, and extraction of other shellfish species from natural banks [65]. Shellfish exploitation is of great socioeconomic importance in the whole region under study and chronic blooms of toxin producing microalgae cause considerable damage to the local economy [4].

5.2. Meteorological Data

Data on air temperature, rainfall and wind speed at Vigo airport (Peinador) were obtained from the Spanish Meteorological Agency [66]. Upwelling indexes every 6 h, from the Spanish Institute of Oceanography (IEO) [67], were estimated using model data from the US Navy's Fleet Numerical Meteorology and Oceanography Center (FNMOC) derived from sea level pressure on a grid of approximately $1° \times 1°$ centered at 43° N 11° W, a representative location for the study area (Figure 1B). Description of the timing, variability, intensity, and duration of coastal upwelling in the Galician Rías Baixas during 1990 was made following the model proposed by Bograd et al. [68]. In this model, the Total Upwelling Magnitude Index (TUMI) is estimated as

$$TUMI = \sum_{END}^{STI} CUI(t)$$

where CUI, the Cumulative Upwelling Index, is the sum of the daily mean upwelling index; STI, the Spring Transition Index, is the date on which CUI (integrated from January 1st) reaches its minimum value; and END is the annual maximum of CUI which marks the end of the upwelling season date (autumn transition).

5.3. Satellite Images

Sea surface temperature (SST) images (2 km resolution) from the Advanced Very High Resolution Radiometry (AVHRR) satellite sensor were obtained from NERC (Plymouth, UK). Although both day and night AVHRR data were available, only night time data were used, because these are not affected by reflected solar radiation and geographically varying diurnal warming [69]. It is important to note that remote sensors measure radiance emitted only over the upper optical depth, typically at a depth of ~1 m in coastal waters [70].

5.4. Field Sampling and Phytoplankton Analyses

Weekly sampling of phytoplankton and environmental conditions in the Rías of Vigo and Pontevedra was carried out on board R.V. *Navaz* as part of the IEO monitoring program of potentially toxic phytoplankton and environmental conditions. One pilot station on each ría was visited twice a week. Following recommendations from the International Council for the Exploration of the Sea (ICES) group of experts, water samples for phytoplankton analyses were collected since 1986 with a dividable (0–5 m, 5–10 m, and 10–15 m) hose sampler [71]. This system was recommended to sample patchy populations which may escape detection with bottle sampling at discrete depths. Samples were immediately fixed on board with acidic Lugol's iodine solution [72]. Quantitative analyses of potentially toxic phytoplankton species were carried out according to the Utermöhl [73] method. Lugol-fixed samples were analyzed with a Zeiss Invertoscop inverted microscope (Zeiss, Jena, Germany) using the method described in Utermöhl (1931). Sedimentation columns of 25 or 50 mL were filled with water samples and left to settle for 24 h. Two transects were counted at 250 X magnification to include the smaller and more abundant species. To count larger, less abundant species (including *Dinophysis* spp.), the whole surface of the chamber was scanned at a magnification of X100, so that the detection limit was 40 and 20 cell L^{-1} when samples of 25 and 50 mL respectively were sedimented.

Weekly reports of phytoplankton distributions in 1990 and 2005 at different stations along the northern Portuguese coast (Figure 1B) were obtained from the Portuguese HAB Monitoring Programme. Additional surface water samples were collected with Nansen bottles at fixed long-term monitoring stations in Cascais (Lisbon, Portugal) and off Aveiro and preserved with neutral Lugol's iodine solution and/or buffered formalin. Subsamples of 50–100 mL were allowed to settle for 1.5–3 d.

Sampling on the Galician shelf in 1990 was carried out on board R.V. *Navarro* during three cruises on 13–14 and 27–28 September and 11–12 October, over shelf transects (Figure 1C–E). Water samples for phytoplankton counts, chlorophyll *a* measurements and nutrients analysis were collected with Niskin bottles. Vertical profiles of temperature and salinity where obtained with a SeaBird SBE-19 CTD. In addition, Sippican XBTs were launched along a diagonal transect from Ría de Vigo to the shelf break.

In all cases, monitoring and cruise samples fixed with Lugol's were analyzed within a few days and a few weeks after being collected.

5.5. Mussel Sampling, Processing, and HPLC Analyses of Okadaic Acid (OA)

Mussels (3–5 kg) from a fixed raft in Ría de Pontevedra were collected weekly by a scuba diver, from June 1990 to January 1991, at three depths (2, 7, and 15 m) from a mussel raft rope. Ten mussels were taken at random from each depth sample, and their digestive glands removed, weighed, and kept labeled at −20 °C until analyses.

The DSP toxins extraction was done following the Lee, et al. [74] procedure with slight modifications. For each mussel sample, 1 g of homogenized hepatopancreas was extracted with 4 mL of methanol/water 80:20. After centrifugation, 2.5 mL of the supernatant was extracted twice with 2.5 mL of hexane. One milliliter of water was added to the methanolic extract and this layer was extracted twice with 4 mL of chloroform. The final chloroform extract was made up to 10 mL, and an aliquot of 0.5 mL evaporated to dryness, and reserved for derivatization with ADAM reagent (SERVA) and OA

(Boehringer) was used as standard. Characteristics of the high-performance liquid chromatography (HPLC) system were Hewlett-Packard 1050, reverse-phase Superspher 100, RP-18 (Lichro-Cart 250-4, Merck, Kenilworth, NJ, USA); mobile phase, MeCN:H_2 O (flow 1.1 mL min^{-1}); column temperature 35 °C; fluorimetric detector HP 1046 A, 365 nm excitation, and 412 nm emission wavelength.

5.6. Data Analysis

CTD data analysis and representation were performed using the *oce* package [75] and maps representation using 'maptools' [76], both from the statistical and programming software R 2.1.12 [77] available through the CRAN repository [78]. Pathfinder SST satellite data were processed and visualized using Matlab® (The MathWorks Inc., Natick, MA, USA).

Author Contributions: Conceptualization: B.R., S.F., and P.A.D.; Methodology: S.F.; T.M.; and B.R.; Formal Analysis: P.A.D.; I.B., S.F., T.M., and B.R.; Investigation: P.A.D., I.B., S.F., T.M., M.R.-V., and B.R.; Writing—Original Draft Preparation: PD., B.R., and S.F.; Writing—Review & Editing: P.A.D., I.B., S.F., T.M., M.R.-V., and B.R.; Supervision: B.R.; Project Administration: M.R.-V. and B.R.; Funding Acquisition: M.R.-V.

Funding: This work was funded by project ASIMUTH (EC FP7-SPACE-2010-1 grant agreement number 261860) and the EU Interreg Atlantic Area Project PRIMROSE (EAPA_182/201).

Acknowledgments: Patricio A. Díaz had a PhD student fellowship from BECAS–CHILE, National Commission for Scientific and Technological Research (CONICYT) and is now funded by projects PAI79160065 (The Attraction and Insertion of Advanced Human Capital Program) and REDES170101 (International Cooperation Programme), CONICYT, Chile. This is a contribution to the SCOR and IOC program on "Global Ecology and Oceanography of Harmful Algal Blooms (GEOHAB)", Core Research Projects on "HABs and Stratification", and "HABs in Upwelling Systems".

Conflicts of Interest: The authors declare no conflicts of interest.

References

1. Reguera, B.; Riobó, P.; Rodríguez, F.; Díaz, P.A.; Pizarro, G.; Paz, B.; Franco, J.M.; Blanco, J. *Dinophysis* toxins: Causative organisms, distribution and fate in shellfish. *Mar. Drugs* **2014**, *12*, 394–461. [CrossRef] [PubMed]
2. Van Egmond, H.P. Natural toxins: Risks, regulations and the analytical situation in Europe. *Anal. Bioanal. Chem.* **2004**, *378*, 1152–1160. [CrossRef] [PubMed]
3. Anonymous. Regulation (EC) no. 853/2004 of the European Parliament and of the Council of 29 April 2004. *Off. J. Eur. Communities* **2004**, *L139*, 55–205.
4. Blanco, J.; Correa, J.; Muñíz, S.; Mariño, C.; Martín, H.; Arévalo, F. Evaluación del impacto de los métodos y niveles utilizados para el control de toxinas en el mejillón. *Revista Galega dos Recursos Mariños* **2013**, *3*, 1–55.
5. Vale, P.; Botelho, M.J.; Rodrigues, S.M.; Gomes, S.; Sampayo, M. Two decades of marine biotoxin monitoring in bivalves from Portugal (1986–2006): A review of exposure assessment. *Harmful Algae* **2008**, *7*, 11–25. [CrossRef]
6. Wooster, W.S.; Bakun, A.; McLain, D.R. The seasonal upwelling cycle along the eastern boundary of the North Atlantic. *J. Mar. Res.* **1976**, *34*, 131–141.
7. Fiuza, A.F.G.; Hamann, M.; Ambar, I.; del Río, G.D.; González, N.; Cabanas, J.M. Water masses and their circulation off western Iberia during May 1993. *Deep Sea Res. I* **1998**, *45*, 1127–1160. [CrossRef]
8. Ruiz-Villareal, M.; Gonzalez-Pola, C.; Diaz del Rio, G.; Lavin, A.; Otero, P.; Piedracoba, S.; Cabanas, J.M. Oceanographic conditions in North and Northwest Iberia and their influence on the Prestige oil spill. *Mar. Pollut. Bull.* **2006**, *53*, 220–238. [CrossRef] [PubMed]
9. Frouin, R.; Fiuza, A.F.G.; Ambar, I.; Boyd, T.J. Observations of a poleward surface current off the coasts of Portugal and Spain during winter. *J. Geophys. Res.* **1990**, *95*, 679–691. [CrossRef]
10. Haynes, R.; Barton, E.D. A poleward flow along the atlantic coast of the Iberian Penisula. *J. Geophys. Res.* **1990**, *95*, 11425–11441. [CrossRef]
11. Sordo, I.; Barton, E.D.; Cotos, J.M.; Pazos, Y. An inshore poleward current in the NW of the Iberian Peninsula detected form satellite images, and its relation with *G. catenatum* and *D. acuminata* blooms in the Galician Rias. *Estuar. Coast. Shelf. Sci.* **2001**, *53*, 787–799. [CrossRef]
12. Peliz, A.; Rosa, T.L.; Santos, A.M.P.; Pissarra, J.L. Fronts, currents and counter-flows in the Western Iberian upwelling system. *J. Mar. Syst.* **2002**, *35*, 61–77. [CrossRef]

13. Figueiras, F.G.; Ríos, A.F. Phytoplankton succession, red tides and the hydrographic regime in the Rias Bajas of Galicia. In *Toxic Phytoplankton Blooms in the Sea*; Smayda, T.J., Shimizu, Y., Eds.; Elsevier: Amsterdam, The Netherlands, 1993; pp. 239–244.
14. Tilstone, G.H.; Míguez, B.M.; Figueiras, F.G.; Fermín, E.G. Diatom dynamics in a coastal ecosystem affected by upwelling: Coupling between species succession, circulation and biogeochemical processes. *Mar. Ecol. Prog. Ser.* **2000**, *205*, 23–41. [CrossRef]
15. Nogueira, E.; Figueiras, F.G. The microplankton succession in the Ría de Vigo revisited: Species assemblages and the role of weather-induced, hydrodynamic variability. *J. Mar. Syst.* **2005**, *54*, 139–155. [CrossRef]
16. Álvarez-Salgado, X.A.; Labarta, U.; Fernández-Reiriz, M.J.; Figueiras, F.G.; Rosón, G.; Piedracoba, S.; Filgueira, R.; Cabanas, J.M. Renewal time and the impact of harmful algal blooms on the extensive mussel raft culture of the Iberian coastal upwelling system (SW Europe). *Harmful Algae* **2008**, *7*, 849–855. [CrossRef]
17. Relvas, P.; Barton, E.D.; Dubert, J.; Oliveira, P.B.; Peliz, A.; da Silva, J.C.B.; Santos, A.M.P. Physical oceanography of the western Iberia ecosystem: Latest views and challenges. *Prog. Oceanogr.* **2007**, *74*, 149–173. [CrossRef]
18. Reguera, B.; Bravo, I.; Fraga, S. Autoecology and some life history stages of *Dinophysis acuta* Ehrenberg. *J. Plankton Res.* **1995**, *17*, 999–1015. [CrossRef]
19. Velo-Suárez, L.; Reguera, B.; Garcés, E.; Wyatt, T. Vertical distribution of division rates in coastal dinoflagellate *Dinophysis* spp. populations: Implications for modeling. *Mar. Ecol. Prog. Ser.* **2009**, *385*, 87–96. [CrossRef]
20. Díaz, P.A.; Ruiz-Villarreal, M.; Velo-Suárez, L.; Ramilo, I.; Gentien, P.; Lunven, M.; Fernand, L.; Raine, R.; Reguera, B. Tidal and wind-event variability and the distribution of two groups of *Pseudo-nitzschia* species in an upwelling-influenced Ría. *Deep Sea Res. II* **2014**, *101*, 163–179. [CrossRef]
21. Reguera, B.; Mariño, J.; Campos, J.; Bravo, I.; Fraga, S. Trends in the occurrence of *Dinophysis* spp. in Galician waters. In *Toxic Phytoplankton Blooms in the Sea*; Smayda, T., Shimizu, Y., Eds.; Elsevier Science Publishers B.V.: Amsterdam, The Netherlands, 1993; pp. 559–564.
22. Palma, A.S.; Vilarinho, M.G.; Moita, M.T. Interannual trends in the longshore distribution of *Dinophysis* off the Portuguese coast. In *Harmful Algae*; Reguera, B., Blanco, J., Fernández, M.L., Wyatt, T., Eds.; Xunta de Galicia and IOC of UNESCO: Vigo, Spain, 1998; pp. 124–127.
23. Escalera, L.; Reguera, B.; Pazos, Y.; Moroño, A.; Cabanas, J.M. Are different species of *Dinophysis* selected by climatological conditions? *Afr. J. Mar. Sci.* **2006**, *28*, 283–288. [CrossRef]
24. Moita, M.T.; Silva, A.J. Dynamics of *Dinophysis acuta*, *D. acuminata*, *D. tripos* and *Gymnodinium catenatum* during an upwelling event off the Northwest Coast of Portugal. In *Harmful Algal Blooms 2000*; Hallegraeff, G.M., Blackburn, S.I., Bolch, C.J., Lewis, R.J., Eds.; Intergovernmental Oceanographic Commission of UNESCO: Paris, France, 2001; pp. 169–172.
25. Pitcher, G.C.; Figueiras, F.G.; Hickey, B.M.; Moita, M.T. The physical oceanography of upwelling systems and the development of harmful algal blooms. *Prog. Oceanogr.* **2010**, *85*, 5–32. [CrossRef]
26. Velo-Suárez, L.; González-Gil, S.; Pazos, Y.; Reguera, B. The growth season of *Dinophysis acuminata* in an upwelling system embayment: A conceptual model based on in situ measurements. *Deep Sea Res. II* **2014**, *101*, 141–151. [CrossRef]
27. Díaz, P.A.; Reguera, B.; Ruiz-Villarreal, M.; Pazos, Y.; Velo-Suárez, L.; Berger, H.; Sourisseau, M. Climate variability and oceanographic settings associated with interannual variability in the initiation of *Dinophysis acuminata* blooms. *Mar. Drugs* **2013**, *11*, 2964–2981. [CrossRef] [PubMed]
28. Moita, M.T.; Pazos, Y.; Rocha, C.; Nolasco, R.; Oliveira, P.B. Towards predicting *Dinophysis* blooms off NW Iberia: A decade of events. *Harmful Algae* **2016**, *52*, 17–32. [CrossRef] [PubMed]
29. Moita, M.T.; Sobrinho-Goncalves, L.; Oliveira, P.B.; Palma, S.; Falcao, M. A bloom of *Dinophysis acuta* in a thin layer off North-West Portugal. *Afr. J. Mar. Sci.* **2006**, *28*, 265–269. [CrossRef]
30. Escalera, L.; Reguera, B.; Moita, T.; Pazos, Y.; Cerejo, M.; Cabanas, J.M.; Ruiz-Villarreal, M. Bloom dynamics of *Dinophysis acuta* in an upwelling system: In situ growth versus transport. *Harmful Algae* **2010**, *9*, 312–322. [CrossRef]
31. Trainer, V.L.; Pitcher, G.C.; Reguera, B.; Smayda, T.J. The distribution and impacts of harmful algal bloom species in eastern boundary upwelling systems. *Prog. Oceanogr.* **2010**, *85*, 33–52. [CrossRef]
32. Fraga, S.; Anderson, D.; Bravo, I.; Reguera, B.; Steidenger, K.A.; Yentsch, C.M. Influence of upwelling relaxation on dinoglagellates and shellfish toxicity in Ria de Vigo, Spain. *Estuar. Coast. Shelf. Sci.* **1988**, *27*, 349–361. [CrossRef]

33. Díaz, P.A.; Ruiz-Villarreal, M.; Pazos, Y.; Moita, M.T.; Reguera, B. Climate variability and *Dinophysis acuta* blooms in an upwelling system. *Harmful Algae* **2016**, *53*, 145–159. [CrossRef]
34. Fraga, F.; Bravo, I.; Reguera, B. Poleward surface current at the shelf break and blooms of *Gymnodinium catenatum* in the Ría de Vigo (NW Spain). In *Toxic Blooms in the Sea*; Smayda, T., Shimizu, Y., Eds.; Elsevier: Amsterdam, The Netherlands, 1993; pp. 245–249.
35. Pino-Querido, A.; Álvarez-Castro, J.M.; Guerra-Varela, J.; Toro, M.A.; Vera, M.; Pardo, B.G.; Fuentes, J.; Blanco, J.; Martínez, P. Heritability estimation for okadaic acid algal toxin accumulation, mantle color and growth traits in Mediterranean mussel (*Mytilus galloprovincialis*). *Aquaculture* **2015**, *440*, 32–39. [CrossRef]
36. Cloern, J.E.; Schraga, T.; Lopez, C.; Knowles, N.; Labiosa, R.; Dugdale, R. Climate anomalies generate an exceptional dinoflagellate bloom in San Francisco Bay. *Geophys. Res. Lett.* **2005**, *32*, L14608. [CrossRef]
37. Edwards, M.; Beaugrand, G.; Reid, P.C.; Rowden, A.A.; Jones, M.B. Ocean climate anomalies and the ecology of the North Sea. *Mar. Ecol. Prog. Ser.* **2002**, *239*, 1–10. [CrossRef]
38. Edwards, M.; Johns, D.G.; Leterme, S.C.; Svendsen, E.; Richardson, A.J. Regional climate change and harmful algal blooms in the northeast Atlantic. *Limnol. Oceanogr.* **2006**, *51*, 820–829. [CrossRef]
39. Roelke, D.; Buyukates, Y. The Diversity of Harmful Algal Bloom-Triggering Mechanisms and the Complexity of Bloom Initiation. *Hum. Ecol. Risk Assess.* **2001**, *7*, 1347–1362. [CrossRef]
40. Park, M.; Kim, S.; Kim, H.; Myung, G.; Kang, Y.; Yih, W. First successful culture of the marine dinoflagellate *Dinophysis acuminata*. *Aquat. Microb. Ecol.* **2006**, *45*, 101–106. [CrossRef]
41. Hansen, P.J.; Nielsen, L.T.; Johnson, M.; Berge, T.; Flynn, K.R. Acquired phototrophy in *Mesodinium* and *Dinophysis*—A review of cellular organization, prey selectivity, nutrient uptake and bioenergetics. *Harmful Algae* **2013**, *28*, 126–139. [CrossRef]
42. González-Gil, S.; Velo-Suárez, L.; Gentien, P.; Ramilo, I.; Reguera, B. Phytoplankton assemblages and characterization of a *Dinophysis acuminata* population during an upwelling-downwelling cycle. *Aquat. Microb. Ecol.* **2010**, *58*, 273–286. [CrossRef]
43. Harred, L.B.; Campbell, L. Predicting harmful algal blooms: A case study with *Dinophysis ovum* in the Gulf of Mexico. *J. Plankton Res.* **2014**, *36*, 1434–1445. [CrossRef]
44. Reguera, B.; Velo-Suárez, L.; Raine, R.; Park, M. Harmful *Dinophysis* species: A review. *Harmful Algae* **2012**, *14*, 87–106. [CrossRef]
45. Margalef, R. Life forms of phytoplankton as survival alternatives in an unstable environment. *Oceanol. Acta* **1978**, *1*, 493–509.
46. Smayda, T. Adaptations and selection of harmful and other dinoflagellate species in upwelling systems. 2. Motility and migratory behaviour. *Prog. Oceanogr.* **2010**, *85*, 71–91. [CrossRef]
47. Smayda, T. Adaptations and selection of harmful and other dinoflagellate species in upwelling systems 1. Morphology and adaptive polymorphism. *Prog. Oceanogr.* **2010**, *85*, 53–70. [CrossRef]
48. Rial, P.; Laza-Martínez, A.; Reguera, B.; Raho, N.; Rodríguez, F. Origin of cryptophyte plastids in *Dinophysis* from Galician waters: Results from field and culture experiments. *Aquat. Microb. Ecol.* **2015**, *76*, 163–174. [CrossRef]
49. García-Portela, M.; Riobó, P.; Reguera, B.; Garrido, J.; Blanco, J.; Rodríguez, F. Comparative ecophysiology of *Dinophysis acuminata* and *D. acuta*: Effect of light intensity and quality on growth, cellular toxin content and photosynthesis. *J. Phycol.* **2018**. [CrossRef]
50. García-Portela, M.; Reguera, B.; Ribera d'Alcalà, M.; Rodríguez, F.; Montresor, M. The turbulent life of *Dinophysis*. In Proceedings of the 18 International Conference on Harmful Algae, Nantes, France, 21–26 October 2018; Abstracts Book. p. 64.
51. Moita, M.T. Development of toxic dinoflagellates in relation to upwelling patterns off Portugal. In *Toxic Phytoplankton Blooms in the Sea*; Smayda, T., Shimizu, Y., Eds.; Elsevier Science Publishers B.V.: Amsterdam, The Netherlands, 1993; pp. 299–304.
52. Moita, M.T.; Oliveira, P.B.; Mendes, J.C.; Palma, A.S. Distribution of chlorophyll a and *Gymnodinium catenatum* associated with coastal upwelling plumes off central Portugal. *Acta Oecol.* **2003**, *24*, S125–S132. [CrossRef]
53. Ruiz-Villarreal, M.; García-García, L.; Cobas, M.; Díaz, P.A.; Reguera, B. Modeling the hydrodynamic conditions associated with *Dinophysis* blooms in Galicia (NW Spain). *Harmful Algae* **2016**, *53*, 40–52. [CrossRef] [PubMed]

54. Farrell, H.; Gentien, P.; Fernand, L.; Lunven, M.; Reguera, B.; González-Gil, S.; Raine, R. Scales characterising a high density thin layer of *Dinophysis acuta* Ehrenberg and its transport within a coastal jet. *Hamrful Algae* **2012**, *15*, 36–46. [CrossRef]
55. Raine, R.; Cosgrove, S.; Fennell, S.; Gregory, C.; Barnett, M.; Purdie, D.; Cave, R. Origins of *Dinophysis* blooms which impact Irish aquaculture. In *Marine and Fresh-Water Harmful Algae, Proceedings of the 17th International Conference on Harmful Algae, Santa Catarina, Brazil, 9–14 October 2016*; Proença, L.A.O., Hallegraeff, G.M., Eds.; International Society for the Study of Harmful Algae and Intergovernmental Oceanographic Commission of UNESCO: Paris, France, 2017; pp. 46–49.
56. Swan, S.C.; Turner, A.D.; Bresnan, E.; Whyte, C.; Paterson, R.F.; McNeill, S.; Mitchell, E.; Davidson, K. *Dinophysis acuta* in Scottish coastal waters and its influence on Diarrhetic Shellfish Toxin profiles. *Toxins* **2018**, *10*, 399. [CrossRef]
57. Smayda, T. Turbulence, watermass stratification and harmful algal blooms: An alternative view and frontal zones as "pelagic seed banks". *Harmful Algae* **2002**, *1*, 95–112. [CrossRef]
58. Reguera, B.; Díaz, P.A.; Escalera, L.; Ramilo, I.; Cabanas, J.M.; Ruiz-Villarreal, M. Winter distributions of *Dinophysis* populations: Do they help predict the onset of the bloom? In *Marine and Freshwater Harmful Algae 2014, Proceedings of the 16th International Conference on Harmful Algae, Wellington, New Zealand, 27–31 October 2014*; MacKenzie, L.A., Ed.; Cawthron Institute: Nelson, New Zealand, the International Society for the Study of Harmful Algae (ISSHA); 2014; pp. 128–131.
59. Reguera, B.; Bravo, I.; Marcaillou-le, C.; Masselin, P. Monitoring of *Dinophysis spp.* and vertical distribution of okadaic acid on mussel rafts in Ría de Pontevedra (NW Spain). In *Toxic phytoplankton Blooms in the Sea*; Smayda, T., Shimizu, Y., Eds.; Elsevier Science Publishers B.V.: Amsterdam, The Netherlands, 1993; pp. 553–558.
60. Lee, J.S.; Igarashi, T.; Fraga, S.; Dahl, E.; Hovgaard, P.; Yasumoto, T. Determination of diarrhetic shellfish toxins in various dinoflagellate species. *J. Appl. Physiol.* **1989**, *1*, 147–152. [CrossRef]
61. Hu, T.; Doyle, J.; Jackson, D.; Marr, J.; Nixon, E.; Pleasance, S.; Quilliam, M.; Walter, J.; Wright, J. Isolation of a new diarrhetic shellfish poison from Irish mussels. *J. Chem. Soc. Chem. Commun.* **1992**, *54*, 39–41. [CrossRef]
62. Fernández, M.L.; Míguez, A.; Martínez, A.; Moroño, A.; Arévalo, F.; Pazos, Y.; Salgado, C.; Correa, J.; Blanco, J.; González-Gil, S.; et al. First report of pectenotoxin-2 in phytoplankton net-hauls and mussels from the Galician Rías Baixas during proliferations of *Dinophysis acuta* and *D. caudata*. In *Molluscan Shellfish Safety*; Villalba, A., Reguera, B., Romalde, J., Beiras, R., Eds.; Consellería de Pesca e Asuntos Marítimos da Xunta de Galicia and Intergovernmental Oceanographic Commission of UNESCO: Santiago de Compostela, Spain, 2003; pp. 75–83. ISBN 84-453-3638-X.
63. Fernández, M.; Reguera, B.; González-Gil, S.; Míguez, A. Pectenotoxin-2 in single-cell isolates of *Dinophysis caudata* and *Dinophysis acuta* from the Galician Rías (NW Spain). *Toxicon* **2006**, *48*, 477–490. [CrossRef]
64. Díaz, P.A.; Ruiz-Villarreal, M.; Rodriguez, F.; Garrido, J.L.; Mouriño-Carballido, B.; Riobó, P.; Reguera, B. Fine scale physical-biological interactions in a *Dinophysis acuminata* population during an upwelling-relaxation transition. In *Marine and Fresh-Water Harmful Algae, Proceedings of the 17th International Conference on Harmful Algae, Santa Catarina, Brazil, 9–14 October 2016*; Proença, L.A.O., Hallegraeff, G.M., Eds.; ISSHA and IOC of UNESCO: Paris, France, 2017; pp. 50–53. ISBN 978-87-990827-6-6.
65. Natural banks. Available online: www.fao.org (accessed on 30 October 2018).
66. Spanish Meteorological Agency. Available online: www.aemet.es (accessed on 30 July 2018).
67. Spanish Institute of Oceanography (IEO). Available online: www.indicedeafloramiento.ieo.es (accessed on 30 July 2018).
68. Bograd, S.T.; Schroeder, I.; Sarkar, N.; Qiu, X.; Sydeman, W.J.; Schwing, F.B. Phenology of coastal upwelling in the California Current. *Geophys. Res. Lett.* **2009**, *36*, L01602. [CrossRef]
69. Rayner, N.A.; Parker, D.E.; Horton, E.B.; Folland, C.K.; Alexander, L.V.; Rowell, D.P.; Kent, E.C.; Kaplan, A. Global analyses of sea surface temperature, sea ice, and night marine air temperature since the late nineteenth century. *J. Geophys. Res.* **2003**, *108*, 4407. [CrossRef]
70. Gordon, H.R.; McCluney, W.R. Estimation of the depth of sunlight penetration in the sea for remote sensing. *Appl. Opt.* **1975**, *14*, 413–416. [CrossRef] [PubMed]
71. Lindahl, O. *A Dividable Hose for Phytoplankton Sampling*; Report of the Working Group on Phytoplankton and Management of Their Effects; International Council for the Exploration of the Sea: Copenhagen, Denmark, 1986; C.M.1986/L: 26, Annex III.

72. Lovegrove, T. An improved form of sedimentation apparatus for use with an inverted microscope. *ICES J. Mar. Sci.* **1960**, *25*, 279–284. [CrossRef]
73. Utermöhl, H. Zur Vervollkomnung der quantitativen phytoplankton-Methodik. *Mitt. Int. Ver. Limnol.* **1958**, *9*, 1–38.
74. Lee, J.S.; Yanagi, T.; Kenma, R.; Yasumoto, T. Fluorometric determination of diarrhetic shellfish toxins by High-Performance Liquid Chomatography. *Agric. Biol. Chem.* **1987**, *51*, 877–881.
75. Kelley, D. *Oce: Analysis of Oceanographic Data*, R package Version 0.9-14; 2014. Available online: http://CRAN.R-project.org/package=oce (accessed on 5 May 2018).
76. Bivand, R. *Maptools: Tools for Reading and Handling Spatial Objects*, R package version 0.9-2; 2017. Available online: https://CRAN.R-project.org/package=maptools/ (accessed on 15 September 2018).
77. R Development Core Team. *R: A Language and Environment for Statistical Computing*; R Foundation for Statistical Computing: Vienna, Austria, 2013; ISBN 3-900051-07-0. Available online: http://www.r-project.org/ (accessed on 15 September 2018).
78. CRAN repository. Available online: www.r-project.org (accessed on 15 September 2018).

toxins

MDPI

Article

Diel Variations in Cell Abundance and Trophic Transfer of Diarrheic Toxins during a Massive *Dinophysis* Bloom in Southern Brazil

Thiago Pereira Alves [1,2,*] and Luiz Laureno Mafra Jr. [1,*]

1 Center for Marine Studies, Federal University of Paraná. Av. Beira-mar s/n, P.O. Box: 61, Pontal do Paraná PR 83255-976, Brazil

2 Federal Institute of Santa Catarina, Av. Ver. Abraão João Francisco, 3988, Ressacada, Itajaí SC 88307-303, Brazil

* Correspondence: thiago.alves@ifsc.edu.br (T.P.A.); mafrajr@gmail.com (L.L.M.J.); Tel.: +55-(47)-3390-1200 (T.P.A.); +55-(41)-3511-8669 (L.L.M.J.); Fax: +55-(41)-3511-8648 (L.L.M.J.)

Received: 10 May 2018; Accepted: 4 June 2018; Published: 6 June 2018

Abstract: *Dinophysis* spp. are a major source of diarrheic toxins to marine food webs, especially during blooms. This study documented the occurrence, in late May 2016, of a massive toxic bloom of the *Dinophysis acuminata* complex along the southern coast of Brazil, associated with an episode of marked salinity stratification. The study tracked the daily vertical distribution of *Dinophysis* spp. cells and their ciliate prey, *Mesodinium* cf. *rubrum*, and quantified the amount of lipophilic toxins present in seston and accumulated by various marine organisms in the food web. The abundance of the *D. acuminata* complex reached 43×10^4 cells·L^{-1} at 1.0 m depth at the peak of the bloom. Maximum cell densities of cryptophyceans and *M.* cf. *rubrum* (>500×10^4 and 18×10^4 cell·L^{-1}, respectively) were recorded on the first day of sampling, one week before the peak in abundance of the *D. acuminata* complex. The diarrheic toxin okadaic acid (OA) was the only toxin detected during the bloom, attaining unprecedented, high concentrations of up to 829 µg·L^{-1} in seston, and 143 ± 93 pg·cell^{-1} in individually picked cells of the *D. acuminata* complex. Suspension-feeders such as the mussel, *Perna perna*, and barnacle, *Megabalanus tintinnabulum*, accumulated maximum OA levels (up to 578.4 and 21.9 µg total OA·Kg^{-1}, respectively) during early bloom stages, whereas predators and detritivores such as Caprellidae amphipods (154.6 µg·Kg^{-1}), *Stramonita haemastoma* gastropods (111.6 µg·Kg^{-1}), *Pilumnus spinosissimus* crabs (33.4 µg·Kg^{-1}) and a commercially important species of shrimp, *Xiphopenaeus kroyeri* (7.2 µg·Kg^{-1}), only incorporated OA from mid- to late bloom stages. Conjugated forms of OA were dominant (>70%) in most organisms, except in blenny fish, *Hypleurochilus fissicornis*, and polychaetes, *Pseudonereis palpata* (up to 59.3 and 164.6 µg total OA·Kg^{-1}, respectively), which contained mostly free-OA throughout the bloom. Although algal toxins are only regulated in bivalves during toxic blooms in most countries, including Brazil, this study indicates that human seafood consumers might be exposed to moderate toxin levels from a variety of other vectors during intense toxic outbreaks.

Keywords: harmful algal bloom; Diarrheic Shellfish Poisoning; okadaic acid; toxin accumulation; toxin vectors; trophic transfer; Brazil

Key Contribution: A massive toxic bloom of the *Dinophysis acuminata* complex associated with salinity stratification; Daily vertical distribution of *Dinophysis* spp. and *Mesodinium* cf. *rubrum* cells, and toxin in seston; Unprecedentedly high toxin cell quota in *D. acuminata* complex; Transfer of lipophilic toxins in the marine food web.

1. Introduction

The frequency, duration and severity of *Dinophysis* blooms have increased worldwide over the past two decades [1], leading to numerous episodes of massive shellfish contamination by lipophilic toxins in Europe [2,3], Africa [4,5], Asia [6], North America [7], and South America [8–10]. Although scientific evidence indicates that the increase in harmful algal blooms may be correlated with meso- and large-scale physico-chemical processes, i.e., artificial eutrophication [11–14], and global climate change [15,16], possible causes for an apparent increase in *Dinophysis* blooms are less comprehended.

Neritic and oceanic *Dinophysis* spp. are frequently observed in offshore waters along the southern coast of Brazil [17]. In 2007, the first large-scale bloom of *Dinophysis acuminata* complex ever reported in this region caused intoxication of at least 170 human consumers of contaminated shellfish (mainly *Perna perna* mussels [18,19]) and led managers and regulators to issue a first-time ban for bivalve mollusk harvesting and commercialization. Recurrent small to medium-scale *Dinophysis* blooms in Brazil have been reported along the coasts of Paraná and Santa Catarina states since then [20,21]. In many cases, episodes of bivalve contamination have been reported based on Diarrheic Shellfish Poisoning (DSP) mouse bioassays [18,22]. Additionally, diarrheic toxins such as okadaic acid (OA) and their congeners dinophysistoxins (DTXs) have been detected by chemical analytical methods in plankton and marine fauna [20,22]. The current Brazilian national monitoring program for harmful algae and phycotoxins uses bivalves (especially brown mussels, *Perna perna*) as sentinel organisms for the presence of toxins in shellfish farming areas, and harvesting bans are issue anytime the regulatory toxin levels are surpassed, i.e., 160 $\mu g \cdot Kg^{-1}$ in the case of diarrheic toxins [23].

Dinophysis spp. are a recurrent threat to shellfish aquaculture areas worldwide (reviewed by Reguera et al., [24]), where bloom initiation depends not only on favorable abiotic conditions, but also on the availability of ciliate prey [25]. Mixotrophy via the sequestration and retention of plastids from the ciliate *Mesodinium* cf. *rubrum* is now considered a key process enabling the development of *Dinophysis* populations both in the laboratory and in the field (e.g., [26,27]). Recent studies have focused on describing the feeding mechanism of *Dinophysis* spp., and elucidating the possible ecological roles of diarrheic toxins and other bioactives produced by the dinoflagellate [27–29]. A number of nutritional and trophic aspects related to toxic *Dinophysis* spp. blooms, such as small-scale interactions with *M.* cf. *rubrum* and possibly with other prey items in the field, however, remain unclear.

During *Dinophysis* blooms, lipophilic toxins can be transferred via several trophic pathways [30]. Toxins can be accumulated not only by bivalves, but also by polychaetes and ascidians [31], fish [32,33], octopuses [20] and crabs [34,35]. *Dinophysis* toxins may also be related to the death of monk seals off the coast of the western Sahara [36], although the implications of toxin incorporation for marine organisms remain poorly known. An understanding of small-scale trophic relationships underlying the initiation and development of *Dinophysis* blooms, as well as the fate of diarrheic toxins in marine food webs, are essential for the evaluation of their associated risks. The main objectives of this study are to (a) determine the diel vertical distribution of *Dinophysis* spp. and their prey in a shallow inlet, and (b) quantify the levels of lipophilic toxins present in seston and in marine organisms representative of different trophic levels, during a massive bloom of the *Dinophysis acuminata* complex in southern Brazil.

2. Results

2.1. Plankton and Toxins in the Water Column

Depth-averaged water temperature and salinity decreased gradually during the first half of the bloom period, from 26 May to 3 June, when the minimum salinities were recorded (mean ± standard deviation (SD) = 24.2 ± 0.55; n = 6). The water temperature continued to decrease thereafter, attaining a minimum of 16.8 ± 0.1 °C on the last sampling day, 16 June (Figure 1A,B). Secchi depth (Figure 1C,D) ranged from 1.8 to 2.8 m during the first half of the bloom and then gradually increased, attaining up to 3.6 m by the end of bloom. Chlorophyll-*a* concentrations were relatively low (0.47 ± 0.17 SD $mg \cdot m^{-3}$) throughout the study, and reached a maximum of 1.1 mg·m^{-3} on 3 June, coinciding with the maximum peak of *Dinophysis* abundance. Decreasing concentrations of mean DIN (±SD), especially those of nitrate (2.3 ± 0.9 μM) and ammonium (2.5 ± 0.7 μM) (Figure 1E), were associated with a concurrent decrease in salinity and temperature, and an increase in the abundance of *M.* cf. *rubrum*. Silicate and phosphate exhibited a marked increase during later stages of the bloom and attained the highest concentration range (39.6–88.7 μM and 1.3–6.3 μM, respectively) by the end of the study period (Figure 1F).

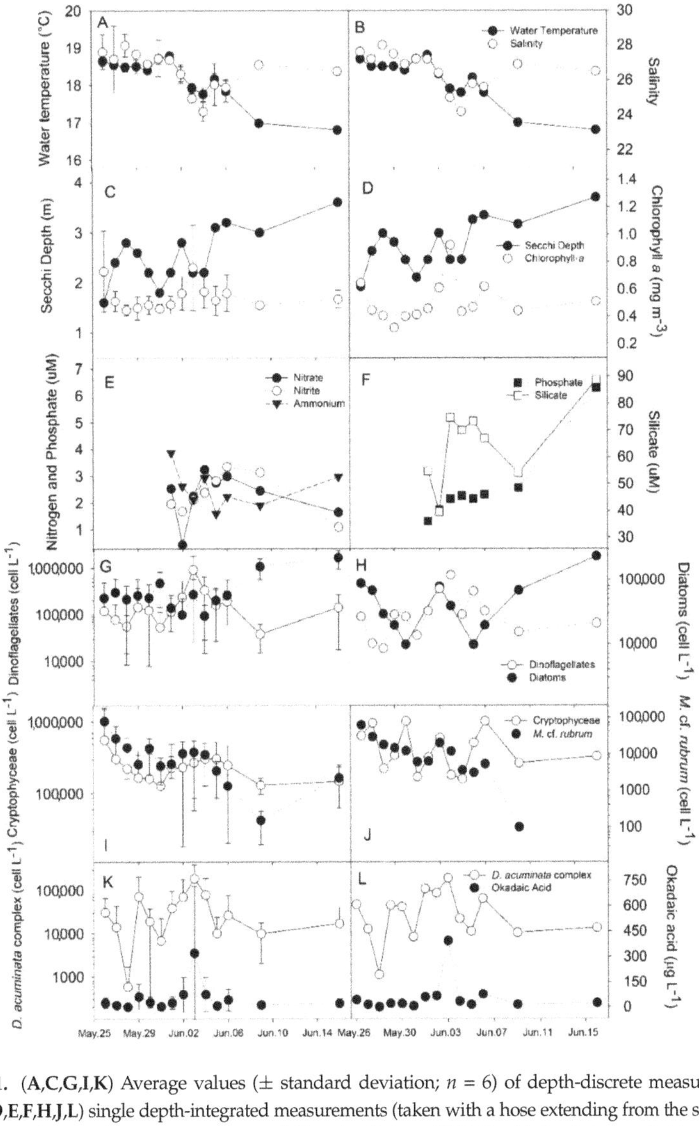

Figure 1. (**A**,**C**,**G**,**I**,**K**) Average values (± standard deviation; n = 6) of depth-discrete measurements, and (**B**,**D**,**E**,**F**,**H**,**J**,**L**) single depth-integrated measurements (taken with a hose extending from the surface to the bottom) for: (**A**,**B**) water temperature (°C) and salinity ; (**C**,**D**) Secchi depth (m) and chlorophyll-*a* concentration (mg·m^{-3}); (**E**,**F**) concentration of dissolved inorganic nutrients (μM); (**G**,**H**) numerical abundance (on log-scale) of dinoflagellates and diatoms (cells·L^{-1}); (**I**,**J**) abundance of cryptophyceans and *Mesodinium* cf. *rubrum* (cells·L^{-1}); (**K**,**L**) abundance of the *Dinophysis acuminata* spp. complex (cells·L^{-1}) and concentration of free okadaic acid (OA) in suspended particulate matter (μg·L^{-1}).

Diatom abundance remained at low to moderate levels (<9 × 10^4 cells·L^{-1}) during the first half of the bloom, rising up to 19 ± 6.2 × 10^4 cells·L^{-1} by the end of the sampling period, when they finally dominated the micro-phytoplankton assemblage (Figure 1H). Dinoflagellates were detected at cell densities comparable to those of diatoms during the first half of the study, attaining a maximum of 90 ± 31.9 × 10^4 cells·L^{-1} and becoming dominant over diatoms on 3 June (Figure 1H). *Dinophysis* species found during this bloom included the taxonomic complex composed by *D. acuminata* and *D. ovum* (referred to as *D. acuminata* complex hereafter), and *D. caudata*. This last species was frequently observed in plankton net samples during the first half of the bloom, although no cells were detected in most cell counts (LOD: 50 cells·L^{-1}), except on 28 and 30 May (100 cells·L^{-1}; not shown). The *Dinophysis acuminata* complex comprised the most abundant dinoflagellate cells and the main component of the total micro-phytoplankton assemblage throughout the study. Their depth-averaged cell density increased from 7.1 ± 13.4 × 10^4 cells·L^{-1} on the first sampling day to 18.7 ± 20.1 × 10^4 cells·L^{-1} (max. 43 × 10^4 cells·L^{-1} at 1.0 m depth) on 3 June (Figure 1K), coinciding with a gradual decrease in the abundance of the ciliate *M.* cf. *rubrum* (Figure 1I). At the beginning of the bloom, average cell densities of cryptophyceans decreased at a rate comparable to that of *M.* cf. *rubrum*, and then increased slightly by the mid-bloom period, when *M.* cf. *rubrum* abundance reached minimum values (Figure 1I).

Water temperature (Kruskal-Wallis test statistic H = 69.4; $p = 0.01$), Secchi depth (H = 79.0; $p = 0.01$), salinity (H = 55.5; $p = 0.01$) and abundance of diatoms (H = 34.3; $p = 0.01$) all varied significantly during the study period. When depth layers were compared over time, however, there was no detectable difference in water temperature (H = 0.24; $p = 0.99$) or diatom abundance values (H = 6.6; $p = 0.25$) over time at any specific depth. The depth layer marking salinity stratification (H = 14.8; $p = 0.01$) ranged from 2 to 3 m over the course of the bloom. Although peaks in the abundance of targeted taxa were clearly identified in time and space/depth, there were no statistically significant differences in the cell density of dinoflagellates, cryptophyceans, *M.* cf. *rubrum* and the *D. acuminata* complex, or in the concentrations of chl-*a* and OA in SPM over time. Chlorophyll-*a* concentrations (H = 45.0; $p < 0.01$), and the abundance of dinoflagellates (H = 51.7; $p < 0.01$), cryptophyceans (H = 56.4; $p < 0.01$), *M.* cf. *rubrum* (H = 31.6; $p < 0.01$), and the *D. acuminata* complex (H = 53.4; $p < 0.01$) all differed significantly between 0–2 m and 3–5 m depth, with higher values found in the upper water layer. In general, depth-integrated samples (those taken with a hose extending from surface to bottom), yielded very similar values to those calculated as the average of depth-discrete measurements, except for the abundance of cryptophyceans (H = 20.3; $p < 0.01$), which was typically greater when estimated from integrated samples (Figure 1I,J).

The onset of the bloom (on 26 May) was marked by pronounced surface stratification in salinity and water temperatures around 18 °C (Figure 2). After 2–3 days, salinity stratification was disrupted and the temperature increased by 1.0 °C, decreasing thereafter to a minimum of 17 °C by the 10th day (4 June), when the water column again became salinity-stratified (Figure 2). Water temperature ranged from 17 to 19.5 °C and salinity from 23 to 29 over time. The relatively high Secchi-depth values (>2.0 m) obtained during the study indicate that the euphotic zone always reached the bottom in the sampling area.

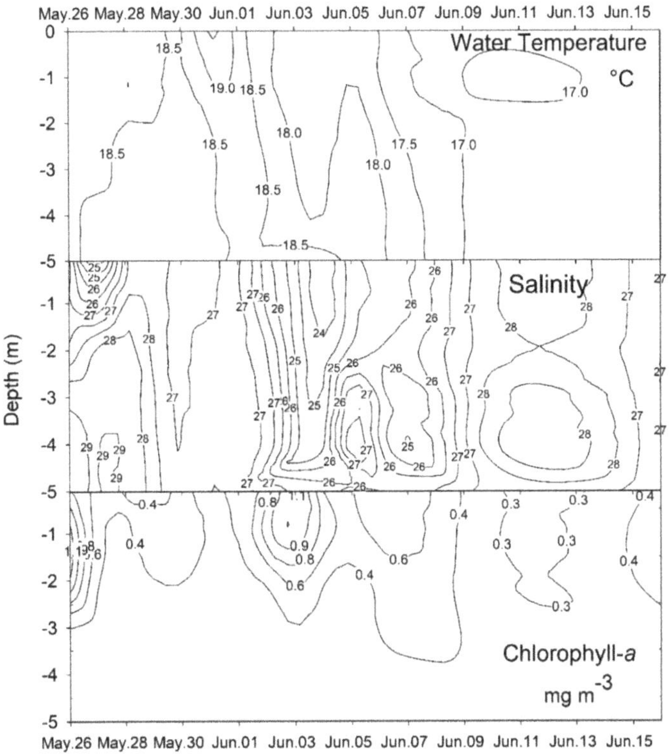

Figure 2. Interpolated depth-discrete measurements of water temperature (°C), salinity, and chlorophyll *a* concentration (mg·m^{-3}), over the course of the study.

Chlorophyll-*a* concentrations were higher during periods of salinity stratification. Values $\geq$1.0 mg·m^{-3} were attained on two occasions, on the 1st and the 9th day of sampling (26 May and 3 June), with a third peak (>0.6 mg·m^{-3}) a few days later (Figures 1D and 2). In all cases, higher concentrations were restricted ($H = 0.45$; $p < 0.01$) to the surface layer (0–2 m). Likewise, the abundance of the main taxa investigated–cryptophyceans, *M.* cf. *rubrum* and *Dinophysis*–also varied vertically, exhibiting higher values in the upper water layer. Maximum values for cryptophyceans and *M.* cf. *rubrum* (>500 $\times$ 10^4 and 18 $\times$ 10^4 cell·L^{-1}, respectively) were measured on the first day of sampling. During subsequent days, their abundance decreased concomitantly with a rapid increase of the *D. acuminata* complex cell density, reaching >20 $\times$ 10^4 cells·L^{-1} on 29 May and >40 $\times$ 10^4 cells·L^{-1} on 3 June, one week following the initial peak in *M.* cf. *rubrum* abundance (Figure 3), and coincident with the second episode of salinity stratification. Higher cell abundances of the *D. acuminata* complex were restricted to the surface layer (>2 m), where concentrations of free-OA >600 µg·L^{-1} were simultaneously detected in the SPM (>0.45-µm particles). During the period of maximum dinoflagellate cell density, the OA cellular quota, as measured from individually-picked cells of the *D. acuminata* complex ranged from 48 $\pm$ 31 SD pg·cells^{-1} (n = 137–208 cells per sample) on 2 June to 143 $\pm$ 93 pg·cell^{-1} (n = 141–220) on 3 June.

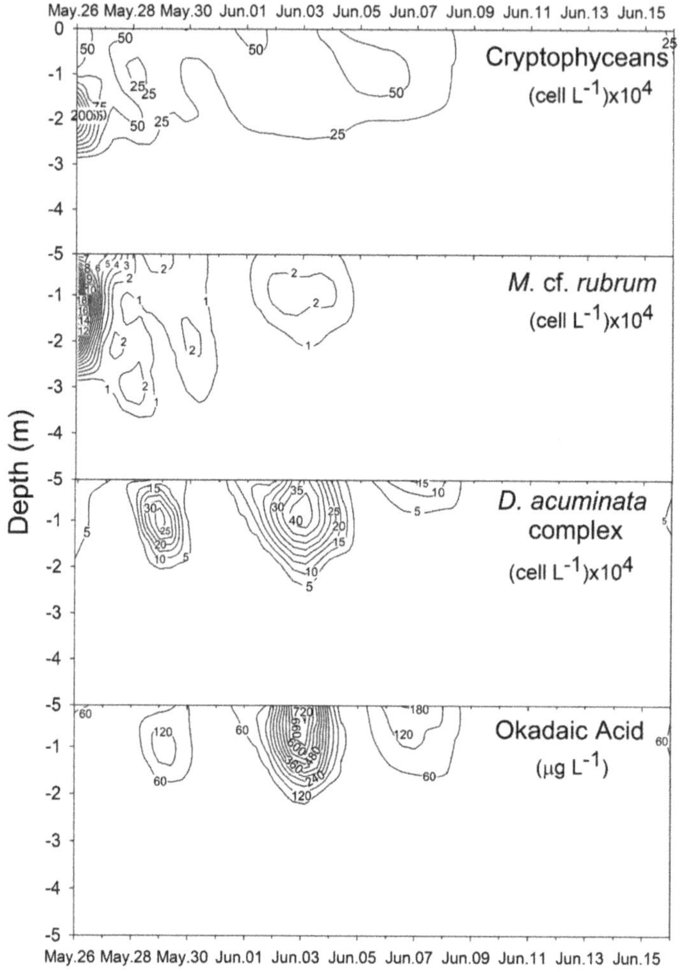

Figure 3. Depth profile of the cell abundance of the main plankton taxonomic groups (cell·L^{-1} × 10^{4}) (top three panels) and the concentration of okadaic acid (μg·L^{-1}) in suspended particulate matter (bottom panel) during the study period.

2.2. Diarrheic Toxins in Marine Fauna

All selected marine faunal components accumulated detectable OA levels during the study. Toxin levels were directly associated with the presence of *D. acuminata* complex cells in the water column; maximum values depended on the species and trophic position of the organisms. Suspension-feeding mussels and barnacles were the first to accumulate detectable levels of OA in their tissues and the only ones to contain detectable toxin levels during the entire sampling period. Mussels accumulated the highest OA concentrations among all organisms analyzed, with toxin levels gradually increasing following an increase in cell density of the *D. acuminata* complex. They attained a maximum of 549.6 μg total OA·Kg^{-1} (wet tissue weight) on 4 June (Figure 4), only one day after the peak abundance of the dinoflagellate. Polychaete worms (max. = 164.5 μg total OA·Kg^{-1}), amphipods (max. = 153.7 μg total OA·Kg^{-1}) and gastropods (max. = 111.6 μg total OA·Kg^{-1}) also retained relatively high toxin amounts, but not before the mid-bloom stage. Amphipods and to some extent fish (max. = 56.2 µg total OA·Kg^{-1}), remained contaminated for shorter periods, i.e., only when OA concentrations in the SPM were maximal (early to mid-bloom period). In contrast, gastropods, polychaetes, crabs (max. = 33.3 µg total OA·Kg^{-1}) and shrimp (max. = 7.2 µg total OA·Kg^{-1}) accumulated detectable toxin levels from the mid- to late bloom stage, after OA peaked in suspension (Figure 4).

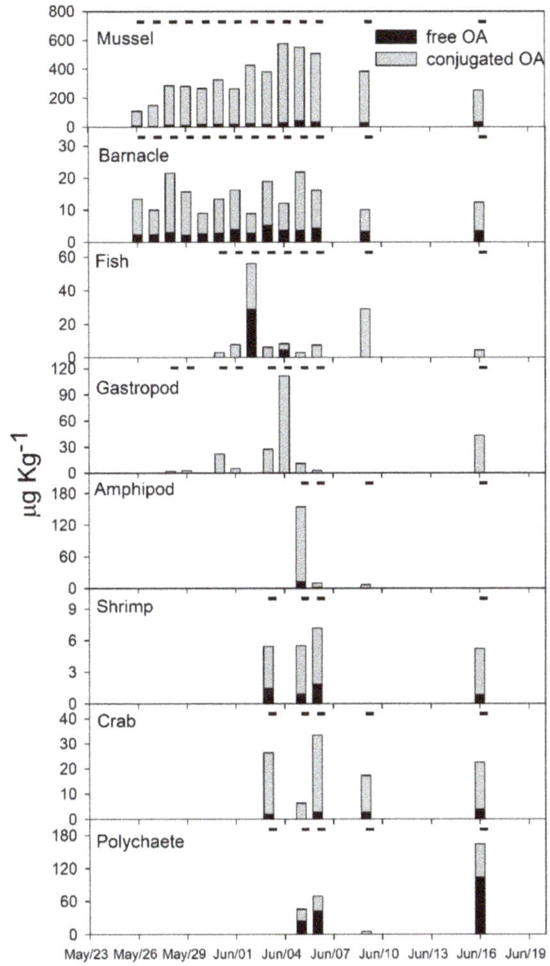

Figure 4. Concentration of okadaic acid (OA, µg·kg^{-1}), in its free (black bars) and conjugated (gray bars) forms, accumulated in different marine organisms during the bloom of the *Dinophysis acuminata* spp. complex. Dashes above the composite bars denote the sampling dates when each marine organism was available.

Fish and polychaetes accumulated the greatest proportions of OA in its free form. The proportion of free-OA was slightly higher in fish (54 ± 7%) at the peak of the bloom, but still did not match that of polychaetes (64 ± 5%). The latter seemed to possess the least efficient detoxification mechanism, given the high proportions of free-OA and the constantly increasing total OA levels measured (Figure 4). Conversely, the conjugated forms of OA were dominant in all other organisms, including barnacles

(76 ± 7% SD), shrimp (79 ± 5%), amphipods (87 ± 5%), crabs (90 ± 7%), mussels (94 ± 2%) and gastropods, which never accumulated detectable levels of free-OA (i.e., exhibited 100% of OA as conjugated forms).

2.3. Correlations

As assessed by principal component analysis, salinity was strongly and inversely correlated with both the abundance of the *D. acuminata* complex and the concentration of OA in suspension (Figure 5). This grouping was also inversely, but less obviously associated with ammonium concentration and the abundance of cryptophyceans, and even less obviously with Secchi depth, phosphate concentration and the abundance of diatoms (Figure 5). These last three variables, as well as the concentration of silicate, were inversely correlated to *M.* cf. *rubrum* abundance, which, in turn, was strongly and directly associated with the abundance of cryptophyceans and the concentrations of nitrite and nitrate.

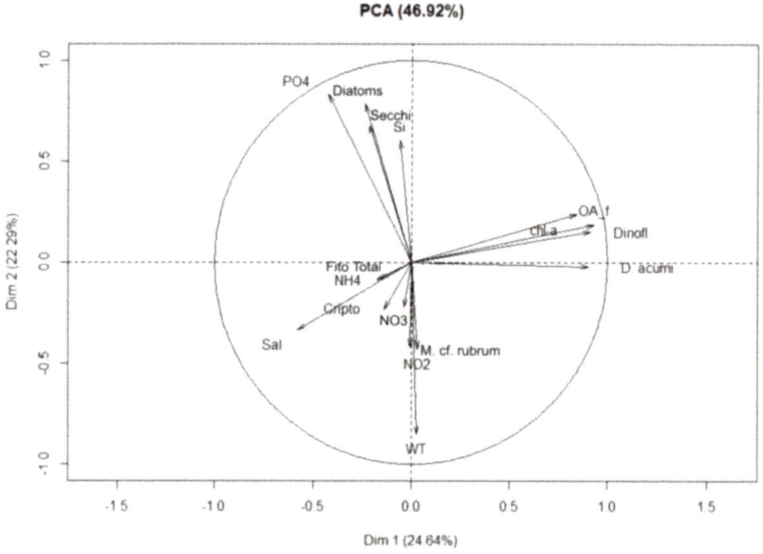

Figure 5. Principal Component Analysis (PCA) of discrete-depth measurements of the following variables: water temperature (WT), Salinity (Sal), Transparency (Secchi depth), Chlorophyll-*a* (chl-*a*), Diatoms (Diatoms), Dinoflagellates (Dinofl), Cryptophyceans (Cripto), total micro-phytoplankton (Fito Total), *Mesodinium* cf. *rubrum* (*M.* cf. *rubrum*), *D. acuminata* complex (*D. acumi*), free okadaic acid (AO_f), Phosphate (PO4), Nitrate (NO3), Nitrite (NO2), Ammonium (NH4), and Silicate (Si) concentrations.

3. Discussion

3.1. Bloom Development and Trophic Relationships

In late May 2016, an episode of marked salinity stratification was associated with the onset of what can be considered the most intense bloom of the *Dinophysis acuminata* complex ever recorded along the Brazilian coast. The bloom only lasted for a few weeks along the coast of Santa Catarina State. It was then transported northward to Paraná State, where it reached even higher cell densities, causing massive contamination of marine fauna and intoxication of human seafood consumers [37]. Although results of the present study indicated that bivalves were also contaminated with unsafe OA levels in Santa Catarina, actions taken in the context of the local HAB monitoring and management program prevented cases of intoxication in this region. More importantly, however, the present study also documents the accumulation of diarrheic toxins in several other marine organisms associated with farmed mussels, some of them for the first time, indicating that multiple toxin vectors and transfer routes should be considered during massive *Dinophysis* blooms.

Blooms of *Dinophysis* spp. are usually associated with marked thermohaline stratification of the water column [10,38–40]. The ciliate prey of *Dinophysis* spp., frequently reported as *Mesodinium rubrum*, usually benefits from vertical water stratification as well [41,42], although blooms of the ciliate may also occur along horizontal thermohaline gradients in shallow estuaries [43].

About one week preceding the maximum *Dinophysis* cell density recorded in Armação do Itapocoroy inlet during this study, high abundances of *M.* cf. *rubrum* and their cryptophycean prey (10^5 to 10^6 cells·L^{-1}, respectively) were observed in the upper water layer associated with lower salinities and strong stratification at 2 m depth. On the following 4–5 days, the abundance of cryptophyceans decreased rapidly, followed by a more gradual decrease in *M.* cf. *rubrum* cell density, as the abundance of cells belonging to the *D. acuminata* complex began to increase in the same surface layer. One week later, a second cryptophycean-ciliate-*Dinophysis* succession cycle occurred once water became stratified again. Although daily variations in the abundance of these three taxa may be partially linked to local advection, what was not the subject of this study; the succession pattern reported herein confirms that the trophic relationships documented in prior laboratory observations [27,28,44–46] may also occur on a similar temporal scale under natural field conditions and sustain massive blooms of the toxic dinoflagellate. On other occasions (i.e., under lower availability of *M.* cf. *rubrum* cells), alternative prey items may provide *Dinophysis* spp. with an additional source of nutrients, as suggested for *D. caudata* preying upon the benthic ciliate *Mesodinium coatsi* [47].

The development of *Dinophysis* blooms in other geographical areas may also be linked to the intrusion of less saline water masses and/or to disturbances in physico-chemical water column structure, although the underlying processes might be different and sometimes occur on a wider spatio-temporal scale. Blooms may thus be either associated to upwelling, as verified in Sweden [48], Galicia (Spain) and Portugal [25], or to river plumes, as found in Tunisia [40] and Scotland [3]. They may also be associated with seasonal changes in wind patterns and the precipitation regime such as those recorded in Ireland [49], Greece [50] and Argentina [9,51]. On the eastern coast of South America, the water mass associated with the La Plata River plume promotes important large-scale changes in the physico-chemical characteristics of the water column along the coasts of NE Argentina, Uruguay and southern Brazil during fall and winter [52,53], when massive *Dinophysis* blooms are usually observed in this region [54,55]. This suggests that the La Plata water plume (PWP) may be one of the main factors controlling the development of large-scale *Dinophysis* blooms in southwestern Atlantic coastal waters.

Chlorophyll-*a* concentrations did not vary substantially over time in the present study, and did not attain values exceeding the historical average for the region [56,57]. This could be explained by the uncommon prevailing phytoplankton succession, whereby one dominant taxon preys upon and acquires the plastids (and the pigments) from its precursor, rather than synthesizing its own pigment quota during a gradual competitive exclusion process. Whereas phosphate concentrations remained relatively high and even increased during the final bloom stage, those of dissolved nitrogen compounds, notably ammonium and nitrate, decreased over the course of the bloom, especially during the period of maximum cell abundance of the *D. acuminata* complex.

Both water sampling strategies used in this study (single integrated samples and multiple depth-discrete sampling) allowed adequate tracking of bloom development, yielding similar abundance values for both the toxic dinoflagellate and its prey, *M.* cf. *rubrum*. Therefore, as demonstrated in other areas such as Spain [58], depth-integrated sampling, undertaken with a hose extending from the surface to the bottom, provided a rapid and reliable early-warning tool in HAB monitoring and risk assessment in shallow waters affected by *Dinophysis* blooms along the southern coast of Brazil. However, special attention is required when applying the technique to ecological studies, as the abundance of cryptophyceans and perhaps other small-celled algal groups can be underestimated. Likewise, vertical migration and cell aggregation processes can be missed as a result of the "diluting" effect introduced by this sampling strategy. More importantly, adoption of *Dinophysis* cell abundance as early warning for DSP should be used conservatively, i.e., the threshold value should be kept cautiously low when integrated samples are used in HAB monitoring programs. One of the main ecological features of *Dinophysis* cells is their ability to aggregate in thin water layers, as reported in this and other studies [59], such that toxin food web transfer may be heterogeneous throughout the water column.

3.2. Fate of Diarrheic Toxins during the Bloom

Cells of the *D. acuminata* complex contained exclusively OA during the bloom described in this study, contrasting with a more complex toxin profile reported during previous blooms in Argentina [10,60] and Chile [61], where *D. acuminata* and *D. tripos*, the species involved in the blooms, produced pectenotoxin-2 (PTX-2) and DTX-1 in addition to OA. It is noteworthy that DTX-1 has been reported in different southern Brazilian estuaries when lower *Dinophysis* spp. cell abundances (<2 × 10^4 cell·L^{-1}) occur, but rarely when only cells of the *D. acuminata* complex are detected, in which case OA usually becomes the single diarrheic toxin present [32]. Similarly, in late summer 2015, one year before the event reported in this study, an extremely dense bloom of the *Dinophysis acuminata* complex affected the coast of Uruguay and only OA was detected by LC-MS/MS [32]. This further suggests that there may be interconnectivity between Uruguayan and southern Brazilian populations of the *D. acuminata* complex, perhaps driven by the northward transport of PWP from late summer to winter. This possibility remains to be addressed in future studies.

All marine organisms collected in the upper water layer (0–1 m) at the sampling site were consistently contaminated with varying amounts of OA. This is the first record of diarrheic toxin accumulation in amphipods (Caprellidae), shrimp (*X. kroyeri*), Nereidae polychaetes and blenny fish (Blenniedae). The only previous records of OA content in fish included carnivorous flounders, *Platichthys flesus* [33], and filter-feeding anchovies, *Cetengraulis edentulus* [32]. Results of the present study demonstrated that the combtooth blenny, *Hypleurochilus fissicornis*, can accumulate moderate OA levels in their viscera during *Dinophysis* blooms, but are able to rapidly eliminate the toxin. Therefore, this fish species may act as a temporary vector of diarrheic toxins for other species, including commercially important species of Serranidae and Lutjanidae, which prey upon small fish like blennies [62]. *Hypleurochilus fissicornis* is widely distributed in the southwest Atlantic; adults feed primarily on isopods and amphipods [63], that were likely an important–although probably not the sole–toxin source for the fish during the bloom, as the peak in OA levels occurred later for amphipods than for *H. fissicornis* in the present study. Amphipods accumulated relatively high OA levels (up to ~150 μg OA·Kg^{-1}) at the peak of the bloom. Although most amphipods are detritivores/scavengers, caprellids such as the ones sampled in our study are omnivorous and may feed not only on detritus, but also on microalgae, protozoans, smaller amphipods and crustacean larvae [64]. Caprellids are frequent and abundant organisms associated with suspended mussel farms, living on substrates such as mussel sleeves and ropes, and may thus be important toxin vectors to several organisms that search for shelter and food within the mussel longlines in aquaculture areas.

Mussels accumulated the greatest OA levels during the bloom, exceeding by 4-fold the 160-μg·Kg^{-1} Brazilian regulatory seafood safety level [65]. *Perna perna* mussels are the sentinel species in HAB monitoring programs in Brazil and, like other mussel species, are able to rapidly incorporate high levels of several marine biotoxins and contaminants [66–70]. Indeed, along with barnacles, mussels were the only organisms exhibiting detectable OA levels during the entire sampling period. They consistently and promptly reflected the abundance of the *D. acuminata* complex (i.e., they attained maximum OA levels only one day after the peak in cell abundance). Considering the high *Dinophysis* cell abundance reported during this bloom, however, OA levels in *P. perna* were not as high as expected, what may be related to its fast toxin elimination rates as reported in previous laboratory experiments [21]. Besides mussels, non-edible polychaetes (*P. palpata*) and amphipods were the only organisms to accumulate total OA levels approaching or surpassing this regulatory level in the present study. Toxin contents in barnacles were 8 to 48 × lower–and less clearly related to *Dinophysis* cell density–than those of mussels. Barnacles colonize hard substrates, rocks, bivalve shells and mooring structures, living in clusters of around a dozen individuals that actively capture food particles from the surrounding water [71]. In the present study, barnacles were collected from the shells of the same mussels sampled for OA analysis, so that the differential toxin accumulation reported here for these two suspension-feeding taxa can only be attributed to distinct feeding mechanisms and toxin uptake/elimination capacity. The consistently greater proportions of conjugated OA in mussels (>90%) reflect their efficient mechanisms of toxin metabolism and elimination. Likewise, Caprellidae amphipods, small crabs (*P. spinosissimus*), shrimp (*X. kroyeri*) may have ingested toxins from the grazers or their organic matter produced [72,73], and carnivorous gastropods (*S. haemastoma*) also accumulated very limited to undetectable free-OA levels. This finding at least partly suggests that these organisms ingested already metabolized (i.e., conjugated) toxin, either incorporated into mussel and barnacle tissues (gastropods, shrimp and crabs) or from detrital origin (in the case of amphipods and crabs). High toxin levels were found in seston during this study and in particles >60 µm (L. Mafra, unpublished data), suggesting that not only *Dinophysis* cells but also toxin-containing organic particles and zooplankton organisms may contribute to the transfer of diarrheic toxins along the foodweb. Therefore, although zooplankton (e.g., copepods) may exert significant grazing impact and contribute considerably to control population growth of *Dinophysis* spp. [74], contaminated individuals will act as vectors of DSP-toxins to higher trophic levels.

Transfer of lipophilic toxins in the marine food web is still poorly understood. Although they represent only a small fraction of the sinking organic material, zooplankters such as the copepod *Temora longicornis*, might contribute in maintaining toxin availability for other organisms via production of toxic faecal pellets following ingestion of *Dinophysis* cells [73]. Inter- and intraspecific differences in the capacity of uptake and elimination of phycotoxins, as reported for suspension-feeding grazers such as oysters, clams and mussels [21,75–77], may ultimately determine the bioavailability of these compounds for other organisms during and after a bloom. In this study, polychaetes, which exhibited the highest proportions of free-OA and whose total OA levels continued to increase through the end of the sampling period, proved to be slow in eliminating OA. They may thus be an important toxin vector during late bloom stages, by prolonging toxin availability in the trophic web even after bloom termination.

To date, potential vectors of diarrheic toxins to human consumers have been restricted to several bivalve species (reviewed by FAO/WHO [78]), a couple of fish species [32,33], octopuses [20] and crabs [34,35]. The present study indicates that seabob shrimp (*X. kroyeri*) can represent a novel vector for toxin transfer to humans during massive dinoflagellate blooms. Although these shrimp accumulated the lowest OA levels ($\leq$7 $\mu g \cdot Kg^{-1}$) of all investigated faunal species and thus cannot be classified as a risk for acute food intoxication among seafood consumers, frequent consumers of this valuable fishery resource may be chronically exposed to low toxin levels during prolonged blooms. Seabob shrimp catches may reach 170 tons per year only in the Armação do Itapocoroy area [79], our study site, and the seabob shrimp fishing season coincides with the usual period of *Dinophysis* blooms in southern Brazil (winter to spring; [80]). Additionally, shrimp and, to some extent crabs and blenny fish, are highly motile. Their frequent vertical migration throughout the water column or on mussel ropes and sleeves may thus help to accelerate toxin transfer from pelagic to benthic compartments, and to spread diarrheic toxins over a more complex trophic web.

4. Materials and Methods

4.1. Study Area

Armação do Itapocoroy is a shallow [mean depth = 8 m; maximum (max.) = 15 m] inlet in Santa Catarina State, southern Brazil (26°47′ S, 48°37′ W). Surrounded by hills (up to 250 m high), its geographic SE-NE orientation provides natural shelter from prevailing waves and winds, especially the stronger ones coming from the south. Due to these favorable attributes, Armação do Itapocoroy (Figure 6) harbors the major marine aquaculture (~360 hectares) operations in the country, mainly used for the cultivation of mussels, but also of oysters and scallops. The location experiences semi-diurnal, micro-tidal cycles and is affected by the Itajaí-Açu River plume, that maintains high levels of local primary production and brings high loads of suspended particulate matter (SPM) mainly during rainy periods such as the austral summer (December–March) [81–83].

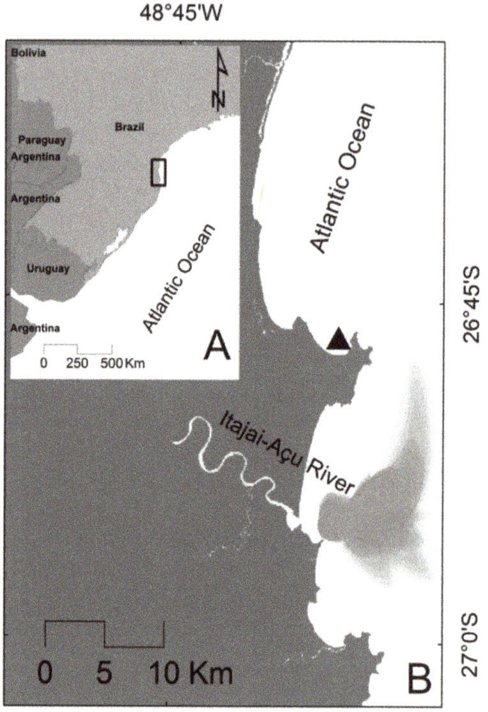

Figure 6. Map showing the location of the study area, Armação do Itapocoroy inlet (triangle in (**B**)), on the southern coast of Brazil (rectangle in (**A**)). A schematic representation of the prevailing direction and influence area of the Itajaí-Açu River plume is also presented, based on Trochimczuk-Fo and Schettini (2003) [83].

4.2. Sampling Design

An intensive sampling effort was conducted between late May and mid-June 2016, when the Santa Catarina coastal zone was affected by a dense *Dinophysis* bloom. Seawater sampling was carried out from a floating platform, anchored at a depth of 4.5 ± 0.5 m and deployed 200 m from the low tide level. Samples (~1.5 L) were taken every meter along a vertical profile, from the surface to the bottom, using an EN-470 manual diaphragm pump (Emifran®, São Paulo, SP, Brazil) equipped with anti-reflux valves and coupled to a 20 mm-diameter hose. Daily samples were taken over 12 days, followed by two sampling operations after 3- and 10-day intervals of the 12th sampling day. Additionally, single depth-integrated water samples (2.0 L) were taken with a 5 m long hose, to compare the efficiency of both sampling strategies for monitoring of extreme bloom events. Plankton net (20-µm mesh size) samples were also collected, and water temperature and salinity were measured along a vertical profile, at 0.5 m intervals from surface to bottom, using a multiparameter YSI Professional Plus probe. Secchi depth was used to estimate water column light penetration or transparency.

In parallel, bivalve mollusks (*Perna perna*; $n > 5$), gastropods (*Stramonita haemastoma*; $n > 2$), barnacles (*Megabalanus tintinnabulum*; $n > 10$), amphipods (Caprellidae; ~10 g of wet weight), crabs

(*Pilumnus spinosissimus*; $n > 3$), shrimp (*Xiphopenaeus kroyeri*; $n > 5$), polychaetes (*Pseudonereis palpate*; $n > 3$) and fish (*Hypleurochilus fissicornis*–Blenniidae; $n > 2$) were manually collected from raft mooring cables at 0–1 m depth, for quantification of the toxin levels incorporated in their tissues. The species collected and sampling frequency depended on their availability in the environment during the study period. Whenever possible, at least two individuals of each species were collected, packed in 50 mL plastic tubes and immediately immersed in an ice bath until return to the laboratory. Before freezing, soft tissues of mussels, barnacles and gastropods were removed from their shells. Fish muscles (flesh) and viscera were dissected and individually stored at −18 °C. The remaining organisms were frozen and analyzed whole.

4.3. Processing of Samples

Water samples: Aliquots (300 mL) of both depth-discrete and integrated samples were fixed with 1% Lugol's iodine solution, and used for quantitative phytoplankton analysis. Plankton net samples, fixed with a 4% formalin solution (final concentration), were used for analysis of cell morphology and phytoplankton identification. In the laboratory, additional 300 mL aliquots of each sample were gently vacuum-filtered in duplicate and immediately frozen. One fiberglass filter (Marcherey-Nagel®, Düren, Germany, model 85/70BF; 47 mm diameter and 0.45 µm nominal retention capacity) was allocated for the analysis of photosynthetic pigments, and the second one to determine the amount of lipophilic toxins contained in SPM. In an ice bath, each filter sample was soaked in HPLC grade methanol (99.5%) and exposed to an ultra-sonic probe (Cole Parmer, Vernon Hills, IL, USA, CPX130) for 30 s. The extract was then passed through a 13 mm × 0.22 µm PVDF syringe filter (Analitica®, São Paulo, SP, Brazil) to remove any cell debris, and the filtrate collected into plastic microtubes (1.5 mL), which were maintained frozen. Aliquots (400 mL) of the filtrate from depth-integrated samples collected from 1 May on were stored frozen in plastic bottles for future spectrophotometric determination of dissolved inorganic nutrient (DIN) concentrations.

Samples of marine fauna: The protocol for toxin extraction was adapted from the official analytical method harmonized by the European Union [84]. Methanol (99.5%; HPLC grade) was added in the ratio of 1:9 (*v*:*v*) to 1.0 ± 0.5 g of homogenate from selected tissues or whole body, exposed to an ultra-sonic probe (Cole Parmer, CPX130) until complete tissue disruption, and centrifuged at 2000× *g* for 10 min. The supernatant was filtered through a 0.22-µm syringe filter directly into a 2.0 mL glass vial, and kept frozen for the analysis of diarrheic toxins in their free form. Subsequently, 1 mL aliquots of the extract were subjected to alkaline hydrolysis by the addition of 2.5 M sodium hydroxide in a 76 °C thermal bath for 40 min, followed by the addition of 2.5 M hydrochloric acid to neutralize the solution and convert the conjugated (metabolized) toxins into their free toxin forms. The amount of conjugated toxins was obtained by subtracting the concentration of free toxins initially measured in the non-hydrolyzed extract from the total concentration of toxins obtained in the hydrolyzed extract.

4.4. Phytoplankton Identification and Enumeration

Counting of *Dinophysis* spp. and *M.* cf. *rubrum* cells was performed using a 20 mL aliquot of the Lugol-fixed sample, after settling the particles for 24 h in a Utermöhl chamber [85]. Cell counting was then performed by scanning the whole chamber under an inverted optical microscope at 200× magnification (limit of detection, LOD: 50 cell·L^{-1}). Other phytoplankton groups (total cryptophytes, diatoms, and dinoflagellates) were quantified in volumes ranging from 10 to 20 mL (depending on sample turbidity) by counting all cells contained in 5–10 random microscope fields of view (LOD: 2100–8400 cell·L^{-1}) after 24-h settlement. Additionally, a minimum of 100 cells of *Dinophysis* spp. were picked with a micropipette from *in natura* plankton net samples at the bloom apex (2 and 3 June; n = 5 samples each day), and placed into 1.5 mL plastic microtubes containing methanol 99.5% (HPLC grade) for determination of the toxin cellular quota.

4.5. Spectrophotometric Analysis of Dissolved Inorganic Nutrients

Aliquots (25 mL) of the filtrate samples were used to determine the concentrations of phosphate (P-PO_4^{3-}), nitrite (N-NO_2^-), nitrate (N-NO_3^-), ammonium (N-NH_4^+), and silicate (SiO_2^-) using colorimetric methods [86]. The concentrations were determined from a linear regression obtained from successive dilutions of the respective analytical standards (coefficient of determination, $r^2 > 0.90$).

4.6. Analysis of Photosynthetic Pigments by LC-DAD

The methanolic extracts were injected (100 µL) into a Chromaster liquid chromatography (LC) system (Hitachi®, Tokyo, Japan), composed of a quaternary gradient pump, an automatic thermostat injector, a column oven (set at 40 °C) and a photodiode detector (DAD). Samples were eluted in a mixture of (A) methanol:acetone:pyridine (50:25:25) and (B) acetonitrile:acetone (80:20), at 1.0 mL·min^{-1}. The proportion of B increased from 0 to 40% in 18 min, and then to 100% within the following 4 min of analysis, remaining at 100% for an extra 16 min before returning to the initial conditions (0% B) for an additional 2 min period (40 min in total). Pigment identification was performed by evaluating retention times after the chromatographic separation in a Waters Symmetry® C8 column (150 × 4.6 mm, 3.5 µm particles), as well as the absorbance spectrum (350–750 nm scan), following methods of Zapata et al. [87]. The chlorophyll-*a* (chl-*a*) concentration was calculated using a linear regression obtained from successive dilutions of the analytical standard (Sigma-Aldrich, Saint Louis, MO, USA) (0.78, 1.56, 3.12, 6.25, 12.50, and 25.00 ng·mL^{-1}) with $r^2 > 0.98$.

4.7. Analysis of Diarrheic Toxins by LC-MS/MS

Toxins were measured using a 1260 LC system (Agilent Technologies®, Santa Clara, CA, USA) coupled to a triple quadrupole mass spectrometer, MS (AB Sciex®, Framingham, MA, USA, qTRAP 3200) equipped with a turbo ion spray ionization source, following the EURLMB protocol [84]. Briefly, 5 to 15 µL of each sample were eluted by the mobile phase, consisting of a mixture of (A) 100% ultra-pure water and (B) 95% acetonitrile, both with the addition of ammonium formate (2 mM) and formic acid (50 mM). At a 0.3 mL·min^{-1} flow rate, the initial proportion of 80:20% (A:B) increased to 100% B during the first 8 min of analysis, thus remaining for 3.5 min, and returning to the initial condition by the end of the analysis (13 min). Compounds were separated on a C18 column (Agilent Poroshell®, Santa Clara, CA, USA, 50 × 2.1 mm, 2.7 µm particles), maintained at 20 °C. Identification of individual toxins was achieved from their retention time and the mass spectra of the transition ions present in the samples in relation to the same parameters obtained for the analytical standards. High-purity nitrogen, heated up to 500 °C, was used as the nebulizing gas. The electron spray (ESI) ion source operated in negative mode, and toxins were scanned for transition ions (Q1 → Q3) of characteristic mass/charge (m/z) ratios. Optimized MS parameters were selected for each toxin of interest (Table 1).

Table 1. Conditions of the tandem mass spectrometry system (MS/MS). Q1: quadrupole 1, Q3: quadrupole 3, DP: declustering potential, EP: entrance potential, CEP: collision cell entrance potential, CE: collision energy and CXP: collision cell exit potential.

Toxins	Q1 (*m/z*)	Q3 (*m/z*)	DP (v)	EP (v)	CEP (v)	CE (v)	CXP (v)
OA	803.5	255.0	−129	−10	−40.1	−82	−2
OA	803.5	113.0	−129	−10	−41.5	−64	−2
DTX-2	803.5	255.0	−129	−10	−40.6	−64	−2
DTX-2	803.5	113.0	−129	−10	−41.5	−84	−2
DTX-1	817.5	255.0	−129	−10	−41.5	−62	−2
DTX-1	817.5	113.0	−120	−10	−51.7	−82	−2
DTX-3	1041.6	255.0	−129	−10	−47.9	−76	−2

Toxin quantification was carried out using an external standard from a calibration curve generated with certified reference material (IMB-NRC, Canada) dissolved in methanol for OA, and in mussel tissue matrix (CRM-DSP-Mus-b) for DTX-1. Quantification of OA was based on the equation obtained by fitting a linear regression ($r^2 > 0.95$) to the following concentrations: 3.49, 13.96, 55.86, and 223.44 ng·mL^{-1}.

4.8. Data Analysis

Graphs were constructed in SigmaPlot® v11.0 (Systat Software Inc., London, UK), using the statistical package for preliminary analysis. Data were statistically analyzed with R studio software [88], using the Kruskal-Wallis non-parametric test (H) followed by the Dunn test (with the software package dunn.test; [89]) for comparative analyses within and among water column depths, between discrete and integrated samples, and for analysis of temporal variation. Principal components analysis (PCA) (with the FactoMiner package; [90]) allowed quantification of the degree of association among water temperature, Secchi depth, salinity, numerical abundance of main taxonomic groups, concentration of dissolved inorganic nutrients and seston toxin content.

Author Contributions: Both authors contributed equally to the study conceptualization, sampling design, LC-MS/MS analysis and manuscript writing; T.P.A. conducted the sampling, plankton analysis, toxin extraction and carried out the data analysis; L.L.M.J. supervised the activities, administrated the project and acquired funding.

Acknowledgments: The authors thank the bivalve growers affiliated with the Association of Marine Farmers of Paulas (AMAP), and personnel involved in HAB monitoring programs in Santa Catarina State, including those from the Agricultural Research and Rural Extension Company of Santa Catarina (EPAGRI), Integrated Company of Agricultural Development Santa Catarina (CIDASC), and the Agricultural and Livestock Defense Secretary (SDA) of the Ministry of Agriculture, Livestock and Food Supply (MAPA). This study was partially funded by CNPq (Grant # 610012/2011-8) through the Brazilian National Institute of Science and Technology (INCT-Mar-COI).

Conflicts of Interest: The authors declare no conflict of interest.

References

1. Reguera, B.; Velo-Suárez, L.; Raine, R.; Park, M.G. Harmful *Dinophysis* species: A review. *Harmful Algae* **2012**, *14*, 87–106. [CrossRef]
2. García-Altares, M.; Casanova, A.; Fernández-Tejedor, M.; Diogène, J.; de la Iglesia, P. Bloom of *Dinophysis* spp. dominated by *D. sacculus* and its related diarrhetic shellfish poisoning (DSP) outbreak in Alfacs Bay (Catalonia, NW Mediterranean Sea): Identification of DSP toxins in phytoplankton, shellfish and passive samplers. *Reg. Stud. Mar. Sci.* **2016**, *6*, 19–28. [CrossRef]
3. Whyte, C.; Swan, S.; Davidson, K. Changing wind patterns linked to unusually high *Dinophysis* blooms around the Shetland Islands, Scotland. *Harmful Algae* **2014**, *39*, 365–373. [CrossRef]
4. Pitcher, G.C.; Krock, B.; Cembella, A.D. Accumulation of diarrhetic shellfish poisoning toxins in the oyster *Crassostrea gigas* and the mussel *Choromytilus meridionalis* in the southern Benguela ecosystem. *Afr. J. Mar. Sci.* **2011**, *33*, 273–281. [CrossRef]
5. Aissaoui, A.; Dhib, A.; Reguera, B.; Ben Hassine, O.K.; Turki, S.; Aleya, L. First evidence of cell deformation occurrence during a *Dinophysis* bloom along the shores of the Gulf of Tunis (SW Mediterranean Sea). *Harmful Algae* **2014**, *39*, 191–201. [CrossRef]
6. Li, A.; Sun, G.; Qiu, J.; Fan, L. Lipophilic shellfish toxins in *Dinophysis caudata* picked cells and in shellfish from the East China Sea. *Environ. Sci. Pollut. Res.* **2015**, *22*, 3116–3126. [CrossRef] [PubMed]
7. Hattenrath-Lehmann, T.K.; Marcoval, M.A.; Berry, D.L.; Fire, S.; Wang, Z.; Morton, S.L.; Gobler, C.J. The emergence of *Dinophysis acuminata* blooms and DSP toxins in shellfish in New York waters. *Harmful Algae* **2013**, *26*, 33–44. [CrossRef]
8. Martínez, A.; Nacional, D.; Acuáticos, D.R.; Fabre, A. Intensification of marine dinoflagellates blooms in Uruguay Intensificación de floraciones de dinoflagelados marinos en Uruguay Intensification of marine dinoflagellates blooms in Uruguay. *Rev. Lab. Tecnol. Urug.* **2017**, *13*, 19–25.
9. Sar, E.A.; Sunesen, I.; Goya, A.B.; Lavigne, A.S.; Tapia, E.; García, C.; Lagos, N. First Report of Diarrheic Shellfish Toxins in Mollusks from Buenos Aires Province (Argentina) associated with *Dinophysis* spp.: Evidence os okadaic acid, dinophysistoxin-1 and their acyl-derivates. *Biol. Soc. Argent. Bot.* **2012**, *47*, 5–14.

10. Villalobos, L.G.; Santinelli, N.; Sastre, V.; Krock, B.; Esteves, J.L. *Dinophysis* Species Associated with Diarrhetic Shellfish Poisoning Episodes in North Patagonian Gulfs (Chubut, Argentina). *J. Shellfish Res.* **2015**, *34*, 1141–1149. [CrossRef]
11. Smayda, T.J. Complexity in the eutrophication–harmful algal bloom relationship, with comment on the importance of grazing. *Harmful Algae* **2008**, *8*, 140–151. [CrossRef]
12. Lewitus, A.J.; Brock, L.M.; Burke, M.K.; DeMattio, K.A.; Wilde, S.B. Lagoonal stormwater detention ponds as promoters of harmful algal blooms and eutrophication along the South Carolina coast. *Harmful Algae* **2008**, *8*, 60–65. [CrossRef]
13. Heisler, J.; Glibert, P.M.; Burkholder, J.M.; Anderson, D.M.; Cochlan, W.; Dennison, W.C.; Dortch, Q.; Gobler, C.J.; Heil, C.A.; Humphries, E.; et al. Eutrophication and harmful algal blooms: A scientific consensus. *Harmful Algae* **2008**, *8*, 3–13. [CrossRef] [PubMed]
14. Buskey, E.J. How does eutrophication affect the role of grazers in harmful algal bloom dynamics? *Harmful Algae* **2008**, *8*, 152–157. [CrossRef]
15. Hallegraeff, G.M. Ocean climate change, phytoplankton community responses, and harmful algal blooms: A formidable predictive challenge. *J. Phycol.* **2010**, *46*, 220–235. [CrossRef]
16. O'Neil, J.M.; Davis, T.W.; Burford, M.A.; Gobler, C.J. The rise of harmful cyanobacteria blooms: The potential roles of eutrophication and climate change. *Harmful Algae* **2012**, *14*, 313–334. [CrossRef]
17. Haraguchi, L.; Odebrecht, C. Dinophysiales (Dinophyceae) no extremo Sul do Brasil (inverno de 2005, verão de 2007). *Biota Neotrop.* **2010**, *10*, 101–114. [CrossRef]
18. Proença, L.A.O.; Schramm, M.A.; da Silva Tamanaha, M.; Alves, T.P. Diarrhoetic shellfish poisoning (DSP) outbreak in Subtropical Southwest Atlantic. *Harmful Algae News* **2007**, 1–28.
19. Rosa, C.M.A.; Philippi, J.M.S. Perfil epidemiologico de surtos de DTA por moluscos bivalves em Santa Catarina, Brasil, em 2007 e 2008. *Hig. Aliment.* **2009**, *23*, 570.
20. Mafra, L.L.; Lopes, D.; Bonilauri, V.C.; Uchida, H.; Suzuki, T. Persistent Contamination of Octopuses and Mussels with Lipophilic Shellfish Toxins during Spring *Dinophysis* Blooms in a Subtropical Estuary. *Mar. Drugs.* **2015**, *13*, 3920–3935. [CrossRef] [PubMed]
21. Mafra, L.L.; Ribas, T.; Alves, T.P.; Proença, L.A.O.; Schramm, M.A.; Uchida, H.; Suzuki, T. Differential okadaic acid accumulation and detoxification by oysters and mussels during natural and simulated *Dinophysis* blooms. *Fish. Sci.* **2015**, *81*, 749–762. [CrossRef]
22. Proença, L.A.; Schmitt, F.; Costa, T.; Rorig, L. Evidences of diarrhetic shellfish poisoning in Santa Catarina—Brazil. *J. Braz. Assoc. Advant. Sci.* **1998**, *50*, 459–462.
23. BRASIL. *Instrução Normativa Interministerial 7 de 8 de Maio de 2012*; Governo do Estado do Tocantins: Brasília, Brasil, 2012; pp. 55–59.
24. Reguera, B.; Riobó, P.; Rodríguez, F.; Díaz, P.A.; Pizarro, G.; Paz, B.; Franco, J.M.; Blanco, J. *Dinophysis* toxins: Causative organisms, distribution and fate in shellfish. *Mar. Drugs.* **2014**, *12*, 394–461. [CrossRef] [PubMed]
25. Moita, M.T.; Pazos, Y.; Rocha, C.; Nolasco, R.; Oliveira, P.B. Toward predicting *Dinophysis* blooms off NW Iberia: A decade of events. *Harmful Algae* **2016**, *53*, 17–32. [CrossRef] [PubMed]
26. Kim, M.; Nam, S.W.; Shin, W.; Coats, D.W.; Park, M.G. *Dinophysis caudata* (dinophyceae) sequesters and retains plastids from the mixotrophic ciliate prey *Mesodinium rubrum*. *J. Phycol.* **2012**, *48*, 569–579. [CrossRef] [PubMed]
27. Giménez Papiol, G.; Beuzenberg, V.; Selwood, A.I.; MacKenzie, L.; Packer, M.A. The use of a mucus trap by *Dinophysis acuta* for the capture of *Mesodinium rubrum* prey under culture conditions. *Harmful Algae* **2016**, *58*, 1–7. [CrossRef] [PubMed]
28. Mafra, L.L.; Nagai, S.; Uchida, H.; Tavares, C.P.S.; Escobar, B.P.; Suzuki, T. Harmful effects of *Dinophysis* to the ciliate *Mesodinium rubrum*: Implications for prey capture. *Harmful Algae* **2016**, *59*, 82–90. [CrossRef] [PubMed]
29. Ojamäe, K.; Hansen, P.J.; Lips, I. Mass entrapment and lysis of *Mesodinium rubrum* cells in mucus threads observed in cultures with *Dinophysis*. *Harmful Algae* **2016**, *55*, 77–84. [CrossRef] [PubMed]
30. Jiang, T.J.; Wang, D.Z.; Niu, T.; Xu, Y.X. Trophic transfer of paralytic shellfish toxins from the cladoceran (*Moina mongolica*) to larvae of the fish (*Sciaenops ocellatus*). *Toxicon* **2007**, *50*, 639–645. [CrossRef] [PubMed]
31. Reizopoulou, S.; Strogyloudi, E.; Giannakourou, A.; Pagou, K.; Hatzianestis, I.; Pyrgaki, C.; Granéli, E. Okadaic acid accumulation in macrofilter feeders subjected to natural blooms of *Dinophysis acuminata*. *Harmful Algae* **2008**, *7*, 228–234. [CrossRef]

32. Mafra, L.L.; dos Santos Tavares, C.P.; Schramm, M.A. Diarrheic toxins in field-sampled and cultivated *Dinophysis* spp. cells from southern Brazil. *J. Appl. Phycol.* **2014**, *26*, 1727–1739. [CrossRef]
33. Sipiä, V.; Kankaanpää, H.; Meriluoto, J.; Høisæter, T. The first observation of okadaic acid in flounder in the Baltic Sea. *Sarsia.* **2000**, *85*, 471–475. [CrossRef]
34. Jiang, T.J.; Niu, T.; Xu, Y.X. Transfer and metabolism of paralytic shellfish poisoning from scallop (*Chlamys nobilis*) to spiny lobster (*Panulirus stimpsoni*). *Toxicon* **2006**, *48*, 988–994. [CrossRef] [PubMed]
35. Vale, P.; Sampayo, M.A.D.M. First confirmation of human diarrhoeic poisonings by okadaic acid esters after ingestion of razor clams (*Solen marginatus*) and green crabs (*Carcinus maenas*) in Aveiro lagoon, Portugal and detection of okadaic acid esters in phytoplankton. *Toxicon* **2002**, *40*, 989–996. [CrossRef]
36. Hernández, M.; Robinson, I.; Aguilar, A.; González, L.M.; López-Jurado, L.F.; Reyero, M.I.; Cacho, E.; Franco, J.; López-Rodas, V.; Costas, E. Did algal toxins cause monk seal mortality? *Nature* **1998**, *393*, 28–29. [CrossRef] [PubMed]
37. Mafra, L.L.; Nolli, P.K.; Luz, L.F.; Leal, J.G.; Sobrinho, B.F.; Pimenta, B.; Escobar; Juraczky, L.; Gonzalez, A.R.M.; Mota, L.E.; et al. Okadaic acid contamination during an exceptionally massive *Dinophysis* cf. *acuminata* bloom in southern Brazil. In Proceedings of the Abstracts of the 17th International Conference of Harmful Algae, Florianópolis, Brazil, 9–14 October 2016; p. 212.
38. Díaz, P.; Molinet, C.; Cáceres, M.A.; Valle-Levinson, A. Seasonal and intratidal distribution of *Dinophysis* spp. in a Chilean fjord. *Harmful Algae* **2011**, *10*, 155–164. [CrossRef]
39. Alves-de-Souza, C.; Varela, D.; Contreras, C.; de La Iglesia, P.; Fernández, P.; Hipp, B.; Hernández, C.; Riobó, P.; Reguera, B.; Franco, J.M.; et al. Seasonal variability of *Dinophysis* spp. and *Protoceratium reticulatum* associated to lipophilic shellfish toxins in a strongly stratified Chilean fjord. *Deep. Res. Part II Top. Stud. Oceanogr.* **2014**, *101*, 152–162. [CrossRef]
40. Aissaoui, A.; Armi, Z.; Turki, S.; Hassine, O.K. Ben Seasonal dynamic and in situ division rates of the dominant *Dinophysis* species in Punic harbors of Carthage (Gulf of Tunis, South Mediterranean). *Environ. Monit. Assess.* **2013**, *185*, 9361–9384. [CrossRef] [PubMed]
41. Van den Hoff, J.; Bell, E. The ciliate *Mesodinium rubrum* and its cryptophyte prey in Antarctic aquatic environments. *Polar Biol.* **2015**, *38*, 1305–1310. [CrossRef]
42. Crawford, D.W.; Lindholm, T. Some observations on vertical distribution and migration of the phototrophic ciliate *Mesodinium rubrum* (=*Myrionecta rubra*) in a stratified brackish inlet. *Aquat. Microb. Ecol.* **1997**, *13*, 267–274. [CrossRef]
43. Johnson, M.D.; Stoecker, D.K.; Marshall, H.G. Seasonal dynamics of *Mesodinium rubrum* in Chesapeake Bay. *J. Plankton Res.* **2013**, *35*, 877–893. [CrossRef]
44. Kim, M.; Kim, S.; Yih, W.; Park, M.G. The marine dinoflagellate genus *Dinophysis* can retain plastids of multiple algal origins at the same time. *Harmful Algae* **2012**, *13*, 105–111. [CrossRef]
45. Stern, R.F.; Amorim, A.L.; Bresnan, E. Diversity and plastid types in *Dinophysis acuminata* complex (Dinophyceae) in Scottish waters. *Harmful Algae* **2014**, *39*, 223–231. [CrossRef]
46. Wisecaver, J.H.; Hackett, J.D. Transcriptome analysis reveals nuclear-encoded proteins for the maintenance of temporary plastids in the dinoflagellate *Dinophysis acuminata*. *BMC Genom.* **2010**, *11*, 366. [CrossRef] [PubMed]
47. Kim, M.; Nam, S.W.; Shin, W.; Coats, D.W.; Park, M.G. Fate of green plastids in *Dinophysis caudata* following ingestion of the benthic ciliate *Mesodinium coatsi*: Ultrastructure and psbA gene. *Harmful Algae* **2015**, *43*, 66–73. [CrossRef]
48. Lindahl, O.; Lundve, B.; Johansen, M. Toxicity of *Dinophysis* spp. in relation to population density and environmental conditions on the Swedish west coast. *Harmful Algae* **2007**, *6*, 218–231. [CrossRef]
49. Raine, R. A review of the biophysical interactions relevant to the promotion of HABs in stratified systems: The case study of Ireland. *Deep. Res. Part II Top. Stud. Oceanogr.* **2014**, *101*, 21–31. [CrossRef]
50. Koukaras, K. *Dinophysis* blooms in Greek coastal waters (Thermaikos Gulf, NW Aegean Sea). *J. Plankton Res.* **2004**, *26*, 445–457. [CrossRef]
51. Fabro, E.; Almandoz, G.O.; Ferrario, M.E.; Hoffmeyer, M.S.; Pettigrosso, R.E.; Uibrig, R.; Krock, B. Co-occurrence of *Dinophysis tripos* and pectenotoxins in Argentinean shelf waters. *Harmful Algae* **2015**, *42*, 25–33. [CrossRef]
52. Möller, O.O.; Piola, A.R.; Freitas, A.C.; Campos, E.J.D. The effects of river discharge and seasonal winds on the shelf off southeastern South America. *Cont. Shelf Res.* **2008**, *28*, 1607–1624. [CrossRef]

53. Piola, A.R.; Romero, S.I.; Zajaczkovski, U. Space–time variability of the Plata plume inferred from ocean color. *Cont. Shelf Res.* **2008**, *28*, 1556–1567. [CrossRef]
54. Méndez, S.; Martínez, A.; Fabre, A. Extreme abundant bloom of Dinophysis ovum associated to positive SST anomalies in Uruguay. In Proceedings of the 17th International Conference of Harmful Algae, Florianópolis, Brazil, 9–14 October 2016; Proença, L.A.O., Hallegraeff, G.M., Eds.; International Society for the Study of Harmful Algae: Florianópolis, Brazil, 2016; pp. 22–25.
55. Méndez, S.; Rodriguez, F.; Reguera, B.; Franco, J.M.; Riobo, P.; Fabre, A. Characterization of Dinophysis ovum as the causative agent of the exceptional DSP event in Uruguay during 2015. In Proceedings of the 17th International Conference on Harmful Algae, Florianópolis, Brazil, 9–14 October 2016; Proença, L.A.O., Hallegraeff, G.M., Eds.; International Society for the Study of Harmful Algae: Florianópolis, Brazil, 2016; pp. 26–29.
56. Proença, L.A.O. Clorofila a do fitoplâncton em seis enseadas utilizadas para o cultivo de moluscos bivalves no litoral de Santa Catarina. *Braz. J. Aquat. Sci. Technol.* **2002**, *6*, 33–44. [CrossRef]
57. Ferreira, J.F.; Besen, K.; Wormsbecher, A.G.; Santos, R.F. Physical-Chemical Parameters of Seawater Mollusc Culture Sites in Santa Catarina—Brazil. *J. Coast. Res.* **2006**, 1122–1126.
58. Escalera, L.; Pazos, Y.; Doval, M.D.; Reguera, B. A comparison of integrated and discrete depth sampling for monitoring toxic species of *Dinophysis*. *Mar. Pollut. Bull.* **2012**, *64*, 106–113. [CrossRef] [PubMed]
59. Farrell, H.; Gentien, P.; Fernand, L.; Lunven, M.; Reguera, B.; González-Gil, S.; Raine, R. Scales characterising a high density thin layer of *Dinophysis acuta* Ehrenberg and its transport within a coastal jet. *Harmful Algae* **2012**, *15*, 36–46. [CrossRef]
60. Aune, T.; Larsen, S.; Aasen, J.A.B.; Rehmann, N.; Satake, M.; Hess, P. Relative toxicity of dinophysistoxin-2 (DTX-2) compared with okadaic acid, based on acute intraperitoneal toxicity in mice. *Toxicon* **2007**, *49*, 1–7. [CrossRef] [PubMed]
61. Blanco, J.; Álvarez, G.; Uribe, E. Identification of pectenotoxins in plankton, filter feeders, and isolated cells of a *Dinophysis acuminata* with an atypical toxin profile, from Chile. *Toxicon* **2007**, *49*, 710–716. [CrossRef] [PubMed]
62. Froese, R.; Pauly, D. FishBase. Available online: http://fishbase.org (accessed on 25 January 2018).
63. Menezes, N.A.; Figueiredo, J.L. *Manual de Peixes Marinhos do Sudeste do Brasil. V. Teleostei (4)*; University of São Paulo: São Paulo, Brasil, 1985.
64. Caine, E.A. Caprellid amphipods: fast food for the reproductively active. *J. Exp. Mar. Bio. Ecol.* **1991**, *148*, 27–33. [CrossRef]
65. Brasil. *Portaria No 204, de 28 de Junho de 2012*; Ministério da Pesca e Aquicultura: Brasília-DF, Brazil, 2012; pp. 2–5.
66. Penna, A.; Bertozzini, E.; Battocchi, C.; Galluzzi, L.; Giacobbe, M.G.; Vila, M.; Garces, E.; Luglie, A.; Magnani, M. Monitoring of HAB species in the Mediterranean Sea through molecular methods. *J. Plankton Res.* **2006**, *29*, 19–38. [CrossRef]
67. Higman, W.A.; Algoet, M.; Stubbs, B.; Lees, D. Overview of developments of the algal biotoxin monitoring programme in England, Scotland and Wales. In Proceedings of the 6th International Conference on Molluscan Shellfish Safety, Blenheim, Marlborough, New Zealand, 18–23 March 2007; pp. 41–45.
68. Vale, P.; Botelho, M.J.; Rodrigues, S.M.; Gomes, S.S.; Sampayo, M.A.D.M. Two decades of marine biotoxin monitoring in bivalves from Portugal (1986–2006): A review of exposure assessment. *Harmful Algae* **2008**, *7*, 11–25. [CrossRef]
69. Brooks, S.; Harman, C.; Soto, M.; Cancio, I.; Glette, T.; Marigómez, I. Integrated coastal monitoring of a gas processing plant using native and caged mussels. *Sci. Total Environ.* **2012**, *426*, 375–386. [CrossRef] [PubMed]
70. Trainer, V.L.; Hardy, F.J. Integrative monitoring of marine and freshwater harmful algae in Washington State for public health protection. *Toxins.* **2015**, *7*, 1206–1234. [CrossRef] [PubMed]
71. Doyle, P.; Mather, A.E.; Bennett, M.R.; Bussell, M.A. Miocene barnacle assemblages from southern Spain and their palaeoenvironmental significance. *Lethaia* **1996**, *29*, 267–274. [CrossRef]
72. Turner, J.T. Planktonic marine copepods and harmful algae. *Harmful Algae* **2014**, *32*, 81–93. [CrossRef]
73. Maneiro, I.; Guisande, C.; Frangópulos, M.; Riveiro, I. Importance of copepod faecal pellets to the fate of the DSP toxins produced by *Dinophysis* spp. *Harmful Algae* **2002**, *1*, 333–341. [CrossRef]

74. Kozlowsky-Suzuki, B.; Carlsson, P.; Rühl, A.; Granéli, E. Food selectivity and grazing impact on toxic *Dinophysis* spp. by copepods feeding on natural plankton assemblages. *Harmful Algae* **2006**, *5*, 57–68. [CrossRef]
75. Armi, Z.; Turki, S.; Trabelsi, E.; Ceredi, A.; Riccardi, E.; Milandri, A. Occurrence of diarrhetic shellfish poisoning (DSP) toxins in clams (*Ruditapes decussatus*) from Tunis north lagoon. *Environ. Monit. Assess.* **2012**, *184*, 5085–5095. [CrossRef] [PubMed]
76. Dumbauld, B.R.; Ruesink, J.L.; Rumrill, S.S. The ecological role of bivalve shellfish aquaculture in the estuarine environment: A review with application to oyster and clam culture in West Coast (USA) estuaries. *Aquaculture.* **2009**, *290*, 196–223. [CrossRef]
77. García-Mendoza, E.; Sánchez-Bravo, Y.A.; Turner, A.; Blanco, J.; O'Neil, A.; Mancera-Flores, J.; Pérez-Brunius, P.; Rivas, D.; Almazán-Becerril, A.; Peña-Manjarrez, J.L. Lipophilic toxins in cultivated mussels (*Mytilus galloprovincialis*) from Baja California, Mexico. *Toxicon* **2014**, *90*, 111–123. [CrossRef] [PubMed]
78. Food and Agriculture Organization of the United Nations (FAO); World Health Organization (WHO). *Technical Paper on Toxicity Equivalency Factors for Marine Biotoxins Associated with Bivalve Molluscs*; FAO: Roman, Italy; WHO: Geneva, Switzerland, 2016.
79. Branco, J.O. Biologia e pesca do camarão sete-barbas *Xiphopenaeus kroyeri* (Heller) (Crustacea, Penaeidae), na Armação do Itapocoroy, Penha, Santa Catarina, Brasil. *Rev. Bras. Zool.* **2005**, *22*, 1050–1062. [CrossRef]
80. Alves, T.P.; Schramm, M.A.; Proença, L.A.O.; Pinto, T.O.; Mafra, L.L. Interannual variability in *Dinophysis* spp. abundance and toxin accumulation in farmed mussels (*Perna perna*) in a subtropical estuary. *Environ. Monit. Assess.* **2018**. [CrossRef] [PubMed]
81. Trochimczuk-Fo, A.; Schettini, C.A.F. Avaliação da dispersão espacial da pluma do estuário do rio Itajaí-Açu em diferentes períodos de descarga. *Braz. J. Aquat. Sci. Technol.* **2003**, *7*, 83–96. [CrossRef]
82. Schettini, C.A.F.; Carvalho, J.L.B.; Truccolo, E.C. Aspectos Hidrodinâmicos da Enseada da Armação de Itapocoroy, SC. *Braz. J. Aquat. Sci. Technol.* **1999**, *3*, 99. [CrossRef]
83. Schettini, C.A.F.; Resgalla, C., Jr.; Pereira-Fo, J.; Silva, M.A.C.; Truccolo, E.C.; Rörig, L.R. Variabilidade temporal das características oceanográficas e ecológicas da região de influência fluvial do rio Itajaí-Açu. *Braz. J. Aquat. Sci. Technol.* **2005**, *9*, 93–102. [CrossRef]
84. EURLMB EU-Harmonised Standard Operating Procedure for Determination of Lipophilic Marine Biotoxins in Molluscs by LC-MS/MS, Version 5. 2015, pp. 1–31. Available online: www.aesan.msps.es/en/CRLMB/web/home.shtml (accessed on 7 May 2017).
85. Edler, L.; Elbrächter, M. The Utermöhl method for quantitative phytoplankton analysis. *Microsc. Mol. Methods Quant. Phytoplankt. Anal.* **2010**, 13–20. [CrossRef]
86. Grasshoff, K.; Kremling, K.; Ehrhardt, M. *Methods of Seawater Analysis*, 3rd ed.; Grasshoff, K., Kremling, K., Ehrhardt, M., Eds.; Wiley-VCH: Weinheim, Germany; New York, NY, USA; Chiester, UK; Brisbane, Australia; Singapore; Toronto, ON, Canada, 1999; Volume 7, ISBN 3-527-25998-8.
87. Zapata, M.; Rodríguez, F.; Garrido, J.L. Separation of chlorophylls and carotenoids from marine phytoplankton: A new HPLC method using a reversed phase C8column and pyridine-containing mobile phases. *Mar. Ecol. Prog. Ser.* **2000**, *195*, 29–45. [CrossRef]
88. R Core Team. *R: A Language and Environment for Statistical Computing*; R Foundation for Statistical Computing: Vienna, Austria, 2017.
89. Dinno, A. *Dunn's Test of Multiple Comparisons Using Rank Sums*; The Comprehensive R Archive Network: Portland, OR, USA, 2017.
90. Lê, S.; Josse, J.; Husson, F. FactoMineR: An R Package for Multivariate Analysis. *J. Stat. Softw.* **2008**, *25*. [CrossRef]

toxins

MDPI

Article

Prey Lysate Enhances Growth and Toxin Production in an Isolate of *Dinophysis acuminata*

Han Gao [1,2], Mengmeng Tong [2,*], Xinlong An [3] and Juliette L. Smith [1]

1 Virginia Institute of Marine Science, College of William & Mary, Gloucester Point, VA 23062, USA; gghanbing@zju.edu.cn (H.G.); jlsmith@vims.edu (J.L.S.)
2 Ocean College, Zhejiang University, Zhoushan 316000, China
3 Ocean College, Agricultural University of Hebei, Qinhuangdao 066000, China; axlqhd@126.com
* Correspondence: mengmengtong@zju.edu.cn; Tel.: +86-188-5816-0402

Received: 22 November 2018; Accepted: 14 January 2019; Published: 21 January 2019

Abstract: The physiological and toxicological characteristics of *Dinophysis acuminata* have been increasingly studied in an attempt to better understand and predict diarrhetic shellfish poisoning (DSP) events worldwide. Recent work has identified prey quantity, organic nitrogen, and ammonium as likely contributors to increased *Dinophysis* growth rates and/or toxicity. Further research is now needed to better understand the interplay between these factors, for example, how inorganic and organic compounds interact with prey and a variety of *Dinophysis* species and/or strains. In this study, the exudate of ciliate prey and cryptophytes were investigated for an ability to support *D. acuminata* growth and toxin production in the presence and absence of prey, i.e., during mixotrophic and phototrophic growth respectively. A series of culturing experiments demonstrated that the addition of ciliate lysate led to faster dinoflagellate growth rates (0.25 ± 0.002/d) in predator-prey co-incubations than in treatments containing (1) similar levels of prey but without lysate (0.21 ± 0.003/d), (2) ciliate lysate but no live prey (0.12 ± 0.004/d), or (3) monocultures of *D. acuminata* without ciliate lysate or live prey (0.01 ± 0.007/d). The addition of ciliate lysate to co-incubations also resulted in maximum toxin quotas and extracellular concentrations of okadaic acid (OA, 0.11 ± 0.01 pg/cell; 1.37 ± 0.10 ng/mL) and dinophysistoxin-1 (DTX1, 0.20 ± 0.02 pg/cell; 1.27 ± 0.10 ng/mL), and significantly greater total DSP toxin concentrations (intracellular + extracellular). Pectenotoxin-2 values, intracellular or extracellular, did not show a clear trend across the treatments. The addition of cryptophyte lysate or whole cells, however, did not support dinoflagellate cell division. Together these data demonstrate that while certain growth was observed when only lysate was added, the benefits to *Dinophysis* were maximized when ciliate lysate was added with the ciliate inoculum (i.e., during mixotrophic growth). Extrapolating to the field, these culturing studies suggest that the presence of ciliate exudate during co-occurring dinoflagellate-ciliate blooms may indirectly and directly exacerbate *D. acuminata* abundance and toxigenicity. More research is required, however, to understand what direct or indirect mechanisms control the predator-prey dynamic and what component(s) of ciliate lysate are being utilized by the dinoflagellate or other organisms (e.g., ciliate or bacteria) in the culture if predictive capabilities are to be developed and management strategies created.

Keywords: *Dinophysis acuminata*; *Mesodinium rubrum*; lysate; organic matter; diarrhetic shellfish poisoning; okadaic acid; dinophysistoxin; pectenotoxins

Key Contribution: The addition of ciliate lysate, but not cryptophyte lysate, to co-incubations led to increased *Dinophysis* growth rate and biomass, maximum DSP toxin quotas and extracellular toxin concentrations, and significantly greater total DSP toxins.

1. Introduction

The dinoflagellate *Dinophysis* spp. has been associated with diarrhetic shellfish poisoning (DSP) events worldwide due to human exposure to the toxin okadaic acid (OA) and its derivatives, dinophysistoxins (DTXs) [1,2]. These lipophilic compounds can accumulate in filter-feeding bivalves and adversely affect humans and other animal consumers. As strong inhibitors of serine and threonine protein phosphatases, DSP toxins can promote potent tumors [3], induce intestinal distress such as vomiting and diarrhea [2,4], and limit the growth of phytoplankton competitors [5,6]. Many toxigenic *Dinophysis* spp. also synthesize pectenotoxins (PTXs), a class of bioactive, polyether lactones. While not a contributor to DSP, some pectenotoxins are acutely toxic to vertebrate models via intraperitoneal injection [7,8], and therefore, the toxin class is regulated in the European Union [9].

With the threat of DSP appearing to be on a rise globally and emerging in new regions, e.g., U.S. coastlines, investigations into the possible drivers of *Dinophysis* spp. growth and toxin production have become a growing area of research in the last decade. This important work was made possible through the revolutionary discovery by Park et al. [10]: to grow in culture, *Dinophysis* spp. must be fed ciliates, *Mesodinium rubrum*, that previously grazed upon cryptophytes of the *Teleaulax/Geminigera* clade [11]. Molecular evidence supports the need for this multi-stage culturing scheme, as *Dinophysis* and *Mesodinium* plastids have been shown to originate from cryptophytes [12–16] and *Dinophysis* cells have been found in the field to concurrently contain plastids originating from different strains of cryptophyte [17]. More specifically, ciliates of the genus *Mesodinium* capture, sequester, and regulate the nuclear genome of its cryptophyte prey [11,15,16], after which, *Dinophysis* consumes the plastids in the ciliates by kleptoplasty via a peduncle. Stemming from this advancement in culturing, numerous *D. acuminata* isolates [10,18–26] and isolates of other *Dinophysis* spp. [21,27–31] have been successfully established, allowing now for comparisons between geographical strains and species.

Prior to the multi-stage culturing technique put forth by Park et al. [10], however, multiple types of organic material, in both dissolved and particulate form, were trialed in an attempt to culture *Dinophysis* as a monoculture, including dissolved organic materials (soil extract, humic acid, dextrans, urea, glutamic acid, hypoxanthine, gibberellic acid, indol acetic acid, kinetin, polyamines, lectins of *Phaseolus* and porcine blood platelets) [32], and live prey (bacteria, pico- and nanoplankton, and yeast) [33]. None of these trials with organic materials supported *Dinophysis* spp. growth enough to allow for successful isolation of the genera and the establishment of cultures, leading to the assumption that *Dinophysis* could not directly utilize organic compounds.

Recent studies with isolates, however, demonstrate that a variety of organic materials, and some inorganics, may benefit *Dinophysis* by indirectly or directly supporting growth and/or toxin production. Toxin production, but not growth, increased when a non-axenic monoculture of *D. acuminata* was supplemented with lysed ciliates and cell debris during a preliminary study [21], and *D. acuminata* growth in monocultures and predator-prey co-incubations was enhanced with the addition of urea, glutamine, or waste water organic matter [24]. With respect to inorganic nutrients, three recent studies have confirmed that *D. acuminata* does not readily utilize nitrate to support growth [24,34,35] or toxin production [34,35], but that the ciliate prey rapidly assimilates nitrate to promote its own division, thereby indirectly supporting *D. acuminata* [35]. Ammonium, interestingly, was shown to likely play a direct role in *D. acuminata* growth, bloom development, and toxin production, through uptake of this inorganic compound by the dinoflagellate [24,34,36,37]. What's improved in these later culturing studies, as compared to Nagai et al. [21], is that compounds of interest were added to *Dinophysis* with and without prey as a food source, examining therefore, growth and toxin production during mixotrophic and phototrophic growth.

By including prey in a treatment with possible nutrient sources, additional questions can be asked regarding the combined roles of ciliates and nutrients in dinoflagellate growth and toxin production. More specifically, a pairing of prey cells and prey exudate or lysate seems more environmentally relevant than testing in solidarity, as the two are likely found in conjunction within a system. Co-occurrence of cells and released internal components, for example, may occur throughout a bloom, due to such processes as sloppy feeding or cell division; however, the presence of these compounds likely increases in the surrounding waters near the termination of a ciliate bloom when cells may be experiencing aging and membrane permeability, parasitic lysis, or cell death. This progression has been demonstrated in the laboratory for endotoxins OA and DTX1 [21,38]. Additionally, ciliates should be considered in this relationship as laboratory studies [10,39–41] have indicated prey abundance as an important controller of *Dinophysis* growth and/or toxin production, and *Dinophysis* spp. have been found to bloom immediately after and co-occur with ciliate prey in the field [42], suggesting that factors controlling ciliate abundance and distribution are important to down-stream DSP events. Further research is now needed to further understand how inorganic and organic compounds interact with prey and a variety of *Dinophysis* spp. and isolates if predictive capabilities are to be developed and management strategies created.

Building on a previous study [21], mixotrophic *D. acuminata* was investigated for its ability to utilize organic material released from the ciliate, *M. rubrum* in the presence or absence of the ciliate as a food source, i.e., during mixotrophic vs. phototrophic growth, respectively. We supplemented a *D. acuminata* culture, comprising of f/6-Si medium [43], with ciliate lysate (derived from probe-sonification of ciliate culture), ciliate lysate and live ciliates, or live ciliates alone at two initial cell concentrations (Table 1). To determine if any measured effect on *D. acuminata* growth or toxin production was unique to the ciliate lysate, we also amended *D. acuminata* culture with cryptophyte lysate or live cryptophytes. All treatments were compared to a monoculture control of *D. acuminata* with no organic amendments, and cultures of *D. acuminata* were starved, in the light, for two weeks before the experiment to ensure that any responses measured in the dinoflagellate were due to the amendments, and not sustained growth or divisions using internal reserves. While the main objective of this study was to begin investigating, in the laboratory, if organic matter derived from a co-occurring bloom of ciliates could support *Dinophysis* growth and toxin production either directly or indirectly, the information may also have implications for future *D. acuminata* isolation attempts. If lysate, for example, promotes *D. acuminata* growth, then this may be a mechanism to increase the likelihood of isolation success.

Table 1. Prey, lysate, or a mixture of the two were provided as nourishment during culturing experiments with a *Dinophysis acuminata* isolate after dinoflagellates were starved for two weeks in the light. Treatments included the addition of live prey and/or probe-sonified lysate of the ciliate, *Mesodinium rubrum*, delivered at two initial cell concentrations or equivalents (eq.). The cryptophyte, *Teleaulax amphioxeia*, was also provided in two treatments: live prey or lysate. Treatments were compared to a *Dinophysis* monoculture control where no prey or lysate were added, and instead an equivalent volume was replaced with additional fresh f/6-Si medium. Mean (±standard error) measurements of *Dinophysis* growth rate and biomass are provided.

Treatment ID	Prey/Lysate Species	Prey Initial Conc. (Cells/mL)	Lysate Initial Conc. (Cell eq./mL)	*Dinophysis* Growth [1]		
				Exponential Growth Rate (/d)	Period of Exponential Growth (d)	Max Biomass (cells/mL)
$Prey_{ciliate}^{3000}$	*M. rubrum*	3000	-	0.21 (±0.003)	12	2508 (±162)
$Prey_{ciliate}^{1500}$	*M. rubrum*	1500	-	0.16 (±0.007)	15	2252 (±110)
$Prey + Lysate_{ciliate}^{3000}$	*M. rubrum*	1500	1500	0.25 (±0.002)	12	3902 (±234)
$Lysate_{ciliate}^{3000}$	*M. rubrum*	-	3000	0.12 (±0.004)	3	302 (±8)
$Prey_{crypto}$	*T. amphioxeia*	15,000	-	-	-	170 (±8)
$Lysate_{crypto}$	*T. amphioxeia*	-	15,000	-	-	193 (±7)
Control	none	-	-	-	-	187 (±5)

[1] Dinophysis initial cell concentration was equal for all 6 treatments and the control, 150 cells/mL. The symbol "-" indicates zero.

2. Results

2.1. Lysate Size Characterization

Particles ($n = 185$) in the ciliate lysate were photographed and measured under a light microscope at 100×. The mean size of lysate particles was 3.41 ± 0.13 µm (mean ± standard error) in diameter and 9.17 ± 0.73 μm^2 in area. Attempts were also made to characterize particles in the cryptophyte lysate; however, particles were not large enough to quantify using supplied magnification and software.

2.2. Growth of Dinoflagellate, Ciliate, and Cryptophyte

Dinoflagellates grew exponentially in the four treatments that were fed live ciliates (1500 or 3000 cells/mL), a 1:1 mixture of living ciliates and lysate (equivalent to 3000 cells/mL), and only ciliate lysate (equivalent to 3000 cells/mL). More specifically, growth rates were 0.16 ± 0.007, 0.21 ± 0.003, 0.25 ± 0.002, and 0.12 ± 0.004/d for treatments $Prey_{ciliate}^{1500}$, $Prey_{ciliate}^{3000}$, Prey + $Lysate_{ciliate}^{3000}$, and $Lysate_{ciliate}^{3000}$, respectively (Table 1, Figure 1). When compared across treatments providing the same concentration of ciliates, 3000 cell eq./mL, *Dinophysis* grew faster when provided prey or a combination of prey and lysate (treatments $Prey_{ciliate}^{3000}$ and Prey + $Lysate_{ciliate}^{3000}$), than when provided only lysate ($Lysate_{ciliate}^{3000}$) (t-test, $p < 0.05$). Similarly, when provided both ciliate prey and lysate (Prey + $Lysate_{ciliate}^{3000}$), *Dinophysis* reached a higher maximum, final biomass (3900 cell/mL) at plateau phase than when it was provided with only living ciliates ($Prey_{ciliate}^{3000}$), 2500 cells/mL, or only lysate ($Lysate_{ciliate}^{3000}$), 302 cells/mL (Table 1, Figure 1). The average maximum biomass of *Dinophysis* in the $Lysate_{ciliate}^{3000}$ treatment was significantly greater than the maximum biomass measured in the monoculture control, showing that growth was supported for three days on materials liberated from the ciliate lysate (after two weeks of starvation in the light). When comparing between treatments providing live ciliates, *Dinophysis* grew significantly faster during exponential growth in the 3000 cells/mL treatment ($Prey_{ciliate}^{3000}$) than in the 1500 cells/mL treatment ($Prey_{ciliate}^{1500}$); however, *Dinophysis* in the latter treatment grew steadily for a longer period, resulting in no detectable difference in maximum biomass between treatments (Table 1). The dinoflagellates in treatments that were provided with either living cryptophytes ($Prey_{crypto}$), cryptophyte lysate ($Lysate_{crypto}$), or no additions (Control, growth rate = 0.01 ± 0.007/d) did not show evidence of exponential growth over the experimental period (Table 1, Figure 1).

The cell concentrations of ciliates and cryptophytes were also monitored in the co-incubations. The cell concentration of the ciliate quickly decreased over time as *Dinophysis* fed during exponential growth. More specifically, ciliates were completely consumed by days 15–18 in the two treatments to which they were added without lysate: $Prey_{ciliate}^{1500}$ and $Prey_{ciliate}^{3000}$ (Figure 1). The prey in the Prey + $Lysate_{ciliate}^{3000}$ treatment were depleted from the co-incubation by day 12, however, transitioning *Dinophysis* into a prey-limited phase earlier than the other two treatments with live ciliates. The cryptophytes that were co-incubated with *Dinophysis* ($Prey_{crypto}$) grew exponentially for 12 days, reaching a maximum concentration of 600,000 cells/mL during the experimental period (data not shown).

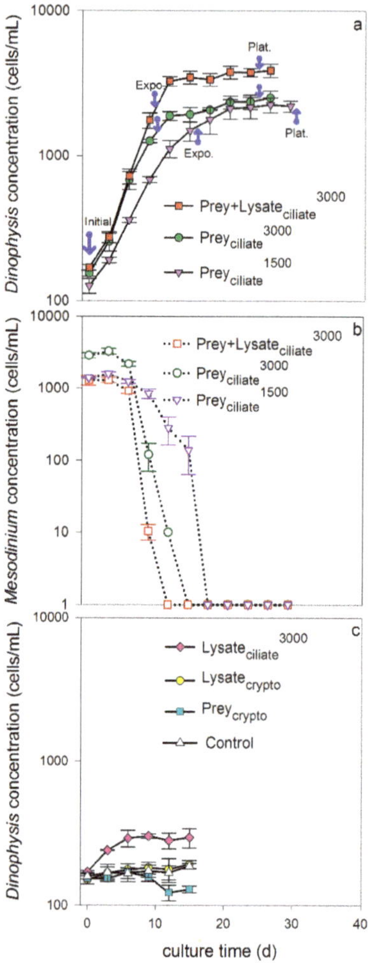

Figure 1. Growth response of *Dinophysis acuminata* (**a**,**c**) and ciliates, *M. rubrum* (**b**), in different treatments after being starved, in the light, for two weeks before the experiment to ensure the prey were fully consumed from the medium and that any responses measured in *Dinophysis* were due to the amendments and not sustained growth or divisions using internal reserves. Treatments include $\text{Prey}_{\text{ciliate}}^{3000}$: with ciliates at 3000 cells/mL; Prey + $\text{Lysate}_{\text{ciliate}}^{3000}$: with ciliates at 1500 cells/mL + ciliate lysate equivalent to 1500 cells/mL; $\text{Prey}_{\text{ciliate}}^{1500}$: with ciliates at 1500 cells/mL (**a**,**b**); $\text{Lysate}_{\text{ciliate}}^{3000}$: with ciliate lysate equivalent to 3000 cells/mL; $\text{Lysate}_{\text{crypto}}$: with cryptophyte lysate equivalent to 15,000 cells/mL; $\text{Prey}_{\text{crypto}}$: with cryptophytes at 15,000 cells/mL; and Control: with no prey or lysate addition (**c**). Initial concentration of *D. acuminata* was 150 cells/mL for all treatments. Mean values and standard deviations are plotted (n = 3). Blue arrows in (**a**) indicate when samples were initially harvested for toxin analysis, and then during exponential (Expo.) and plateau (Plat.) growth phases.

2.3. Toxin Quota, Concentration, and Production

Cells and media of *Dinophysis* were harvested separately and analyzed for toxin during two growth phases, exponential and plateau, for three treatments: $\text{Prey}_{\text{ciliate}}^{1500}$, $\text{Prey}_{\text{ciliate}}^{3000}$, and Prey + $\text{Lysate}_{\text{ciliate}}^{3000}$. Initial toxin samples were also collected and analyzed from the inoculum

Dinophysis cultures for comparison. Toxin data are not reported for the other four treatments, because growth rates and final biomass were significantly lower when *Dinophysis* was grown with only ciliate lysate, grown with cryptophytes that were living or lysed, or grown as a monoculture control. More specifically, *Dinophysis* in these latter treatments (1) produced insufficient biomass to reach toxin detection limits, and/or (2) did not progress through typical growth phases, i.e., lag, exponential, and plateau, during the experimental period, making the toxin data incomparable to the high-growth treatments.

We calculated the potential loss of *D. acuminata* during the harvesting process for toxin samples, i.e., sieving. Only 1% of the harvested cells were potentially lost during harvesting; possible mechanisms include being trapped in/on the sieve, loss of small cells, and/or artificial cell lysis during processing. This error was found to be minimal and constant over growth phases, and therefore, considered irrelevant to this study.

Toxin quotas (intracellular toxin) and concentrations (extracellular toxins) measured during exponential and plateau phases were compared to the initial toxin levels in the maintenance *Dinophysis* culture that was used for inoculation (taken in late plateau phase) to demonstrate increases in toxin relative to initial conditions. As a general trend, intracellular levels of OA, DTX1, and PTX2 remained minimal, i.e., similar to initial levels, during exponential growth, but increased during plateau phase (Figure 2a–c). Exceptions were observed, however, whereby *Dinophysis* that was provided ciliate prey at an initial concentration of 3000 cells/mL ($Prey_{ciliate}{}^{3000}$) did not increase their OA toxin quota, relative to initial conditions, over the entire experimental period. Additionally, *Dinophysis* fed the lower initial concentration of ciliate ($Prey_{ciliate}{}^{1500}$) did not increase their internal quotas of DTX1 or PTX2 above initial conditions over the entire experimental period. Maximum average toxin quotas were reached during plateau phase for OA, 0.11 ± 0.01 pg OA/cell (Prey + $Lysate_{ciliate}{}^{3000}$); DTX1, 0.20 ± 0.02 pg/cell (Prey + $Lysate_{ciliate}{}^{3000}$); and PTX2, 28.38 ± 5.02 pg/cell ($Prey_{ciliate}{}^{3000}$).

As seen with intracellular toxin quotas, extracellular toxin concentrations of OA, DTX1, and PTX2 in the culture medium of the three treatments remained low, relative to initial toxin concentrations, through exponential growth, but significantly increased by plateau phase (Figure 2d–f). Maximum, average extracellular toxin concentrations were reached during plateau growth phase for OA, 1.37 ± 0.01 ng/mL (Prey + $Lysate_{ciliate}{}^{3000}$) DTX1, 1.27 ± 0.10 ng/mL (Prey + $Lysate_{ciliate}{}^{3000}$); and PTX2, 22.37 ± 0.54 ng/mL ($Prey_{ciliate}{}^{1500}$). Once the intracellular quotas were converted to intracellular toxin concentrations per milliliter of culture and combined with extracellular toxin concentrations to yield total toxin concentrations (Figure 2g–i), it became apparent that total toxin concentration showed the same overall pattern across treatments; total toxins increased over the aging of the culture and reach maximum levels by plateau phase. DSP toxins, OA and DTX1, were more associated with the extracellular fraction, <15 μm, while PTX2 was associated with the cells and particulates, ≥15 μm.

Total toxin concentrations, toxin quotas, and extracellular concentrations were also compared across treatments during plateau phase to look for any effect from the different organic amendments (Figure 2). Overall, the total toxin concentrations of OA and DTX1 were significantly greater in the Prey + $Lysate_{ciliate}{}^{3000}$ treatment, as compared to the treatments with only live ciliates added ($Prey_{ciliate}{}^{1500}$, $Prey_{ciliate}{}^{3000}$). When evaluating intra and extracellular toxins separately, the same trend remained: the mean OA toxin quota and DTX1 extracellular concentration were significantly greater than treatments with live prey. Okadaic acid extracellular concentrations (Figure 2d) and DTX1 intracellular toxin quotas (Figure 2b), however, were indistinguishable between the two treatments with lysate (Prey + $Lysate_{ciliate}{}^{3000}$) and the higher prey abundance ($Prey_{ciliate}{}^{3000}$). In all cases, Prey + $Lysate_{ciliate}{}^{3000}$ and the higher prey abundance $Prey_{ciliate}{}^{3000}$ contained more OA or DTX1 in the intra or extra cellular fractions than the treatment with the lowest prey abundance ($Prey_{ciliate}{}^{1500}$). Pectenotoxin-2 levels did not follow a distinguishable trend across treatments or toxin measurements, but values were more than a magnitude greater than OA and DTX1 combined.

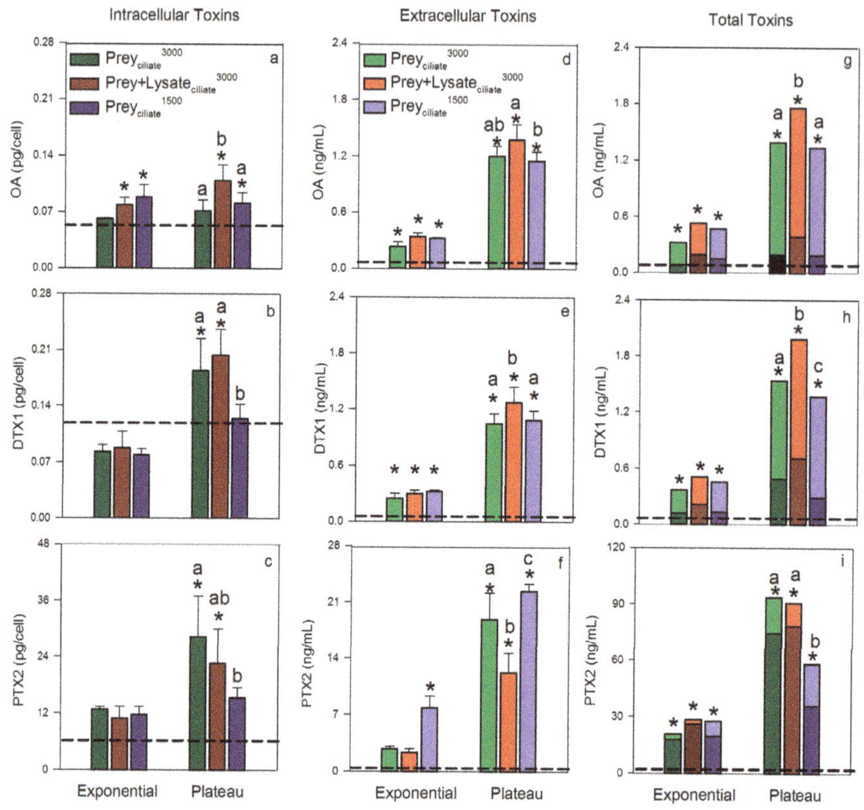

Figure 2. Toxin levels in *Dinophysis acuminata* cells and medium over two growth phases: exponential and plateau for three treatments. (**a–c**, Mean ± SD, n = 3) intracellular toxin quotas, (**d–f**, Mean ± SD, n = 3) extracellular toxin concentrations in the cultures, and (**g–i**) total toxin concentration in *D. acuminata* cultures with ciliate prey and/or lysate (Mean, n = 3). Intracellular toxins are indicated with darker color bars, while extracellular toxins are represented using the lighter color bars. Toxins quantified include okadaic acid (OA), dinophysistoxin-1 (DTX1), and pectenotoxin-2 (PTX2). Dashed horizontal line in each panel indicates the mean initial toxin level at the start of the experimental period. Asterisks '*' indicate that a treatment was significantly greater at that growth phase as compared to the initial toxin level, and letters that are uncommon show significant difference ($p < 0.05$) in toxin levels between treatments during plateau phase, within that respective panel only.

The rate of intracellular toxin production (OA, DTX, or PTX2) by *Dinophysis* was greater during exponential growth phase than as cells transitioned into plateau phase (Table 2). Toxin production rates of OA, DTX1, and PTX2 were significantly faster ($p < 0.05$) when *Dinophysis* was provided with a mixture of prey and lysate (Prey + Lysate$_{\text{ciliate}}^{3000}$) than when provided the same concentration of prey, but no lysate (Prey$_{\text{ciliate}}^{1500}$). Toxin production in the mixed treatment and higher prey treatment (Prey$_{\text{ciliate}}^{1500}$) were more comparable. Toxin production occurred during the transition from exponential to plateau phase as well; however, rates of OA, DTX1, and PTX2 production were reduced (Table 2).

Table 2. Mean (±standard error) calculations of *Dinophysis* toxin production rate over two growth phases, exponential (expo.) and plateau (plat.). The duration of days used to represent each growth phase, and therefore calculate net toxin production rate (R_{tox}), are included for reference. Statistical differences are indicated by uncommon lowercase letters (Two-Way Repeated Measures ANOVA with alpha set to 0.05, n = 3).

Treatment ID	Duration of Each Growth Phase (d)		*Dinophysis* R_{tox} (fg/cell/d)					
			Initial to Exponential			Exponential to Plateau		
	Expo.	Plat.	OA	DTX1	PTX2	OA	DTX1	PTX2
$Prey_{ciliate}^{3000}$	10	15	46 (±4) ^{a}	56 (±4) ^{a}	3747 (±177) ^{ab}	40 (±4) ^{a}	44 (±2) ^{a}	2837 (±241) ^{a}
$Prey_{ciliate}^{1500}$	16	16	39 (±1) ^{a}	37 (±1) ^{b}	2723 (±234) ^{b}	24 (±1) ^{b}	26 (±2) ^{b}	920 (±58) ^{b}
Prey + $Lysate_{ciliate}^{3000}$	10	15	65 (±3) ^{b}	63 (±5) ^{a}	4171 (±573) ^{a}	30 (±1) ^{ab}	37 (±4) ^{ab}	1662 (±372) ^{b}

OA, okadaic acid. DTX1, dinophysistoxin-1. PTX2, pectenotoxin-2.

3. Discussion

Mixotrophic *Dinophysis acuminata* was investigated for its ability to utilize organic material released from the ciliate, *Mesodinium rubrum*, or the cryptophyte, *Teleaulax amphioxeia*. As such, an isolate of *D. acuminata* was grown in the presence of live cells, lysate, live cells and lysate, or no amendments except fresh culture medium. Overall, the addition of ciliate lysate, but not cryptophyte lysate, to co-incubations of predator and prey led to significantly higher *Dinophysis* growth rate, biomass, OA toxin quotas, DTX1 extracellular toxin concentrations, and DSP total toxins (Figures 1 and 2, and Tables 1 and 2). It is important to note, that the addition of ciliate lysate to co-incubations increased growth and toxigenicity above similar treatments where *Dinophysis* was provided with the same or more live ciliate prey (1500 and 3000 cells/mL, respectively) or the same amount of overall ciliate biomass as lysate (3000 cell eq/mL). Together these results demonstrate that the organic matter from the lysed ciliates provided the necessary nutrition to *Dinophysis* (directly or indirectly) to support growth (phototrophic or mixotrophic, respectively) and toxin production by the dinoflagellate.

3.1. Ciliate Lysate in Support of Growth

Early culturing experiments proposed that *Dinophysis acuminata* required both prey and light to grow in culture [10,22,39–41]; however, more recently, *D. acuminata* has been shown to undergo phototrophic growth, in the presence of ammonium and urea, and the absence of prey, but that growth occurs at a slower rate than during mixotrophy [34,36]. Similarly, in the present study, an isolate of *D. acuminata* from Eel Pond, USA, grew for 3 days and reached significantly higher biomass when provided only ciliate lysate as an amendment beyond medium ($Lysate_{ciliate}^{3000}$, Figure 1) as compared to a monoculture control that showed no growth or change in biomass over the same period. These dinoflagellate cultures were starved for two weeks in the light prior to the experiment to ensure that internal reserves were depleted and that any responses measured in *Dinophysis* were due to the new amendments. While certain growth (photosynthetic + mixotrophic) occurred without prey in the ciliate lysate treatment ($Lysate_{ciliate}^{3000}$), growth rates and final biomass significantly increased once prey were added to *D. acuminata* culture (Prey + $Lysate_{ciliate}^{3000}$, $Prey_{ciliate}^{1500}$, $Prey_{ciliate}^{3000}$) (Table 1), supporting previous findings for faster growth rates during mixotrophic growth. It is unclear whether the dinoflagellate directly and/or indirectly benefitted from the organic materials liberated from the ciliates. Other studies have proposed an indirect link between dissolved nutrients and *Dinophysis* abundance, citing the ciliate's high affinity for dissolved inorganic and organic nutrients and a cascading increase in ciliate abundance and then *Dinophysis* abundance [34,35,44]. Ciliates, however, did not increase in abundance or extend their presence in the co-incubation with the addition of lysate (Figure 1b); this is contrary to what can be expected if the ciliate was the link between the liberated organic materials and increased *Dinophysis* abundance. This result, instead, lends support for an alternative conclusion: *D. acuminata* directly used the liberated materials to enhance total (photosynthetic + mixotrophic) growth on top of mixotrophic growth.

The growth-promoting effect of ciliate lysate also surpassed the effects of doubling ciliate abundance and exceeding prey saturation levels. More specifically, doubling the concentration of live ciliates inoculated into co-incubations from 1500 to 3000 cells/mL ($Prey_{ciliate}^{1500}$, $Prey_{ciliate}^{3000}$, respectively), significantly increased *Dinophysis* growth rate (Figure 1, Table 1). This increase in rate and biomass achieved with more prey, however, was still below that achieved by *D. acuminata* when grown in the presence of lysate and less prey ($Prey + Lysate_{ciliate}^{3000}$). Differences in growth rate between the low and high prey treatments were expected given that the initial prey concentrations, 1500 and 3000 cells/mL respectively, were below and above the published prey saturation threshold: ~2000 cells/mL [39,45]. The design of these treatment levels was intentional in that it allowed for the examination of whether a sub-saturation level of live prey, as seen in treatments $Prey + Lysate_{ciliate}^{3000}$ and $Prey_{ciliate}^{1500}$, would lead to similar maximum *Dinophysis* growth rates and biomass, or if supplementing that sub-saturation level of prey with lysate would allow *D. acuminata* to perform at the level of super-saturation, i.e., equivalent to the high prey treatment, $Prey_{ciliate}^{3000}$. As the latter outcome was observed, i.e., *D. acuminata* grew fastest in the lysate and prey treatment ($Prey + Lysate_{ciliate}^{3000}$), one can conclude that either (1) the ciliate (or associated bacteria) utilized the liberated materials promoting *D. acuminata* growth by making itself more enriched or abundant, or (2) with the addition of ciliate lysate, total (photosynthetic + mixotrophic) growth was enhanced in *D. acuminata* (i.e., direct uptake of liberated materials by dinoflagellate).

Alternatively, the bacteria associated with the ciliate culture inoculum may be indirectly responsible for the measured increase in *D. acuminata* growth in the mixed treatment ($Prey + Lysate_{ciliate}^{3000}$). The three cultures of cryptophyte, ciliate, and dinoflagellate used in this study were non-axenic, and so likely contained heterotrophic bacteria at the time of co-incubation. Bacteria, in general, are well known for their contributions to phytoplankton growth [46–48], and may have remineralized the organic material (dissolved or particulate) into nutrient chemical forms that *D. acuminata* can directly utilize to support cell division, such as ammonium or urea [34,49]. Growth factors, such as essential vitamins and metals, may also be liberated through remineralization of dissolved organic substrates. Therefore, interactions between *Dinophysis*-ciliate-bacteria still need to be evaluated systematically if the link between the dinoflagellate, ciliate, and/or organic compounds or materials is to be realized.

As ciliate lysate was shown to enhance *D. acuminata* growth in the presence of ciliate inoculum (i.e., live ciliates and associated bacteria), then ciliate lysate addition may be a mechanism to increase the likelihood of success during *D. acuminata* isolation. While early attempts to isolate and establish *Dinophysis* cultures with organic matter failed [32,33], more recent studies with field populations and established isolates suggest *Dinophysis* experiences direct or indirect benefits from organic compounds [21,24,34,36] and this study. Given how critical the multi-stage feeding scheme [10] is to the successful isolation of *Dinophysis* spp., we do not recommend replacing prey with ciliate lysate, but instead suggest that in addition to typical *Dinophysis* isolation methods, researchers consider adding equal parts of live ciliates and ciliate lysate to a subset of single-cells in a well plate. Note that the growth-promoting effect of ciliate lysate has only been demonstrated for *D. acuminata* and so it is not known if these results extrapolate to others in the genus. Additionally, ciliates used in this study were maintained by performing a 1:2 dilution with fresh medium (see Materials and Methods), meaning that ciliates were likely conditioned to utilize additional nutrient forms than those that are strictly provided in f/6-Si medium. It is, therefore, unknown if the growth-promoting effect of ciliate lysate, in the present study, was dependent upon the pre-conditioning of ciliates, and therefore *D. acuminata*, to utilize multiple chemical forms.

3.2. Ciliate Lysate in Support of Toxin Production

The addition of a mixture of ciliate lysate and live ciliates to *D. acuminata* cultures significantly increased total toxin concentrations (intracellular + extracellular) of OA and DTX1 relative to both initial levels and the other treatments that provided only ciliates (Figure 2g–h). Pectenotoxin-2 did not show a consistent trend across treatments and toxin fractions, but did significantly increase in the lysate and prey treatment from initial levels (Figure 2c,f,i). These novel findings built upon a previous study by Nagai et al., [21], whereby the authors showed that the addition of lysate alone increased total toxin levels in a monoculture of *D. acuminata*. While the current study cannot ask the same question, i.e., the lysate-only treatment did not produce enough biomass for toxin testing, it is interesting that both studies reported a toxin-promoting effect of lysate. The consistency in results between studies, two geographical isolates, and different prey lines, lends support to this result's validity. Additionally, the earlier depletion of live ciliates from the Prey + $\text{Lysate}_{\text{ciliate}}^{3000}$ treatment (Figure 1b) may have contributed to the enhanced toxin quotas in *D. acuminata* as toxin content has been shown to increase in cultures during the prey-limited phase (52).

Okadaic acid and DTX1 released into the surrounding environment, whether actively or passively, by *D. acuminata* may have detrimental effects on competitors and prey. These toxins have been shown to limit the growth of several microalgae [5,6] and have been proposed to aid in the capture and immobilization of ciliate prey [31,40,50,51]. Ciliates, *M. rubrum*, exhibited abnormal behavior when exposed to high densities of *D. fortii*, such as forming clumps or rotating at the same place, followed by death [51]. Other mechanisms of capture have also been investigated, such as mucus traps [30] and chemical or physical sensing [52,53], in which OA has either been found unimportant to the mechanism or not evaluated as a contributor. The present study suggests a positive feedback may occur, whereby the addition of prey lysate enhances the production and exudation of DSP toxins. The addition of ciliate lysate to co-incubations (Prey + $\text{Lysate}_{\text{ciliate}}^{3000}$) resulted in a significant increase in OA and DTX1 levels to 0.38 and 0.71 ng/mL intracellularly, and 1.37 and 1.27 ng/mL extracellularly by plateau phase, respectively (Figure 2g–h). Mechanisms underlying this feedback, e.g., chemical detection of prey [52], should be further explored as these data suggest that the presence of cells and/or their exudate will enhance extracellular DSP toxin levels.

4. Conclusions

To summarize, an isolate of *D. acuminata* benefitted from the addition of organic matter that was released from *M. rubrum* by probe-sonification. Growth and DSP toxin metrics elevated when the lysate was administered with live prey, suggesting that either total (photosynthetic + mixotrophic) growth of *D. acuminata* was enhanced with the addition of the liberated organic compounds and/or the ciliate (or associated bacteria) was directly utilizing the liberated materials and indirectly providing the benefit to *D. acuminata* through remineralization to bioavailable forms or increasing ciliate enrichment and/or abundance. When provided with ciliate lysate only, however, growth of *D. acuminata* was also observed, lending some support to the conclusion that the dinoflagellate does have some capacity to directly utilize the liberated compounds itself and promote certain growth and toxin production.

Extrapolating to the field, these culturing studies suggest that the co-occurrence of a ciliate-dinoflagellate bloom may exacerbate *D. acuminata* abundance and toxigenicity due to exudate or lysing. The lysate from the cryptophyte, however, did not support *Dinophysis* growth, suggesting this growth-promoting effect may be unique to ciliates. Further studies should be conducted to better understand the interactions between organic compounds and *Dinophysis*-ciliate-bacteria relationships and characterize the nutritional composition of ciliate lysate to identify the beneficial components as those might be important drivers of *D. acuminata* abundance and DSP events in the field.

5. Materials and Methods

5.1. Culture Maintenance

A uni-algal culture of *Dinophysis acuminata* (DAEP01) was previously isolated from Eel Pond, Woods Hole, MA, in September of 2006 [54]. The ciliate *Mesodinium rubrum* (GenBank accession NO. AB364286) and cryptophyte *Teleaulax amphioxeia* (GenBank accession NO. AB364287) were isolated from Inokushi Bay in Oita Prefecture, Japan, in February of 2007 as described in [27]. All cultures were maintained at a salinity of 30 in f/6-Si medium, which was prepared with 1/3 nitrate, 1/3 phosphate, 1/3 metals, and 1/3 vitamins of f/2-Si medium. The three-stage culture system [10] was utilized; the cryptophyte was fed to the ciliate prior to being fed to the dinoflagellate. In detail, every 7 days, 20 mL of *M. rubrum* culture medium was added to 20 mL of fresh f/6-Si medium with 0.5 mL *T. amphioxeia* cultures, providing roughly a 1:2 dilution of ciliate culture. After the cryptophyte cells were consumed, the ciliates were then fed to *Dinophysis* cells at a prey: predator ratio of 3:1. Cultures were maintained at 15 °C with dim light (ca. 20 µmol photons m^{-2} s^{-1}) on a 14 h light: 10 h dark photo cycle.

5.2. Lysate Preparation and Size Characterization

Mesodinium rubrum and *T. amphioxeia* cultures in early plateau phase (11 and 6 days old, respectively) were pretreated by probe sonication to prepare fresh ciliate and cryptophyte lysate for the experiment (Table 1). More specifically, 100 mL of the *M. rubrum* culture (4×10^3 cells/mL) or 50 mL of the *T. amphioxeia* culture (2×10^5 cells/mL) were probe sonified (Scientz JY92-IIN, Ningbo, China) using a repeated pulse cycle (3 s sonify/3 s pause = 90 s of active sonication, power = 400 W) over three minutes to lyse all cells. The duration and amplitude were determined by a preliminary experiment in which time of active sonification was increased from 60 s to 120 s over 200 W to 400 W (data not shown). No intact ciliate or cryptophyte cells were observed under a light microscope at 400 W after 60 s ultrasonic treatment.

Triplicate subsamples of experimental cell lysate were immediately scanned under light microscope using a Sedgewick-Rafter counting chamber to ensure the absence of living or whole cells. Particles of the ciliate lysate were photographed and measured using an Olympus CKX53 inverted microscope (Olympus, Shinjuku, Tokyo) with Infinity Analyze imaging software (Lumenera Corporation, Ottawa, Canada). All particles were evaluated as spheres, and therefore, were fit to a circle and diameter and area measurements collected.

5.3. Experimental Design

Triplicate maintenance cultures of *Dinophysis acuminata* and *Mesodinium rubrum* were starved, in the light, for two weeks before the experiment to ensure the prey were fully consumed from the medium and that any responses measured in *Dinophysis* were due to the amendments and not sustained growth or divisions using internal reserves. To begin the experiment, triplicate 1-L flasks were inoculated with *Dinophysis* monoculture at an initial concentration of 150 cell/mL for all seven treatments (Table 1). Live ciliate prey were then provided to *Dinophysis* at two initial concentrations, 1500 and 3000 cells/mL: the $\text{Prey}_{\text{ciliate}}{}^{1500}$ and $\text{Prey}_{\text{ciliate}}{}^{3000}$ treatments, respectively. To determine if prey was equally supportive of growth and toxin production when provided as organic matter, half of the ciliates were lysed and then fed to *Dinophysis* as a mixture of live prey and lysate, equivalent to 3000 cells/mL: the Prey + $\text{Lysate}_{\text{ciliate}}{}^{3000}$ treatment. Additionally, ciliate lysate equivalent to 3000 cells/mL was offered alone to determine if organic "dead" particles could support *Dinophysis* growth and toxin production: the $\text{Lysate}_{\text{ciliate}}{}^{3000}$ treatment. Prey to predator ratios for all the 1500 cells/mL and 3000 cells/mL ciliate treatments were 10:1 and 20:1, respectively.

Two additional treatments were included to determine if similar growth and toxin production could be achieved by *Dinophysis* through exposure to lysed cryptophytes, $\text{Lysate}_{\text{crypto}}{}^{15000}$, with an equivalent live cryptophyte treatment run in parallel: $\text{Prey}_{\text{crypto}}{}^{15000}$ (Table 1). All treatments were compared to a monoculture *Dinophysis* control in which no prey or lysate was provided, and the triplicate flasks were instead supplemented with fresh f/6-Si medium to reach a similar final volume of 500 mL.

Samples, 1.2 mL, were taken every three days from each flask, fixed with 3% (v/v) formalin solution, and the dinoflagellates, ciliates, and cryptophytes were enumerated microscopically using a Sedgewick-Rafter counting chamber at 100× magnification.

5.4. Toxin Analysis

Culture was harvested and separated into medium and cells of *Dinophysis* once experimental cultures reached two growth phases, exponential and plateau. Initial toxin samples were also collected and analyzed from the *Dinophysis* inoculum cultures. Cells were separated from medium using a 15-μm Nitex sieve affixed to polyvinyl chloride (PVC) pipe and back-washed into a pre-weighed 15-mL centrifuge tube (w_1) using fresh media; the sieved medium was collected into a beaker. As such, intracellular (≥15 μm) and extracellular (<15 μm) fractions of each sample were collected, extracted, and analyzed separately. In order to determine the total number of harvested cells for extraction, 200 μL subsamples were pipetted from the intracellular toxin samples into a 2-mL micro-centrifuge tube containing 1.0 mL filtered seawater and 37 μL formalin solution (3% v/v). The fixed and diluted subsamples were enumerated microscopically to calculate cell concentration using a Sedgewich-Rafter counting chamber at 100× magnification. The 15-mL tube was then reweighed (w_2) to calculate the volume of harvested *Dinophysis* cells (v) using the formula:

$$v = \frac{w_2 - w_1}{\rho_{seawater}} \tag{1}$$

where ρ_{seawater} was set at 1.03 g/mL given the salinity of the culture medium was 30. The volume harvested (v) was then multiplied by the cell concentration to estimate the total number of cells in the tube. Tubes were then frozen at −80 °C for over 24 h before toxin extraction.

Methods of solid phase extraction (SPE) were used as described in [38] to clean up samples prior to analysis. SPE cartridges (Oasis HLB 60 mg; Waters, Milford, MA, USA) were conditioned with 6 mL of methanol and rinsed with 6 mL of Milli-Q water in preparation for cell or media. Culture media (extracellular fraction, <15 μm) was loaded onto the column immediately after separation from cells with no additional processing. Cell samples (intracellular fraction, ≥15 μm), however, underwent a freeze/thaw cycle and bath sonification (KQ-3200E, ultrasonic power = 150 watt, frequency = 40 KHz, Kunshan Ultrasonic Instruments Co., Ltd., Kunshan, China) for 15 min at room temperature, to aid in cell lysis before being loaded onto the conditioned SPE cartridges. The cartridges were then washed with 3 mL of Milli-Q water and toxins were ultimately eluted with 1 mL of methanol into an autosampler vial. Eluates from the samples were heated at 40 °C in a heating block, dried under a stream of high-purity N_2 (HP-S016SY,), and re-suspended in 1 mL of methanol for toxin analysis to remove error associated with varying elution volumes. Eluates were frozen at −20 °C until analysis.

The Dionex UltiMate 3000 liquid chromatrography system (Thermo Scientific™ Dionex™, Waltham, MA, USA) coupled with an AB 4000 mass spectrometer (SCIEX, Framingham, MA, USA) with electrospray ionization (LC-MS/MS) was used for the analysis. Toxins, okadaic acid (OA) and dinophysistoxin-1 (DTX1), were analyzed in negative mode, and pectenotoxin-2 (PTX2) in positive mode. Chromatographic separation for OA and DTX1 was performed using a Waters XBridge™ C18 column (3.0 × 150 mm, 3.5 μm particle size) at 40 °C in negative mode. The mobile phase used during negative mode consisted of phase A, 0.05 v/v % ammonia hydroxide (pH 11) in water and phase B, 0.05 v/v % ammonia hydroxide in 90% acetonitrile, with a flow rate of 0.4 mL/min and 10 μL injection. A linear gradient elution from 10% to 90% B was run for 9 min, held for 3 min at 90% B, decreased to 10% B in 2 min and held at 10% B for 4 min to equilibrate at initial conditions before the next run was started. In positive mode, Waters XBridge™ C18 column (2.1 × 50 mm, 2.5 μm particle size) at 25 °C was performed for chromatographic separation of PTX2. The mobile phase consisted of phase C, water and phase D, 95% acetonitrile, both contain a constant concentration of buffer (2 mM ammonium formate and 50 mM formic acid). A linear gradient from 10% to 80% acetonitrile was run between 0 and 3 min, held at 80% acetonitrile for 2 min, decreased to 10% in 2 min and held another 2 min. The flow rate during positive mode runs was 0.3 mL/min and the injection volume was set to 10 µL.

The mass spectrometer was operated in multiple reaction monitoring (MRM) mode. Transitions of $[M + NH_4^+]$ ion: PTX2, m/z 876.5 > 823.4, $[M\text{-}H^+]$ ions: OA, m/z 803.5 > 255.0 and DTX1, m/z 817.5 > 255.0 were selected for quantitation. The operation conditions were as follows: ion spray voltage (ISV): −4.5 kV, temperature (TEM): 600 °C, nebulizer gas (NEB) 13 psi, curtain gas (CUR): 13 psi, collision gas (CAD): 5 psi in negative mode and ISV: 3 kV, TEM: 650 °C, NEB: 14 psi, CUR: 16 psi, CAD: 5 psi in positive mode. Standards for OA, DTX1, and PTX2 were purchased from the National Research Council, Canada (NRC). Five-point standard curves were generated using NRC reference materials, with concentrations ranging from 1.25 to 20 ng/mL for OA and DTX1, and 6.25 to 100 ng/mL for PTX2.

5.5. Calculations

Dinophysis growth rate was calculated over the entire period of exponential growth phase (Table 1) using the following formula [55]:

$$\mu = \frac{\ln(N_2/N_1)}{t_2 - t_1} \tag{2}$$

where N_1 and N_2 (cells/mL) are the cell concentrations at time 1 and time 2, respectively. Sampling times are represented by t_1 and t_2 with units of day, and µ is the growth rate calculated at the sampling interval with units of day^{-1}.

Toxin data are presented as cellular toxin content or quota (toxin amount per cell), total toxin concentration (intracellular + extracellular, i.e., total toxin in a milliliter of culture), proportion of extracellular toxin (extracellular/ (intracellular + extracellular) × 100%) and net toxin production rate R_{tox} (amount toxin/cell/d). The R_{tox} was calculated using the total toxin concentration (extracellular + intracellular) as described by the authors of [56].

$$R_{tox} = \frac{(T_2 - T_1)}{(\overline{C})(t_2 - t_1)} \tag{3}$$

$$\overline{C} = \frac{C_2 - C_1}{\ln(C_2/C_1)} \tag{4}$$

In these equations, T_1 and T_2 are the total toxin concentrations (intracellular + extracellular, i.e., total toxin per milliliter of culture) at time 1 and time 2, respectively. Toxin production rates were calculated for two periods of time: from initial to exponential growth phase, and then from exponential into plateau phase (Table 2). The concentrations of *Dinophysis* cells at time 1 and time 2 are represented as C_1 and C_2, (cells/mL), respectively.

5.6. Statistical Analysis

Repeated Measures ANOVA (SigmaPlot v12.0, Systat Software Inc., London, UK) was used to analyze for differences in DSP and PTX2 toxin content, total toxin concentrations, and differences of toxin production rates between treatments or over time. Shapiro-Wilk test was used to test for normality. T-tests were used to analyze for any differences in growth rate and biomass of *Dinophysis* between treatments. Alpha was set at 0.05 for all analyses.

Author Contributions: Writing—original draft preparation, H.G. and J.L.S.; Writing—review and editing, J.L.S. and M.T.; Visualization, H.G.; Supervision, M.T.; Project administration, M.T. and X.A.; Funding acquisition, J.L.S. and M.T.

Funding: This research was supported by a National Key R&D Program of China NO. 2016YFC1402104, Research on Public Welfare Technology Application Projects of Zhejiang Province, China NO. 2013C32040, Key Laboratory of Integrated Marine Monitoring and Applied Technologies for Harmful Algal Blooms, Ministry of Natural Resources of the People's Republic of China (MNR), MATHAB201803, the Laboratory of Marine Ecosystem and Biogeochemistry, MNR, LMEB201507, Natural Science Foundation of China (Grant No. 41306095) and Funding for Tang Scholar to M.T. Research completed in the USA was supported by NOAA Sea Grant Aquaculture Initiative NA14OAR4170093 and partial funding from the NOAA National Centers for Coastal Ocean Science ECOHAB Program grant number NA17NOS4780184 to J.L.S. This paper is contribution No. 3803 of the Virginia Institute of Marine Science, College of William & Mary.

Acknowledgments: The authors would like to thank Lei Liu (National Marine Environmental Monitoring Center, China) and Caroline DeMent (VIMS) for their contributions to this work.

Conflicts of Interest: The authors declare no conflict of interest.

References

1. Hallegraeff, G.M. A review of harmful algal blooms and their apparent global increase. *Phycologia* **1993**, *32*, 79–99. [CrossRef]
2. Reguera, B.; Riobo, P.; Rodriguez, F.; Diaz, P.A.; Pizarro, G.; Paz, B.; Franco, J.M.; Blanco, J. *Dinophysis* toxins: Causative organisms, distribution and fate in shellfish. *Mar. Drugs* **2014**, *12*, 394–461. [CrossRef]
3. Zhou, J.; Fritz, L. Okadaic acid antibody localizes to chloroplasts in the DSP-toxin-producing dinoflagellates *Prorocentrum lima* and *Prorocentrum maculosum*. *Phycologia* **1994**, *33*, 455–461. [CrossRef]
4. Marasigan, A.N.; Sato, S.; Fukuyo, Y.; Kodama, M. Accumulation of a high level of diarrhetic shellfish toxins in the green mussel Perna viridis during a bloom of *Dinophysis caudata* and *Dinophysis miles* in Sapian Bay, Panay Island, the Philippines. *Fish. Sci.* **2001**, *67*, 994–996. [CrossRef]
5. Windust, A.J.; Wright, J.L.C.; McLachlan, J.L. The effects of the diarrhetic shellfish poisoning toxins, okadaic acid and dinophysistoxin-1, on the growth of microalgae. *Mar. Biol.* **1996**, *126*, 19–25. [CrossRef]
6. Windust, A.J.; Quilliam, M.A.; Wright, J.L.; McLachlan, J.L. Comparative toxicity of the diarrhetic shellfish poisons, okadaic acid, okadaic acid diol-ester and dinophysistoxin-4, to the diatom *Thalassiosira weissflogii*. *Toxicon* **1997**, *35*, 1591–1603. [CrossRef]
7. Miles, C.O.; Wilkins, A.L.; Munday, R.; Dines, M.H.; Hawkes, A.D.; Briggs, L.R.; Sandvik, M.; Jensen, D.J.; Cooney, J.M.; Holland, P.T.; et al. Isolation of pectenotoxin-2 from *Dinophysis acuta* and its conversion to pectenotoxin-2 seco acid, and preliminary assessment of their acute toxicities. *Toxicon* **2004**, *43*, 1–9. [CrossRef]
8. Ito, E.; Suzuki, T.; Oshima, Y.; Yasumoto, T. Studies of diarrhetic activity on pectenotoxin-6 in the mouse and rat. *Toxicon* **2008**, *51*, 707–716. [CrossRef]
9. Anonymous. Commission regulation (EC) No. 2074/2005 of the European parliament and of the council of 5 December 2005. *Off. J. Eur. Commun.* **2005**, *L338*, 27–59.
10. Park, M.G.; Kim, S.; Kim, H.S.; Myung, G.; Kang, Y.G.; Yih, W. First successful culture of the marine dinoflagellate *Dinophysis acuminata*. *Aquat. Microb. Ecol.* **2006**, *45*, 101–106. [CrossRef]
11. Yih, W.; Kim, H.S.; Jeong, H.A.; Myung, G.; Kim, Y.G. Ingestion of cryptophyte cells by the marine photosynthetic ciliate *Mesodinium rubrum*. *Aquat. Microb. Ecol.* **2004**, *36*, 165–170. [CrossRef]
12. Takishita, K.; Koike, K.; Maruyama, T.; Ogata, T. Molecular evidence for plastid robbery (Kleptoplastidy) in *Dinophysis*, a dinoflagellate causing diarrhetic shellfish poisoning. *Protist* **2002**, *153*, 293–302. [CrossRef] [PubMed]
13. Hackett, J.D.; Maranda, L.; Yoon, H.S.; Bhattacharya, D. Phylogenetic evidence for the cryptophyte origin of the plastid of *Dinophysis* (Dinophysiales, Dinophyceae). *J. Phycol.* **2003**, *39*, 440–448. [CrossRef]
14. Janson, S.; Granéli, E. Genetic analysis of the psbA gene from single cells indicates a cryptomonad origin of the plastid in *Dinophysis* (Dinophyceae). *Phycologia* **2003**, *42*, 473–477. [CrossRef]
15. Johnson, M.D.; Oldach, D.; Delwiche, C.F.; Stoecker, D.K. Retention of transcriptionally active cryptophyte nuclei by the ciliate *Myrionecta rubra*. *Nature* **2007**, *445*, 426–428. [CrossRef] [PubMed]
16. Kim, G.H.; Han, J.H.; Kim, B. Cryptophyte gene regulation in the kleptoplastidic, karyokleptic ciliate *Mesodinium rubrum*. *Harmful Algae* **2016**, *52*, 23–33. [CrossRef] [PubMed]
17. Janson, S. Molecular evidence that plastids in the toxin-producing dinoflagellate genus *Dinophysis* originate from the free-living cryptophyte *Teleaulax amphioxeia*. *Environ. Microbiol.* **2004**, *6*, 1102–1106. [CrossRef] [PubMed]

18. Hackett, J.D.; Tong, M.; Kulis, D.M.; Fux, E.; Hess, P.; Bire, R.; Anderson, D.M. DSP toxin production de novo in cultures of *Dinophysis acuminata* (Dinophyceae) from North America. *Harmful Algae* **2009**, *8*, 873–879. [CrossRef]
19. Kamiyama, T.; Suzuki, T. Production of dinophysistoxin-1 and pectenotoxin-2 by a culture of *Dinophysis acuminata* (Dinophyceae). *Harmful Algae* **2009**, *8*, 312–317. [CrossRef]
20. Kamiyama, T.; Nagai, S.; Suzuki, T.; Miyamura, K. Effect of temperature on production of okadaic acid, dinophysistoxin-1, and pectenotoxin-2 by *Dinophysis acuminata* in culture experiments. *Aquat. Microb. Ecol.* **2010**, *60*, 193–202. [CrossRef]
21. Nagai, S.; Suzuki, T.; Nishikawa, T.; Kamiyama, T. Differences in the production and excretion kinetics of okadaic acid, dinophysistoxin-1, and pectenotoxin-2 between cultures of *Dinophysis acuminata* and *Dinophysis fortii* isolated from western Japan. *J. Phycol.* **2011**, *47*, 1326–1337. [CrossRef] [PubMed]
22. Nielsen, L.T.; Krock, B.; Hansen, P.J. Effects of light and food availability on toxin production, growth and photosynthesis in *Dinophysis acuminata*. *Mar. Ecol. Prog. Ser.* **2012**, *471*, 37–50. [CrossRef]
23. Mafra, L.L.; dos Santos Tavares, C.P.; Schramm, M.A. Diarrheic toxins in field-sampled and cultivated *Dinophysis* spp. cells from southern Brazil. *J. Appl. Phycol.* **2014**, *26*, 1727–1739. [CrossRef]
24. Hattenrath-Lehmann, T.; Gobler, C.J. The contribution of inorganic and organic nutrients to the growth of a North American isolate of the mixotrophic dinoflagellate, *Dinophysis acuminata*. *Limnol. Oceanogr.* **2015**, *60*, 1588–1630. [CrossRef]
25. Tong, M.; Smith, J.L.; Richlen, M.; Steidinger, K.A.; Kulis, D.M.; Fux, E.; Anderson, D.M. Characterization and comparison of toxin-producing isolates of *Dinophysis acuminata* from New England and Canada. *J. Phycol.* **2015**, *51*, 66–81. [CrossRef] [PubMed]
26. Gao, H.; An, X.; Liu, L.; Zhang, K.; Zheng, D.; Tong, M. Characterization of *Dinophysis acuminata* from the Yellow Sea, China, and its response to different temperatures and *Mesodinium* prey. *Oceanol. Hydrobiol. Stud.* **2017**, *46*, 439–450. [CrossRef]
27. Nishitani, G.; Nagai, S.; Sakiyama, S.; Kamiyama, T. Successful cultivation of the toxic dinoflagellate *Dinophysis caudata* (Dinophyceae). *Plankton Benthos Res.* **2008**, *3*, 78–85. [CrossRef]
28. Nishitani, G.; Nagai, S.; Takano, Y.; Sakiyama, S.; Baba, K.; Kamiyama, T. Growth characteristics and phylogenetic analysis of the marine dinoflagellate *Dinophysis infundibulus* (Dinophyceae). *Aquat. Microb. Ecol.* **2008**, *52*, 209–221. [CrossRef]
29. Nielsen, L.T.; Krock, B.; Hansen, P.J. Production and excretion of okadaic acid, pectenotoxin-2 and a novel dinophysistoxin from the DSP-causing marine dinoflagellate *Dinophysis acuta*—Effects of light, food availability and growth phase. *Harmful Algae* **2013**, *23*, 34–45. [CrossRef]
30. Mafra, L.L., Jr.; Nagai, S.; Uchida, H.; Tavares, C.P.; Escobar, B.P.; Suzuki, T. Harmful effects of *Dinophysis* to the ciliate *Mesodinium rubrum*: Implications for prey capture. *Harmful Algae* **2016**, *59*, 82–90. [CrossRef]
31. Papiol, G.G.; Beuzenberg, V.; Selwood, A.I.; MacKenzie, L.; Packer, M.A. The use of a mucus trap by *Dinophysis acuta* for the capture of *Mesodinium rubrum* prey under culture conditions. *Harmful Algae* **2016**, *58*, 1–7. [CrossRef] [PubMed]
32. Maestrini, S.Y.; Berland, B.R.; Grzebyk, D.; Spano, A.M. *Dinophysis* spp cells concentrated from nature for experimental purposes, using size fractionation and reverse migration. *Aquat. Microb. Ecol.* **1995**, *9*, 177–182. [CrossRef]
33. Sampayo, T.J. Trying to cultivate *Dinophysis* spp. In *Toxic Phytoplankton Blooms in the Sea*; Smayda, T.J., Shimizu, Y., Eds.; Elsevier Science Publisher: New York, NY, USA, 1993; pp. 807–811. ISBN O-444-89719-4.
34. Hattenrath-Lehmann, T.K.; Marcoval, M.A.; Mittlesdorf, H.; Goleski, J.A.; Wang, Z.H.; Haynes, B.; Morton, S.L.; Gobler, C.J. Nitrogenous nutrients promote the growth and toxicity of *Dinophysis acuminata* during estuarine bloom events. *PLoS ONE* **2015**, *10*, e0124148. [CrossRef] [PubMed]
35. Tong, M.; Smith, J.L.; Kulis, D.M.; Anderson, D.M. Role of dissolved nitrate and phosphate in isolates of *Mesodinium rubrum* and toxin-producing *Dinophysis acuminata*. *Aquat. Microb. Ecol.* **2015**, *75*, 169–185. [CrossRef] [PubMed]
36. Seeyave, S.; Probyn, T.; Pitcher, G.; Lucas, M.; Purdie, D. Nitrogen nutrition in assemblages dominated by *Pseudo-nitzschia* spp., *Alexandrium catenella* and *Dinophysis acuminata* off the west coast of South Africa. *Mar. Ecol. Prog. Ser.* **2009**, *379*, 91–107. [CrossRef]

37. Hattenrath-Lehmann, T.K.; Marcoval, M.A.; Berry, D.L.; Fire, S.; Wang, Z.; Morton, S.L.; Gobler, C.J. The emergence of *Dinophysis acuminata* blooms and DSP toxins in shellfish in New York waters. *Harmful Algae* **2013**, *26*, 33–44. [CrossRef]
38. Smith, J.L.; Tong, M.; Fux, E.; Anderson, D.M. Toxin production, retention, and extracellular release by *Dinophysis acuminata* during extended plateau phase and culture decline. *Harmful Algae* **2012**, *19*, 125–132. [CrossRef]
39. Kim, S.; Kang, Y.G.; Kim, H.S.; Yih, W.; Coats, D.W.; Park, M.G. Growth and grazing responses of the mixotrophic dinoflagellate *Dinophysis acuminata* as functions of light intensity and prey concentration. *Aquat. Microb. Ecol.* **2008**, *51*, 301–310. [CrossRef]
40. Riisgaard, K.; Hansen, P.J. Role of food uptake for photosynthesis, growth and survival of the mixotrophic dinoflagellate *Dinophysis acuminata*. *Mar. Ecol. Prog. Ser.* **2009**, *381*, 51–62. [CrossRef]
41. Tong, M.; Kulis, D.M.; Fux, E.; Smith, J.L.; Hess, P.; Zhou, Q.; Anderson, D.M. The effects of growth phase and light intensity on toxin production by *Dinophysis acuminata* from the northeastern United States. *Harmful Algae* **2011**, *10*, 254–264. [CrossRef]
42. Harred, L.B.; Campbell, L. Predicting harmful algal blooms: A case study with *Dinophysis ovum* in the Gulf of Mexico. *J. Plankton Res.* **2014**, *36*, 1434–1445. [CrossRef]
43. Anderson, D.M.; Kulis, D.M.; Doucette, G.J.; Gallagher, J.C.; Balech, E. Biogeography of toxic dinoflagellates in the genus *Alexandrium* from the northeastern United-States and Canada. *Mar. Biol.* **1994**, *120*, 467–478. [CrossRef]
44. Sagert, S.; Krause Jensen, D.; Henriksen, P.; Rieling, T.; Schubert, H. Integrated ecological assessment of Danish Baltic Sea coastal areas by means of phytoplankton and macrophytobenthos. *Estuar. Coast. Shelf Sci.* **2005**, *63*, 109–118. [CrossRef]
45. Smith, J.L.; Tong, M.; Kulis, D.; Anderson, D.M. Effect of ciliate strain, size, and nutritional content on the growth and toxicity of mixotrophic *Dinophysis acuminata*. *Harmful Algae* **2018**, *78*, 95–105. [CrossRef]
46. Haines, K.C.; Guillard, R.R. Growth of vitamin b12-requiring marine diatoms in mixed laboratory cultures with vitamin b12-producing marine bacteria. *J. Phycol.* **1974**, *10*, 245–252.
47. Azam, F. Microbial control of oceanic carbon flux: The plot thickens. *Science* **1998**, *280*, 694–696. [CrossRef]
48. Sakami, T.; Nakahara, H.; Chinain, M.; Ishida, Y. Effects of epiphytic bacteria on the growth of the toxic dinoflagellate *Gambierdiscus toxicus* (Dinophyceae). *J. Exp. Mar. Biol. Ecol.* **1999**, *233*, 231–246. [CrossRef]
49. Gao, H.; Hua, C.; Tong, M. Impact of *Dinophysis acuminata* Feeding *Mesodinium rubrum* on Nutrient Dynamics and Bacterial Composition in a Microcosm. *Toxins* **2018**, *10*, 443. [CrossRef]
50. Ojamäe, K.; Hansen, P.J.; Lips, I. Mass entrapment and lysis of *Mesodinium rubrum* cells in mucus threads observed in cultures with *Dinophysis*. *Harmful Algae* **2016**, *55*, 77–84. [CrossRef]
51. Nagai, S.; Nitshitani, G.; Tomaru, Y.; Sakiyama, S.; Kamiyama, T. Predation by the toxic dinoflagellate *Dinophysis fortii* on the ciliate *Myrionecta rubra* and observation of sequestration of ciliate chloroplasts. *J. Phycol.* **2008**, *44*, 909–922. [CrossRef]
52. García-Portela, M.; Reguera, B.; Sibat, M.; Altenburger, A.; Rodríguez, F.; Hess, P. Metabolomic Profiles of *Dinophysis acuminata* and *Dinophysis acuta* Using Non-Targeted High-Resolution Mass Spectrometry: Effect of Nutritional Status and Prey. *Mar. Drugs* **2018**, *16*, 143. [CrossRef]
53. Jiang, H.; Kulis, D.M.; Brosnahan, M.L.; Anderson, D.M. Behavioral and mechanistic characteristics of the predator-prey interaction between the dinoflagellate *Dinophysis acuminata* and the ciliate *Mesodinium rubrum*. *Harmful Algae* **2018**, *77*, 43–54. [CrossRef]
54. Tong, M.; Zhou, Q.; David, K.M.; Jiang, T.; Qi, Y.; Donald, A.M. Culture techniques and growth characteristics of *Dinophysis acuminata* and its prey. *Chin. J. Oceanol. Limnol.* **2010**, *28*, 1230–1239. [CrossRef]
55. Guillard, R.R.L. Division rates. In *Handbook of Phycological Methods: Culture Methods and Growth Measurements*; Stein, J.R., Ed.; Cambridge University Press: Cambridge, UK, 1973; pp. 289–312. ISBN 10: 0521200490.
56. Anderson, D.M.; Kulis, D.M.; Sullivan, J.J.; Hall, S.; Lee, C. Dynamics and physiology of saxitoxin production by the dinoflagellates *Alexandrium* spp. *Mar. Biol.* **1990**, *104*, 511–524. [CrossRef]

toxins

MDPI

Article

Impact of *Dinophysis acuminata* Feeding *Mesodinium rubrum* on Nutrient Dynamics and Bacterial Composition in a Microcosm

Han Gao, Chenfeng Hua and Mengmeng Tong *

Ocean College, Zhejiang University, No 1 Zheda Road, Zhoushan 316000, Zhejiang, China; gghanbing@zju.edu.cn (H.G.); verahcf@zju.edu.cn (C.H.)
* Correspondence: mengmengtong@zju.edu.cn

Received: 14 September 2018; Accepted: 25 October 2018; Published: 30 October 2018

Abstract: The development of *Dinophysis* populations, producers of diarrhetic shellfish toxins, has been attributed to both abiotic (e.g., water column stratification) and biotic (prey availability) factors. An important process to consider is mixotrophy of the *Dinophysis* species, which is an intensive feeding of the *Mesodinium* species for nutrients and a benefit from kleptochloroplasts. During the feeding process, the nutritional status in the environment changes due to the preference of *Mesodinium* and/or *Dinophysis* for different nutrients, prey cell debris generated by sloppy feeding, and their degradation by micro-organisms changes. However, there is little knowledge about the role of the bacterial community during the co-occurrence of *Mesodinium* and *Dinophysis* and how they directly or indirectly interact with the mixotrophs. In this study, laboratory experiments were performed to characterize the environmental changes including those of the prey present, the bacterial communities, and the ambient dissolved nutrients during the co-occurrence of *Mesodinium rubrum* and *Dinophysis acuminata*. The results showed that, during the incubation of the ciliate prey *Mesodinium* with its predator *Dinophysis*, available dissolved nitrogen significantly shifted from nitrate to ammonium especially when the population of *M. rubrum* decayed. Growth phases of *Dinophysis* and *Mesodinium* greatly affected the structure and composition of the bacterial community. These changes could be mainly explained by both the changes of the nutrient status and the activity of *Dinophysis* cells. *Dinophysis* feeding activity also accelerated the decline of *M. rubrum* and contamination of cultures with okadaic acid, dinophysistoxin-1, and pectenotoxin-2, but their influence on the prokaryotic communities was limited to the rare taxa (<0.1%) fraction. This suggests that the interaction between *D. acuminata* and bacteria is species-specific and takes place intracellularly or in the phycosphere. Moreover, a majority of the dominant bacterial taxa in our cultures may also exhibit a metabolic flexibility and, thus, be unaffected taxonomically by changes within the *Mesodinium-Dinophysis* culture system.

Keywords: DSP toxins; pectenotoxins; *Dinophysis acuminata*; *Mesodinium rubrum*; bacterial community; high throughput sequencing

Key Contribution: toxin levels; nutrient dynamics and changes in bacterial communities during *Dinophysis acuminata* feeding on *Mesodinium rubrum*; interactions among toxin-producing *Dinophysis* species; bloom-forming *Mesodinium rubrum* and heterotrophic bacteria were discussed; *Dinophysis-Mesodinium* predator prey interactions.

1. Introduction

The cosmopolitan dinoflagellate species *Dinophysis acuminata* is responsible for diarrhetic shellfish poisoning (DSP) events all around the world [1,2]. Okadaic acid (OA) and its derivatives known as dinophysistoxins (DTXs) and/or pectenotoxins (PTXs) are the dominant components in the toxin profile of *D. acuminata*. As strong inhibitors of serine and threonine protein phosphatases in eukaryotic organisms, OA and DTXs are capable of promoting potent tumors [3], inducing typical diarrhetic symptoms [2,4], and even acting as lethal agents to mammals. Recent transcriptomics analysis also revealed that OA and DTX-1 may induce hypoxia-related pathways or processes, unfolded protein response (UPR), and endoplasmic reticulum (ER) stress [5]. PTXs are generally not responsible for unpleasant gastrointestinal symptoms but are potentially involved in acute toxicity [6].

D. acuminata is a mixotrophic species that primarily requires phototrophic metabolism and plastid retention for long-term maintenance in the laboratory [7–9]. The *Dinophysis–Mesodinium*–cryptophyte is so far the only known food chain for *Dinophysis* growth. *Dinophysis* blooms are very much related to the distribution and abundance of *Mesodinium* [10–12]. Therefore, the nutritional status of prey and the surrounding environment may have a critical impact on the growth and toxin production of *Dinophysis* [13–17]. The feeding process of the latter involves not only the direct uptake of the prey organelles through a feeding peduncle (myzocytosis) and secretion of mucus traps but also the intense lysis of the ciliate cells [18–20]. Cell debris and organic substances originating from prey were reported to induce the DSP toxin release from *Dinophysis* [21]. The suspected harmful compounds (e.g., free polyunsaturated fatty acids) were not the shellfish toxins [22]. Additionally, "sloppy feeding" behavior generates a substantial amount of dissolved and particulate materials in the surrounding environment. This pool of biological organic matter combined with the extracellular toxin fraction may also function as a source of nutrients available to the heterotrophic bacterial community and, in turn, for *Dinophysis* cells after regeneration [21,23,24] or other biochemical pathways [25]. However, few studies have been conducted to assess the contribution and availability of these nutritional sources.

The role of algal–bacterial interactions during harmful algal bloom (HAB) has received attention in recent years [26–28]. The supply of dissolved organic substances through cell exudation or cell lysis is hypothesized to be a major interaction between phytoplankton and the associated bacterial community [24,25,29]. The influence of bacteria on the toxigenic properties of photosynthetic microalgae (mainly *Alexandrium* spp. producing paralytic shellfish toxins) has been widely examined (Reference [26] and literature therein). The "obligate" relationship between bacteria and mixotrophic *Dinophysis* species has been explored in terms of cell abundance and carbon equivalents, which show a possible dependence on bacteria-produced vitamin B_{12} and, to a lesser extent, the potential of bacterivory for *Dinophysis* growth [23], which was otherwise confirmed in the case of *Mesodinium rubrum* [30]. Recently [31], the cluster of Alteromonadales have been identified as the unique prokaryotic microbiome associated with *D. acuminata* blooms in Northport Harbor, New York. This finding highlighted the importance of biogeochemical conditions in shaping the microbial consortia.

Mixotrophs may become the major players in an aquatic ecosystem due to their substantial contribution to the energy cycles and to nutrient cycles where heterotrophic bacteria control most of the pathways [32,33]. However, more compelling evidence is needed to explain the interactions between specific heterotrophic bacteria and nutrient dynamics mediated by the mixotrophy of *Dinophysis* species. Therefore, in this study, we focused on the bacterial community associated with the mixotrophic *D. acuminata* feeding on the mixotrophic *M. rubrum* in laboratory culture conditions. By tracking the changes of the bacterial assemblages and the nutritional status of the culture medium, we aimed to (i) study the nutrient dynamics mediated by mixotrophy through the different growth phases of *Dinophysis* feeding *Mesodinium* and the possible consequences for the ambient microbial community and (ii) identify the prevailing interactions among deterministic factors, the bacterial community, and DSP toxin dynamics during the feeding process. In the context of its mixotrophic nature, we hypothesized that an ingestion-derived nutrient shift combined with the activities of the toxin-producing *Dinophysis* could lead to niche separation of the microbial community.

2. Results

2.1. Predator-Prey Population Dynamics and Environmental Changes

The simulation started with an initial density of *M. rubrum* of 6740 ± 1379.3 (mean ± SD, Group A) cells mL^{-1} and 7902 ± 373.0 (Group B) cells mL^{-1} (Figure 1). The *M. rubrum* population developed until the 5th day when *Dinophysis* cells were inoculated (Group A). The ciliate cell-density gradually declined under an average ingestion rate of 3.25 ± 0.38 prey cells $predator^{-1}$ day^{-1} during 16 days while the *Mesodinium* population in the control group (Group B) doubled in 4 days and then significantly declined to 4833 ± 378.6 cell mL^{-1} from days 5 to 16. *Dinophysis* exponential growth lasted 15 days (from T1 to T3) and reached a maximal density of 1302 ± 282.1 cells mL^{-1} on the 20th day and remained in a plateau phase thereafter (Figure 1). The bacterial abundance also changed during the feeding process (Group A) and the growth of *M. rubrum* (Group B).

Environmental characteristics varied differently over the course of the growth curve (Table 1). Based on our design, inorganic nitrogen (mainly comprised of NO_3^-) and phosphate PO_4^{3-} concentrations at T0 (45.95 ± 5.77 and 2.90 ± 0.85 μM, respectively) were much lower than those in f/20 medium. As the population developed, a sharp increase of NH_4^+ was observed from T1 to T2 while NO_3^- became undetectable (Table 1). PO_4^{3-} also decreased but at a relatively slower rate. Accordingly, particulate phosphorus exhibited an opposite pattern and slightly declined after 30 days of incubation. Dissolved organic carbon (DOC) increased along with the rise and cell maxima of *M. rubrum*. Thereafter, DOC content was generally reduced with fluctuations. Particulate organic carbon (POC) remained constant for the first 5 days and decreased as the population declined (Table 1 and Figure 1). A separate trend of POC, however, was observed for T3 when this compound continued declining in Group B but gradually accumulated in Group A. In addition, toxins accumulated in the culture medium as the *Dinophysis* population increased at the expense of *Mesodinium* in Group A. OA and DTX1 were presented together in the summary and in the following analysis due to the fact that they share the same chemical backbone (Table 1). Total OA + DTX1 and PTX2 contents in the culture medium were shown to increase over the growth curve and reached a concentration of 4109.58 ± 621.79 pg mL^{-1} and 26.74 ± 0.73 ng mL^{-1}, respectively, by the end of the experiment (Table 1).

2.2. Composition and Structure of the Microbial Community throughout the Growth Curve

Bacteria samples were also harvested six times throughout the entire growth curve. The composition and structure of the microbial community was demonstrated at the class and order levels, according to the DNA results (Figure 2), and analyzed statistically using unweighted (structure) and weighted (composition) NMDS (Figure 3) and UniFrac dissimilarity (Figure 4).

During the molecular analysis, a total of 93 OTUs were observed throughout all the samples after being rarefied to an even depth of 25,396 reads (Table 2). A Good's coverage index of over 0.999 and the high validity of clean tags indicated that the sequencing had covered almost all the species in the samples and the results were convincing. Alpha diversity indexes (Simpson, Shannon Wiener, and Chao1) indicated that there were no significant differences (ANOVA, $p > 0.05$) of the bacterial community between the two treatments in each crucial time period (Table 2). Proteobacteria (relative abundance = 74.3%) and Bacteroidetes (relative abundance = 21.1%) were the two dominant bacterial phyla in all samples. The majority of Proteobacteria were Alphaproteobacteria (97.8%) and a small fraction of Gammaproteobacteria (2.1%). Bacteroidetes and Sphingobacteria only attributed to the Sphingobacteriales accounted for 14.2% of the total microbial assemblage (Figure 2a). At the order level, Rhodobacterales and Cellvibrionales, which are representative of Alphaproteobacteria and Gammaproteobacteria, respectively, were dominant (Figure 2b).

Table 1. Summary of environmental variables in the *Dinophysis* + *Mesodinium* culture (A) and in the *Dinophysis*-free control (B) over the predator-prey growth curves. Data are presented as mean ± SD. POP and POC stand for particulate organic phosphate and particulate organic carbon, respectively.

Samples	POP (µM)	DIP (PO_4^{3-}) (µM)	DIN ($NH4^+$) (µM)	DIN (NO_3^-) (µM)	DOC (µM)	POC (µM)	OA + DTX1 (pg mL^{-1})	PTX2 (ng mL^{-1})
T0	1.21 ± 0.05	2.90 ± 0.85	2.86 ± 2.02	45.95 ± 5.77	633.61 ± 74.23	792.80 ± 133.67	-	-
T1	1.26 ± 0.06	2.80 ± 0.37	2.62 ± 0.82	9.76 ± 5.77	977.85 ± 283.32	789.13 ± 124.75	99.33 ± 5.71	0.43 ± 0.03
T2 (A)	1.51 ± 0.12	2.47 ± 0.19	54.29 ± 1.89	2.50 ± 2.53	606.24 ± 211.48	666.22 ± 22.08	559.88 ± 23.09	6.87 ± 1.46
T2 (B)	1.31 ± 0.32	2.26 ± 0.32	30.36 ± 6.89	0.48 ± 0.41	463.64 ± 118.71	659.62 ± 30.02	-	-
T3 (A)	1.68 ± 0.03	2.37 ± 0.37	62.62 ± 11.79	LOD	693.88 ± 124.99	661.13 ± 23.72	1001.08 ± 163.95	13.45 ± 2.11
T3 (B)	1.45 ± 0.14	2.26 ± 0.32	50.24 ± 4.76	0.71 ± 0.71	764.90 ± 56.27	580.10 ± 16.55	-	-
T4 (A)	1.75 ± 0.17	2.15 ± 0.19	50.36 ± 2.51	LOD	614.06 ± 111.31	739.42 ± 53.55	2494.61 ± 526.41	18.71 ± 2.74
T4 (B)	1.65 ± 0.25	2.15 ± 0.19	57.86 ± 2.58	2.86 ± 2.02	636.20 ± 69.36	510.67 ± 56.38	-	-
T5 (A)	1.63 ± 0.19	2.04 ± 0.19	55.48 ± 17.04	LOD	391.74 ± 63.33	866.42 ± 70.63	4109.58 ± 621.79	26.74 ± 0.73
T5 (B)	1.35 ± 1.16	2.04 ± 0.19	72.38 ± 9.10	LOD	479.49 ± 36.14	409.98 ± 137.61	-	-

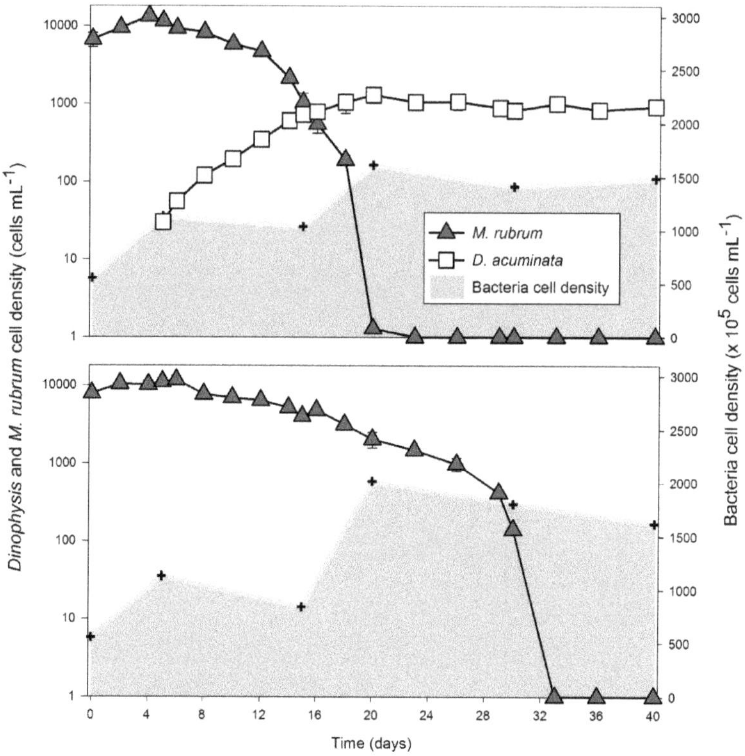

Figure 1. Cell density of *Mesodinium rubrum* and *Dinophysis acuminata* in Group A and Group B (control group without *Dinophysis* cells) over the growth curve. The shaded area indicates the bacterial concentration and the hex symbol shows the time point when subsamples were retrieved for nutrients analysis, bacterial counts, and analysis of the bacterial community.

Table 2. The validity of tags and alpha diversity indexes in *Dinophysis* present (A) and *Dinophysis*-free control (B) at the six growth phases (T0–T5). Triplicate subsamples were harvested for each treatment and phase. One subsample failed to produce the 16S rRNA gene amplification ("T1-2").

Sample ID	Valid Tags	Valid%	Goods Coverage	OTU Counts	Simpson	Shannon Wiener	Chao1
T0-1	35,860	91.37%	0.9995	57	1.31	0.51	64.8
T0-2	37,205	89.24%	0.9995	79	1.75	0.56	83.4
T0-3	36,596	91.55%	0.9994	57	1.69	0.59	81.0
T1-1	25,396	85.29%	0.9996	81	1.93	0.57	85.0
T1-2	-	-	-	-	-	-	-
T1-3	38,153	92.66%	0.9994	49	1.24	0.50	67.2
T2-1 (A)	38,611	92.30%	0.9996	52	1.84	0.61	56.0
T2-2 (A)	34,985	90.78%	0.9998	51	1.99	0.64	52.3
T2-3 (A)	33,591	87.98%	0.9992	55	1.29	0.47	82.1
T2-1 (B)	34,373	89.63%	0.9995	54	1.65	0.56	63.8
T2-2 (B)	36,081	91.48%	0.9995	48	1.60	0.54	59.0
T2-3 (B)	35,202	87.22%	0.9996	40	1.71	0.57	46.0
T3-1 (A)	38,304	92.79%	0.9995	59	1.55	0.53	65.6
T3-2 (A)	35,826	91.63%	0.9996	43	1.25	0.44	49.0
T3-3 (A)	36,145	92.71%	0.9997	47	1.52	0.51	51.7
T3-1 (B)	37,516	91.71%	0.9998	42	1.38	0.49	43.9
T3-2 (B)	35,153	90.96%	0.9995	44	1.16	0.42	63.5

Table 2. *Cont.*

Sample ID	Valid Tags	Valid%	Goods Coverage	OTU Counts	Simpson	Shannon Wiener	Chao1
T3-3 (B)	36,480	91.28%	0.9996	41	1.56	0.51	44.3
T4-1 (A)	35,231	91.41%	0.9998	42	1.56	0.51	43.7
T4-2 (A)	37,869	90.60%	0.9995	47	1.68	0.53	66.5
T4-3 (A)	36,610	92.61%	0.9995	53	1.62	0.52	66.0
T4-1 (B)	38,995	93.12%	0.9997	47	1.37	0.47	50.5
T4-2 (B)	35,561	87.96%	0.9996	45	1.85	0.60	49.5
T4-3 (B)	34,364	90.38%	0.9996	47	1.36	0.43	56.2
T5-1 (A)	33,756	88.31%	0.9996	46	1.86	0.62	55.2
T5-2 (A)	37,201	88.99%	0.9995	51	1.66	0.54	64.0
T5-3 (A)	36,041	89.82%	0.9995	57	1.70	0.56	65.7
T5-1 (B)	36,348	91.57%	0.9993	48	1.42	0.46	86.3
T5-2 (B)	36,231	90.09%	0.9994	48	1.78	0.59	63.2
T5-3 (B)	29,843	86.83%	0.9995	70	1.88	0.56	77.3

NMDS also demonstrated the difference of structure (Figure 3a) and composition (Figure 3b) of the bacterial community in Groups A and B. The unweighted (Figure 3a) and weighted (Figure 3b) UniFrac distances represent the structure and composition of the microbial assemblage, respectively. The patterns of structural differences (Figure 3a) in both treatments were not as clear as the patterns of composition differences (Figure 3b) within the growth phases (T0–T5). In fact, growth phases (*Dinophysis* in Group A and *Mesodinium* in Group B) had a great effect on shaping the bacterial structure (ANOSIM $r = 0.37$, $p = 0.001$) and composition (ANOSIM $r = 0.257$, $p = 0.004$) of the communities regardless of whether *Dinophysis* cells were present or not (ANOSIM, unweighted $r = -0.015$, $p = 0.544$ and weighted $r = -0.06$, $p = 0.933$). The same results were also found in UniFrac dissimilarities analysis, which showed that the composition and structure of the bacterial community significantly changed during *Dinophysis* growth (Figure 4a) and *M. rubrum* decay (Figure 4b) by using the dissimilarity indexes and the generalized, unweighted, and weighted UniFrac distances. As for the difference between the two treatments (Figure 4c), only a minor increase in an unweighted distance analysis was observed and an opposite trend was observed when the abundance of bacterial taxa was considered (generalized and weighted UniFrac distance), which suggests that the presence and proliferation of the *Dinophysis* population or the consequences of its association with *Mesodinium* decay may not influence the composition and structure of the dominant bacterial species.

To better identify the interactions between the microbiome and the biotic or abiotic factors characterized in the growth curve, we manually defined the bacteria into three groups, which include the abundant (Ab) group, the moderately abundant (M) group, and the rare (R) taxa group. These groups stand for a relative abundance above 1%, between 0.1% and 1%, and below 0.1%, respectively. In summary, out of the 93 identified OTUs, 5 OTUs were assigned to the abundant (Ab) group, 83 OTUs met the criterion of rare taxa (R), and 5 OTUs belonged to the moderate (M) group.

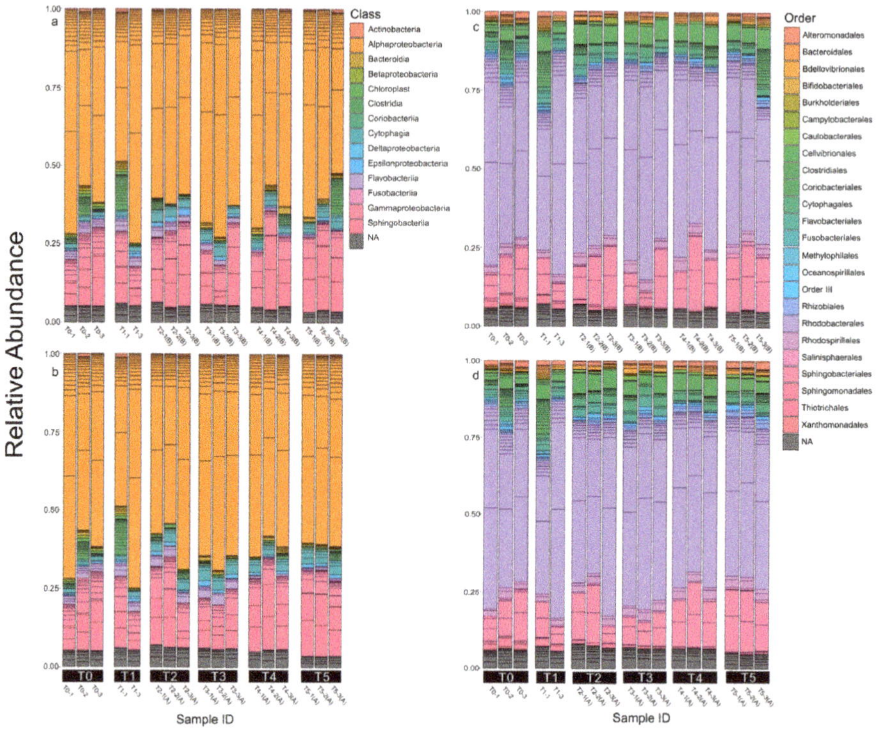

Figure 2. Microbial community compositions across all the samples are shown. Above the sample IDs, the time series of those samples were identified (T0–T5). The color key represents bacterial taxa at class (**a**,**b**) and order level (**c**,**d**).

The response of the microbial communities to the environmental changes was further investigated by the Mantel test (Table 3) and the most related factors were selected by the BIOENV procedure (Table 4). The results showed that all three assemblages were significantly correlated ($p < 0.01$) to the environmental matrix (Table 1) especially the M and R ($r > 0.5$), which suggests that the selected parameters had a better interpretation on a relatively lower abundance of bacterial assemblages. Cell density of *M. rubrum* and *D. acuminata* were also included in the "environmental matrix" (Table 1) for interpretation through the BIOENV procedure (Table 4). Out of the 11 parameters, eight were finally selected by BIOENV for the best correlation models to interpret the Bray–Curtis distance matrices of bacterial communities. They were *M. rubrum* density, *Dinophysis* cell density, DOC, PO_4^{3-}, NH_4^+, POP, OA + DTX1, and PTX2. Similarly, the selected parameters were more powerful in representing the M and R taxa (Table 4).

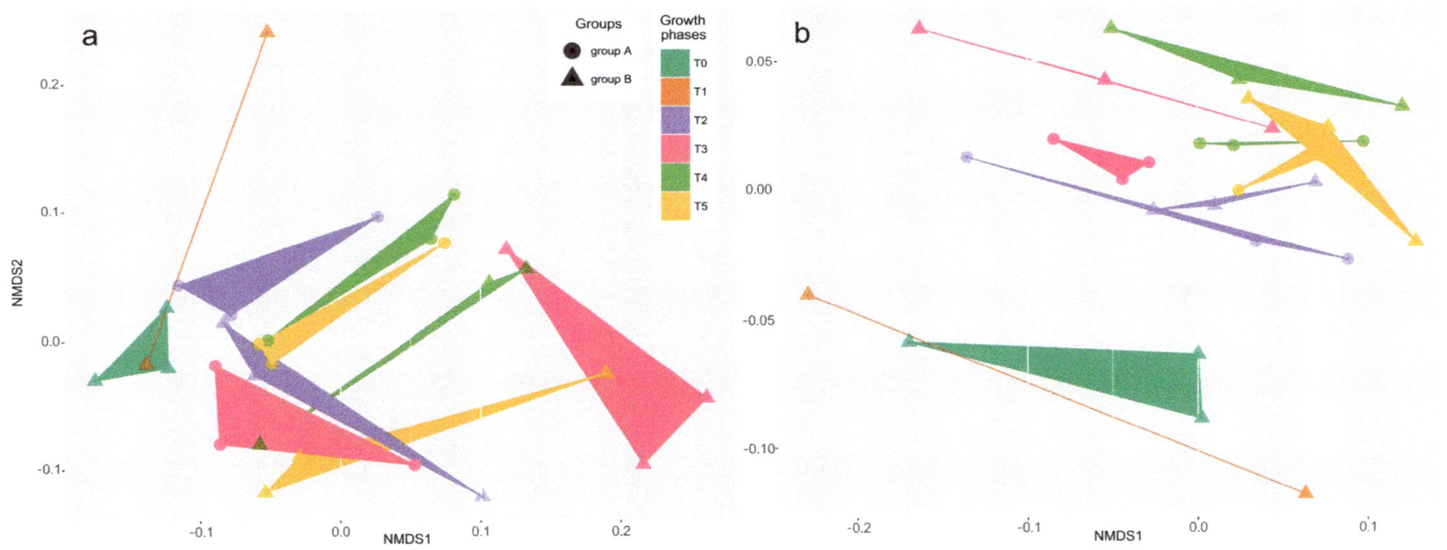

Figure 3. NMDS plot based on unweighted (**a**) and weighted (**b**) UniFrac distances. Sample points are shaded by growth phases and their shape represents groups. Growth phases seem to be more powerful in shaping the composition (ANOSIM, r = 0.257, $p = 0.004$) and structure (ANOSIM, r = 0.37, $p = 0.001$) of the communities compared to the presence/absence of *Dinophysis* cells (ANOSIM, unweighted r = −0.015, $p = 0.544$ and weighted r = −0.06, $p = 0.933$).

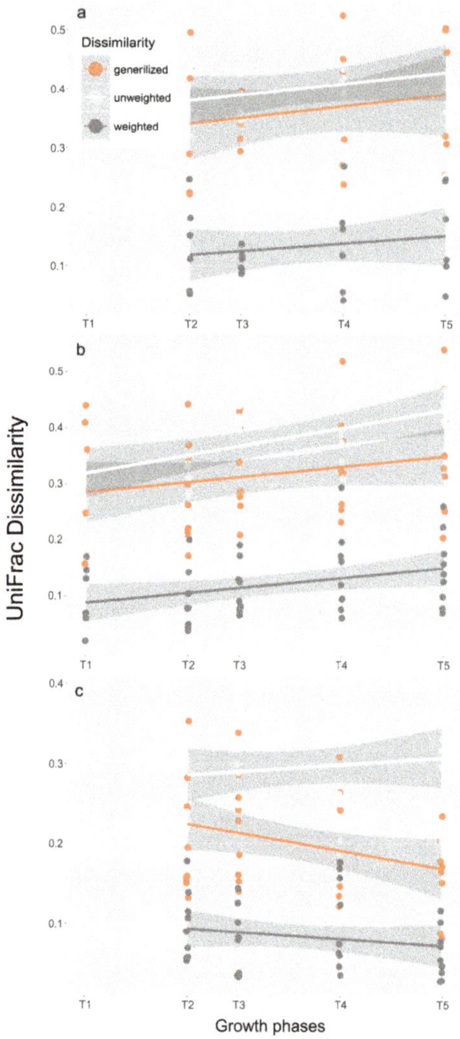

Figure 4. UniFrac dissimilarities between the onset and each of the following growth phases in (**a**) *Dinophysis* group (since *Dinophysis* cells were added at T1, calculations were carried out from T2) and (**b**) *M. rubrum* control group, and (**c**) dissimilarities between the two groups at the same phase were also plotted against growth phases. Three measures (unweighted, weighted, and generalized) were color-coded and liner fitted with a 95% confidence interval.

Table 3. The Mantel test on the relationship between the bacterial community and environmental factors.

Mantel Test	Pearson Correlation		Spearman Correlation	
	Statistic r	*p* Value	Statistic r	*p* Value
Ab taxa	0.361	0.002	0.363	0.001
M taxa	0.593	0.001	0.575	0.001
R taxa	0.520	0.001	0.542	0.001

Table 4. BIOENV procedure on the relationship between the bacterial community and environmental factors.

BIOENV	Pearson Correlation	Parameters in Best Model	Spearman Correlation	Parameters in Best Model
Ab taxa	0.340	DOC, OA + DTX1, PTX2, *M. rubrum*, *Dinophysis*	0.287	PO_4^{3-}, DOC, OA + DTX1, *M. rubrum*, *Dinophysis*
M taxa	0.756	PO_4^{3-}, NH_4^+, OA + DTX1, PTX2, *M. rubrum*, *Dinophysis*	0.729	PO_4^{3-}, NH_4^+, OA + DTX1, PTX2, *M. rubrum*, *Dinophysis*
R taxa	0.661	POP, PO_4^{3-}, NH_4^+, PTX2, *M. rubrum*	0.670	POP, PO_4^{3-}, NH_4^+, PTX2, *M. rubrum*

Furthermore, Bray–Curtis dissimilarities were used to interpret the differences of the three assemblages of microbial communities during the growth phases of *Dinophysis* (Figure 5a) and *Mesodinium* (Figure 6a) and with the surrounding environment in a mixed culture (Figure 5b–i) as well as in a control treatment (Figure 6b–f). In detail, during *Dinophysis* growth (Group A), the dissimilarity between the M and R taxa varied significantly ($p < 0.01$) since the culture aged while the abundant taxa showed no differences (Figure 5a). As for the environmental factors, the M and R taxa also showed a more active response than the Ab taxa. These two assemblages positively correlated ($p < 0.05$) with changes of *M. rubrum* density (Figure 5b) and particulate organic phosphorus (Figure 5e) but showed no difference with ammonium (Figure 5c), dissolved the inorganic phosphate (PO_4^{3-}, Figure 5d), dissolved organic carbon (DOC, Figure 5f), or *Dinophysis* changes (Figure 5i). Interestingly, accumulation of both OA + DTX1 and PTX2 led to a significant partition of those bacterial taxa in moderate and low abundance (Figure 5g,h), which indicates the potential effects of the exposure to a high-toxin-concentration environment when the culture aged. The Ab taxa did not change with any of the environmental parameters. The response of the bacterial community in the *Mesodinium* control (Group B) was highly active. The correlations between Bray–Curtis dissimilarities of the bacterial community and days of cultivation were significant ($p < 0.05$) in all fractions (Figure 6a), *M. rubrum* cell density (Figure 6b), and variances of ammonium concentration (Figure 6c), which suggests that the bacterial community in the *M. rubrum* population, free of *Dinophysis*, would possibly be associated with the decline of the dominant species (*M. rubrum*) and biogeochemical characteristics mediated by the nutrient ammonium. Similar to the *Dinophysis-Mesodinium* co-culture treatment (Group A), PO_4^{3-} (Figure 6e) showed a positive correlation with bacteria of the M and R taxa, which suggests the similar function of phosphate in the *Dinophysis* and *Mesodinium* predator-prey interaction. DOC may be critical in the variance of the bacterial community over time, but the interaction was limited to the R taxa (Figure 6f). The dominant prokaryotes in our artificial culture system were not sensitive to the changes of organic carbon levels.

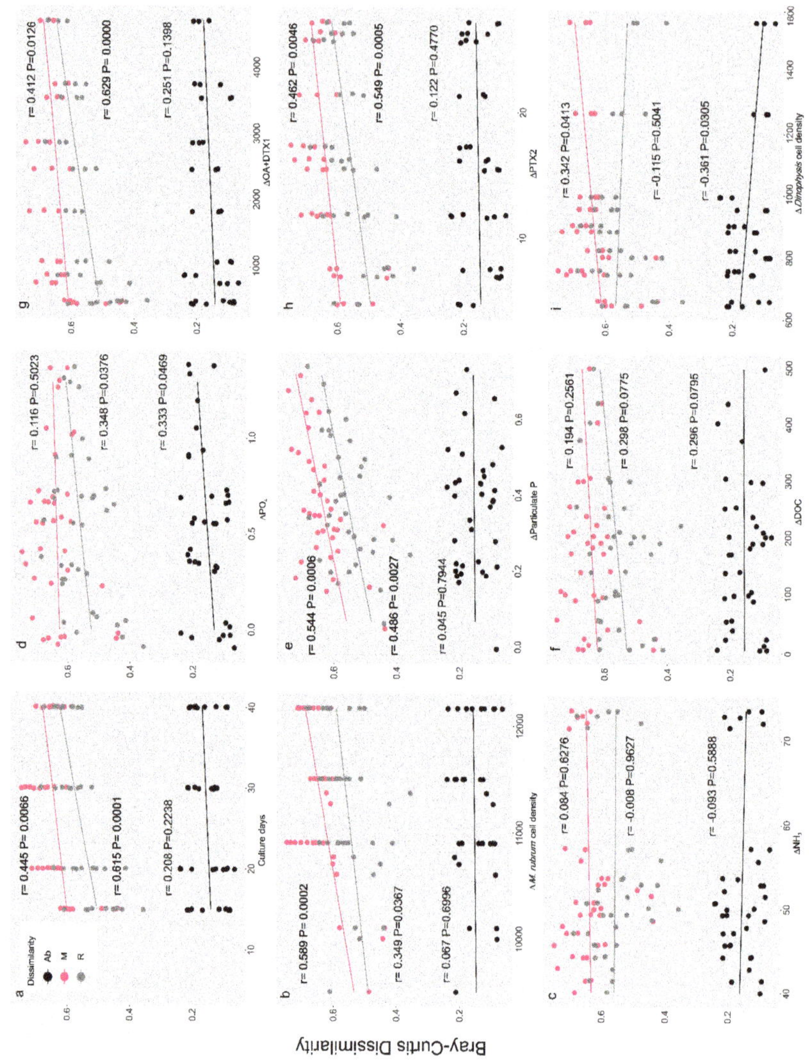

Figure 5. Bray–Curtis dissimilarities of the bacterial community between the onset (T1) and each of the following growth phases (T2–T5) against culture days (**a**) and variance of BIOENV-selected environmental factors (**b**–**i**) in the *Dinophysis* treatment.

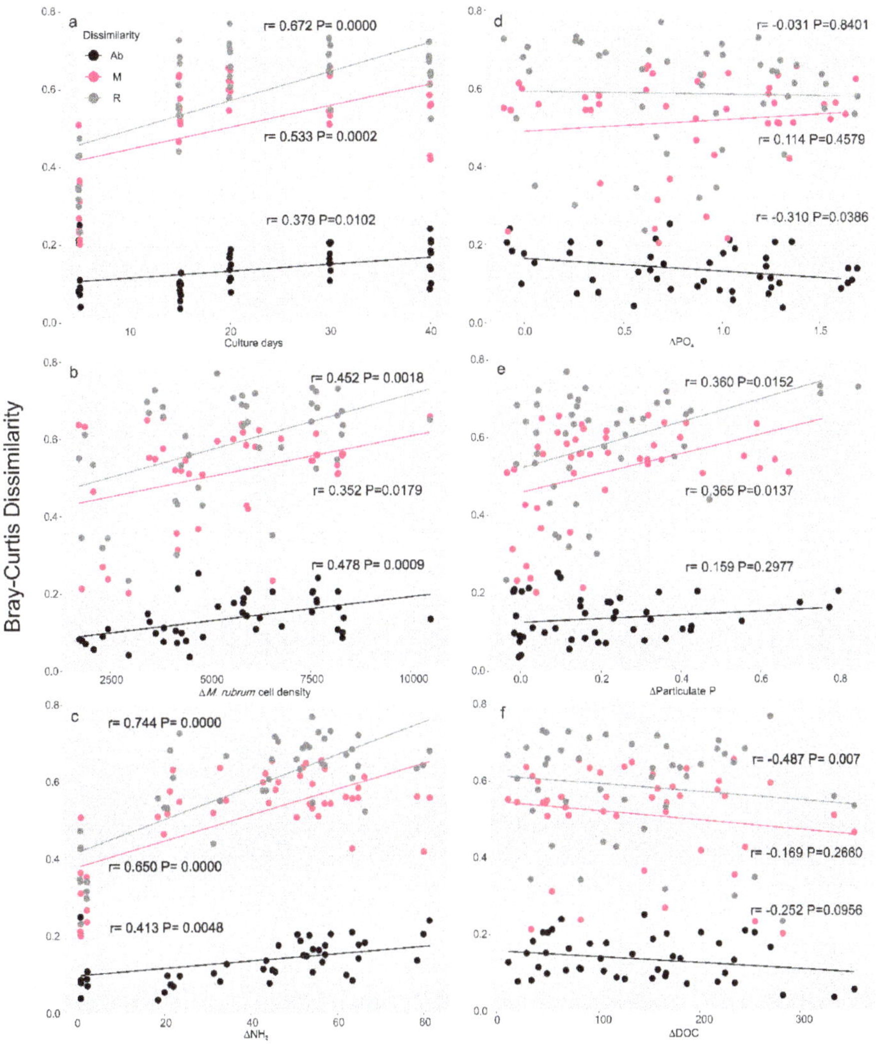

Figure 6. Bray–Curtis dissimilarities of the bacterial community between the onset (T0) and each of the following growth phases (T1–T5) against culture days (**a**) and variance of BIOENV-selected environmental factors (**b**–**f**) in the *M. rubrum* control.

Lastly, dissimilarities of the bacterial communities under the two treatments with the growth phases (Figure 7a) and all the selected factors (Figure 7b–f) were compared. Results of dissimilarities over time (Figure 7a) were consistent with the UniFrac distance plot (Figure 4c) where generalized distances generally implied OTUs of moderate abundance. Considering the resemblance of environmental factors between the two groups (Table 1), the significant decrease in distance of the 0.1–1% fraction (Figure 7a, r = −0.567, p = 0.0003) may be mostly attributed to the approaching environmental variables. Therefore, the previously detected deleterious effect of *Dinophysis* activity (Figure 5g,h) may be limited to the R taxa fraction in the culture medium. The differences of the selected factors did not appear to be responsible for the differences in the bacterial community (Figure 7c–f) except for the *M. rubrum* cell density effect with which the M taxa significantly varied (Figure 7b). The impact of *M. rubrum* cells on the M taxa was partly responsible for the decrease in dissimilarity over culture days (Figure 7a) and the largest differences of ciliate density were actually observed in the early phases of the *Mesodinium* growth curve (Figure 1). In summary, dissimilarities of the R taxa between the two groups (Figure 7) were generally higher than those of M and Ab taxas compared to the results within each group (Figures 5 and 6), which leads to our assumption that the influence of *Dinophysis* and the toxins it produces may affect those R bacterial taxa.

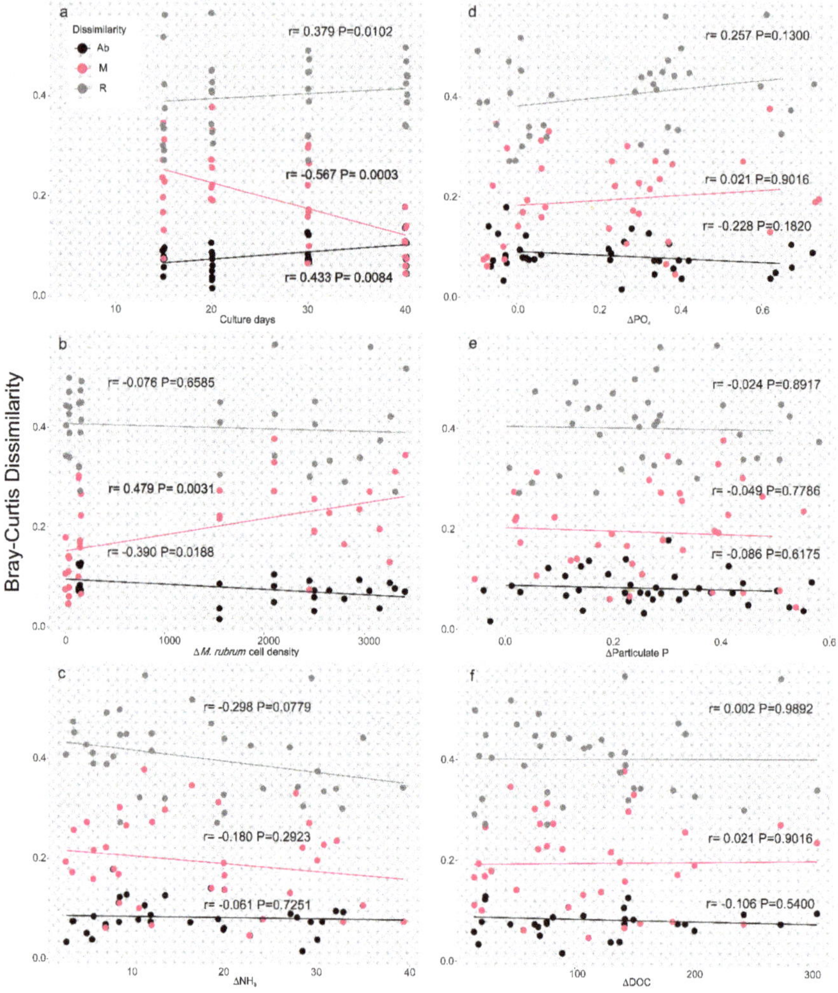

Figure 7. Bray–Curtis dissimilarities of the bacterial community between the two Groups at each growth phases (T2–T5) against the time of cultures (**a**) and variance of BIOENV-selected environmental factors (**b**–**f**).

3. Discussion

The algal–bacterial interaction has been shown to have a critical effect on bloom dynamics, but much of the research on this subject has been limited to photosynthetic algal species [34–36]. Due to their mixotrophic nature, *Dinophysis* species need to ingest *Mesodinium*, which is the sole determined prey [37,38], for population growth. Field populations of the ciliate usually aggregate in the subsurface water layers and perform diurnal vertical migration [39]. At the same time, *Dinophysis* species normally represent a small proportion of the phytoplankton community with a minor importance in relation to major biogeochemical cycles [25,40,41]. Thus, *Dinophysis* blooms and the time period from *Dinophysis* initiation to the *M. rubrum* decline is difficult to capture [10]. In the current study, we simulated an ideal predator-prey microcosms study to estimate the biogeochemical consequences of their co-occurrence and identify the ecological niche of bacterial communities developed during *Dinophysis* growth and *Mesodinium* decline.

We found that the *M. rubrum-Dinophysis* system intensively altered the biogeochemical status of the culture medium (Table 1). *Dinophysis* feeding activities accelerated the decline of the *M. rubrum* population (Figure 1). The differences in microbial communities between Groups A and B were mainly ascribed to the presence of *Dinophysis* cells (up to 1300 cells per mL^{-1}) and the accumulation of toxins or other compounds produced by *Dinophysis*. In addition, considering that the influence of *Dinophysis* was restricted to the taxa in relatively low abundance, the dissimilarity may mainly consist of intracellular or phycosphere bacteria given that *Dinophysis* cells could function as particulate vectors or as hosts of certain bacterial species [42]. This assumption was also shown by the increased particulate organic carbon in this study (Table 1) as well as previous experiments [14]. Furthermore, in a study on bacterial assemblages associated with *Dinophysis*, it was also found that the addition of *Dinophysis* culture filtrate caused no significant changes in their relative abundance while the prokaryotic genera directly associated with *Dinophysis* were found in the >20-μm size fraction [31]. Species-specific grazing or deleterious effects of *Dinophysis* cells may also gradually shape the structure of the bacterial community. In a recent study [23], the potential contribution of bacterivory and bacterial remineralization to the growth of *Dinophysis* was calculated. It was concluded that neither of these processes were quantitatively relevant in order to support the increased biomass observed in the study.

Changes in nutrients and carbon content were observed in the *M. rubrum–D. acuminata* culture (Group A) (Figure 1 and Table 1), but the pattern was quite similar to of *M. rubrum* population dynamic itself (Group B, the control group), which indicates that ingestion by *Dinophysis* was unable to integrate most of the nutrients and carbon compounds derived from the *M. rubrum* population. Enhancement of secondary metabolite (DSP toxins) production was verified in *Dinophysis* cells [21] and in heterotrophic microbes [32] when exposed to *M. rubrum* living cells as well as cell lysate, but no direct evidence has emerged to decipher the associations among *Dinophysis*, microbes, and detritus in terms of nutrient cycling [37,43]. Tong et al. [14] estimated that *D. acuminata* was able to assimilate 65% and 25% of the particulate nitrogen and phosphate through predation, respectively. In the current study, the ingestion rate (ca. 3.25 prey cells $predator^{-1}$ day^{-1}) approached the highest level of the calculated growth rate where the predator: prey ratio was considered saturated [44]. The ingestion rate may not able to reach a higher value due to the low growth rate of the prey. However, the amount of ingested carbon calculated from a recently published paper [15] was about 2466.7 pg C $cell^{-1}$ d^{-1}, which is already beyond *Dinophysis* needs to maintain growth [8]. Field studies also found that the *Dinophysis* population preferred savaging on their prey in a short period of time [10,45].

After the *M. rubrum* population collapsed, the nutritional status of the culture medium was remarkably affected, which is expressed by the elevated levels of prey ammonium and fluctuant DOC and forms a hotspot of biogeochemical activities for the *Dinophysis* [40,46] and also the heterotrophic bacteria therein [47–50]. In this case, ammonium became the key component in the nitrogen cycle *Mesodinium* decline. NH_4^+ concentration remained constant until the addition of *Dinophysis* (T1, Table 1). A sharp increase was noticed due to a possible consequence of bacterial ammonification when *M. rubrum* decayed (Figure 1). Then NH_4^+ was significantly low at the late plateau phase of *Dinophysis* (T4 and T5, Table 1, Mann–Whitney Rank Sum Test, $p = 0.041$) when compared to the *Mesodinium* control. This finding is consistent with previous results showing that ammonium may lead to an increase of field populations of *Dinophysis* [51] and could be assimilated, which enhances the growth of *Dinophysis* at certain levels [23]. As for the other forms of nitrogen, nitrate with a moderate level (~50 μM) was dominant in our initial culture system but was used up in the first five days (Table 1, phase T1). When a high concentration of nitrate, e.g., up to 200 μM, is available in the culture medium, the availability of ammonium at lower concentrations (<2 μM) may be undetected or compensated [14]. The decay of the *M. rubrum* population seems unrelated to the nutrient limitation given the availability of both nitrogen (ammonium and nitrate) and phosphate in the culture medium [32,37].

Characterized as a plastidic-specific non-constitutive mixotroph [52], *Dinophysis* cells mainly retain chloroplasts from their prey and perform photosynthesis by those kleptoplastids as a carbon source. At the same time, marine heterotrophic bacteria play a major role in incorporating, respiring, and degrading dissolved organic carbon. However, changes of DOC concentration in this study hardly demonstrated the dissimilarities of the microbial community (Figures 5–7), which suggests that the heterotrophic bacteria assemblages in our culture system may exhibit a metabolic versatility at least within the range of our DOC measurement. Moreover, bacterial communities at large phylogenetic group levels may exhibit general outcomes when exposed to high DOC concentrations [24]. Therefore, variation of DOC during phytoplankton dynamics may not taxonomically drive the shift of the major microbial community. Bacterial assemblages of M taxa (>0.1% and <1% of relative abundance) seem to be the most sensitive portion to changing the environmental nutrient conditions (Figures 5–7). High-throughput sequencing revealed that this portion is composed of bacterial taxa assigned to the Rhodospirillaceae, Cytophagaceae, Flavobacteriaceae, and CHAB-XI-27 at family-level resolution. According to the 16s rDNA sequencing, Proteobacteria (Alphaproteobacteria-Rhodobacterales and Gammaproteobacteria-Cellvibrionales dominated) and Bacteroidetes (Sphingobacteria-Sphingobacteriales dominated) constituted more than 90% of the relative abundance of the microbial community in the culture medium cumulatively. These results are not surprising since only a limited number of heterotrophic bacterial lineages dominate those eukaryotic phytoplankton-associated communities [48]. Furthermore, these bacteria lineages cover those groups responsible for both monomer (such as amino acids) and polymer (such as chitin and protein) degradation in the ocean [53]. Less than 100 bacterial OTUs were assigned in our culture system, which is far less than previous field studies [45,54]. Bacterial community results from laboratory cultures show a lower diversity of bacterial assemblages because long-term maintenance may have eliminated those species that had already been overwhelmed and laboratory studies could avoid invasion of accidental species that are common in field studies. This is also the reason for which some studies exclude those rare species in their analysis [54]. The only study addressing the interaction between a *Dinophysis* bloom and the microbial community revealed that, even during the peak of a *Dinophysis acuminata* bloom (cell density ~1300 cell mL^{-1}), the *Dinophysis* cells only accounted for 29% of the phytoplankton community [31]. Thus, the comparison of the bacterial community between our two groups could merely be attributed to the influence of the *D. acuminata* population. Our finding that only a low abundance of bacterial species was altered during *Dinophysis* intensive feeding activities indicated that, even though intense mixotrophy could remarkably drive biogeochemical dynamics, changes of the phytoplankton population may not be reflected by changes in those abundant bacterial phylotypes or in metabolic generalists. Moreover, connections may exist between specific species of bacteria and *Dinophysis* cells. Locating these connections by using metabolite and meta-transcriptome analysis may give us a further understanding for how these organisms interact with each other. Establishing an axenic culture of *Dinophysis* and comparing physiologies with non-axenic cultures over long-term periods may offer more robust evidence of the dependence of *Dinophysis* on bacteria [25]. However, attempts to purify *Dinophysis* and *M. ruburm* cells by using antibiotic treatment were not successful either in our laboratory or after efforts devoted by other groups [31]. Novel approaches to generate axenic algae cultures have been tested on the cyst-forming species *Gymnodinium catenatum* starting from resting cysts [55] and freshwater species by using fluorescence-activated cell sorting [56]. Yet, the methods proposed may not be universal and transferable considering that *Dinophysis* and *M. rubrum* cells are oddly shaped and fragile. More efforts are needed in the future to come up with appropriate approaches to initiate axenic *Dinophysis* cultures or elegant methods to directly target specific interactions between *Dinophysis* and associated bacteria.

4. Materials and Methods

4.1. Cultures

A unicellular algal culture of *D. acuminata* (DAYS01) was established from cells previously isolated from Xiaoping Island (121.53° E 38.83° N), the Yellow Sea, China in July 2014 [13]. The ciliate *M. rubrum* (AND-A0711) and the cryptophyte, *Teleaulax amphioxeia* (AND-A0710) were isolated from coastal waters off Huelva, Southern Spain in 2007 [57]. All cultures were routinely inoculated based on the cryptophyte–*M. rubrum*–*Dinophysis* food chain [7,13] in f/6-Si medium, which was prepared with 1/3 nitrate, 1/3 phosphate, 1/3 metals, and 1/3 of the vitamins concentrations in the f/2-Si medium. Cultures were maintained at 15 °C under a light intensity of 3000 lux and a 14 h light:10 h dark photo cycle.

4.2. Batch Culture Setup

A mono-algal culture of *M. rubrum* was maintained for a few days and gradually eaten by *Dinophysis* cultures. High ambient nutrient concentrations may obscure the detection of nutritional flows within the microbial loop. Therefore, *M. rubrum* were first inoculated from f/6 medium to f/10 and then to f/20. Then six *M. rubrum* replicates with an initial concentration of 6000 cells mL^{-1} were prepared in 5-L glass flasks to start this batch culture experiment. *Dinophysis* cells were pre-starved over 14 days, filtered onto 15-µm Nitex sieves, and gently rinsed with fresh artificial seawater to minimize carryover free living bacteria. The cells were then re-suspended in 90 mL of artificial seawater. After 5 days of inoculation of the *M. rubrum* cultures, 30 mL of the previously rinsed *Dinophysis* were added into three out of the six flasks (Group A). The other three *M. rubrum* cultures with the addition of 30 mL of artificial seawater were designated as Group B or control. The whole experiment was conducted at 15 °C under a light intensity of 3000 lux on a 14 h light:10 h dark photo cycle.

Dinophysis and/or the ciliate subsamples were taken every 2 or 3 days and fixed with 3% (*v/v*) formalin solution for microscopic enumeration in a Sedgewick-Rafter counting chamber at 100× magnification. For bacterial analysis, the formalin-preserved samples (1 mL) were stained with 2 µL of 4′,6-diami-dino-2-phenylindole (DAPI) solution (1 mg mL^{-1}) and filtered onto a black polycarbonate filter (pore size: 0.22 µm, diameter: 25 mm, Millipore, Burlington, MA, USA). Then the filters were gently removed onto a glass slide and observed at 600× by using fluorescence microscopy (DMi8, Leica Microsystems, Buffalo Grove, IL, USA) under UV excitation.

4.3. Nutrient Sample Collection and Preparation

The growth curve was manually divided into six different growth phases. Six sampling spots were set up to collect nutrient and toxin samples, which are, hereafter, referred to as T0—at the very beginning of the incubation, T1—early phase following inoculation of *Dinophysis*, T2—the middle of the exponential growth of *Dinophysis*, T3—the end of the exponential growth of *Dinophysis*, T4—the depletion of *M. rubrum*, and T5—the end of *Dinophysis* growth.

For nutrients, 30-mL culture medium were filtered through pre-combusted GF/F filters (25 mm, Whatman, Maidstone, UK) for particulate organic carbon (POC) and particulate organic phosphate (POP) collection, respectively. The filters for POC were dried in a 60 °C oven for 24 h, stored at −20 °C, and analyzed on an elemental Analyzer (EA3000, EuroVector S.p.A, Milan, Italy). The particulate phosphate was converted to orthophosphate (PO_4^{3-}) by first hydrolyzing it by the addition of 5 mL of 5% potassium persulfate and 10 mL of Milli-Q water and then autoclaving it (121 °C) for 20 min. The filtrate was used for quantifying the dissolved inorganic nutrients (DIN and DIP) and dissolved organic carbon (DOC). Nitrate, ammonium, and phosphate were analyzed by SKALAR SAN^{++} Autoanalyser (SKALAR, Breda, The Netherlands). DOC concentration was determined by using a TOC Analyzer (Multi C/N 3100, Analytik Jena, Jena, Germany). All analyses were conducted following the protocols of the manufacturers.

4.4. *Toxin Analysis*

Dinophysis cells and culture medium were separated for toxin analysis. Between 10 and 30 mL of culture medium was harvested and analyzed for toxins since the inoculation day (T1) of *Dinophysis* cells. The medium was kept in 50-mL centrifuge tubes and stored at −20 °C before extraction. Solid-phase extraction (SPE) was employed [13,58] for the extraction of cells or medium samples. The SPE column (Oasis HLB 60 mg, Waters, Milford, MA, USA) was preconditioned with 6 mL of methanol and 6 mL of Milli-Q water. Once the cells or medium samples were loaded, the cartridge was washed with 3 mL of Milli-Q water and then blow-dried and eluted with 1 mL of methanol to collect the toxins into an HPLC vial. Eluates from the samples were then heated at 40 °C in a heating block (HP-S016SY), dried under a stream of N_2, and re-suspended in 1 mL of 100% methanol for toxin analysis.

Toxin analysis was performed on an UltiMate 3000 LC (Thermo Scientific^{TM} Dionex^{TM}, Waltham, MA, USA) and an AB 4000 mass spectrometer system (SCIEX, Framingham, MA, USA) with electrospray ionization. PTX2 was analyzed in positive mode, while OA and DTX1 were analyzed in negative mode. Chromatographic separation was performed by using a Waters XBridgeTM C18 column (3.0 × 150 mm, 3.5-μm particle size) (Milford, MA, USA) at 40 °C for a negative mode. The mobile phase consisted of phase A, 0.05 *v/v* % ammonia hydroxide in water, and phase B, 0.05 *v/v* % ammonia hydroxide in 90% acetonitrile with a flow rate of 0.4 mL min^{-1} and 10 μL injection. A linear gradient elution from 10% to 90% B was run for 9 min, held for 3 min at 90% B, decreased to 10% B for 2 min, and held at 10% B for 4 min to equilibrate at the initial conditions before the next run. In a positive mode, a Waters XBridgeTM C18 column (2.1 × 50 mm, 2.5-μm particle size) at 25 °C was used for chromatographic separation. A linear gradient from 10% to 80% acetonitrile containing a constant concentration of buffer (2 mM ammonium formate and 50 mM formic acid) was run between 0 min and 9 min and held at 80% acetonitrile for 2 min at a flow rate of 0.3 mL min^{-1}. Standards for OA, DTX1, and PTX2 were purchased from the National Research Council, Canada.

4.5. *DNA Extraction and Illumine Sequencing*

At each time spot, a 120 to 150 mL culture medium was retrieved and filtered by using a 0.22-μm cellulose filter. Then the filters were folded and stored at −80 °C. Total genome DNA was extracted by using GenJET Genomic DNA Purification Kits (Thermo Scientific, Waltham, WA, USA) following the protocols of the manufacturer. Bacterial amplicons were produced by targeting the 16S V3-V4 hypervariable region with universal primers 343F (5′-TACGGRAGGCAGCAG-3′) and 798R (5′-AGGGTATCTAATCCT-3′). The amplicon quality was visualized by using gel electrophoresis, which was purified with AMPure XP beads (Agencourt) and amplified for another round of PCR. After being purified with the AMPure XP beads again, the final amplicon was quantified by using Qubit dsDNA assay kits. Equal amounts of purified amplicons were pooled for subsequent sequencing. The amplicon libraries were then sequenced on an Illumina MiSeq platform (Shanghai OE Biotechnology Co., Ltd., Shanghai, China).

4.6. *Bioinformatics Analysis*

Paired-end reads were preprocessed by using Trimmomatic software [59] to detect and cut off the ambiguous bases (N), barcodes, primers, and low-quality sequences. After trimming, paired-end reads were assembled by using FLASH [60]. Valid tags were subjected to clustering to generate operational taxonomic units (OTUs) using VSEARCH software (Version 2.4.2) at a 97% similarity setting [61]. The representative sequence of each OTU was selected by using the QIIME package. Representative reads were annotated and blasted against the Silva database (Version 123) using the ribosome database project (RDP) classifier with a confidence threshold of 70%. Sequences were submitted to the NCBI Sequence Read Archive with the accession number SRR6048156.

Package *phyloseq* [62] in R (http://www.Rproject.org, v. 3.3.3) was used to perform alpha and beta diversity calculations and to visualize the results of dimensional reduction approaches (nonmetric multidimensional scaling, NMDS). UniFrac distance matrices (weighted, unweighted, and generalized) were calculated with the R package *GUniFrac* [63] based on the OTU table and the phylogenetic tree. Note that the OTU table was square-root transformed and the explanatory matrix was z-score-transformed in R before the statistic procedures. To characterize the potential functions of different bacteria groups, we defined "abundant" (Ab) and "rare" (R) OTUs with the criteria of the average relative abundance across all the samples above 1% and below 0.1%, respectively [64]. The rest of the bacterial lineages (>0.1% and <1%) were assigned to a "moderately abundant" (M) group. The BIOENV procedure was implemented to identify the subset of a set of explanatory variables (nutrients profile, toxin content, and mixotrophs density). The Euclidean distance matrix of this correlates maximally with the Bray–Curtis compositional dissimilarity matrix of the OTU table. The Mantel test was also run with 999 permutations to check whether the subset of explanatory variables was able to capture the variation of bacterial communities from the three fractions. The BIOENV procedure and Mantel test on the three matrices (abundant, moderately-abundant, and rare fraction) were achieved by using relevant functions in the R package *vegan* [65]. Bray–Curtis dissimilarities of abundant (Ab), moderately abundant (M), and rare taxa (R) among samples were plotted against differences of explanatory variables (subtraction between samples) selected via BIOENV.

Author Contributions: H.G. and C.H. conducted the experiment setup, cell counting, nutrients analysis, toxin extraction. H.G. carried out the data management and analysis. M.T. revised the manuscript, supervised the experiment, and administrated the project and funding.

Funding: National Key R&D Program of China NO. 2016YFC1402104, Key Laboratory of Integrated Marine Monitoring and Applied Technologies for Harmful Algal Blooms, SOA, MATHAB201803, the Laboratory of Marine Ecosystem and Biogeochemistry, SOA, LMEB201507, the Key Laboratory of Marine Ecology and Environmental Science and Engineering, SOA MESE-2015-05, NSF Grant of China No. 41306095, 41501514, Fundamental Research Funds for the Central Universities, N172304046, and State Key Laboratory of Satellite Ocean Environment Dynamics Foundation (Grant No. SOED1701).

Conflicts of Interest: The author declares no conflict of interest.

References

1. Hallegraeff, G.M. A review of harmful algal blooms and their apparent global increase. *Phycologia* **1993**, *32*, 79–99. [CrossRef]
2. Reguera, B.; Riobo, P.; Rodriguez, F.; Diaz, P.A.; Pizarro, G.; Paz, B.; Franco, J.M.; Blanco, J. *Dinophysis* toxins: Causative organisms, distribution and fate in shellfish. *Mar. Drugs* **2014**, *12*, 394–461. [CrossRef] [PubMed]
3. Fujiki, H.; Suganuma, M. Tumor promotion by inhibitors of protein phosphatase 1 and 2A: The okadaic acid class of compounds. *Adv Cancer Res.* **1993**, *61*, 143–194. [PubMed]
4. Marasigan, A.N.; Sato, S.; Fukuyo, Y.; Kodama, M. Accumulation of a high level of diarrhetic shellfish toxins in the green mussel Perna viridis during a bloom of *Dinophysis caudata* and *Dinophysis miles* in Sapian bay, Panay island, the Philippines. *Fish. Sci.* **2001**, *67*, 994–996. [CrossRef]
5. Bodero, M.; Hoogenboom, R.; Bovee, T.F.H.; Portier, L.; de Haan, L.; Peijnenburg, A.; Hendriksen, P.J.M. Whole genome mRNA transcriptomics analysis reveals different modes of action of the diarrheic shellfish poisons okadaic acid and dinophysistoxin-1 versus azaspiracid-1 in Caco-2 cells. *Toxicol. In Vitro* **2017**, *46*, 102–112. [CrossRef] [PubMed]
6. Miles, C.O.; Wilkins, A.L.; Munday, R.; Dines, M.H.; Hawkes, A.D.; Briggs, L.R.; Sandvik, M.; Jensen, D.J.; Cooney, J.M.; Holland, P.T.; et al. Isolation of pectenotoxin-2 from *Dinophysis acuta* and its conversion to pectenotoxin-2 seco acid, and preliminary assessment of their acute toxicities. *Toxicon* **2004**, *43*, 1–9. [CrossRef] [PubMed]
7. Park, M.G.; Kim, S. First successful culture of the marine dinoflagellate *Dinophysis acuminata*. *Aquat. Microb. Ecol.* **2006**, *45*, 101–106. [CrossRef]
8. Riisgaard, K.; Hansen, P.J. Role of food uptake for photosynthesis, growth and survival of the mixotrophic dinoflagellate *Dinophysis acuminata*. *Mar. Ecol. Prog. Ser.* **2009**, *381*, 51–62. [CrossRef]
9. Stoecker, D.K.; Hansen, P.J.; Caron, D.A.; Mitra, A. Mixotrophy in the Marine Plankton. *Ann. Rev. Mar. Sci.* **2017**, *9*, 311–335. [CrossRef] [PubMed]

10. Campbell, L.; Olson, R.J.; Sosik, H.M.; Abraham, A.; Henrichs, D.W.; Hyatt, C.J.; Buskey, E.J. First Harmful *Dinophysis* (Dinophyceae, Dinophysiales) bloom in the U.S. Is Revealed by Automated Imaging Flow Cytometry1. *J. Phycol.* **2010**, *46*, 66–75. [CrossRef]
11. Hattenrath-Lehmann, T.K.; Marcoval, M.A.; Berry, D.L.; Fire, S.; Wang, Z.; Morton, S.L.; Gobler, C.J. The emergence of *Dinophysis acuminata* blooms and DSP toxins in shellfish in New York waters. *Harmful Algae* **2013**, *26*, 33–44. [CrossRef]
12. Moita, M.T.; Pazos, Y.; Rocha, C.; Nolasco, R.; Oliveira, P.B. Toward predicting *Dinophysis* blooms off NW Iberia: A decade of events. *Harmful Algae* **2016**, *53*, 17–32. [CrossRef] [PubMed]
13. Gao, H.; An, X.; Liu, L.; Zhang, K.; Zheng, D.; Tong, M. Characterization of *Dinophysis acuminata* from the Yellow Sea, China, and its response to different temperatures and *Mesodinium* prey. *Oceanol. Hydrobiol. Stud.* **2017**, *46*, 439–450. [CrossRef]
14. Tong, M.; Smith, J.L.; Kulis, D.M.; Anderson, D.M. Role of dissolved nitrate and phosphate in isolates of *Mesodinium rubrum* and toxin-producing *Dinophysis acuminata*. *Aquat. Microb. Ecol.* **2015**, *75*, 169–185. [CrossRef] [PubMed]
15. Smith, J.L.; Tong, M.; Kulis, D.; Anderson, D.M. Effect of ciliate strain, size, and nutritional content on the growth and toxicity of mixotrophic *Dinophysis acuminata*. *Harmful Algae* **2018**, *78*, 95–105. [CrossRef] [PubMed]
16. Tong, M.; Kulis, D.M.; Fux, E.; Smith, J.L.; Hess, P.; Zhou, Q.; Anderson, D.M. The effects of growth phase and light intensity on toxin production by *Dinophysis acuminata* from the northeastern United States. *Harmful Algae* **2011**, *10*, 254–264. [CrossRef]
17. Lundgren, V.M.; Glibert, P.M.; Granéli, E.; Vidyarathna, N.K.; Fiori, E.; Ou, L.; Flynn, K.J.; Mitra, A.; Stoecker, D.K.; Hansen, P.J. Metabolic and physiological changes in *Prymnesium parvum* when grown under, and grazing on prey of, variable nitrogen: Phosphorus stoichiometry. *Harmful Algae* **2016**, *55*, 1–12. [CrossRef] [PubMed]
18. Nagai, S.; Nitshitani, G.; Tomaru, Y.; Sakiyama, S.; Kamiyama, T. Predation by the toxic dinoflagellate *Dinophysis fortii* on the ciliate *Myrionecta rubra* and observation of sequestration of ciliate chloroplasts. *J. Phycol.* **2008**, *44*, 909–922. [CrossRef] [PubMed]
19. Ojamäe, K.; Hansen, P.J.; Lips, I. Mass entrapment and lysis of *Mesodinium rubrum* cells in mucus threads observed in cultures with *Dinophysis*. *Harmful Algae* **2016**, *55*, 77–84. [CrossRef] [PubMed]
20. Giménez Papiol, G.; Beuzenberg, V.; Selwood, A.I.; MacKenzie, L.; Packer, M.A. The use of a mucus trap by *Dinophysis acuta* for the capture of *Mesodinium rubrum* prey under culture conditions. *Harmful Algae* **2016**, *58*, 1–7. [CrossRef] [PubMed]
21. Nagai, S.; Suzuki, T.; Nishikawa, T.; Kamiyama, T. Differences in the Production and Excretion Kinetics of Okadaic Acid, Dinophysistoxin-1, and Pectenotoxin-2 between Cultures of *Dinophysis acuminata* and *Dinophysis fortii* Isolated from Western Japan1. *J. Phycol.* **2011**, *47*, 1326–1337. [CrossRef] [PubMed]
22. Mafra, L.L., Jr.; Nagai, S.; Uchida, H.; Tavares, C.P.S.; Escobar, B.P.; Suzuki, T. Harmful effects of *Dinophysis* to the ciliate *Mesodinium rubrum*: Implications for prey capture. *Harmful Algae* **2016**, *59*, 82–90. [CrossRef] [PubMed]
23. Hattenrath-Lehmann, T.; Gobler, C.J. The contribution of inorganic and organic nutrients to the growth of a North American isolate of the mixotrophic Dinoflagellate, *Dinophysis acuminata*. *Limnol. Oceanogr.* **2015**, *60*, 1588–1630. [CrossRef]
24. Sarmento, H.; Morana, C.; Gasol, J.M. Bacterioplankton niche partitioning in the use of phytoplankton-derived dissolved organic carbon: Quantity is more important than quality. *ISME J.* **2016**, *10*, 2582. [CrossRef] [PubMed]
25. Amin, S.A.; Hmelo, L.R.; van Tol, H.M.; Durham, B.P.; Carlson, L.T.; Heal, K.R.; Morales, R.L.; Berthiaume, C.T.; Parker, M.S.; Djunaedi, B.; et al. Interaction and signaling between a cosmopolitan phytoplankton and associated bacteria. *Nature* **2015**, *522*, 98–101. [CrossRef] [PubMed]
26. Jauzein, C.; Evans, A.N.; Erdner, D.L. The impact of associated bacteria on morphology and physiology of the dinoflagellate *Alexandrium tamarense*. *Harmful Algae* **2015**, *50*, 65–75. [CrossRef]
27. Park, B.S.; Kim, J.-H.; Kim, J.H.; Gobler, C.J.; Baek, S.H.; Han, M.-S. Dynamics of bacterial community structure during blooms of *Cochlodinium* polykrikoides (Gymnodiniales, Dinophyceae) in Korean coastal waters. *Harmful Algae* **2015**, *48*, 44–54. [CrossRef] [PubMed]

28. Park, B.S.; Joo, J.-H.; Baek, K.-D.; Han, M.-S. A mutualistic interaction between the bacterium *Pseudomonas asplenii* and the harmful algal species *Chattonella marina* (Raphidophyceae). *Harmful Algae* **2016**, *56*, 29–36. [CrossRef] [PubMed]
29. Buhmann, M.T.; Schulze, B.; Forderer, A.; Schleheck, D.; Kroth, P.G. Bacteria may induce the secretion of mucin-like proteins by the diatom *Phaeodactylum tricornutum*. *J. Phycol.* **2016**, *52*, 463–474. [CrossRef] [PubMed]
30. Myung, G.; Yih, W.; Kim, H.S.; Park, J.S.; Cho, B.C. Ingestion of bacterial cells by the marine photosynthetic ciliate *Myrionecta rubra*. *Aquat. Microb. Ecol.* **2006**, *44*, 175–180. [CrossRef]
31. Hattenrath-Lehmann, T.K.; Gobler, C.J. Identification of unique microbiomes associated with harmful algal blooms caused by *Alexandrium fundyense* and *Dinophysis acuminata*. *Harmful Algae* **2017**, *68*, 17–30. [CrossRef] [PubMed]
32. Herfort, L.; Peterson, T.D.; Prahl, F.G.; McCue, L.A.; Needoba, J.A.; Crump, B.C.; Roegner, G.C.; Campbell, V.; Zuber, P. Red Waters of *Myrionecta rubra* are Biogeochemical Hotspots for the Columbia River Estuary with Impacts on Primary/Secondary Productions and Nutrient Cycles. *Estuaries Coasts* **2012**, *35*, 878–891. [CrossRef]
33. Mitra, A.; Flynn, K.J.; Burkholder, J.M.; Berge, T.; Calbet, A.; Raven, J.A.; Granéli, E.; Glibert, P.M.; Hansen, P.J.; Stoecker, D.K.; et al. The role of mixotrophic protists in the biological carbon pump. *Biogeosciences* **2014**, *11*, 995–1005. [CrossRef]
34. Krabberød, A.K.; Bjorbækmo, M.F.M.; Shalchian-Tabrizi, K.; Logares, R. Exploring the oceanic microeukaryotic interactome with metaomics approaches. *Aquat. Microb. Ecol.* **2017**, *79*, 1–12. [CrossRef]
35. Ward, C.S.; Yung, C.M.; Davis, K.M.; Blinebry, S.K.; Williams, T.C.; Johnson, Z.I.; Hunt, D.E. Annual community patterns are driven by seasonal switching between closely related marine bacteria. *ISME J.* **2017**, *11*, 1412–1422. [CrossRef] [PubMed]
36. Needham, D.M.; Fuhrman, J.A. Pronounced daily succession of phytoplankton, archaea and bacteria following a spring bloom. *Nat. Microbiol.* **2016**, *1*, 16005. [CrossRef] [PubMed]
37. Hansen, P.J.; Nielsen, L.T.; Johnson, M.; Berge, T.; Flynn, K.J. Acquired phototrophy in *Mesodinium* and *Dinophysis*—A review of cellular organization, prey selectivity, nutrient uptake and bioenergetics. *Harmful Algae* **2013**, *28*, 126–139. [CrossRef]
38. Kim, M.; Nam, S.W.; Shin, W.; Coats, D.W.; Park, M.G. Fate of green plastids in *Dinophysis caudata* following ingestion of the benthic ciliate *Mesodinium coatsi*: Ultrastructure and psbA gene. *Harmful Algae* **2015**, *43*, 66–73. [CrossRef]
39. Reguera, B.; Velo-Suárez, L.; Raine, R.; Park, M.G. Harmful *dinophysis* species: A review. *Harmful Algae* **2012**, *14*, 87–106. [CrossRef]
40. Osterholz, H.; Singer, G.; Wemheuer, B.; Daniel, R.; Simon, M.; Niggemann, J.; Dittmar, T. Deciphering associations between dissolved organic molecules and bacterial communities in a pelagic marine system. *ISME J.* **2016**, *10*, 1717. [CrossRef] [PubMed]
41. Lundgaard, A.S.B.; Treusch, A.H.; Stief, P.; Thamdrup, B.; Glud, R.N. Nitrogen cycling and bacterial community structure of sinking and aging diatom aggregates. *Aquat. Microb. Ecol.* **2017**, *79*, 85–99. [CrossRef]
42. Lucas, I.A.; Vesk, M. The fine structure of two photosynthetic species of *Dinophysis* (Dinophysiales, Dinophyceae). *J. Phycol.* **1990**, *26*, 345–357. [CrossRef]
43. Hansen, P.J.; Ojamae, K.; Berge, T.; Trampe, E.C.; Nielsen, L.T.; Lips, I.; Kuhl, M. Photoregulation in a Kleptochloroplastidic Dinoflagellate, *Dinophysis acuta*. *Front. Microbiol.* **2016**, *7*, 785. [CrossRef] [PubMed]
44. Kim, S.; Kang, Y.G.; Kim, H.S.; Yih, W.; Coats, D.W.; Park, M.G. Growth and grazing responses of the mixotrophic dinoflagellate *Dinophysis acuminata* as functions of light intensity and prey concentration. *Aquatic Microb. Ecol.* **2008**, *51*, 301–310. [CrossRef]
45. Seeyave, S.; Probyn, T.A.; Pitcher, G.C.; Lucas, M.I.; Purdie, D.A. Nitrogen nutrition in assemblages dominated by *Pseudo-nitzschia* spp., *Alexandrium catenella* and *Dinophysis acuminata* off the west coast of South Africa. *Mar. Ecol. Prog. Ser.* **2009**, *379*, 91–107. [CrossRef]
46. Harred, L.B.; Campbell, L. Predicting harmful algal blooms: A case study with *Dinophysis ovum* in the Gulf of Mexico. *J. Plankton Res.* **2014**, *36*, 1434–1445. [CrossRef]

47. Landa, M.; Cottrell, M.T.; Kirchman, D.L.; Blain, S.; Obernosterer, I. Changes in bacterial diversity in response to dissolved organic matter supply in a continuous culture experiment. *Aquat. Microb. Ecol.* **2013**, *69*, 157–168. [CrossRef]
48. Buchan, A.; LeCleir, G.R.; Gulvik, C.A.; Gonzalez, J.M. Master recyclers: Features and functions of bacteria associated with phytoplankton blooms. *Nat. Rev. Microbiol.* **2014**, *12*, 686–698. [CrossRef] [PubMed]
49. Riemann, L.; Steward, G.F.; Azam, F. Dynamics of Bacterial Community Composition and Activity during a Mesocosm Diatom Bloom. *Appl. Environ. Microbiol.* **2000**, *66*, 578–587. [CrossRef] [PubMed]
50. Arrieta, J.M.; Herndl, G.J. Changes in bacterial β-glucosidase diversity during a coastal phytoplankton bloom. *Limnol. Oceanogr.* **2002**, *47*, 594–599. [CrossRef]
51. Hattenrath-Lehmann, T.K.; Marcoval, M.A.; Mittlesdorf, H.; Goleski, J.A.; Wang, Z.; Haynes, B.; Morton, S.L.; Gobler, C.J. Nitrogenous nutrients promote the growth and toxicity of *Dinophysis acuminata* during Estuarine bloom events. *PLoS ONE* **2015**, *10*, e0124148. [CrossRef] [PubMed]
52. Mitra, A.; Flynn, K.J.; Tillmann, U.; Raven, J.A.; Caron, D.; Stoecker, D.K.; Not, F.; Hansen, P.J.; Hallegraeff, G.; Sanders, R.; et al. Defining Planktonic Protist Functional Groups on Mechanisms for Energy and Nutrient Acquisition: Incorporation of Diverse Mixotrophic Strategies. *Protist* **2016**, *167*, 106–120. [CrossRef] [PubMed]
53. Cottrell, M.T.; Kirchman, D.L. Natural assemblages of marine proteobacteria and members of the Cytophaga-Flavobacter cluster consuming low-and high-molecular-weight dissolved organic matter. *Appl. Environ. Microbiol.* **2000**, *66*, 1692–1697. [CrossRef] [PubMed]
54. Pearman, J.K.; Casas, L.; Merle, T.; Michell, C.; Irigoien, X. Bacterial and protist community changes during a phytoplankton bloom. *Limnol. Oceanogr.* **2016**, *61*, 198–213. [CrossRef]
55. Bolch, C.J.; Subramanian, T.A.; Green, D.H. The Toxic Dinoflagellate *Gymnodinium Catenatum* (Dinophyceae) Requires Marine Bacteria for Growth. *J. Phycol.* **2011**, *47*, 1009–1022. [CrossRef] [PubMed]
56. Cho, D.-H.; Ramanan, R.; Kim, B.-H.; Lee, J.; Kim, S.; Yoo, C.; Choi, G.-G.; Oh, H.-M.; Kim, H.-S.; Lindell, D. Novel approach for the development of axenic microalgal cultures from environmental samples. *J. Phycol.* **2013**, *49*, 802–810. [CrossRef] [PubMed]
57. Rodríguez, F.; Escalera, L.; Reguera, B.; Rial, P.; Riobó, P.; da Silva, T.D.J. Morphological variability, toxinology and genetics of the dinoflagellate *Dinophysis tripos* (Dinophysiaceae, Dinophysiales). *Harmful Algae* **2012**, *13*, 26–33. [CrossRef]
58. Smith, J.L.; Tong, M.; Fux, E.; Anderson, D.M. Toxin production, retention, and extracellular release by *Dinophysis acuminata* during extended stationary phase and culture decline. *Harmful Algae* **2012**, *19*, 125–132. [CrossRef]
59. Bolger, A.M.; Lohse, M.; Usadel, B. Trimmomatic: A flexible trimmer for Illumina sequence data. *Bioinformatics* **2014**, *30*, 2114–2120. [CrossRef] [PubMed]
60. Reyon, D.; Tsai, S.Q.; Khayter, C.; Foden, J.A.; Sander, J.D.; Joung, J.K. FLASH assembly of TALENs for high-throughput genome editing. *Nat. Biotechnol.* **2012**, *30*, 460–465. [CrossRef] [PubMed]
61. Edgar, R.C. UPARSE: Highly accurate OTU sequences from microbial amplicon reads. *Nat. Methods* **2013**, *10*, 996. [CrossRef] [PubMed]
62. McMurdie, P.J.; Holmes, S. Phyloseq: An R Package for Reproducible Interactive Analysis and Graphics of Microbiome Census Data. *PLoS ONE* **2013**, *8*, e61217. [CrossRef] [PubMed]
63. Chen, J.; Bittinger, K.; Charlson, E.S.; Hoffmann, C.; Lewis, J.; Wu, G.D.; Collman, R.G.; Bushman, F.D.; Li, H. Associating microbiome composition with environmental covariates using generalized UniFrac distances. *Bioinformatics* **2012**, *28*, 2106–2113. [CrossRef] [PubMed]
64. Pedrós-Alió, C. The rare bacterial biosphere. *Ann. Rev. Mar. Sci.* **2012**, *4*, 449–466. [CrossRef] [PubMed]
65. Oksanen, J.; Blanchet, F.G.; Kindt, R.; Legendre, P.; Minchin, P.R.; O'hara, R.; Simpson, G.L.; Solymos, P.; Stevens, M.H.H.; Wagner, H. Package 'vegan'. *Community Ecol. Package* **2013**, *2*, 34–115.

toxins

MDPI

Article

Notes on the Cultivation of Two Mixotrophic *Dinophysis* Species and Their Ciliate Prey *Mesodinium rubrum*

Jorge Hernández-Urcera [1,†], Pilar Rial [1,†], María García-Portela [1], Patricia Lourés [1], Jane Kilcoyne [2], Francisco Rodríguez [1], Amelia Fernández-Villamarín [1] and Beatriz Reguera [1,*]

1. Microalgas Nocivas, Centro Oceanográfico de Vigo, IEO, Subida a Radio Faro 50, 36390 Vigo, Spain; jurcera@iim.csic.es (J.H.-U.); pilar.rial@ieo.es (P.R.); maria.garcia@ieo.es (M.G.-P.); patricia.loures@ieo.es (P.L.); francisco.rodriguez@ieo.es (F.R.); amelia.fernandez@ieo.es (A.F.-V.)
2. Biotoxin Chemistry, Marine Institute, Rinville, Oranmore, Co. Galway H91 R673, Ireland; jane.kilcoyne@marine.ie

* Correspondence: beatriz.reguera@ieo.es; Tel.: +34-986-492111

† These co-first authors contributed equally to this work.

Received: 28 September 2018; Accepted: 26 November 2018; Published: 1 December 2018

Abstract: Kleptoplastic mixotrophic species of the genus *Dinophysis* are cultured by feeding with the ciliate *Mesodinium rubrum*, itself a kleptoplastic mixotroph, that in turn feeds on cryptophytes of the *Teleaulax/Plagioselmis/Geminigera* (TPG) clade. Optimal culture media for phototrophic growth of *D. acuminata* and *D. acuta* from the Galician Rías (northwest Spain) and culture media and cryptophyte prey for *M. rubrum* from Huelva (southwest Spain) used to feed *Dinophysis*, were investigated. Phototrophic growth rates and yields were maximal when *D. acuminata* and *D. acuta* were grown in ammonia-containing K(-Si) medium versus f/2(-Si) or L1(-Si) media. *Dinophysis acuminata* cultures were scaled up to 18 L in a photobioreactor. Large differences in cell toxin quota were observed in the same *Dinophysis* strains under different experimental conditions. Yields and duration of exponential growth were maximal for *M. rubrum* from Huelva when fed *Teleaulax amphioxeia* from the same region, versus *T. amphioxeia* from the Galician Rías or *T. minuta* and *Plagioselmis prolonga*. Limitations for mass cultivation of northern *Dinophysis* strains with southern *M. rubrum* were overcome using more favorable (1:20) *Dinophysis*: *Mesodinium* ratios. These subtleties highlight the ciliate strain-specific response to prey and its importance to mass production of *M. rubrum* and *Dinophysis* cultures.

Keywords: *Dinophysis*; *Mesodinium*; cryptophytes; predator-prey preferences; Diarrhetic Shellfish Toxins (DST); pectenotoxins (PTXs); mixotrophic cultures; mass culture conditions

Key Contribution: Phototrophic growth of *D. acuminata* and *D. acuta* was maximal in ammonia-containing K media; ciliate *M. rubrum* and its cryptophyte prey had higher growth rate and yields with f/2(-Si). Sustained growth and yields in mixotrophic cultures of *Dinophysis* were maximal when *M. rubrum* was grown with the cryptophyte *T. amphioxeia* from the same location as prey; additionally, high growth rates were achieved with high ratios of prey (1:20, *Dinophysis*: *M. rubrum*) grown with *T. minuta* and *P. prolonga*.

1. Introduction

Several mixotrophic species of the genus *Dinophysis* produce one or two groups of lipophilic toxins: (i) okadaic acid (OA) and its derivatives, the dinophysistoxins (DTXs), and (ii) pectenotoxins (PTXs) [1,2]. The OA and DTXs, known as Diarrhetic Shellfish Poisoning (DSP) toxins, are acid polyethers that inhibit protein phosphatase and have diarrheogenic effects in mammals. The PTXs are polyether lactones, some of which are hepatotoxic to mice by intraperitoneal injection [3]. Their toxicity has been questioned, since they do not appear to be toxic when ingested orally [4]. Nevertheless, they are still subject to regulation in the European Union (EU). The two groups of toxins, OA related toxins and PTXs, can now be analyzed with independent analytical methods, which have led the EU to regulate them separately [5].

DSP toxins pose a threat to public health, and together with PTXs, cause considerable losses to the shellfish industry globally [6,7]. Harvest closures are enforced when toxin levels exceed local regulatory limits (RL). *Dinophysis* blooms, in particular those of *D. acuminata* and *D. acuta*, are persistent in western Iberia (Spain and Portugal). Contamination of shellfish with *Dinophysis* toxins above the RL can last up to nine months in the most affected aquaculture sites [8,9]. Harmful algal blooms (HABs), in particular *Dinophysis* blooms, cannot be eliminated, therefore, more detailed knowledge of the conditions affecting *Dinophysis* growth and toxin production is crucial to improve risk forecasting. Forecasts can help the shellfish industry schedule harvest plans and help mitigate the deleterious impacts of such blooms.

Protection of public health and seafood safety control require the implementation of costly monitoring systems; these include frequent toxin analyses of all commercially exploited shellfish species with sophisticated analytical instruments, such as liquid chromatography coupled to tandem mass spectrometry (LC–MS/MS) [8,9]. These chemical methods require pure certified toxin standards for the analyses, which are difficult to obtain or are yet to be developed. Successful cultivation of *Dinophysis* in the laboratory is instrumental for addressing these shortfalls. Of particular importance is the optimization of mass production of *Dinophysis* to allow isolation and purification of toxins. Further, some *Dinophysis* toxins may have a wide spectrum of applications. For example, PTX2 has been found to cause a selective apoptosis of carcinogenic cells [10,11], and currently, protocols for the mass production of *D. acuminata* in Korea to obtain PTX2 for the pharmaceutical industry have been patented [12].

For years, the establishment of *Dinophysis* cultures challenged microalgal physiologists. *Dinophysis* species were found to bear unusual plastids containing pigments—phycoerythrins—and a structure similar to those of cryptophyte microflagellates [13]. Attempts to grow them with conventional culture media used for dinoflagellates, with addition of dissolved organic matter or even with bacteria were unsuccessful [14]. The observation of ciliate remains in the digestive vacuoles of *D. acuminata* and *D. norvegica* confirmed their mixotrophic nature [15]. The next breakthroughs came with the application of molecular tools. DNA sequences of the plastid SSU rRNA gene of *Dinophysis* were found to coincide with those from living cryptophytes closely related to *Geminigera cryophila* [16]. A correlation between *Dinophysis* and cryptophyte cell densities in the field, estimated with molecular probes, was found [17], but attempts to grow *Dinophysis* directly fed with cryptophytes were unsuccessful [18].

Further studies showed that partial sequences of the plastid *psbA* gene and the ribosomal 16S rRNA gene from *Dinophysis* species were identical to the same loci in living cryptophyte *Teleaulax amphioxeia*. These findings raised the suspicion that *Dinophysis* plastids were stolen plastids (kleptoplastids). The key question was whether *Dinophysis* acquired these kleptoplastids through an intermediate organism [19]. A few years earlier, the first culture of the phototrophic ciliate *M. rubrum* to feed the cryptophyte *Geminigera cryophyla* was achieved [20]; its feeding behavior taking up crytophytes (*T. amphioxeia)* through an oral cavity was described [21]. Finally, the first successful culture of *D. acuminata* using the ciliate *M. rubrum*, grown with *T. amphioxeia* as prey was established. *Dinophysis* was found to feed on *M. rubrum* by myzocytosis, a type of phagotrophy where the predator pierces the prey with a feeding peduncle and sucks its content. After the feeding process, *Dinophysis* appeared full of digestive vacuoles, but the prey plastids were retained and used as kleptoplastids [22].

Since then, cultures of several *Dinophysis* species—*D. acuta* [23], *D. caudata* [24], *D. fortii* [25], *D. infundibulus* [26], *D. sacculus* [27], and *D. tripos* [28]—have been established via this three-species chain of serial kleptoplastidy, i.e., cryptophyte plastid acquisition from the TPG clade (*Teleaulax/Plagioselmis/Geminigera)* to *M. rubrum*, which in turn provides plastids to *Dinophysis*. Small-volume cultures, ranging from a few mL in multiwell plates to Erlenmeyer flasks of 250 mL, based on the same kind of mixotrophic nutrition, were set up to carry out physiological, toxinological and genetic studies. These *Dinophysis* species were cultivated with the ciliate *M. rubrum* fed two cryptophytes belonging to the TPG clade (i.e., *Teleaulax amphioxeia* or *Geminigera cryophila*) using full or diluted f/2 [29] or L1 medium [30].

The mass production of *D. acuminata* to obtain pectenotoxins, including production of the ciliate *M. rubrum* and cryptophyte of the genus *Teleaulax* to feed *Dinophysis*, has been addressed and the results patented. Nevertheless, the exact details of the *Teleaulax* species used to feed *M. rubrum* were not provided in the patent description [12]. Maintaining a balance between the three species of the 'cryptophyte–ciliate–dinoflagellate' food chain is difficult, because each has different requirements. These requirements range from the purely autotrophic *T. amphioxeia*, to mixotrophic *M. rubrum* and *Dinophysis* species, which require light and live prey for sustained growth [31–33]. Nevertheless, *M. rubrum* only needs to ingest 1–2% of its daily carbon intake from its prey to attain maximum growth, whereas *Dinophysis* species require ~50% for the same purpose [31]. Both *M. rubrum* and *Dinophysis* species can survive for months in the light without food, and their light preferences are different from the cryptophytes [33].

This work is a compilation of original observations and problems frequently faced in the maintenance and optimization of *Dinophysis*, *M. rubrum*, and cryptophyte cultures. Observations are from strain maintenance in the culture collection and experiments carried out at the IEO-Vigo laboratory, Nantes, France [34] and Naples, Italy [35] where the same *Dinophysis* and *M. rubrum* strains were used. The objectives of this work were: (i) to optimize culture medium for *Dinophysis* (*D. acuminata* and *D. acuta*) from the Galician Rías (northwest Spain), the ciliate prey *M. rubrum* from Huelva (southwest Spain) and different cryptophyte prey species; (ii) to estimate growth and yields of *M. rubrum* grown with cryptophyte species different from *T. amphioxeia*; and (iii) to optimize cryptophyte prey for *M. rubrum* for maximal *Dinophysis* growth and yield.

2. Results

2.1. Optimizing Culture Medium for Phototrophic Growth of D. acuminata and D. acuta

The objective of this experiment was to test which of the three culture media (f/2 [29], L1 [30] and K [36]) was best for the phototrophic growth (no prey added) of *D. acuminata* (VGO1391) and *D. acuta* (VGO1065) from the Galician Rías (northwest Spain), and if the best medium for *Dinophysis* growth coincided with the best for their ciliate prey *M. rubrum* (AND-A071) from Huelva (southwest Spain).

Dinophysis acuminata cell densities increased moderately the first 7–10 days with the three treatments. From day 14 onwards, cultures grown with diluted (1:2) f/2 and L1 media started to decline. Cultures with diluted (1:2) K(-Si) medium showed 7-d stationary phase (day 7 to 14) followed by exponential growth ($\mu = 0.15$ d^{-1}) until day 28, reaching 619 cells mL^{-1}. By day 42, cell density in cultures with K(-Si) medium was 390 cells mL^{-1} (mean), whereas no cells were observed in the cultures with diluted f/2 and L1 media (Figure 1A). Therefore, duration of exponential growth was 14 d longer and the final yield was significantly higher ($p = 1.3 \times 10^{-6}$) in *D. acuminata* cultures with K(-Si) medium.

Regarding *D. acuta*, maximal growth rate—also obtained with K(-Si) medium—was extremely low ($\mu = 0.06$ d^{-1}) and positive growth lasted seven days only. Differences between treatments were not statistically significant ($p = 0.67$) (Figure 1B). Phototrophic (no cryptophyte prey added) growth rates of the prey, *M. rubrum*, with the three different culture media in 250 mL at 15 °C were similar for the duration of the experiment, but the initiation of the exponential decline was later (day 7) and the final yield maximal ($p < 0.02$) with f/2(-Si) medium (Figure 2).

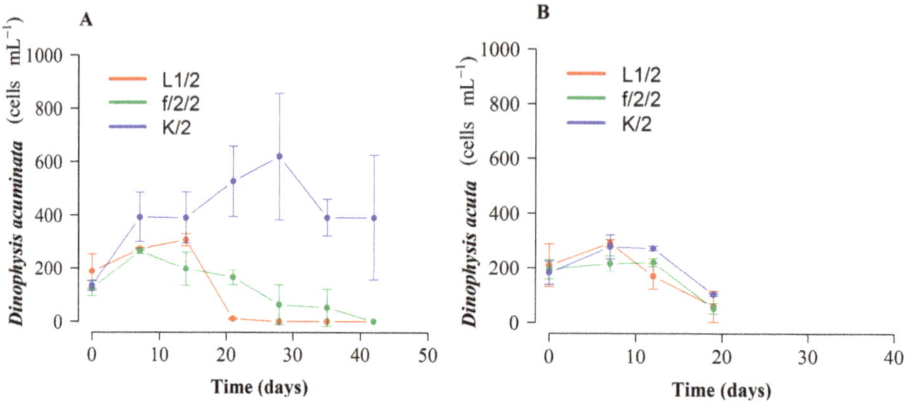

Figure 1. Phototrophic growth (prey-depleted) of *Dinophysis* species with three different diluted (1:2), Si free culture media (L1, f/2 and K). (**A**) *D. acuminata* (VGO1391) and (**B**) *D. acuta* (VGO1065). Bars represent standard error.

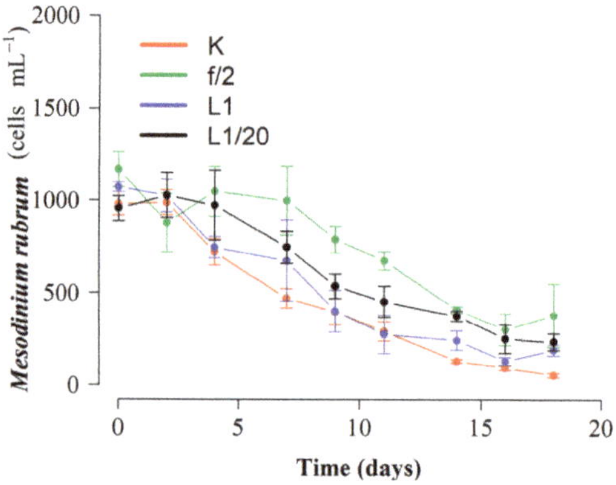

Figure 2. Phototrophic growth (no cryptophyte prey) of *M. rubrum* (AND-A071) cultures (previously fed with *T. minuta*, CR8EHU) with different Si free enrichment media (K, f/2, L1 and diluted, 1:20, L1). Bars represent standard error.

2.2. *Growth and Cell Toxin Quota in 4 L Mixotrophic Cultures of* D. acuminata *and* D. acuta

Scaled-up (4 L) mixotrophic cultures of *D. acuminata* and *D. acuta* with full K(-Si) medium and addition of *M. rubrum* (AND-A071) prey showed maximal growth rates of $\mu = 0.33\ d^{-1}$ and $0.26\ d^{-1}$ respectively in short-term experiments at 19 °C and a 16:8 light:dark cycle. Final yields by day 8 were 2287 cells mL^{-1} for *D. acuminata* and 883 cells mL^{-1} for *D. acuta* (Figure 3). Toxin contents were 9.9 pg OA $cell^{-1}$ in *D. acuminata* and 7.7 pg OA + 2.9 pg DTX2 + 8.2 pg PTX2 $cell^{-1}$ in *D. acuta* (Table 1).

2.3. *Optimization of* M. rubrum *Prey*

Mixotrophic growth of *M. rubrum* from Huelva (southwest Spain), fed with different species of the TPG clade from different Spanish regions was tested. Growth curves of *M. rubrum*, previously grown with *P. prolonga* in K(-Si) medium, showed a lag phase of more than 10 days in mixotrophic cultures while being fed two different strains of cryptophye *T. amphioxeia*: strain AND-A070 from Huelva (southwest Spain) and strain VGO1392 from the Galician Rías (northwest Spain) respectively (Figure 4A). This was followed by a moderate ($\mu = 0.18\ d^{-1}$ between day 16 and 28) exponential growth until day 35, and an abrupt decline after reaching the maximal yield (30–50 × 10^3 cells mL^{-1}) in cultures fed *T. amphioxeia*, strain AND-A070, i.e., from the same area as the ciliate. Final yields in *M. rubrum* cultures fed the same cryptophyte species, *T. amphioxeia* strain VGO1392, but from northwest Spain, were three times smaller. Growth rates with this strain were lower and comparable with those observed in cultures fed with *T. minuta* ($p = 0.02$) (Figure 4B). In fact, the growth curves of *M. rubrum* cultures fed *T. amphioxeia* from northwest Spain and *T. minuta* showed very similar patterns and both reached the maximal yield after three weeks. Cultures fed *P. prolonga* with K(-Si) medium showed a moderate growth ($\mu = 0.17$ d^{-1}) between day 9 and 16, and entered a plateau phase on day 19, followed by a fast decline (Figure 4C). Cultures of *M. rubrum* with *P. prolonga* in diluted (1:20) L1(-Si) medium, used as an internal control, exhibited a maximal yield slightly lower than those fed the same cryptophyte with K(-Si) medium, but growth rate over the first two weeks was very low and it took an additional week to reach the maximal yield.

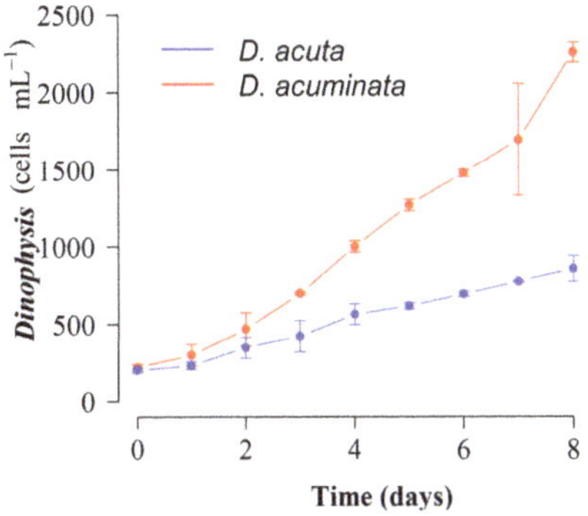

Figure 3. Growth curves of mixotrophic cultures of *D. acuminata* (VGO1391) and *D. acuta* (VGO1065) (fed *M. rubrum*, AND-A071) grown with *P. prolonga*, CR10EHU) with K(-Si) medium in 4 L flasks at 19 °C and a 16L:8D cycle. Bars represent standard error ($n = 9$).

2.4. *Optimal Cryptophyte Prey for* M. rubrum *and* Dinophysis:Mesodinium *(D:M) Ratio for Highest* Dinophysis *Growth and Survival*

Dinophysis acuminata was able to grow with *M. rubrum* fed four cryptophyte species growing in diluted (1:20) L1 medium. Growth rate, and in particular final yield of *D. acuminata* achieved with *M. rubrum* fed *T. amphioxeia*, strain AND-A070 ($\mu = 0.36$ d^{-1}; 1.11 × 10^3 cells mL^{-1}), were higher than those with *T. minuta* ($\mu = 0.33$ d^{-1}; 0.82 × 10^3 cells mL^{-1}), *T. gracilis* ($\mu = 0.27$ d^{-1}; 0.68 × 10^3 cells mL^{-1}), and *P. prolonga* ($\mu = 0.30$ d^{-1}; 0.81 × 10^3 cells mL^{-1}) ($p = 0.016$) (Figure 5A). Differences were more marked in the case of *D. acuta* grown with *M. rubrum* fed *T. amphioxeia* (AND-070). These cultures showed four weeks of sustained exponential growth phase ($\mu = 0.2$ d^{-1}), from day 10 to 38, and a final yield of 1.21 × 10^3 cells mL^{-1}. In contrast, shorter exponential growth phase and about half the final yield were achieved in cultures with the same species fed: *T. amphioxeia* (VGO1392) ($\mu = 0.26$ d^{-1}; yield: 0.43 × 10^3 cells mL^{-1}), *P. prolonga* (CR10EHU) grown with full K(-Si) medium ($\mu = 0.23$ d^{-1}; 0.54 × 10^3 cells mL^{-1}) and *P. prolonga* with diluted (1:20) L1 ($\mu = 0.22$ d^{-1}; 0.5 × 10^3 cells mL^{-1}) ($p = 1.3 \times 10^{-15}$) (Figure 5B). Thus, a longer exponential phase and a 2-fold higher yield were obtained in *D. acuta* cultures with *M. rubrum* fed the *T. amphioxeia* (AND-A070) from the same location. Results from *D. acuta* cultures with *M. rubrum* fed *P. prolonga* were about the same whether the ciliate + cryptophyte had been growing with K(-Si) medium or with diluted (1:20) L1(-Si) medium.

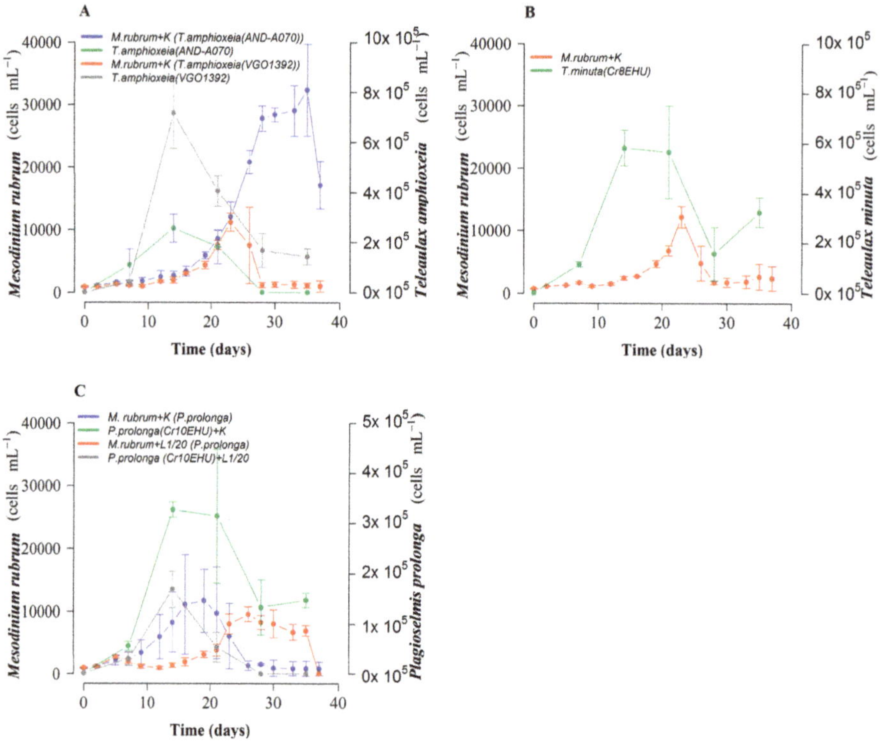

Figure 4. Growth of *M. rubrum* (AND-A071) fed three cryptophyte species with K(-Si) medium: (**A**) *T. amphioxeia* strains from Vigo (VGO1392) and Huelva (AND-A070); (**B**) *T. minuta* (Cr8EHU), and (**C**) *P. prolonga* (Cr10EHU) from the Basque Country, north Spain, with K(-Si) and L1/20 (-Si) culture media. Bars represent standard error.

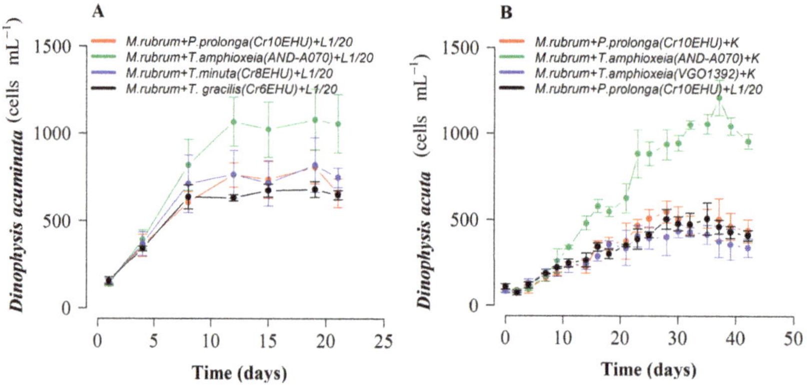

Figure 5. Growth of *Dinophysis* species with *M. rubrum* (AND-A071) fed different crytptophyte species. (**A**) *D. acuminata* with *M. rubrum* fed *T.amphioxeia* (AND-A070), *T. minuta* (Cr8EHU), *T. gracilis* (Cr6EHU), and *P. prolonga* (Cr10EHU). (**B**) *D. acuta* with *M. rubrum* fed two crytptophyte species: *T. amphioxeia* (AND-A070, VGO1392) and *P. prolonga* (Cr10EHU). Bars represent standard error.

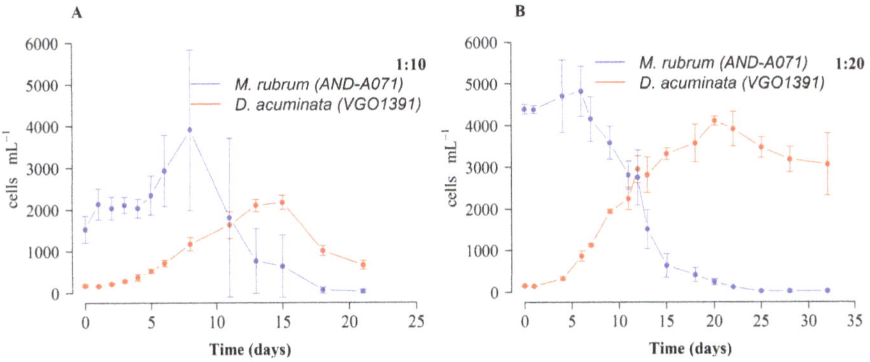

Figure 6. Growth of *D. acuminata* (VGO1391) fed *M. rubrum* (AND-A071) grown with *T. minuta* (CR8EHU) and K(-Si) medium with different predator:prey ratio. (**A**) *D. acuminata:M.rubrum* 1:10 and (**B**) *D. acuminata:M. rubrum* 1:20. Bars represent standard error.

Dinophysis acuminata cultures fed *M. rubrum* (which in turn was fed *T. minuta*) with a 1:20 D:M ratio, showed a higher growth rate ($\mu = 0.28\ d^{-1}$), a two-fold higher final yield (4000 cells mL^{-1}), and seven more days of sustained exponential growth as compared with the same strain of *D. acuminata* ($\mu = 0.21\ d^{-1}$) fed with a 1:10 D:M ratio (Figure 6).

2.5. *Mass Cultivation and Total Toxin Yield of* Dinophysis *in 30 L Photobioreactors*

A final yield of 0.77×10^3 cells mL^{-1} of *D. acuminata* was obtained after 20 d of culture with a final volume of 18 L. Maximal growth rate achieved, between days 6 and 8 was 0.28 d^{-1} (Figure 7). LC–MS/MS analysis of total toxins (particulate and dissolved) adsorbed with the Diaion®resins revealed a content of 22.3 ng OA mL^{-1}, corresponding to 770 cell mL^{-1} of *D. acuminata* and the extracellular toxins released in the culture medium.

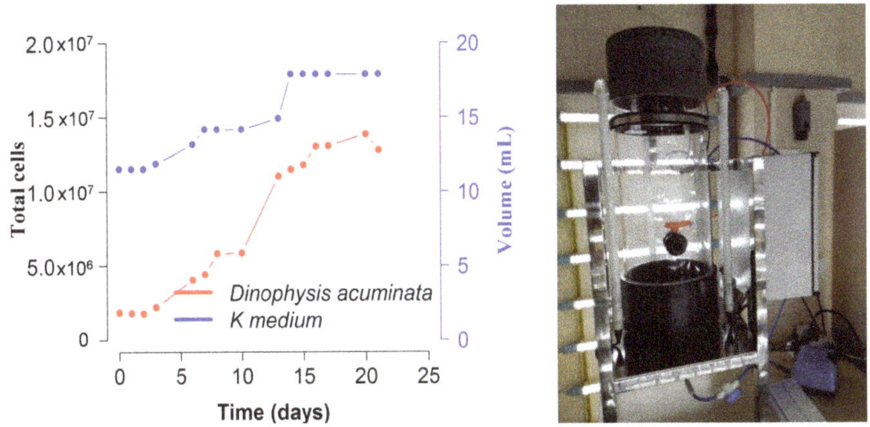

Figure 7. Cultures of *D. acuminata* with *M. rubrum* fed *T. amphioxeia* in a 30 L photobioreactor (right hand picture) with K(-Si) medium at 18 °C. Blue line indicates changes in volume in the photobioreactor.

Table 1. Intracellular (particulate, pg cell^{-1}) and total toxin (particulate + dissolved, pg mL^{-1}cell^{-1}, marked with *) contents in cultures of *D. acuta* (VGO1065) and *D. acuminata* (VGO1391) from this work and from other experiments carried out with the same strains isolated in Vigo. Abbreviations: Ref. = reference; ES = *M. rubrum* strain from Huelva, Spain, or DK = from Denmark, V = volume, T = temperature; sta = stationary phase; exp = exponential phase; L:D = light:dark; OA = okadaic acid; DTX2 = dinophysistoxin 2; PTX2 = pectenotoxin 2.

Species	Ref.	Experimental Conditions	V (mL)	T (°C)	L:D Cycle (h)	Medium	OA (pg cell^{-1})	DTX2 (pg cell^{-1})	PTX2 (pg cell^{-1})
D. acuta	[34]	Well-fed (ES)	250	15	12:12	L1-Si/20	12.2 ± 2.3	4.4 ± 0.9	22.2 ± 9.4
	[34]	Well-fed (ES)	150	17	14:10	L1-Si/20	41.0 ± 4.9	17.4 ± 4.1	38.0 ± 8.2
		Prey-limited (ES)	150	17	14:10		74.1 ± 8.2	32.4 ± 3.8	59.3 ± 11.8
	[34]	Well-fed (DK)	150	17	14:10	L1-Si/20	35.9 ± 7.07	16.5 ± 0.8	70.0 ± 0.8
		Prey-limited (DK)	150	17	14:10		38.6 ± 4.5	19.0 ± 2.3	43.6 ± 6.2
	[33]	Low light	250	15	12:12	L1-Si/40	3.3 ± 1.6	2.2 ± 0.1	71.5 ± 14.2
		High light	250	15	12:12		50.2 ± 20.1	35.4 ± 17.4	187.8 ± 104.1
	This work	Mass culture-sta	1450	15	12:12	L1-Si/20	30.2 *	7.3 *	48.2 *
		Mass culture-sta	3500	15	12:12	K-Si	15.5 *	5.2 *	50.5 *
		Mass culture-exp	4000	19	16:8	K-Si	7.7	2.9	8.2
		Mass culture-sta	5000	15	12:12	L1-Si/20	61.5 *	20.3 *	3 *
D. acuminata	[34]	Well-fed (ES)	250	15	12:12	L1-Si/20	35.2 ± 6.8		
	[34]	Well-fed (ES)	150	17	14:10	L1-Si/20	6.0 ± 2.8		
		Prey-limited (ES)	150	17	14:10		21.5 ± 0.7		
	[34]	Well-fed (DK)	150	17	14:10	L1-Si/20	9.8 ± 1.7		
		Prey-limited (DK)	150	17	14:10		32.3 ±4.7		
	[33]	Low light	250	15	12:12	L1-Si/40	14.7 ± 12.1		
		High light	250	15	12:12		41.4 ± 4		
	This work	Mass culture-sta	2200	15	12:12	L1-Si/20	33.3 *		
		Mass culture-sta	2700	15	12:12	L1-Si/20	122.2 *		
		Mass culture-exp	4000	19	16:8	K-Si	9.9		
		Mass culture-sta	4500	15	12:12	K-Si	20.3 *		
		Mass culture-sta	17,900	15	12:12	K-Si	28.9 *		

2.6. Dinophysis *Vertical Distribution in the Culture Vessels*

In small- (≤250 mL) and medium- (several L) volume cultures of *Dinophysis*, cells were usually distributed in the bottom of the container. When depleted prey was replenished, observation of the cultures with the inverted microscope showed that *Dinophysis* cells swam upwards to catch *M. rubrum*. Otherwise, in samples collected after a gentle but thorough shaking of the containers to estimate cell densities, it was common to observe prey cells still attached to *Dinophysis* through a feeding peduncle. In contrast, in the large volume (up to 25 L) cultures in the bioreactor, *Dinophysis* cells could be observed in the water column forming patches above the level of the black plastic ring that protects the base of the metacrylate bioreactor (Figure 7) and in the air–water interface.

2.7. *Nanoflagellate Contamination*

Not infrequently, mixotrophic cultures of *Dinophysis* appeared contaminated with a tiny (~10 µm) nanoflagellate. Its growth became out of control and smothered *M. rubrum* cultures when either full f/2 or L1 media were used. The use of diluted (1:20) L1(-Si) medium, often used to control overgrowth of the cryptophyte in mixotrophic cultures of *M. rubrum*, proved to be effective in controlling the contaminating nanoflagellate. Mass cultures of *Dinophysis* became contaminated sometimes with it. In those cases, *Dinophysis* toxins from the cells and culture medium were cropped with the adsorbing Diaion®resins before the culture started to decline. The contaminating nanoflagellate was established in culture, sequenced, and identified as an undetermined chrysophyte species of the genus *Ochromonas*.

2.8. *Sequencing and Phylogenetic Analysis*

Partial plastid 23S rDNA sequences (373 base pairs, bp) of *T. amphioxeia* (strains AND-A070 from Huelva and VGO1392 from Vigo) and *P. prolonga* (CR10EHU, north Spain) cultures, *M. rubrum* (cultivated strains AND-A071 from Huelva and isolated field specimens from Vigo) and *Mesodinium major* and *Dinophysis* isolated specimens from the Galician Rías (see isolation dates in Table 2) were almost identical (Table 2). In fact, a single base pair (bp) difference (out of the 373) was found in the amplified region between the plastids of *M. rubrum* and *T. amphioxeia* from Huelva versus those from the Galician specimens (*M. rubrum*, *M. major*, and *T. amphioxeia*). *Plagioselmis prolonga*, from the Basque country, differed in one additional base pair from these organisms (Figure 8).

Table 2. Alignment of the first 100 bp from the partial (373 bp) plastid 23S rDNA of *T. amphioxeia* (strains from Huelva and Vigo) and *P. prolonga* (Basque Country, north Spain) cultures, *M. rubrum* (cultivated strains from Huelva and isolated cells from Vigo), *M. major*, and *Dinophysis* cells isolated from water samples collected in Ría de Vigo and Ria de Pontevedra (Galician Rias Baixas, northwest Spain). The whole 373 bp partial plastid sequence was identical except in positions 79 and 90 shown here. These correspond to positions 2123 and 2134 in the whole plastid 23S rRNA gene (referred to *Rhodomonas salina*, NCBI Reference Sequence: NC_009573.1).

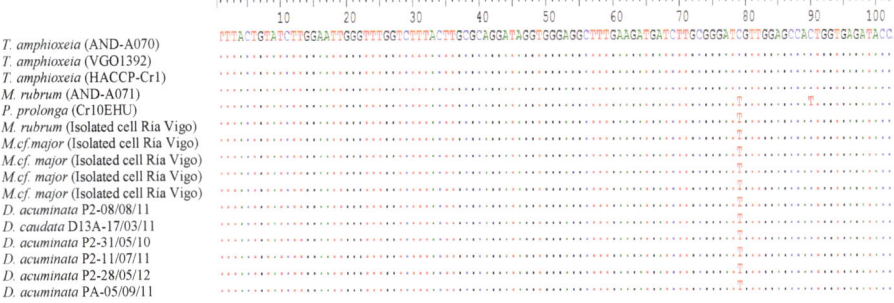

	10 20 30 40 50 60 70 80 90 100
T. amphioxeia (AND-A070)	TTTACTGTATCTTGGAATTGGGTTTGGTCTTTACTTGCGCAGGATAGGTGGAGGCTTTGAAGATGATCTTGCGGGATCGTTGGAGCCACTGGTGAGATACC
T. amphioxeia (VGO1392)	....
T. amphioxeia (HACCP-Cr1)	....
M. rubrum (AND-A071)	....
P. prolonga (Cr10EHU)	....T..........T...........
M. rubrum (Isolated cell Ría Vigo)	....T......................
M.cf.major (Isolated cell Ría Vigo)	....T......................
M.cf. major (Isolated cell Ría Vigo)	....T......................
M.cf. major (Isolated cell Ría Vigo)	....T......................
M.cf. major (Isolated cell Ría Vigo)	....T......................
D. acuminata P2-08/08/11	....T......................
D. caudata D13A-17/03/11	....T......................
D. acuminata P2-31/05/10	....T......................
D. acuminata P2-11/07/11	....T......................
D. acuminata P2-28/05/12	....T......................
D. acuminata PA-05/09/11	....T......................

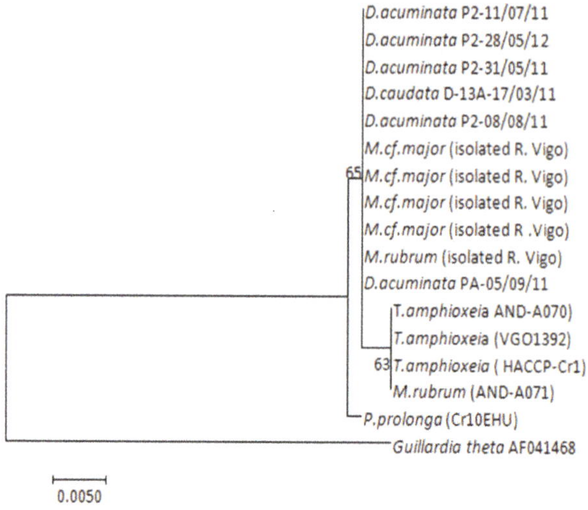

Figure 8. Maximum-likelihood (ML) tree inferred from partial plastid 23S rDNA sequences of *D. acuminata, D. caudata, T. amphioxeia, M. rubrum, P. prolonga*, and *M. cf. major*. Support at internal nodes is based on bootstrap values of ML methods with 1000 resamplings. *Guillardia theta* was added as outgroup to root the tree. Scale bar indicates number of substitutions per site.

3. Discussion

3.1. *K(-Si) Medium Best for* Dinophysis *Growth*

The most recent research with *Dinophysis* cultures has been carried out using full or diluted f/2 medium [29] for the dinoflagellate, the ciliate, and the cryptophytes, and in a few cases, L1 medium [30]. These enrichment media have only nitrate as a nitrogen source. Earlier studies showed that inorganic nutrients (nitrates and phosphates) provided in the culture medium were not used by *D. acuminata* and led to the conclusion that this species fulfilled its nitrogenous and phosphorous needs from ingested ciliate prey [37]. Incubation of field populations during a *D. acuminata* bloom in the Benguela upwelling system, South Africa, with radiolabeled (N^{15}) nitrogenous compounds had shown this species had a great affinity for regenerated N compounds, such as ammonium and urea [38]. Culture incubations confirmed *D. acuminata* preference for ammonia, urea, and other organic forms of nitrogen rather than nitrate (new production) [39]. Recent studies found similar results and an apparent inability to use nitrate in cultures of the *D. acuminata* and *D. acuta* strains used in the present study [40]. These results led us to test K(-Si) medium [36] for *Dinophysis* cultivation, because it is the only one, among the commonly used culture media for dinoflagellates, which includes ammonium in the form of ammonium chloride (NH_4Cl) as a nitrogen source. This better explains the results obtained, in terms of growth rate and yield, in phototrophic cultures of *D. acuminata* when using this culture medium (Figure 1A).

Growth rate ($\mu < 0.1$ d^{-1}) and yields (<400 cells mL^{-1}) obtained in phototrophic cultures of *D. acuta* grown with K(-Si) medium (experiment 1) were very poor (maximum of one doubling of the population), and slightly higher than with f/2 and L1 media (Figure 1B). This strain of *D. acuta* (VGO1065) had shown lower division rates than *D. acuminata* in all previous studies [40]. But the same strain of *D. acuta* showed a much higher growth ($\mu = 0.26$ d^{-1}) in the second experiment, where ciliate prey was supplied (mixotrophic growth), temperature (19 °C) was 4 °C higher, and the cycle had 4 h additional light. There is not enough information available to reach definitive conclusions, but a preliminary interpretation is that *D. acuta*, a late summer species in Western Europe, grows better with higher temperatures. Additionally, it can be speculated that heterotrophic growth is more important in *D. acuta* than in *D. acuminata*. This last hypothesis agrees with results obtained by García-Portela et al. [33], who found *D. acuta* had a much higher survival (30% of the initial population) than *D. acuminata* (10%) after four weeks in dark conditions. This hypothesis implies that *D. acuta* will suffer more from lack of prey than *D. acuminata*. In addition, the same D:M ratio was provided, in all the experiments, to the two species, although *D. acuta* is three times larger in terms of biovolume [33].

To date, culture experiments have grown both the ciliate *M. rubrum* and its cryptophyte prey in f/2 medium [41–46]. In our work, cellular yields of *M. rubrum* were similar with K and f/2 media. The three culture media tested here (f/2(-Si), L1(-Si), and K(-Si)) have extremely high (880 µM) concentrations of nitrates. This excess of inorganic nutrients favors the autotrophic cryptophytes (e.g., *Teleaulax*), with a much higher growth rate than *M. rubrum* and *Dinophysis*. A frequent problem is that *Teleaulax* overgrows and even smothers *M. rubrum* cultures. This problem is exacerbated when the cryptophyte species/strain chosen is not the best ciliate's prey and grazing rates are lower [42,43]. This explains the common use of diluted f/2 medium in *Dinophysis* and *M. rubrum* culture experiments [33,34,41] in an attempt to prevent *Teleaulax* taking over.

In summary, K(-Si) is the best enrichment medium for growing *Dinophysis*, whether in small containers or in medium-scale volumes in photobioreactors. The use of diluted (1:20) L1(-Si) medium seems a good choice for long-term maintenance of *M. rubrum* and *Dinophysis* cultures. Despite showing lower cell densities than with full strength media, *Dinophysis* cells continue to grow and the risk of proliferation of *Ochromonas* and other contaminating small flagellates is reduced.

3.2. Optimal Cryptophyte Prey for M. rubrum *Growth*

M. rubrum cultures showed different lag phase patterns in response to the different cryptophyte prey provided. The *M. rubrum* culture used as inoculum had been fed with *P. prolonga* before three weeks of starvation preceding the experiment. Our initial interpretation is that *M. rubrum* inoculum was still adapted to grow with its most recent *P. prolonga* prey. It has been shown that *M. rubrum* can grow with different species belonging to the TPG clade, and that old plastids are replaced when a new prey species is provided [44,45]. Plastid replacement from *T. amphioxeia* to *T. acuta* took approximately two weeks in an earlier study and occurred when *M. rubrum* was fed with only the other *Teleaulax* species [44]. Thus, after a period of adaptation *M. rubrum* plastids reflect those of the new prey [44,45], but the length of the adaptation period will vary with different cryptophyte prey provided. Therefore, the inoculum cells of *M. rubrum* probably had all their plastids replaced from *P. prolonga* when experiment 3 began. This would explain the better performance of *M. rubrum* cultures fed *P. prolonga* in the first two weeks while in the other cultures, *M. rubrum* specimens were progressively replacing their old *P. prolonga* plastids with those from the new cryptophyte prey provided. But after *M. rubrum* replaced its plastids with those from the new prey, there was a remarkable change of trends. Thus, cultures of *M. rubrum* with *P. prolonga* (CR10EHU), *T. minuta* (CR8EHU), and the *T. amphioxeia* strain (VGO1392) from the Galician Rías reached similar final yields on day 23. In the meantime, *M. rubrum* cultures fed *T. amphioxeia* (AND-A071) from the same region as *M. rubrum* continued a sustained exponential growth ($\mu = 0.18\ d^{-1}$) for at least 12 more days, and reached a final yield 3-fold higher (up to 5×10^4 cell mL^{-1}) than the cell maxima attained with the other cryptophyte prey. These results agree with those reported by other authors who showed higher yields and growth rates for *M. rubrum* fed *T. amphioxeia* compared to other cryptophyte species [42,44].

It is worth highlighting that *M. rubrum* reached a much higher growth rate and final yield in cultures fed *T. amphioxeia* (AND-A070) from Huelva (southwest Spain) than with the same species, *T. amphioxeia* (VGO1392), with an identical partial plastid sequence, but from a different geographic area (Figure 8). The strain of *M. rubrum* (AND-A071) used in all the experiments was also isolated from Huelva. It has been claimed that *M. rubrum* exhibits genus-level but not species-level cryptophyte prey selection [44]. In the present work *M. rubrum* was grown with different species of *Teleaulax* and *Plagioselmis*, but best growth and yield were attained with the *T. amphioxeia* strain from the same location as the ciliate. It is possible that local adaptation allows a predator to recognize prey from the same geographical area. Alternatively, the two strains, despite having identical partial plastid sequences, may have other genetic differences that the southern strain of *M. rubrum* is able to recognize.

Attempts to establish cultures of our local strains of *M. rubrum* and *M. major* from the Galician Rías to test these hypotheses have been unsuccessful. But we must note here that some of the densest *Dinophysis* cultures cited in the literature [22,24,47] are fed with *M. rubrum* and its *T. amphioxeia* prey isolated from the same locality as the dinoflagellate. The partial plastid 23S rDNA sequence from the Galician *Mesodinium* species (*M. rubrum* and *M. major*) coincides with that from field specimens of *Dinophysis*, and is 1 bp different from *T. amphioxeia* [45]. This sequence does not coincide with any other from the TPG cryptophytes known in the region. It is quite possible that we will not be able to establish successful cultures of our local strains of *Mesodinium* until we isolate a *Teleaulax*-like cryptophyte with the same partial plastid 23S rDNA sequence.

3.3. *Best Results with Mass Production of* Dinophysis *and Other Considerations*

Some of the best results so far attained with *D. acuminata* cultures in our laboratory, in terms of sustained exponential growth (3 weeks) and high yields, were obtained using *M. rubrum* fed *T. minuta*, with a very favorable (1:20) predator:prey ratio (Figure 6). This fact suggests that the lack of our own optimal cryptophyte prey may be to some extent compensated by using a high *M. rubrum:Dinophysis* ratio. Until now, most laboratory studies applied a D:M ratio of 1:10 [41,42,46]. However, in the experiments reported by these authors, *M. rubrum* was added to the cultures every three to 14 days, while in our experiments *M. rubrum* was all added the first day of the experiment.

To our knowledge, this is the first report of a *D. acuminata* culture in a photobioreactor. *Dinophysis acuminata* numbers increased 7-fold in 20 days (from 2×10^6 to 13.8×10^6). These are not very high values and they could have been improved had our production of *Mesodinium* been better at that moment. But results from earlier studies confirmed here have shown that a good (1:10) D:M ratio is a key factor to achieve high dinoflagellate yields [41,42]. There is limited literature regarding the distribution of *Dinophysis* cells through the culture vessel. In our study, *D. acuminata* cells were aggregated at the base of the small-scale culture flasks but were swimming in the water column forming patches in the photobioreactor. This response may reflect a difference in the availability of light between the two culture systems. By design, the photobioreactors are light limited at the base (Figure 7), which may have triggered a phototropic response of the cells, resulting in vertical migration towards the upper illuminated layers.

3.4. *Variability in* Dinophysis *Cell Toxin Quota and Culture Strategies*

This work was focused on the growth of two species of *Dinophysis* and *M. rubrum* in culture. However, often the purpose of high biomass cultures is to have a clean and reliable source of toxins needed to prepare standards for chemical analyses in monitoring programs. Earlier studies in the Swedish fjords and the Galician Rias showed changes of one order of magnitude in the toxin content of the same species throughout their growing season [48,49]. Maximal toxin per cell was usually found at the stationary phase, both in the field [48–50] and laboratory experiments [51,52], due to an imbalance between toxin production and reduced division. This imbalance resulted in an increased toxin per-cell (particulate) accumulation but also to higher levels of extracellular toxins. The latter could represent a very high percentage of the total amount of toxins produced by the cells in the field [50] and in laboratory experiments [51,52].

Values of toxin per cell observed under different experimental conditions, working with the same strains of *D. acuminata* and *D. acuta* (this work and other studies discussed below), also revealed a large variability (Table 1). In addition to the already cited imbalance between growth and toxin production, leading to the highest cell toxin quota, some other factors can be envisaged from the values depicted in Table 1. For example, prey-limited cells of *D. acuminata* and *D. acuta* had higher toxin per cell than the parallel treatment with well-fed cells in experiments detailed by Portela et al. [34]. Lack of food (or the excess of it) has been already highlighted by other authors as a key factor promoting fast (well fed) or reduced (prey-limited) division [41,46]. Another striking observation is the high values of toxin per cell in well illuminated cultures versus those in low light conditions (Table 1). In that case, light seems to have had a strong and direct positive effect on toxin production. This effect would act presumably through the enhancement of photosynthetic activity required to generate reduction power to synthesize secondary metabolites (i.e., toxins) [41,47]. Some of the lowest values correspond to cells that were grown at the maximal temperature (19 °C) and light hours (16L:8D cycle) in experiment 3 of this work. These conditions favored a maximal division rate in *D. acuminata* and *D. acuta* cultures that were harvested for toxins extraction on day 6, during early exponential growth. It is well known that higher temperature (within a species-specific range) and hours of light promote higher division rates in *Dinophysis* cultures (33,41,47). Increased division "dilutes" the cell toxin quota. In other words, there is a negative correlation between division and toxin accumulation rates. The origin of the *Mesodinium* prey, i.e., a *M. rubrum* strain from Denmark versus the strain from southwest Spain used in this work, was also found to have an effect on *Dinophysis* growth and toxin accumulation [34,53].

Some extremely high values of cell toxin quota were observed in cultures growing in suboptimal conditions and with a very low division rate. That was the case with *D. acuta* fed a Danish strain of *M. rubrum* [34]. The record values of total toxin (particulate + dissolved, marked with an * in Table 1) per cell were observed in some mass cultures of *D. acuminata* grown for toxins sourcing and harvested with DIAON®adsorbing resins (Table 1 in bold). They corresponded to a slow growing, low-density (320 cells L^{-1}) culture of *D. acuminata* that was harvested at the stationary phase when nanoflagellate contamination was detected. Values of toxin per cell estimated when total toxins (harvested with resins) are measured are misleading. The dissolved toxins detected have been accumulated from the toxins released by cells growing in the preceding exponential phase of the culture, and which may have already died and contributed to the dissolved toxins pool. In these cases, it is more appropriate to express toxin content per unit of culture volume.

The development of passive samplers for in situ detection of lipophilic toxins with "solid-phase adsorption toxin tracking" (SPATT) resins provided a valuable new tool for the toxin dynamic studies [54]. Before that, extracellular toxins released by the cells in the water were not quantified. There is controversy on the advantages of the SPATT resins for early warning of *Dinophysis* blooms, but their value for research on physiology and toxin production dynamics is unquestionable [50]. The predominance of dissolved versus particulate toxins, detected with SPATT resins, has been reported in the stationary phase during blooms of *D. acuta* in New Zealand [54] and in laboratory experiments with the same species [52]. This observation led to the deployment of in situ toxin-harvesting devices as an alternative to cultures for toxins sourcing [55].

All the above observations give hints on the appropriate strategies to follow in order to get high numbers of toxic cells. *Dinophysis* cultures can be produced following two stages, with a different set of conditions promoting either growth or toxin accumulation. The first "production stage", will aim to reach the maximal cell density (yield) through good division rates. This will be supported by a high temperature (≥19 °C), favorable D:M ratio (20:1) using the preferred prey, and optimal light intensity according to each species/strain of *Dinophysis*. The second "seasoning stage", will aim to reach maximal values of toxin per cell and extracellular toxins This situation will be triggered via *Dinophysis* starvation, lowering the temperature and any additional factor contributing to an arrest of cellular division, i.e., forcing the imbalance between division and toxin production rates in favor of the latter.

4. Conclusions

Dinophysis acuminata and *D. acuta* exhibited higher growth rates when grown in K(-Si) medium, likely reflecting the presence of ammonia which is the preferred N source. *M. rubrum* showed a strain-specific growth response to the cryptophyte prey supplied: enhanced growth with *T. amphioxeia* isolated from the same geographic area (Huelva, southwest Spain) as compared with the same species from the Galician Rías (northwest Spain). Maximal growth rates in *D. acuminata* and *D. acuta* cultures were achieved with *M. rubrum* fed *T. amphioxeia* from the same region, therefore "what is better for *M. rubrum* is better for *Dinophysis*". The use of diluted L1 and f/2 media can be helpful for maintenance of *M. rubrum* and cryptophytes by keeping excessive cryptophyte growth and undesirable contaminants at bay. A favorable (1:20) D:M ratio, the key factor to high division rates, combined with the use of K(-Si) medium, may alleviate the lack of the optimal local cryptophye strain (of the *Teleaulax/Plagioselmis/Geminigera* clade), to produce mass cultures of *Dinophysis*. Galician *Mesodinium* and *Dinophysis* partial plastid 23S rDNA sequences differ by just one nucleotide from those in southern Spain specimens. This difference seems to suggest some degree of variability between those organisms affecting the growth of the southern *Mesodinium* with the northern cryptophyte prey. The lack of cultures of local strains of *Teleaulax*-like cryptophytes with the same partial 23S rDNA sequence could also explain unsuccesful attempts to establish cultures of the local *Mesodinium* species (*M. rubrum* and *M. major*) in the Galician Rías with the southern strains of *T. amphioxeia*. Practical recommendations for mass production of *Dinophysis* with high toxin content are given.

5. Materials and Methods

5.1. Cultures, Culturing Conditions, and Single-Cell Isolated Field Specimens

Dinophysis cultures were established from water samples from the Galician Rías Baixas (northwest Spain). *Dinophysis acuminata* (strain VGO1391) was isolated from Ría de Vigo in July 2016 and *D. acuta* (VGO1065) from Ría de Pontevedra in October 2010, both rías being part of the Galician Rías Baixas (northwest Spain). The ciliate *M. rubrum* (AND-A071) was isolated in 2007 from samples collected off Huelva (southwest Spain). Cryptophytes used in the culture experiments were from three different regions in Spain. *Teleaulax amphioxeia* (AND-A070) was isolated from samples off Huelva in 2007; another strain of *T. amphioxeia* (VGO1392) was isolated from Ría de Vigo (northwest Spain) in 2017, and the cryptophyte strains *Plagioselmis prolonga* (CR10EHU), *Teleaulax gracilis* (CR6EHU), and *Teleaulax minuta* (CR8EHU) from the Nervión River estuary, Bay of Biscay (north Spain). These cryptophytes have been found to be eaten by *M. rubrum* and plastid replacement in the ciliate with those of the new prey, demonstrated with partial sequencing of their 23S rDNA [45]. All cultures were grown with diluted (1:20) f/2 [29] or L1 medium [30] culture media prepared with autoclaved seawater at pH 8.00 ± 0.02 and salinity of 32 psu. They were kept in a temperature controlled room at 15 ± 1 °C and provided ~150 μmol photons m^2 s^{-1} PAR (photosynthetically active radiation) on a 12 h light:12 h dark cycle. Irradiance was delivered by Osram LED 30W-cold light, 6400 °K, tubes (OSRAM GmbH, Munich, Germany). All cultures were non-axenic.

A second species of *Mesodinium*, *M. major*, common in Galician coastal waters during blooms of *Dinophysis*, was considered in this study. Attempts to cultivate local strains of the two species of *Mesodinium*, *M. rubrum* and *M. major*, have been unsuccessful. Field specimens of *M. rubrum* and *M. major* were isolated from water samples from the Galician Rías for partial sequencing of their plastid gene 23S rDNA to compare it with those from cultivated *M. rubrum* (AND-A071), and with the local cultivated strains of *D. acuminata* (VGO1391), *D. acuta* (VGO1065), and *T. amphioxeia* (VGO1392). Cells were picked manually, one by one, with a capillary pipette under a Zeiss Invertoscop D (Karl Zeiss, Jena, Germany) microscope, washed in 3 drops of sterile distilled water and transferred to PCR tubes (see Section 5.8). Species identification of *Dinophysis* and *Mesodinium* species was based on morphological characteristics observed by light microscopy. A graphic diagram with the names of the species used in different experiments and their trophic interactions is shown in Figure 9.

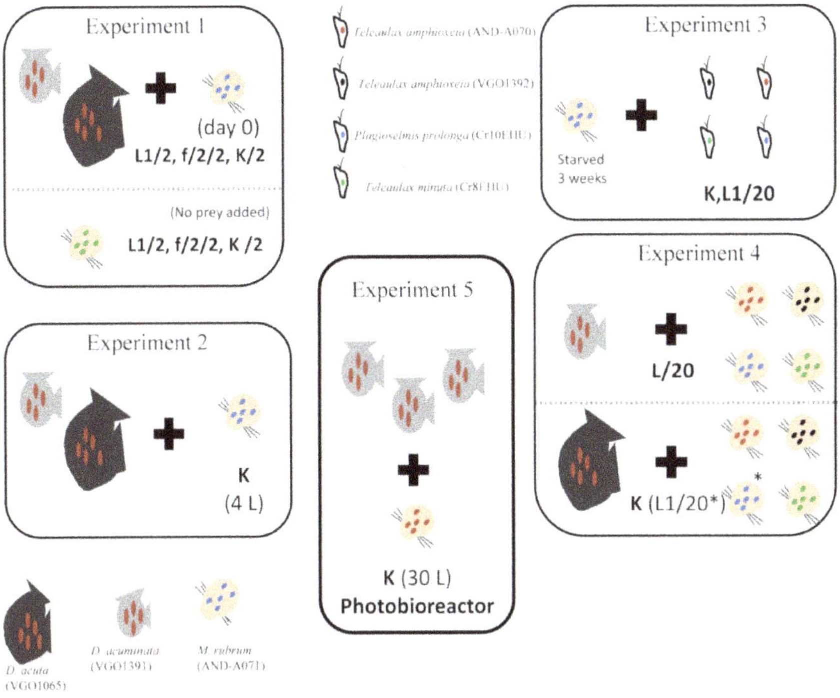

Figure 9. Graphic summary of the species/strains used in the experiments and trophic interactions investigated. Experiment 1: Phototrophic growth of *D. acuminata*, *D. acuta*, and *M. rubrum* with different culture media. Experiment 2: Scaling up mixotrophic cultures of *D. acuminata* and *D. acuta* with K medium. Experiment 3: Mixotrophic growth of *M. rubrum* with different cryptophytes. Experiment 4. Optimal cryptophyte prey for *M. rubrum* and best *M. rubrum* ratio to feed *Dinophysis*. All media were Si free and diluted (1:2). * indicates one treatment using L1 medium with a 1:20 dilution.

5.2. Cell Counts and Growth Rate Estimates

To estimate cell densities, specimens in 2 mL subsamples from 3 aliquots were fixed with acidic Lugol's solution (0.5%) and counted. *Dinophysis* species and *M. rubrum* were counted in a 1 mL Sedgwick-Rafter (Pyser-SGI S50, Pyser Optics, Kents, UK) counting chamber with a Zeiss Invertoscope D microscope at 100× or 250× magnification. Cryptophyte species were counted either in a 1 mL Sedgwick-Rafter chamber or in a Neubauer-type hemocytometer (depending on the cell density) at 200×.

Specific growth rates (μ) were calculated from

$$\mu = (\ln N_2 - \ln N_1 / t_2 - t_1)$$

where N_1 and N_2 denote cell numbers (cell mL^{-1}) recorded at time t_1 and t_2 (days), respectively.

A one-way ANOVA was used to identify significant differences in cell densities among treatments. Values of $p < 0.05$ were considered statistically significant. Statistical analyses were carried out with the RStudio, version 3.3.2, (RStudio, Boston, MA, USA).

5.3. Experiment 1. Phototrophic Growth of D. acuminata, D. acuta, and M. rubrum with Different Culture Media

Culture experiments were set up to compare phototrophic growth of *D. acuminata* and *D. acuta* grown in autoclaved seawater enriched with diluted (1:2) L1(-Si) [30], f/2(-Si) [29], and K(-Si) [36] culture media. To observe phototrophic growth of *Dinophysis*, without interferences from mixotrophic feeding, *M. rubrum*, previously fed *P. prolonga*, was added as prey only on day 0. Initial *Dinophysis* (D) cell concentrations were adjusted to approximately 150 and 200 cells mL^{-1} for *D. acuminata* and *D. acuta* respectively and *M. rubrum* (M) concentrations were adjusted to have a 1:10 D:M ratio.

To observe phototrophic growth of *M. rubrum*, cultures of the ciliate fed *T. minuta*, were deprived of prey for 3 weeks and the absence of cryptophyte cells confirmed by light microscopy observations. Thereafter, an experiment was run to compare phototrophic growth of *M. rubrum* in autoclaved seawater enriched with L1(-Si), f/2(-Si), and K(-Si) media. Experiments were carried out in triplicate in 250 mL Erlenmeyer flasks and the same conditions described in 5.1. Samples were collected every 2 d except in the case of the experiment with *D. acuta* (once a week) due to the already known very slow growth of this species when prey is not added [33].

5.4. Experiment 2. Scaling up Mixotrophic Cultures of D. acuminata *and* D. acuta *Cultures with K(-Si) Medium*

Dinophysis acuminata and *D. acuta* cultures volume was scaled-up from 100 mL to medium-scale volume (4 L) cultures. Mixotrophic cultures of *D. acuminata* and *D. acuta* were carried out three times in triplicate 4 L flasks with K(-Si) medium at 19 °C and provided 150–200 µmol photons m^2 s^{-1} PAR on a 16 h L:8 h D cycle. *Dinophysis* and *M. rubrum* cells, grown in autoclaved seawater enriched with K(-Si) medium, were previously acclimated to the culture parameters. The initial *Dinophysis* cell concentrations were adjusted to 200 cells mL^{-1} and the D:M ratio to 1:10 and then adjusted to 1:5 every 2 days.

Therefore, *D. acuminata* and *D. acuta* culture volumes were scaled-up periodically with *M. rubrum* grown with the cryptophyte *P. prolonga*. Samples were taken every day. On day 6, cultures were filtered through 25 mm GF/D glass microfiber filters (Cole-Parmer Instrument, Filter-Lab, Vernon, IL, USA), the filter with the filtered material placed in 15 mL centrifuge tubes and filled with MeOH (analytical grade) and kept in the deep-freeze at −20 °C until extraction for liquid chromatography coupled to tandem mass spectrometry (LC–MS/MS) analysis (see Sections 5.10 and 5.11).

5.5. Experiment 3. Mixotrophic Growth of M. rubrum *with Different Cryptophytes*

Mixotrophic growth of *M. rubrum* fed different cryptophyte species was studied. *M. rubrum* fed *P. prolonga* with K(-Si) medium was starved for 3 weeks and the absence of cryptophyte cells was confirmed with the light microscope before the experiment. Thereafter, three cryptophyte species, *T. amphioxeia* (strains AND-A070 and VGO1392), *T. minuta* (CR8EHU), and *P. prolonga* (CR10EHU), were given on day 0 to *M. rubrum* grown with K(-Si) medium to identify the optimal prey for the ciliate. The initial *M. rubrum* cell concentrations were adjusted to 10^3 cells mL^{-1} and a *M. rubrum:cryptophyte* (M:C) ratio of 1:10. Cultures of *M. rubrum* with *P. prolonga* and diluted (1:20) L1(-Si) medium were used as an internal control. All cultures were carried out in triplicate 250 mL Erlenmeyer flasks and the same conditions described in Section 5.1. Samples were taken every 2 days.

5.6. Experiment 4. Optimal Cryptophyte Prey for M. rubrum *and Best* M. rubrum *Ratio to Feed* Dinophysis

The next step was to investigate if the optimal prey for *M. rubrum* was also the best to feed *Dinophysis*. *M. rubrum* cultures, each one grown with different cryptophyte species (*T. amphioxeia*, AND-A070 and VGO1392; *T. minuta*, CR8EHU; *T. gracilis*, CR6EHU; and *P. prolonga*, CR10EHU) were provided as prey to *D. acuminata*, grown with L1/20(-Si) medium. Likewise, *M. rubrum* fed *T. amphioxeia* (AND-A070 and VGO1392), and *P. prolonga* (CR10EHU) was given to *D. acuta* (grown with K(-Si) and L1/20(-Si) medium) at day 0, to determine the optimal cryptophyte prey for *M. rubrum* to be used as prey for this species. The initial *Dinophysis* cell concentrations were adjusted to 150 cells mL^{-1} and the D:M ratio was 1:10. In addition, two culture experiments were carried out to compare *D. acuminata* mixotrophic growth in autoclaved seawater enriched with K(-Si) medium with *M. rubrum*, fed *T. minuta* (CR8EHU), added as prey only on day 0 and D:M ratios adjusted to 1:10 and 1:20 respectively. Cultures were carried out in triplicate 250 mL Erlenmeyer flasks and the same conditions described in Section 5.1. Samples were taken every 2 days.

5.7. Experiment 5. Mass Production of D. acuminata in 30 L Photobioreactors

Mixotrophic growth of *D. acuminata* in large volumes was studied in a photobioreactor. This photobioreactor, model AIS1316 from Aqualgae (Aqualgae S.L., A Coruña, Spain), has a polymethyl metacrylate (PPM), 250 mm diameter, and 30 L column supported on a stainless steel structure. Light is provided by 3 vertical LED tubes (cold light, 6400 °K); light intensity, photoperiod, temperature, and pH are controlled by an automatic mini-pic sensor (Siemens AG, Munich, Germany). Cultures in the photobioreactor were initiated with a volume of 12.5 L and a density of 160 cells mL^{-1} of *D. acuminata* in K(-Si) medium. No aeration was provided. *Dinophysis* (D) were fed *M. rubrum* (M) grown with *T. amphioxeia* (AND-A070) at a D:M ratio 1:1, 2–3 times a week. This ratio was readjusted to 1:5 D:M when a density of 500 cells mL^{-1} of *Dinophysis* was reached. Then it was adjusted to a 1:5 (D:M) ratio. Aliquots for cell counts were taken with a 5 mL pipette at the center of the water column after gentle circular agitation of the bioreactor. When the experiment finished, particulate and dissolved toxins were collected from the bioreactor with DIAON resins (see Section 5.10).

5.8. DNA Extraction, PCR Amplification and Sequencing

Field specimens isolated by micromanipulation (see Section 5.1) of *D. acuminata*, *D. acuta*, *M. rubrum*, and *M. cf. major* from the Galician Rías were transferred to 200 µL PCR tubes and kept at −20 °C for 24 h before direct amplification. For DNA extraction of species already in culture, 1 mL of each cryptophyte species used in the experiments, and of *M. rubrum* (AND-A071) were centrifuged for 5 min at ×12,000 *g* in a mini Spin Eppendorf centrifuge (Eppendorf AG, Hamburg, Germany), pellets rinsed in MilliQ water, centrifuged again, and then DNA was extracted using Chelex® 100 (Bio-Rad, Hercules, CA, USA) following the extraction procedure of Richlen & Barber [56]. For amplification of partial plastid 23S rDNA sequences, universal primers p23Sr_f1 (5′-GGA CAG AAA GAC CCT ATG AA-3′), and 23Sr_r1 (5′-TCA GCC TGT TAT CCC TAG AG-3′) [57] were used. The PCR reactions were performed using a thermocycler (Eppendorf AG, Hamburg, Germany), following the conditions detailed by these authors. PCR reaction mixtures (25 µL) contained 1 to 3 *Dinophysis* cells each, 1 mM $MgCl_2$, 2.5 µL 10× PCR buffer, 125 nM of each primer, 25 nM dNTPs, and 0.65 units Taq DNA polymerase (Bioline Reagents Ltd., London, UK). The PCR products were analyzed by 1.5% agarose gel electrophoresis. The amplified products were purified using an ExoSAP-IT (USB Corporation, Cleveland, OH, USA). Finally, the PCR products obtained were sequenced using the ABI PRISM BigDye Terminator Cycle Sequencing Ready Reaction Kit and an Applied Biosystems ABI 310 automated sequencer (CACTI, University of Vigo, Vigo, Pontevedra, Spain).

5.9. Phylogenetic Analysis

The partial sequences of plastid 23S rDNA (373bp) were aligned using CLUSTAL W [58] in Bioedit [59]. Phylogenetic analyses of 23S rDNA were performed using Tamura-Nei model [60]. Evolutionary analyses were conducted in MEGA 7, version 7.0. (Microsoft Windows applications, graphical user interface) [61]. Maximum likelihood (ML) phylogenetic analyses were conducted. The phylogenetic tree was represented using the ML method with bootstrap values ($n = 1000$). The tree with the highest log likelihood (−639.0779) was shown. The percentage of trees in which the associated taxa clustered together was shown next to the branches. Initial tree(s) for the heuristic search were obtained automatically by applying Neighbor-Joining and BioNJ algorithms to a matrix of pairwise distances estimated using the Maximum Composite Likelihood (MCL) approach, and then selecting the topology with superior log likelihood value. The tree was drawn to scale, with branch lengths measured in the number of substitutions per site. The analysis involved 17 sequences. Codon positions included were 1st + 2nd + 3rd + Noncoding. All positions containing gaps and missing data were eliminated.

5.10. *Harvesting and Total Toxin Extraction from* Dinophysis *Cultures*

Both particulate and extracellular toxins released in the culture medium from mass cultures produced to extract and biorefine toxins were harvested with polyaromatic adsorbent resin Diaion™ HP-20SS resin, Ø 75–150 µm SUPELCO (Bellefonte, PA, USA). First, *Dinophysis* cells were lysed by addition of acetone (final concentration 7%). Then the Diaion™ HP-20SS resin had to be activated before use, as described in MacKenzie et al. [54] and applied by Pizarro et al. [49,50]. In short, batches of adsorbent resin were washed several times with at least 10 volumes (10 solvent: 1 resin) of MeOH, to remove fines and leachable material; then, hydrated by soaking in MilliQ water, and drained through a 95 mm mesh sieve. Activated resin (2 g HP-2055 per L of culture) was added to the lysed-cells culture and stirred with a magnetic bar at low speed, very gently, for 24 h to ensure resuspension of the particles in the water column. After incubation, the resin retained by filtration over a mesh (20 µm), thoroughly rinsed with MilliQ water to remove salts from the culture medium, was transferred to a glass Petri dish. This was dried in an oven (3 h, 50 °C) and then kept at −20 °C until analysis.

5.11. *Toxin Analyses*

Toxin analyses were carried out at the Marine Institute in Galway, Ireland. The resin was transferred into a glass beaker and extracted by sonication with MeOH for 1 h. The extract was filtered through a SPE cartridge (empty with frit) and transferred into a volumetric flask. The remaining resin was further sonicated in MeOH several times until LC–MS/MS indicated that >95% of the toxin was extracted, with each extract decanted into the same volumetric flask which was then made up to volume with MeOH. Samples were filtered through a plugged (with cotton wool) glass pipette into HPLC vials for analysis. Next, they were hydrolyzed (to convert any OA group esters back to the parent compounds) by adding 125 µL 2.5 M NaOH to 1 mL of sample, placed in a water bath set at 76 °C for 10 min, cooled and then neutralized with 2.5 M HCl. Both the unhydrolyzed and the hydrolyzed samples were analyzed by LC–MS/MS to determine the level of esters present in the samples.

LC–MS/MS analysis of the resin extracts was carried out with a Waters Acquity UPLC system coupled to a Xevo G2-S QToF monitoring in MS^e mode in both positive and negative modes (m/z 100−1200), using leucine enkephalin as the reference compound. The cone voltage was 40 V, collision energy was 50 V, the cone and desolvation gas flows were set at 100 and 1000 L/h, respectively, and the source temperature was 120 °C. Analytical separation was performed on an Acquity UPLC BEH C18 (50 × 2.1 mm, 1.7 µm) column (Waters, Wexford, Ireland). Binary gradient elution was used, with phase A consisting of H_2O and phase B of CH_3CN (95%) in H_2O (both containing 2 mM ammonium formate and 50 mM formic acid). The injection volume was 2 µL and the column and sample temperatures were 25 °C and 6 °C, respectively.

In positive mode the gradient was from 30% to 90% B over 5 min at 0.3 mL/min, held for 0.5 min, and returned to the initial conditions and held for 1 min to equilibrate the system. Processing of results was performed using Waters Targetlynx software pulling out the masses for PTX2 (m/z 876.51 + 881.46). In negative mode the gradient was from 5% to 90% B over 2 min at 0.3 mL/min, held for 1 min, and returned to the initial conditions and held for 1 min to equilibrate the system.. Processing of results was performed using Waters Targetlynx software pulling out the mass for OA and DTX2 (m/z 803.45). PTX2, OA and DTX2 were quantitated using certified reference materials from the National Research Council, Canada.

Author Contributions: Conceptualization: J.H.-U., P.R., and B.R. Culture experiments: J.H.-U., P.R., M.G.-P., P.L., and A.F.-V. Toxin analysis: J.K. Formal analysis: J.H.-U., P.R., and M.G.-P. Funding acquisition: B.R. and F.R. Investigation: J.H.-U., P.R., M.G.-P., F.R., and B.R. Visualization: J.H.-U., P.R., and B.R. Writing—Original draft: J.H.-U., P.R., and B.R. Writing—Review and editing: J.H.-U., P.R., B.R., F.R., and J.K.

Funding: This research was funded by the MARBioFEED project which is supported by the first call for transnational research projects within the Marine Biotechnology ERA-NET; project no. 604814. ("Enhanced Biorefining Methods for the Production of Marine Biotoxins and Microalgae Fish Feed") and by Spanish project PCIN-2015-252, International Cooperation Programme, Ministry of Economy, Industry and Competition (MINEICO). M.G.-P. was supported by a MINEICO-PhD contract (BES-2014-067832).

Acknowledgments: We thank David Jaén (LCCRRPP, Huelva, Spain) for the kind supply of *M. rubrum* (AND-A0711) and *T. amphioxeia* (AND-A0710) from Huelva (western Andalucía, southwest Spain) and to Aitor Laza-Martínez for cryptophyte strains *P. prolonga* (CR10EHU), *T. gracilis* (CR6EHU), and *T. minuta* (CR8EHU) from the Nervión River estuary, Basque Country (North Spain).

Conflicts of Interest: The authors declare no conflicts of interest.

References

1. Yasumoto, T.; Murata, M.; Oshima, Y.; Sano, M.; Matsumoto, G.; Glardy, J. Diarrhetic Shellfish Toxins. *Tetrahedron* **1985**, *41*, 1019–1025. [CrossRef]
2. Reguera, B.; Pizarro, G. Planktonic dinoflagellates which produce polyether toxins of the old "DSP Complex". In *Seafood and Freshwater Toxins: Pharmacology, Physiology and Detection*, 2nd ed.; Botana, L.M., Ed.; Taylor & Francis: London, UK, 2008; pp. 257–284.
3. Domínguez, H.P.; Paz, B.; Daranas, A.H.; Norte, M.; Franco, J.M.; Fernández, J.J. Dinoflagellate polyether within the yessotoxin, pectenotoxin and okadaic acid toxin groups: Characterization, analysis and human health implications. *Toxicon* **2010**, *56*, 191–217. [CrossRef] [PubMed]
4. Miles, C.O.; Wilkins, A.L.; Munday, R.; Dines, M.H.; Hawkes, A.D.; Briggs, L.R.; Sandvik, M.; Jensen, D.J.; Cooney, J.M.; Holland, P.T.; et al. Isolation of pectenotoxin-2 from *Dinophysis acuta* and its conversion to pectenotoxin-2 seco acid, and preliminary assessment of their acute toxicities. *Toxicon* **2004**, *43*, 1–9. [CrossRef] [PubMed]
5. Anonymous. Regulation (EC)N°853/2004 of the European Parliament and of the Council of 29 April 2004 laying down specific hygiene rules for food of animal origin. *Off. Eur. Commun* **2004**, *139*, 55.
6. Reguera, B.; Riobó, P.; Rodríguez, F.; Díaz, P.; Pizarro, G.; Paz, B.; Franco, J.M.; Blanco, J. *Dinophysis* Toxins: Causative Organisms, Distribution and Fate in Shellfish. *Mar. Drugs* **2014**, *12*, 394–461. [CrossRef] [PubMed]
7. van Egmond, H.P.; Aune, T.; Lassus, P.; Speijers, G.J.A.; Waldock, M. Paralytic and diarrhoeic shellfish poisons: Occurrence in Europe, toxicity, analysis and regulation. *J. Nat. Toxins* **2004**, *2*, 41–82.
8. Vale, P.; Botelho, M.J.; Rodrigues, S.M.; Gomes, S.S.; Sampayo, M.A.M. Two decades of marine biotoxin monitoring in bivalves from Portugal (1986–2006): A review of exposure assessment. *Harmful Algae* **2008**, *7*, 11–25. [CrossRef]
9. Blanco, J.; Correa, J.; Muñiz, S.; Mariño, C.; Martín, H.; Arévalo, A. Evaluación del impacto de los métodos utilizados para el control de toxinas en el mejillón. *Revista Galega dos Recursos Mariños (Art. Inf. Technol.)* **2013**, *3*, 1–55.
10. Kim, G.Y.; Kim, W.J.; Choi, Y.H. Pectenotoxin-2 from Marine Sponges: A Potential Anti-Cancer Agent—A Review. *Mar. Drugs* **2011**, *9*, 2176–2187. [CrossRef] [PubMed]
11. Hwang, B.S.; Kim, H.S.; Jeong, E.J.; Rho, J.R. Acuminolide A: Structure and bioactivity of a new polyether macrolide from dinoflagellate *Dinophysis acuminata*. *Org. Lett.* **2014**, *16*, 5362–5365. [CrossRef] [PubMed]
12. Yih, W.; Rho, J.-R.; Kim, H.-S.; Kang, H.J. Methods for Massive Culture of Dinophysis acuminata and Isolation of Pectenotoxin-2. U.S. Patent No. US008247213B2, 21 August 2012.
13. Schnepf, E.; Elbrächter, M. Cryptophycean-like double membrane-bound chloroplast in the dinoflagellate *Dinophysis* Ehrenb.: Evolutionary, phylogenetic and toxicological implications. *Bot. Acta* **1998**, *101*, 196–203. [CrossRef]
14. Maestrini, S.Y. Bloom dynamics and ecophysiology of *Dinophysis* spp. In *Physiological Ecology of Harmful Algal Blooms*; Anderson, D.M., Cembella, A.D., Hallegraeff, G.M., Eds.; NATO ASI Series, Series G, Ecological Science; Springer: Berlin/Heidelberg, Germany; New York, NY, USA, 1998; pp. 243–266.
15. Jacobson, D.M.; Andersen, R.A. The discovery of mixotrophy in photosynthetic species of *Dinophysis* (Dinophyceae): Light and electron microscopical observations of food vacuoles in *Dinophysis acuminata*, *D. norvegica* and two heterotrophic dinophysoid dinoflagellates. *Phycologia* **1994**, *33*, 97–110. [CrossRef]
16. Takishita, K.; Koike, K.; Maruyama, T.; Ogata, T. Molecular Evidence for Plastid Robbery (Kleptoplastidy) in *Dinophysis*, a Dinoflagellate causing Diarrhetic Shellfish Poisoning. *Protist* **2002**, *153*, 293–302. [CrossRef] [PubMed]

17. Takahashi, Y.; Takishita, K.; Koike, K.; Maruyama, T.; Nakayama, T.; Kobiyama, A.; Ogata, T. Development of molecular probes for *Dinophysis* (Dinophyceae) plastid: A tool to predict blooming and explore plastid origin. *Mar. Biotechnol.* **2005**, *7*, 95–103. [CrossRef] [PubMed]
18. Nishitani, G.; Miyamura, K.; Imai, I. Trying to cultivation of *Dinophysis caudata* (Dinophyceae) and the appearence of small cells. *Plankton Biol. Ecol.* **2003**, *50*, 31–36.
19. Janson, S. Molecular evidence that plastids in the toxin-producing dinoflagellate genus *Dinophysis* originate from the free-living cryptophyte *Teleaulax amphioxeia*. *Environ. Microbiol.* **2004**, *6*, 1102–1106. [CrossRef] [PubMed]
20. Gustafson, J.D.E.; Stoecker, D.K.; Johnson, M.D.; Van Heukelem, W.F.; Sneider, K. Cryptophyte algae are robbed of their organelles by the marine ciliate *Mesodinium rubrum*. *Nature* **2000**, *405*, 1049–1052. [CrossRef] [PubMed]
21. Yih, W.; Kim, H.S.; Jeong, H.J.; Myung, G.; Kim, Y.G. Ingestion of cryptophyte cells by the marine photosynthetic ciliate *Mesodinium rubrum*. *Aquat. Microb. Ecol.* **2004**, *36*, 165–170. [CrossRef]
22. Park, M.G.; Kim, S.; Kim, H.S.; Myung, G.; Kang, Y.G.; Yih, W. First successful culture of the marine dinoflagellate *Dinophysis acuminata*. *Aquat. Microb. Ecol.* **2006**, *45*, 101–106. [CrossRef]
23. Jaen, D.; Mamán, L.; Domínguez, R.; Martín, E. First report of *Dinophysis acuta* in culture. *Harmful Algae News* **2009**, *39*, 1–2.
24. Nishitani, G.; Nagai, S.; Sakiyama, S.; Kamiyama, T. Successful cultivation of the toxic dinoflagellate *Dinophysis caudata* (Dinophyceae). *Plankton Benthos Res.* **2008**, *3*, 78–85. [CrossRef]
25. Nagai, S.; Nitshitani, G.; Tomaru, Y.; Sakiyama, S.; Kamiyama, T. Predation by the toxic dinoflagellate *Dinophysis fortii* on the ciliate *Myrionecta rubra* and observation of sequestration of ciliate chloroplasts. *J. Phycol.* **2008**, *44*, 909–922. [CrossRef] [PubMed]
26. Nishitani, G.; Nagai, S.; Takano, Y.; Sakiyama, S.; Baba, K.; Kamiyama, T. Growth charareristics and phylogenetic analysis of the marine dinoflagellate *Dinophysis infundibulus* (Dinophyceae). *Aquat. Microb. Ecol.* **2008**, 209–221. [CrossRef]
27. Riobó, P.; Reguera, B.; Franco, J.M.; Rodríguez, F. First report of the toxin profile of *Dinophysis sacculus* Stein from LC–MS analysis of laboratory cultures. *Toxicon* **2013**, *76*, 221–224. [CrossRef] [PubMed]
28. Rodríguez, F.; Escalera, L.; Reguera, B.; Rial, P.; Riobó, P.; de Jesús da Silva, T. Morphological variability, toxinology and genetics of the dinoflagellate *Dinophysis tripos* (Dinophysiaceae, Dinophysiales). *Harmful Algae* **2012**, *13*, 26–33. [CrossRef]
29. Guillard, R.R.L.; Ryther, J.H. Studies of marine planktonic diatoms. I. *Cyclotella nana* Hustedt and *Detonula confervacea* (Cleve). *Can. J. Microbiol.* **1962**, *8*, 229–239. [CrossRef] [PubMed]
30. Guillard, R.R.L.; Hargraves, P.E. *Stichochrysis immobilis* is a diatom, not a Chrysophyte. *Phycologia* **1993**, *32*, 234–236. [CrossRef]
31. Hansen, P.J.; Nielsen, L.T.; Johnson, M.; Berge, T.; Flynn, K.J. Acquired phototrophy in *Mesodinium* and *Dinophysis*–A review of cellular organization, prey selectivity, nutrient uptake and bioenergetics. *Harmful Algae* **2013**, *28*, 126–139. [CrossRef]
32. Mitra, A.; Flynn, K.J.; Tillmann, U.; Raven, J.A.; Caron, D.; Stoecker, D.K.; Not, F.; Hansen, P.J.; Hallegraeff, G.; Sanders, R.; et al. Defining Planktonic Protist Functional Groups on Mechanism for Energy and Nutrient Acquisition: Incorporation of Diverse Mixotrophic Strategies. *Protist* **2016**, *167*, 106–120. [CrossRef] [PubMed]
33. García-Portela, M.; Riobó, P.; Reguera, B.; Garrido, J.; Blanco, J.; Rodríguez, F. Comparative ecophysiology of *Dinophysis acuminata* and *D. acuta*: Effect of light intensity and quality on growth, cellular toxin content and photosynthesis. *J. Phycol.* [CrossRef]
34. García-Portela, M.; Reguera, B.; Sibat, M.; Altenburger, A.; Rodríguez, F.; Hess, P. Metabolomic profiles of *Dinophysis acuminata* and *Dinophysis acuta* using non-targeted high-resolution mass espectrometry: Effect of nutritional status and prey. *Mar. Drugs* **2018**, *16*, 143–168. [CrossRef] [PubMed]
35. García-Portela, M.; Reguera, B.; Ribera d'Alcalà, M.; Rodríguez, F.; Montresor, M. The turbulent life of *Dinophysis*. In Proceedings of the 18th International Conference on Harmful Algae, Nantes, France, 21–26 October 2018; Book of Abstracts O-051. p. 64.
36. Keller, M.D.; Selvin, R.C.; Claus, W.; Guillard, R.R. Media for the culture of oceanic ultraphytoplankton. *J. Phycol.* **1987**, *23*, 633–638. [CrossRef]

37. Tong, M.; Smith, J.L.; Kulis, D.M.; Anderson, D.M. Role of dissolved nitrate and phosphate in isolates of *Mesodinium rubrum* and toxin-producing *Dinophysis acuminata*. *Aquat. Microb. Ecol.* **2015**, *75*, 169–185. [CrossRef] [PubMed]
38. Seeyave, S.; Probyn, T.A.; Pitcher, G.C.; Lucas, M.I.; Purdie, D.A. Nitrogen nutrition in assemblages dominated by *Pseudo-nitzschia* spp., *Alexandrium catenella* and *Dinophysis acuminata* off the west coast of South Africa. *Mar. Ecol. Prog. Ser.* **2009**, *379*, 91–107. [CrossRef]
39. Hattenrath-Lehmann, T.; Gobler, C.J. The contribution of inorganic and organic nutrients to the growth of a North American isolate of the mixotrophic dinoflagellate, *Dinophysis acuminata*. *Limnol. Oceanogr.* **2015**, *60*, 1588–1603. [CrossRef]
40. García-Portela, M. Comparative Ecophysiology of Two Mixotrophic Species of *Dinophysis* Producers of Lipophilic Toxins. Ph.D Thesis, Univerdidad de Vigo, Vigo, Spain, 2018.
41. Smith, M.; Hansen, P.J. Interaction between *Mesodinium rubrum* and its prey: Importance of prey concentration, irradiance and pH. *Mar. Ecol. Prog. Ser.* **2007**, *338*, 61–70. [CrossRef]
42. Park, J.S.; Myung, G.; Kim, H.S.; Cho, B.C.; Yih, W. Growth responses of the marine photosynthetic ciliate *Myrionecta rubra* to different cryptomonad strains. *Aquat. Microb. Ecol.* **2007**, *48*, 83–90. [CrossRef]
43. Myung, G.; Kim, H.S.; Park, J.S.; Park, M.G.; Yih, W. Population growth and plastid type of *Myrionecta rubra* depend on the kinds of available cryptomonad prey. *Harmful Algae* **2011**, *10*, 536–541. [CrossRef]
44. Peltomaa, E.; Johnson, M.D. *Mesodinium rubrum* exhibits genus-level but not species-level cryptophyte prey selection. *Aquat. Microb. Ecol.* **2017**, *78*, 147–159. [CrossRef]
45. Rial, P.; Laza-Martínez, A.; Reguera, B.; Raho, N.; Rodríguez, F. Origin of cryptophyte plastids in *Dinophysis* from Galician waters: Results from field and culture experiments. *Aquat. Microb. Ecol.* **2015**, *76*, 163–174. [CrossRef]
46. Gao, H.; Hua, C.; Tong, M. Impact of *Dinophysis acuminata* feeding *Mesodinium rubrum* on nutrient dynamics and bacterial composition in a microcosm. *Toxins* **2018**, *10*, 443. [CrossRef] [PubMed]
47. Nielsen, L.T.; Krock, B.; Hansen, P.J. Effects of light and food availability on toxin production, growth and photosynthesis in *Dinophysis acuminata*. *Mar. Ecol. Prog. Ser.* **2012**, *471*, 37–50. [CrossRef]
48. Lindahl, O.; Lundve, B.; Johansen, M. Toxicity of *Dinophysis* spp. in relation to population abundance and environmental condition on the Swedish west coast. *Harmful Algae* **2007**, *6*, 218–231. [CrossRef]
49. Pizarro, G.; Paz, B.; González-Gil, S.; Franco, J.M.; Reguera, B. Seasonal variability of lipophilic toxins during a *Dinophysis acuta* bloom in Western Iberia: Differences between picked cells and plankton concentrates. *Harmful Algae* **2009**, *8*, 926–937. [CrossRef]
50. Pizarro, G.; Moroño, A.; Paz, B.; Franco, J.M.; Reguera, B. Evaluation of passive samples as a monitoring tool for early warning of *Dinophysis* toxins in shelfish. *Mar. Drugs* **2013**, *11*, 3823–3845. [CrossRef] [PubMed]
51. Tong, M.M.; Kulis, D.M.; Fux, E.; Smith, J.L.; Hess, P.; Zhou, Q.X.; Anderson, D.M. The effects of growth phase and light intensity on toxin production by *Dinophysis acuminata* from the northeastern United States. *Harmful Algae* **2011**, *10*, 254–264. [CrossRef]
52. Nielsen, L.T.; Krock, B.; Hansen, P.J. Production and excretion of okadaic acid, pectenotoxin-2 and a novel dinophysistoxin from the DSP-causing marine dinoflagellate *Dinophysis acuta*—Effects of light, food availability and growth phase. *Harmful Algae* **2013**, *23*, 34–45. [CrossRef]
53. Smith, J.L.; Tong, M.; Kulis, D.; Anderson, D.M. Effect of ciliate strain, size, and nutritional content on the growth and toxicity of mixotrophic *Dinophysis acuminata*. *Harmful Algae* **2018**, *78*, 95–105. [CrossRef] [PubMed]
54. MacKenzie, L.; Beuzenberg, V.; Holland, P.; McNabb, P.; Selwood, A. Solid phase adsorption toxin tracking (SPATT): A new monitoring tool that simulates the biotoxin contamination of filter feeding bivalves. *Toxicon* **2004**, *44*, 901–918. [CrossRef] [PubMed]
55. Rundberget, T.; Sandvik, M.; Larsen, K.; Pizarro, G.M.; Reguera, B.; Castberg, T.; Gustad, E.; Loader, J.I.; Rise, F.; Wilkins, A.L.; et al. Extraction of microalgal toxins by large-scale pumping of seawater in Spain and Norway, and isolation of okadaic acid and dinophysistoxin-2. *Toxicon* **2007**, *50*, 960–970. [CrossRef] [PubMed]
56. Richlen, M.L.; Barber, P.H. A technique for the rapid extraction of microalgal DNA from single live and preserved cells. *Mol. Ecol. Notes* **2005**, *5*, 688–691. [CrossRef]
57. Sherwood, A.R.; Presting, G.G. Universal primers amplify a 23S rDNA plastid marker in Eukaryotic algae and Cyanobacteria. *J. Phycol.* **2007**, *43*, 605–608. [CrossRef]

58. Thompson, J.D.; Higgins, D.G.; Gibson, T.J. CLUSTAL W:Improving the sensivity of progresive multiple sequence alignement though sequence weighting, position specific gap penalties and matrix choice. *Nucleic Aids Res.* **1994**, *22*, 4673–4680. [CrossRef]
59. Hall, T.A. BioEdit: A user-friendly biological sequence alignment editor and analysis program for Windows 95/98/NT. *Nucl. Acids Symp. Ser.* **1999**, *41*, 95–98.
60. Tamura, K.; Nei, M. Estimation of the number of nucleotide substitutions in the control region of mitochondrial DNA in humans and chimpanzees. *Mol. Biol. Evol.* **1993**, *10*, 512–526. [PubMed]
61. Kumar, S.; Stecher, G.; Tamura, K. MEGA7: Molecular evolutionary Genetics Analysis version 7.0 for bigger datasets. *Mol. Biol. Evol.* **2016**, *33*, 1870–1874. [CrossRef] [PubMed]

toxins

MDPI

Article

Toxin Profiles of Okadaic Acid Analogues and Other Lipophilic Toxins in *Dinophysis* from Japanese Coastal Waters

Hajime Uchida [1], Ryuichi Watanabe [1], Ryoji Matsushima [1], Hiroshi Oikawa [1], Satoshi Nagai [1], Takashi Kamiyama [2], Katsuhisa Baba [3], Akira Miyazono [4], Yuki Kosaka [5], Shinnosuke Kaga [6], Yukihiko Matsuyama [7] and Toshiyuki Suzuki [1,*]

1. National Research Institute of Fisheries Science, Japan Fisheries Research and Education Agency, 2-12-4 Fukuura, Kanazawa-ku, Yokohama, Kanagawa 236-8648, Japan; huchida@affrc.go.jp (H.U.); rwatanabe@affrc.go.jp (R.W.); matsur@affrc.go.jp (R.M.); oikawah@affrc.go.jp (H.O.); snagai@affrc.go.jp (S.N.)
2. National Research Institute of Fisheries and Environment of Inland Sea, Japan Fisheries Research and Education Agency, 2-17-5, Maruishi, Hatsukaichi, Hiroshima 739-0452, Japan; kamiyama@affrc.go.jp
3. Central Fisheries Research Institute, Fisheries Research Department, Hokkaido Research Organization, 238, Hamanakacho, Yoichi-cho, Yoichi-gun, Hokkaido 046-8555, Japan; baba-katuhisa@hro.or.jp
4. Kushiro Fisheries Research Institute, Fisheries Research Department, Hokkaido Research Organization, 4-25, Nakahamacho, Kushiro-city, Hokkaido 085-0027, Japan; miyazono-akira@hro.or.jp
5. Aomori Prefectural Industrial Technology Research Center, Fisheries Research Institute, Hiranai, Higashitsugarugun, Aomori 039-3381, Japan; yuuki_kosaka@aomori-itc.or.jp
6. Iwate Fisheries Technology Center, 3-75-3 Hirata, Kamaishi, Iwate 026-0001, Japan; s-kaga@pref.iwate.jp
7. Seikai National Fisheries Research Institute, Japan Fisheries Research and Education Agency, 1551-8, Taira-machi, Nagasaki-shi, Nagasaki 851-2213, Japan; yukihiko@affrc.go.jp

* Correspondence: tsuzuki@affrc.go.jp; Tel.: +81-45-788-7662; Fax: +81-45-788-5001

Received: 23 September 2018; Accepted: 4 November 2018; Published: 6 November 2018

Abstract: The identification and quantification of okadaic acid (OA)/dinophysistoxin (DTX) analogues and pectenotoxins (PTXs) in *Dinophysis* samples collected from coastal locations around Japan were evaluated by liquid chromatography mass spectrometry. The species identified and analyzed included *Dinophysis fortii*, *D. acuminata*, *D. mitra* (*Phalacroma mitra*), *D. norvegica*, *D. infundibulus*, *D. tripos*, *D. caudata*, *D. rotundata* (*Phalacroma rotundatum*), and *D. rudgei*. The dominant toxin found in *D. acuminata* was PTX2 although some samples contained DTX1 as a minor toxin. *D. acuminata* specimens isolated from the southwestern regions (Takada and Hiroshima) showed characteristic toxin profiles, with only OA detected in samples collected from Takada. In contrast, both OA and DTX1, in addition to a larger proportion of PTX2, were detected in *D. acuminata* from Hiroshima. *D. fortii* showed a toxin profile dominated by PTX2 although this species had higher levels of DTX1 than *D. acuminata*. OA was detected as a minor toxin in some *D. fortii* samples collected from Yakumo, Noheji, and Hakata. PTX2 was also the dominant toxin found among other *Dinophysis* species analyzed, such as *D. norvegica*, *D. tripos*, and *D. caudata*, although some pooled picked cells of these species contained trace levels of OA or DTX1. The results obtained in this study re-confirm that cellular toxin content and profiles are different even among strains of the same species.

Keywords: *Dinophysis*; diarrhetic shellfish poisoning; marine toxins; pectenotoxin; okadaic acid; dinophysistoxin

Key Contribution: Pooled picked cells of *Dinophysis* species collected from locations around Japan were analyzed by liquid chromatography mass spectrometry to determine their toxin content and relative toxin profiles.

1. Introduction

The diarrhetic shellfish toxins (DSTs), okadaic acid (OA) and dinophysistoxins (DTXs), as well as pectenotoxins (PTXs) (Figure 1) [1], are produced by planktonic species of the genus, *Dinophysis* and benthic species of *Prorocentrum* [2]. Bivalves become contaminated with these marine toxins by feeding on toxic *Dinophysis* species. The regulation of DSTs recommended by Codex Alimentarius [3] is 160 ng OA equivalent/g in the edible part of bivalves. The regulation in the European Union (EU) is a total of 160 ng OA/DTX and PTXs/g in the edible part of bivalves [4]. The cellular toxin content and profiles of several *Dinophysis* species have been reported by analyzing field multispecific samples obtained by plankton net hauls, or monospecific cultures [5–18]. However, it remains important to update toxin content and profile information of *Dinophysis* species to improve the prediction of bivalve contamination. The cellular toxin content and profiles of *Dinophysis* species of pooled picked cells reported in previous studies was revised (Table 1) [19–35]. Analysis of individually picked cells was historically the only unambiguous way to ascribe a toxin profile and content information to a *Dinophysis* species, until 2006, when cultures of *D. acuminata* became available [36]. Because the cellular toxin content and profiles are different even among samples of the same species [36,37], it is necessary to clarify cellular toxin contents and profiles of *Dinophysis* spp. present in each bivalve monitoring area.

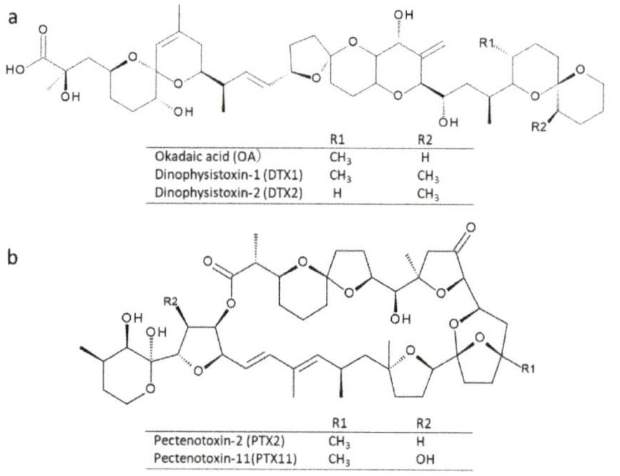

	R1	R2
Okadaic acid (OA)	CH_3	H
Dinophysistoxin-1 (DTX1)	CH_3	CH_3
Dinophysistoxin-2 (DTX2)	H	CH_3

	R1	R2
Pectenotoxin-2 (PTX2)	CH_3	H
Pectenotoxin-11(PTX11)	CH_3	OH

Figure 1. Chemical structure of okadaic acid (OA) and dinophysistoxin (DTX) and pectenotoxin (PTX) analogues found in *Dinophysis* species. (**a**) OA and DTX analogues. (**b**) PTX2 and PTX11.

Historically, DST contamination of bivalves, and associated human poisoning cases, were restricted in the northeastern regions of Japan (Tohoku and Hokkaido area). Therefore, data on the toxin content and profiles of *Dinophysis* from these regions is essential for predicting bivalve contamination. Although *Dinophysis* occurs in the southwestern parts of Japan, no toxin information has been reported for *Dinophysis* species found there. It is interesting that DST positive cases in bivalves obtained with the previous DST official testing method (mouse bioassay) in the southwestern parts of Japan have hardly been reported.

Between 2006 and 2014, pooled picked cells of many *Dinophysis* species were generated from seawater samples taken from many locations around the Japanese coastline. DSTs and PTXs were extracted using a solid phase extraction method [6,19,23], and the extracts kept frozen until analysis. In this study, the presence of DSTs and PTXs in these samples was determined by liquid chromatography triple quadrupole tandem mass spectrometry (LC/MS/MS) [23] and liquid chromatography quadrupole mass spectrometry (LC/MS) [38].

Table 1. Reported toxin content and profiles in pooled picked cell isolates of *Dinophysis* field specimens.

Species	pg/cell				Location	Analysis Method	Reference
	OA	DTX1	DTX2	PTX2			
Dinophysis acuminata	1.6	-	-	-	Le Havre, France	HPLC-FLD	[19]
	Trace	-	-	-	Tokyo Bay, Japan	HPLC-FLD	[19]
	9.1	-	-	-	Gullmar, Sweden	HPLC-FLD	[20]
	9.9–21.7	-	-	-	Galicia, Spain	HPLC-FLD	[21]
	-	-	-	180.0	Bahia Inglesa, Chile	LC/MS/MS	[22]
	-	0.3–0.7	-	10.7–22.4	Abashiri, Japan	LC/MS/MS	[23]
	-	ND–0.7	-	25.9–50.2	Yakumo, Japan	LC/MS/MS	[23]
	ND–0.8	-	-	0.9–8.7	Flødevigen Bay, Noway	LC/MS/MS	[24]
	3.7	-	-	-	Bueu, Spain	LC/MS/MS	[25]
Dinophysis fortii	-	13.0–191.5	-	42.5	Mutsu Bay, Japan	HPLC-FLD	[19]
	23.0	-	-	-	Inland Sea, Japan	HPLC-FLD	[19]
	ND–57.7	ND–16.0	-	-	Ofunato, Japan	HPLC-FLD	[26]
	-	8.4–10.9	-	51.4–63.8	Yakumo, Japan	LC/MS/MS	[23]
Dinophysis acuta	9.4	-	-	-	Vigo, Spain	HPLC-FLD	[19]
	4.0	4.2	-	-	Sogndal, Norway	HPLC-FLD	[19]
	-	6.6	-	-	Gullmar, Sweden	HPLC-FLD	[20]
	58.0	-	78.0	-	Ireland	HPLC-FLD	[27]
	6.3–33.1	-	1.0–22.0	-	Galicia, Spain	HPLC-FLD	[21]
	85.0	-	77.0	14.0	Glandore, Ireland	LC/MS/MS	[28]
	-	-	-	29.1–32.3	Galicia, Spain	LC/MS/MS	[29]
	0.7–9.4	-	0.9–6.6	0.3–3.3	Pontevedra, Spain	LC/MS	[30]
	1.0–8.5	-	-	0.2–3.3	Flødevigen Bay, Noway	LC/MS/MS	[24]
	2.9	-	1.9	1.5	Bueu, Spain	LC/MS/MS	[25]
Dinophysis caudata	0.7	-	-	-	Galicia, Spain	HPLC-FLD	[21]
	7.9–56.5	ND–53.9	-	-	Sapian, Phillipines	HPLC-FLD	[31]
	-	-	-	100.0–127.4	Galicia, Spain	LC/MS/MS	[29]
	0.6	-	2.8	5.0	Moana, Spain	LC/MS/MS	[25]
	-	-	-	2.0–14.5	Day Bay, China	LC/MS/MS	[32]
Dinophysis infundibulus	-	-	-	14.8	Yakumo, Japan	LC/MS/MS	[23]
Dinophysis miles	5.7–20.9	ND–10.7	-	-	Sapian, Phillipines	HPLC-FLD	[31]

Table 1. *Cont.*

Species	pg/cell				Location	Analysis Method	Reference
	OA	DTX1	DTX2	PTX2			
Dinophysis mitra	-	10.0	-	-	Mutsu Bay, Japan	HPLC-FLD	[19]
	-	-	-	-	Yakumo, Japan	LC/MS/MS	[23]
Dinophysis norvegica	-	14.0	-	-	Sogndal, Norway	HPLC-FLD	[19]
	-	-	-	50.8–67.4	Yakumo, Japan	LC/MS/MS	[23]
	ND–0.2	-	-	0.3–1.7	Flødevigen Bay, Noway	LC/MS/MS	[24]
Dinophysis ovum	7.1	-	-	-	Vigo, Spain	LC/MS/MS	[33]
Dinophysis rotundata	ND–0.4	-	ND–0.5	ND–0.3	Bueu, Spain	LC/MS/MS	[34]
	-	101.0	-	-	Mutsu Bay, Japan	HPLC-FLD	[19]
	-	-	-	-	Yakumo, Japan	LC/MS/MS	[23]
	-	-	-	0.8	Flødevigen Bay, Noway	LC/MS/MS	[24]
Dinophysis sacculus	16.5	-	-	-	Le Croisic, France	HPLC-FLD	[35]
	14.0	-	-	-	Morgat, France	HPLC-FLD	[35]
	29.6	-	-	-	Kervel, France	HPLC-FLD	[35]
	12.9	-	-	-	Pont-Aven, France	HPLC-FLD	[35]
Dinophysis skagii	-	-	-	-	Bueu, Spain	LC/MS/MS	[25]
Dinophysis tripos	-	36.0	-	-	Kesennuma, Japan	HPLC-FLD	[19]
	-	-	-	-	Yakumo, Japan	LC/MS/MS	[23]

2. Results

2.1. *Dinophysis acuminata*

The toxin content and profiles of *D. acuminata* obtained in this study are shown in Figure 2 and Table S1. The dominant toxin in *D. acuminata* samples from Yakumo, Saroma, and Shimonoseki was PTX2, and DTX1 was also observed at lower levels in some samples from Yakumo and Saroma. The DTX1 content (4.7 pg/cell) found in *D. acuminata* sample collected in Saroma was greater than the highest value of (0.7 pg/cell) reported in previous studies (Table 1) [23]. The toxin profile and contents found from *D. acuminata* in Yakumo were close to those obtained in a previous study for *D. acuminata* in the same area [23]. It is interesting that *D. acuminata* collected in Uramura did not produce any of the monitored toxins. *D. acuminata* collected in Takada and Hiroshima showed characteristic toxin profiles, with OA exclusively detected in *D. acuminata* collected in Takada, whereas both OA and DTX1, in addition to a higher proportions of PTX2, were detected in *D. acuminata* from Hiroshima.

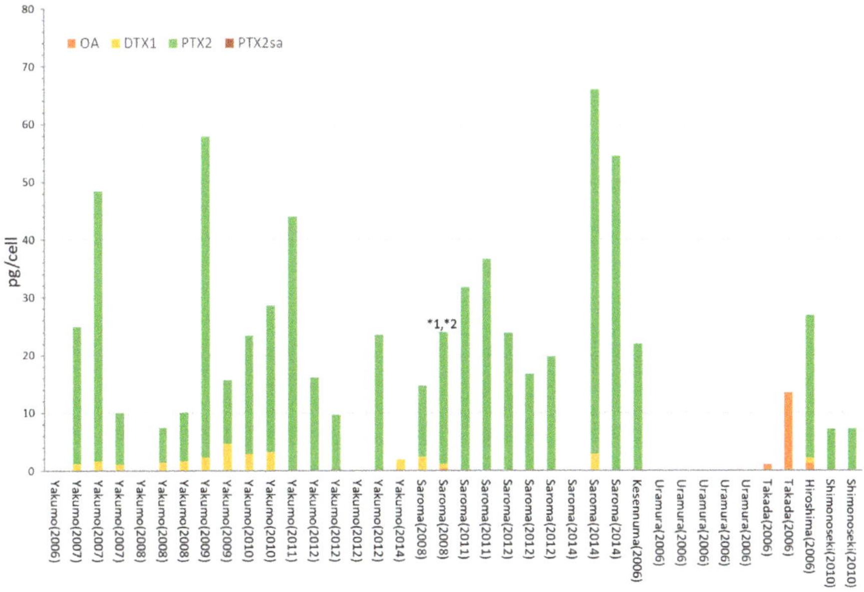

Figure 2. The toxin contents and profiles of *D. acuminata* in Japan. * 1 Trace levels of OA were detected. * 2 Trace levels of DTX1 were detected. The toxin contents, profiles, analyzed cell numbers, and detection limits for negative values are also given in Table S1.

2.2. *Dinophysis fortii*

The toxin content and profiles of *D. fortii* obtained in the present study are shown in Figure 3 and Table S1. Although the dominant toxin observed in *D. fortii* samples was PTX2, some samples also produced DTX1 or OA. The DTX1 content found in many *D. fortii* samples was considerably higher than that in *D. acuminata*. OA was detected as a minor toxin in some samples collected from Noheji and Yakumo. Several *D. fortii* samples from Noheji and Yakumo did not have any of the monitored toxins. PTX2 seco-acid was detected in *D. fortii* collected in Hakata. The PTX2 content (236.0 pg/cell) of *D. fortii* collected in Akita represents the highest value ever reported (Table 1) [23].

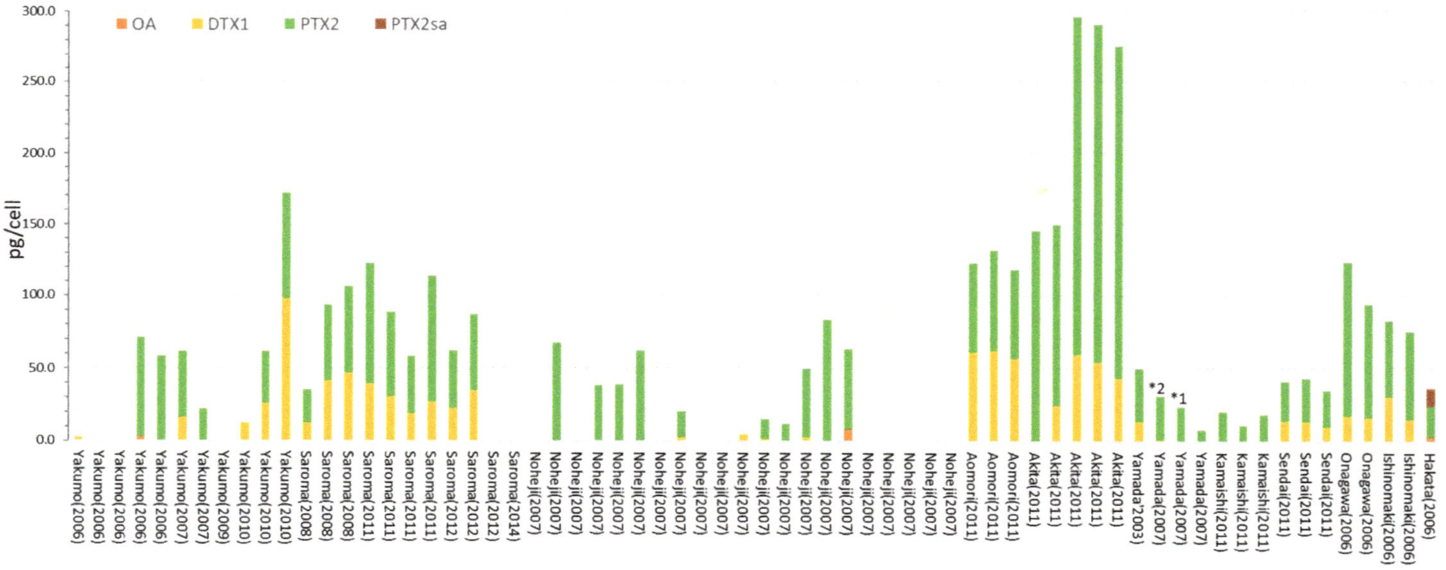

Figure 3. The toxin contents and profiles of *D. fortii* in Japan. * 1 Trace levels of OA were detected. * 2 Trace levels of DTX1 were detected. The toxin contents, the profiles, analyzed cell numbers, and detection limits for negative values are also given in Table S1.

2.3. *Other Dinophysis Species*

PTX2 was the only toxin detected in many other *Dinophysis* species collected and analyzed as part of this study, including *D. norvegica*, *D. tripos*, and *D. caudata*. Trace levels of DTX1 or OA were observed in some of these samples (Figure 4, Table S1). PTX2 was detected for the first time in *D. mitra* from Yakumo (2012) by LC/MS when using selected ion monitoring (SIM) in positive ion mode. The highest PTX2 content per cell of a *D. tripos* found in this study was 467.4 pg/cell, which represents the highest value ever reported (Table 1). It was also interesting that some of the other *Dinophysis* species collected and identified (e.g., *D. rudgei*) did not produce any of the monitored toxins, which aligns with the observations from *D. acuminata* and *D. fortii* isolates. Some *D. mitra* and *D. rotundata* samples, showed trace levels of DTX1 or OA. *D. norvegica* collected in Yakumo also contained a low level of DTX1.

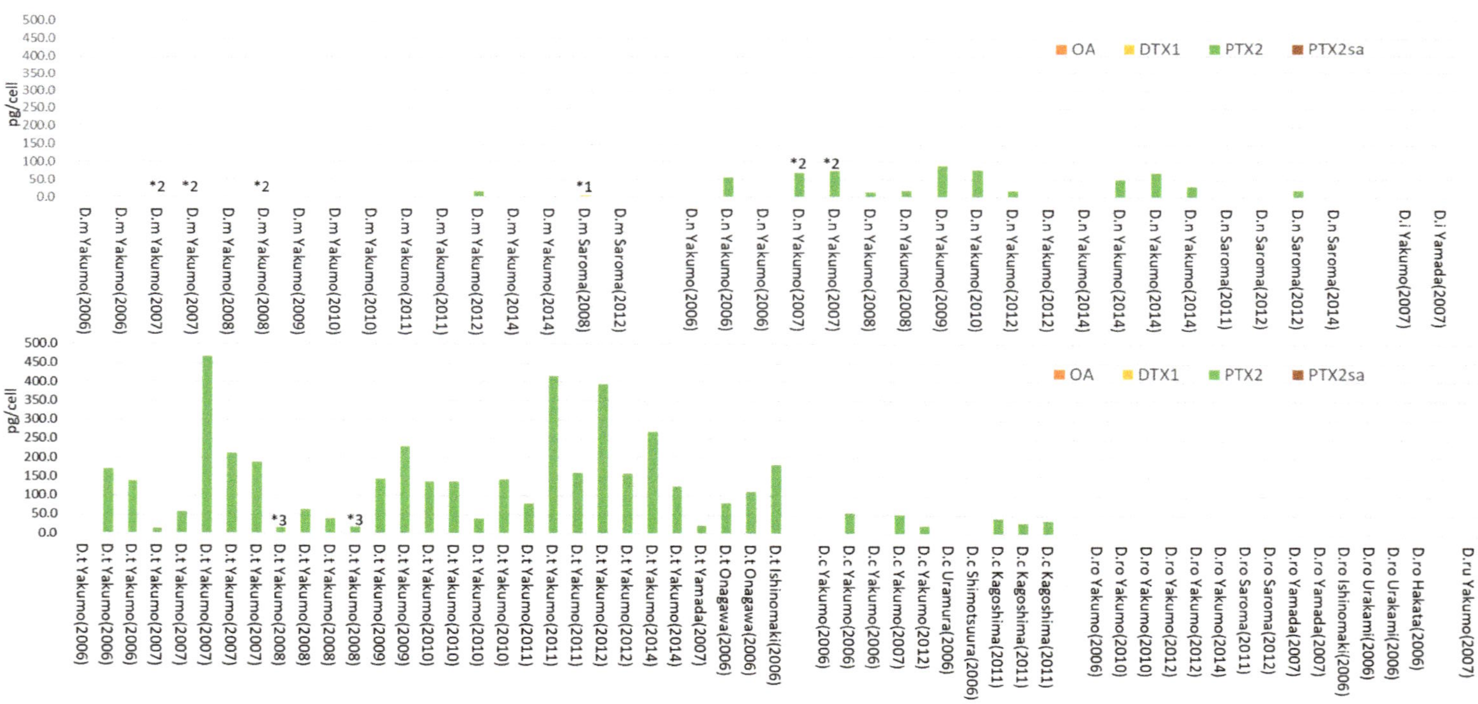

Figure 4. Toxin contents and the profiles of other *Dinophysis* species in Japan. D.m; *D. mitra*, D.n; *D. norvegica*, D.i; *D. infundibulus*, D.t; *D. tripos*, D.c; *D. caudata*, D.ro; *D. rotundata*, D.ru; *D. rudgei*. * 1 Trace levels of OA were detected. * 2 Trace levels of DTX1 were detected. * 3 Trace levels of PTX2 were detected. The toxin contents, profiles, analyzed cell numbers, and detection limits for negative values are also given in Table S1.

3. Discussion

In this study, the toxin content and profiles of *Dinophysis* species collected around the Japanese coastline were determined. Novel findings include the detection of DTX1 in *D. norvegica* and PTX2 in *D. caudata*. OA or DTX1 have been reported in *D. norvegica* from coastal waters in other countries [19,24]. Detection of PTX2 in pooled picked cells of *D. caudata* in Japan reported for the first time, however, it has been detected in Spanish and Chinese strains of this species [25,29,32]. Detection of PTX2 in pooled picked cells of *D. tripos* and *D. mitra* is also a novel observation, although PTX2 has been detected in cultures of *D. tripos* isolated from Japan [14]. Due to the very low concentration of PTX2 observed in the *D. mitra* samples, its presence was not confirmed by LC/MS/MS fragment ions, and further confirmation will be required.

LC-MS analyses of picked cells of *Phalacroma rotundatum* (*D. rotundata*) showed small amounts of the same toxins (OA, DTXs, PTXs) present in the co-occurring *Dinophysis* species or no toxins at all. These observations led to the hypothesis that the heterotrophic *P. rotundatum* is not a de novo toxin-producer, but a vector of DSP toxins taken up from its tintinnid prey. [36]. The small amount of DTX1 observed in *D. rotundata*, and heterotroph that feedss on tintinids collected and analyzed as part of our study might be derived from DTX1 produced by other co-occurring *Dinophysis* species present in the area.

This study determined that the most dominant toxin produced by *Dinophysis* species in Japan is PTX2, except for some samples of *D. acuminata*, *D. fortii*, *D. rotundata*, and *D. mitra* that produced only OA or DTX1. PTX11, which had been detected in *D. acuta* from Spain and New Zealand [8,9,39], was not detected in any *Dinophysis* samples from Japan. This indicates that, in Japan, there is little risk of bivalves being contaminated with PTX11. It was interesting that there were non-toxic *Dinophysis* samples even within the same species. This demonstrates the difficulty in predicting contamination of bivalves with DSTs or PTXs by monitoring *Dinophysis* cell densities. Monitoring of DSTs and PTXs in plankton net samples or SPATT devices [40] by LC/MS/MS methods could be useful for early warnings of bivalve contamination with these toxins.

In Japan, the LC/MS/MS method [38] for OA/DTX analogues has been introduced as the official testing method for DSTs since 2015 [41]. In terms of early warning of bivalve contamination with DSTs, *D. fortii* could be regarded as the most important *Dinophysis* species to monitor because the DTX1 contents of *D. fortii* were relatively higher than those found in other *Dinophysis* species. It is interesting that sampling sites that showed DTX1-containing *D. fortii* coincided well with the historical human poisoning cases of DSP [42–44]. When the percentages of DTX1 and OA from *D. fortii* samples in Japan were compared, those of DTX1 are greater. This result is consistent with the fact that the dominant OA analogue in Japanese bivalves is DTX1 and 7-*O*-acyl-DTX1 [45,46]. It is also noteworthy that *D. acuminata* from Takada produces a relatively high amount of OA. Although there have been no human DSP cases in this area, attention should be payed to prevent future cases when high cell densities of *D. acuminata* were observed in this area.

Monitoring of DSP in Japanese bivalves has historically been performed using the mouse bioassay (MBA). This methodology was implemented as the official testing method for the DSP monitoring program established in the 1980s [47]. Although the presence of *Dinophysis* had been confirmed in southeastern regions (Tokai, Kinki, Shikoku, Sanyo, Sanin, Kyusyu regions), in Japan, there had been a few MBA positive cases in bivalves from those regions. This could be explained by the results of this study showing the dominant toxin in *Dinophysis* collected in the southwestern regions (Hakata, Shimonoseki, Kagoshima, Hiroshima) is PTX2, which is then converted to a MBA non-toxic PTX2SA in many bivalve species (Pacific oyster, manila clam, etc.). The exception to this is Japanese scallops, *Patinopecten yessoensis* (*Mizuhopecten yessoensis*), cultured in northeastern Japan [37,48]. However, as *D. acuminata* collected in Takada produces a sufficiently high amounts of OA, there is a risk of human poisoning by DSTs when there is high cell densities of *D. acuminata* in this region. Therefore, continuous monitoring of DSP in bivalves around the coastline of Japan is necessary.

4. Materials and Methods

4.1. Chemicals

Okadaic acid (OA) and dinophysistoxin-1 (DTX1), pectenotoxin (PTX-1, 2, 6), and yessotoxin (YTX) were produced by the Japanese reference material project [49]. PTX-11 was isolated from *D. acuta* collected in New Zealand [8]. Methanol and acetonitrile, and formic acid of LC/MS grade were purchased from Kanto chemical co., Tokyo, Japan And ammonium formate of analytical grade was purchased from Nacalai tesque co., Tokyo, Japan. Distilled water was prepared by milli-Q Reference (Merck Millipore, Burlington, MA, USA).

4.2. Sampling Locations and Dinophysis Sample Preparation

Seawater samples were collected from various locations around the Japanese coastline (Figure 5). Using a light microscope, 50 individual cells of *Dinophysis* species identified in the seawater samples were carefully selected using a glass capillary to exclude non-targeted microorganisms. The cells were identified by their morphological characteristics. Isolated *Dinophysis* cells that had been taxonomically identified were combined in a single vessel filled with filtered seawater and stored frozen until extraction. Detailed information on the sampling is shown in Table S1.

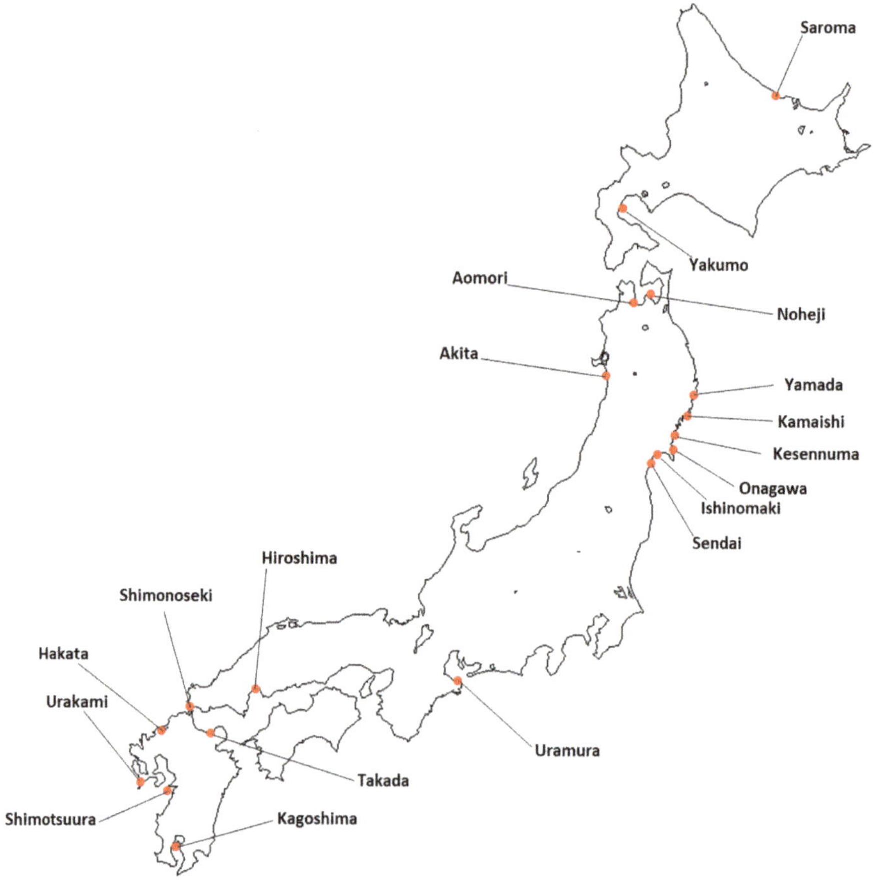

Figure 5. *Dinophysis* sampling locations around Japan.

4.3. Extraction

Toxins were extracted from cells of *Dinophysis* species by solid phase extraction (SPE) (Sep pak C18 plus, Waters co., Milford, MA, USA) as reported in previous studies [6,19,23]. Toxin extracts were dissolved in 200 μL of methanol for LC/MS/MS analysis.

4.4. LC/MS/MS and LC/MS Analysis

LC/MS/MS analysis was carried out according to a previous method [23]. The LC/MS/MS system was an Agilent 1100 series of high performance liquid chromatograph (HPLC) (Agilent technologies, Lexington, MA, USA) coupled with a 3200 Qtrap triple quadrupole MS/MS system (Sciex, Framingham, MA, USA). Separations were performed on Quicksilver cartridge columns (50 mm × 2.1 mm i.d) packed with 3 μm Hypersil-BDS-C8 (Keystone Scientific, Bellefonte, PA, USA) and maintained at 20 °C. Eluent A was water and B was acetonitrile–water (95:5), both containing 2 mM ammonium formate and 50 mM formic acid [50,51]. A linear gradient elution from 20% to 100% B was performed over 10 min and then held at 100% B for 15 min, followed by re-equilibration with 20% B (13 min). The flow rate was 0.2 mL/min and the injection volume was 10 μL. MRM LC/MS/MS analysis for the targeted toxins were carried out using the following ions; $[M - H]^-$ (OA, DTX1, 7-*O*-palmitoyl-DTX1, DTX2, PTX6, PTX2sa, YTX, 45OHYTX) and $[M + HCOOH - H]^-$ (PTX1, PTX2, PTX11) as the target parent ions in Q1 and particular fragment ions of each toxin in Q3 as reported in a previous study [40]. SIM LC/MS analysis for toxins were carried out using the $[M + NH_4]^+$ (OA, DTX1, DTX2, PTX1, PTX2, PTX6, PTX11) as the target ions in Q1.

Supplementary Materials: The following are available online at http://www.mdpi.com/2072-6651/10/11/457/s1, Table S1: Toxin profiles of *Dinophysis* species collected from around the coast of Japan.

Author Contributions: H.U. and T.S. performed sample analysis by LC/MS/MS. S.N., T.K., K.B., A.M., Y.K., S.K., and Y.M. performed sampling and cleanup of sample for LC/MS/MS. R.W., R.M., and H.O. contributed on experimental design, providing several assistances in laboratory facilities for LC/MS analyses. H.U. and T.S. performed data evaluation, important discussion, paper writing as well as experimental design.

Funding: This research was partly conducted by a research project for marine toxin safety measures funded by Japanese Ministry of Agriculture, Forestry, and Fisheries.

Acknowledgments: The authors deeply appreciate Tim Harwood for his kind help for corrections of our English manuscript.

Conflicts of Interest: The authors declare no conflict of interest.

References

1. Yasumoto, T.; Murata, M. Marine Toxins. *Chem. Rev.* **1993**, *93*, 1897–1909. [CrossRef]
2. Yasumoto, T.; Oshima, Y.; Sugawara, W.; Fukuyo, Y.; Oguri, H.; Igarashi, T.; Fujita, N. Identification of *Dinophysis fortii* as the causative organism of diarrhetic shellfish poisoning. *Bull. Jpn. Soc. Fish.* **1980**, *46*, 1405–1411. [CrossRef]
3. FAO and WHO. Standard for Live and Raw Bivalve Molluscs. Codex Stan 292-2008. 2008, pp. 1–9. Available online: http://www.fao.org/fao-who-codexalimentarius/codex-texts/list-standards/en/ (accessed on 5 November 2018).
4. Scientific Opinion of the Panel on Contaminants in the Food Chain. Marine biotoxins in shellfish—Summary on regulated marine biotoxins. *EFSA J.* **2009**, *1306*, 1–23.
5. Draisci, R.; Lucentini, L.; Giannetti, L.; Boria, P.; Poletti, R. First report of pectenotoxin-2 (PTX-2) in algae (*Dinophysis fortii*) related to seafood poisoning in Europe. *Toxicon* **1996**, *34*, 923–935. [CrossRef]
6. Suzuki, T.; Mitsuya, T.; Imai, M.; Yamasaki, M. DSP toxin contents in *Dinophysis fortii* and scallops collected at Mutsu Bay, Japan. *J. Appl. Phycol.* **1997**, *8*, 509–515. [CrossRef]
7. James, K.J.; Bishop, A.G.; Healy, B.M.; Roden, C.; Sherlock, I.R.; Twohig, M.; Draisci, R.; Giannetti, L.; Lucentini, L. Efficient isolation of the rare diarrhoeic shellfish toxin, dinophysistoxin-2, from marine phytoplankton. *Toxicon* **1999**, *37*, 343–357. [CrossRef]

8. Suzuki, T.; Walter, J.A.; LeBlanc, P.; MacKinnon, S.; Miles, C.O.; Wilkins, A.L.; Munday, R.; Beuzenberg, V.; MacKenzie, A.L.; Jensen, D.J.; et al. Identification of pectenotoxin-11 as 34 S-hydroxypectenotoxin-2, a new pectenotoxin analogue in the toxic dinoflagellate *Dinophysis acuta* from New Zealand. *Chem. Res. Toxicol.* **2006**, *19*, 310–318. [CrossRef] [PubMed]
9. Pizarro, G.; Paz, B.; Franco, J.M.; Suzuki, T.; Reguera, B. First detection of Pectenotoxin-11 and confirmation of OA-D8 diol-ester in *Dinophysis acuta* from European waters by LC–MS/MS. *Toxicon* **2008**, *52*, 889–896. [CrossRef] [PubMed]
10. Kamiyama, T.; Suzuki, T. Production of dinophysistoxin-1 and pectenotoxin-2 by a culture of *Dinophysis acuminata* (Dinophyceae). *Harmful Algae* **2009**, *8*, 312–317. [CrossRef]
11. Morton, S.L.; Vershinin, A.; Smith, L.L.; Leighfield, T.A.; Pankov, S.; Quilliam, M.A. Seasonality of *Dinophysis* spp. and *Prorocentrum lima* in Black Sea phytoplankton and associated shellfish toxicity. *Harmful Algae* **2009**, *8*, 629–636. [CrossRef]
12. Fux, E.; Smith, J.L.; Tong, M.; Guzman, L.; Anderson, D.M. Toxin profiles of five geographical isolates of *Dinophysis* spp. from North and South America. *Toxicon* **2011**, *57*, 275–287. [CrossRef] [PubMed]
13. Nagai, S.; Suzuki, T.; Nishikawa, T.; Kamiyama, T. Differences in the production and excretion kinetics of okadaicacid, dinophysistoxin-1, and pectenotoxin-2 between cultures of *Dinophysis acuminata* and *Dinophysis fortii* isolated from western japan. *J. Phycol.* **2011**, *47*, 1326–1337. [CrossRef] [PubMed]
14. Nagai, S.; Suzuki, T.; Kamiyama, T. Successful cultivation of the toxic dinoflagellate *Dinophysis tripos* (Dinophyceae). *Plankton Benthos Res.* **2013**, *8*, 171–177. [CrossRef]
15. Blanco, E.P.; Karlsson, C.; Pallon, J.; Yasumoto, T.; Granéli, E. Cellular nutrient content measured with the nuclear microprobe and toxins produced by *Dinophysis norvegica* (Dinophyceae) from the Trondheim fjord (Norway). *Aquat. Microb. Ecol.* **2015**, *75*, 259–269. [CrossRef]
16. Mafra, L.L., Jr.; Lopes, D.; Bonilauri, V.C.; Uchida, H.; Suzuki, T. Persistent contamination of octopuses and mussels with lipophilic shellfish toxins during spring *Dinophysis* blooms in a subtropical estuary. *Mar. Drugs* **2015**, *13*, 3920–3935. [CrossRef] [PubMed]
17. Basti, L.; Uchida, H.; Matsushima, R.; Watanabe, R.; Suzuki, T.; Yamatogi, T.; Nagai, S. Influence of Temperature on Growth and Production of Pectenotoxin-2 by a Monoclonal Culture of *Dinophysis caudata*. *Mar. Drugs* **2015**, *13*, 7124–7137. [CrossRef] [PubMed]
18. Nielsen, L.T.; Hansen, P.J.; Krock, B.; Vismann, B. Accumulation, transformation and breakdown of DSP toxins from the toxic dinoflagellate *Dinophysis acuta* in blue mussels, Mytilus edulis. *Toxicon* **2016**, *117*, 84–93. [CrossRef] [PubMed]
19. Lee, J.S.; Igarashi, T.; Santiago, F.; Einal, D.; Peter, H.; Yasumoto, T. Determination of diarrhetic shellfish toxins in various dinoflagellate species. *J. Appl. Phycol.* **1989**, *1*, 147–152. [CrossRef]
20. Johansson, N.; Graneli, E.; Yasumoto, T.; Carlsson, P.; Legrand, C. Toxin production by *Dinophysis acuminata* and *D. acuta* cells grown under nutrient sufficient and deficient conditions. In *Harmful and Toxic Algal Bloom*; Yasumoto, T., Oshima, Y., Fukuyo, Y., Eds.; Intergovernmental Oceanographic Comission of UNESCO: Sendai, Japan, 1996; pp. 277–280.
21. Fernández, M.L.; Reguera, B.; Ramilo, I.; Martínez, A. Toxin content of *Dinophysis acuminata, D. acuta, D. caudata* from the Galician Rias Bajas. In *Harmful and Toxic Algal Bloom*; Hallegraeff, G.M., Blackburn, S.I., Bolch, C.J., Lewis, R.J., Eds.; Intergovernmental Oceanographic Comission of UNESCO: Hobart, Tasmania, Australia, 2001; pp. 360–363.
22. Blanco, J.; Álvarez, G.; Uribe, E. Identification of pectenotoxins in plankton, filter feeders, and isolated cells of a *Dinophysis acuminata* with an atypical toxin profile, from Chile. *Toxicon* **2007**, *49*, 710–716. [CrossRef] [PubMed]
23. Suzuki, T.; Miyazono, A.; Baba, K.; Sugawara, R.; Kamiyama, T. LC–MS/MS analysis of okadaic acid analogues and other lipophilic toxins in single-cell isolates of several *Dinophysis* species collected in Hokkaido, Japan. *Harmful Algae* **2009**, *8*, 233–238. [CrossRef]
24. Miles, C.O.; Wilkins, A.L.; Samdal, I.A.; Sandvik, M.; Petersen, D.; Quilliam, M.A.; Naustvoll, L.J.; Rundberget, T.; Torgersen, T.; Hovgaard, P.; et al. A novel pectenotoxin, PTX-12, in *Dinophysis* spp. and shellfish from Norway. *Chem. Res. Toxicol.* **2004**, *17*, 1423–1433. [CrossRef] [PubMed]
25. Pizarro, G.; Moroño, A.; Paz, B.; Franco, J.M.; Pazos, Y.; Reguera, B. Evaluation of Passive Samplers as a Monitoring Tool for Early Warning of Dinophysis Toxins in Shellfish. *Mar. Drugs* **2013**, *11*, 3823–3845. [CrossRef] [PubMed]

26. Sato, S.; Koike, K.; Kodama, M. Seasonal variation of okadaic acid and dinophysistoxin-1 in *Dinophysis* spp. in association with the toxicity of scallop. In *Harmful and Toxic Algal Bloom*; Yasumoto, T., Oshima, Y., Fukuyo, Y., Eds.; Intergovernmental Oceanographic Comission of UNESCO: Sendai, Japan, 1996; pp. 285–288.
27. James, K.J.; Bishop, A.G.; Gillman, M.; Kelly, S.S.; Roden, C.; Draisci, R.; Lucentini, L.; Giannetti, L. The Diarrhoeic Shellfish Poisoning toxins of *Dinophysis acuta*: Identification and isolation of dinophysistoxin-2 (DTX-2). In *Harmful and Toxic Algal Bloom*; Reguera, B., Blanco, J., Fernández, L.M., Wyatt, T., Eds.; Xunta de Galicia and Intergovernmental Oceanographic Comission of UNESCO: Santiago de Compostela, Spain, 1998; pp. 489–492.
28. Puente, P.F.; Sáez, M.J.F.; Hamilton, B.; Furey, A.; James, K.J. Studies of polyether toxins in the marine phytoplankton, *Dinophysis acuta*, in Ireland using multiple tandem mass spectrometry. *Toxicon* **2004**, *44*, 919–926. [CrossRef] [PubMed]
29. Fernández, L.M.; Reguera, B.; González, G.S.; Mguez, A. Pectenotoxin-2 in single-cell isolates of *Dinophysis caudata* and *Dinophysis acuta* from the Galician Rías (NW Spain). *Toxicon* **2006**, *48*, 477–490. [CrossRef] [PubMed]
30. Pizarro, G.; Paz, B.; González, G.S.; Franco, J.M.; Reguera, B. Seasonal variability of lipophilic toxins during a *Dinophysis acuta* bloom in Western Iberia: Differences between picked cells and plankton concentrates. *Harmful Algae* **2009**, *8*, 233–238. [CrossRef]
31. Marasigan, A.N.; Sato, S.; Fukuyo, Y.; Kodama, M. Accumulation of a high level of diarrhetic shellfish toxins in the green mussel Perna viridis during a bloom of *Dinophysis caudata* and *Dinophysis miles* in Sapian Bay, Panay Island, the Philippines. *Fish. Sci.* **2001**, *67*, 994–996. [CrossRef]
32. Jiang, T.; Liu, L.; Li, Y.; Zhang, J.; Tan, Z.; Wu, H.; Jiang, T.; Lu, S. Occurrence of marine algal toxins in oyster and phytoplankton samples in Daya Bay, South China Sea. *Chemosphere* **2017**, *183*, 80–88. [CrossRef] [PubMed]
33. Raho, N.; Pizarro, G.; Escalera, L.; Reguera, B.; Marin, I. Morphology, toxin composition and molecular analysis of *Dinophysis ovum* Schütt, a dinoflagellate of the "*Dinophysis acuminata* complex". *Harmful Algae* **2008**, *7*, 839–848. [CrossRef]
34. González, G.S.; Pizarro, G.; Paz, B.; Velo-Suarez, L.; Reguera, B. Considerations on thetoxigenic nature and prey sources of *Phalacroma rotundatum*. *Aquat. Microb. Ecol.* **2011**, *64*, 197–203. [CrossRef]
35. Masselin, P.; Lassus, P.; Bardouil, M. High performance liquid chromatography analysis of diarrhetic toxins in *Dinophysis* spp. from French coast. *J. Appl. Phycol.* **1992**, *4*, 385–389. [CrossRef]
36. Reguera, B.; Riobó, P.; Rodríguez, F.; Díaz, P.A.; Pizarro, G.; Paz, B.; Franco, J.M.; Blanco, J. Dinophysis Toxins: Causative Organisms, Distribution and Fate in Shellfish. *Mar. Drugs* **2014**, *12*, 394–461. [CrossRef] [PubMed]
37. Reguera, B.; Pizarro, G. Planktonic Dinoflagellates That Contain Polyether Toxins of the Old "DSP Complex". In *Seefood and Freshwater Toxins, Pharmacology, Physiology, and Detection*, 2nd ed.; Luis, M.B., Ed.; CRC Press, Taylor and Francis Group: New York, NY, USA, 2008; pp. 258–276.
38. Suzuki, T.; Quilliam, M.A. LC-MS/MS Analysis of Diarrhetic Shellfish Poisoning (DSP) Toxins, Okadaic Acid and Dinophysistoxin Analogues, and Other Lipophilic Toxins. *Anal. Sci.* **2011**, *27*, 572–584. [CrossRef]
39. MacKenzie, A.L.; Beuzenberg, V.; Holland, P.; McNabb, P.; Suzuki, T.; Selwood, A. Pectenotoxin and okadaic acid-based toxin profiles in *Dinophysis acuta* and *Dinophysis acuminata* from New Zealand. *Harmful Algae* **2005**, *4*, 75–85. [CrossRef]
40. MacKenzie, A.L.; Beuzenberg, V.; Holland, P.; McNabb, P.; Selwood, A. Solid phase adsorption toxin tracking (SPATT): A new monitoring tool that simulates the biotoxin contamination of filter feeding bivalves. *Toxicon* **2004**, *44*, 901–918. [CrossRef] [PubMed]
41. Ministry of Agriculture, Forestry and Fisheries. Guidelines for Risk Management of Shellfish Toxins in Bivalves. 2015. Available online: http://www.maff.go.jp/j/syouan/tikusui/gyokai/g_kenko/busitu/pdf/150306_kaidoku_guide.pdf (accessed on 5 November 2018).
42. Yasumoto, T.; Oshima, Y.; Yamaguchi, M. Occurrence of a New Type of shellfish poisoning in the Tohoku district. *Bull. Jpn. Soc. Fish.* **1978**, *44*, 1249–1255. [CrossRef]
43. Sato, N.; Ishige, M.; Kawase, S.; Tazawa, T.; Nakagawa, T. First cases of Paralytic and Diarrhoetic shellfish poisoning in Hokkaido. *Rep. Hokkaido Inst. Public Health* **1983**, *33*, 78–83.
44. Toda, M.; Uneyama, C.; Toyofuku, H.; Morikawa, K. Trends of Food Poisonings Caused by Natural Toxins in Japan, 1989–2011. *J. Food Hyg. Soc. Jpn.* **2011**, *53*, 105–119. [CrossRef]

45. Suzuki, T.; Jin, T.; Shirota, Y.; Mitsuya, T.; Okumura, Y.; Kamiyama, T. Quantification of lipophilic toxins associated with diarrhetic shellfish poisoning in Japanese bivalves by liquid chromatography–mass spectrometry and comparison with mouse bioassay. *Fish. Sci.* **2005**, *71*, 1370–1378. [CrossRef]
46. Suzuki, T.; Kamiyama, T.; Okumura, Y.; Ishihara, K.; Matsushima, R.; Kaneniwa, M. Liquid-chromatographic hybrid triple–quadrupole linear-ion-trap MS/MS analysis of fatty-acid esters of dinophysistoxin-1 in bivalves and toxic dinoflagellates in Japan. *Fish. Sci.* **2009**, *75*, 1039–1048. [CrossRef]
47. Japanese Ministry of Health and Welfare. *Food Sanitation Research*; Japanese Ministry of Health and Welfare: Toyko, Japan, 1981; Volume 7, p. 60.
48. Suzuki, T.; Mitsuya, T.; Matsubara, H.; Yamasaki, M. Determination of pectenotoxin-2 after solid-phase extraction from seawater and from the dinoflagellate *Dinophysis fortii* by liquid chromatography with electrospray mass spectrometry and ultraviolet detection Evidence of oxidation of pectenotoxin-2 to pectenotoxin-6 in scallops. *J. Chromatogr. A* **1998**, *815*, 155–160. [PubMed]
49. Goto, H.; Igarashi, T.; Sekiguchi, R.; Tanno, K.; Satake, M.; Oshima, Y.; Yasumoto, T. A Japanese project for production and distribution of shellfish toxins as calibrants for HPLC analysis. In *Proc. VIII International Conference on Harmful Algae*; Reguera, B., Blanco, J., Fernández, M.L., Wyatt, T., Eds.; Xunta de Galicia and Intergovernmental Oceanographic Commission of UNESCO: Vigo, Spain, 1998; pp. 216–219.
50. Quilliam, M.A.; Hess, P.; Dell'Aversano, C. Recent developments in the analysis of phycotoxins by liquid chromatography–mass spectrometry. In *Perspective at the Turn of the Millenium, Proceedings of the 10th International IUPAC Symposium on Mycotoxins and Phycotoxins, Guaruja, Brazil, 21–25 May 2000*; De Koe, W.J., Samson, R.A., van Egmond, H.P., Gilbert, J., Sabino, M., Eds.; IRIS: Guaruja, Brazil, 2001; pp. 383–391.
51. Quilliam, M.A. The role of chromatography in the hunt for red tide toxins. *J. Chromatogr. A* **2003**, *1000*, 527–548. [CrossRef]

toxins

MDPI

Article

Anatomical Distribution of Diarrhetic Shellfish Toxins (DSTs) in the Japanese Scallop *Patinopecten yessoensis* and Individual Variability in Scallops and *Mytilus edulis* Mussels: Statistical Considerations

Ryoji Matsushima [1], Hajime Uchida [1], Ryuichi Watanabe [1], Hiroshi Oikawa [1], Izumi Oogida [2], Yuki Kosaka [2], Makoto Kanamori [3], Tatsuro Akamine [1] and Toshiyuki Suzuki [1,*]

1 National Research Institute of Fisheries Science, Japan Fisheries Research and Education Agency, Fukuura 2-12-4, Kanazawa-ku, Yokohama, Kanagawa 236-8648, Japan; matsur@affrc.go.jp (R.M.); huchida@affrc.go.jp (H.U.); rwatanabe@affrc.go.jp (R.W.); oikawah@affrc.go.jp (H.O.); akabe@affrc.go.jp (T.A.)

2 Aomori Prefectural Industrial Technology Research Center, Fisheries Research Institute, Hiranai, Higashitsugarugun, Aomori 039-3381, Japan; izumi_oogida@aomori-itc.or.jp (I.O.); yuuki_kosaka@aomori-itc.or.jp (Y.K.)

3 Hokkaido Research Organization, Fisheries Research Department, Hakodate Fisheries Research Institute, Benten-cho 20-5, Hakodate, Hokkaido 040-0051, Japan; Kanamori-makoto@hro.or.jp

* Correspondence: tsuzuki@affrc.go.jp; Tel.: +81-45-788-7630

Received: 20 August 2018; Accepted: 21 September 2018; Published: 27 September 2018

Abstract: Diarrhetic shellfish toxins (DSTs) are a group of phycotoxins that include okadaic acid (OA)/dinophysistoxin (DTX) analogues. At present, detailed data on the distribution of DST is insufficient, and studies of the appropriate sample sizes are lacking. This study investigated the DST frequency distribution in scallops and mussels by liquid chromatography-tandem mass spectrometry (LC/MS/MS) and a resampling analysis of existing data was carried out. The DST population-interval and the necessary sample size were also estimated. DSTs are localized in the scallop digestive-gland, and the DST concentrations in scallops were water-depth-dependent. DST concentrations in scallops and mussels showed normal distributions, but mussels tended to contain more DSTs than scallops. In the statistical resampling analysis of the acquired data on scallops and mussels, especially that using the bootstrap method, sample size was difficult to estimate when the DST variation was large. Although the DST population-interval could be statistically estimated from the sample standard deviation of three samples, the sample size corresponded to the risk management level, and the use of 13 or more samples was preferable. The statistical methods used here to analyze individual contents and estimate population content-intervals could be applied in various situations and for shellfish toxins other than DSTs.

Keywords: diarrhetic shellfish toxins; accumulation; dinophysistoxin; Japanese scallop; dinophysis; LC/MS/MS; statistical analysis

Key Contribution: This is the first detailed analysis of the distribution of individual concentrations of DSTs in shellfish samples, as well as the first report of a method for analyzing and evaluating the relationship between the individual concentrations and mean population concentrations based on statistical methods.

1. Introduction

Diarrhetic shellfish poisoning (DSP) is a severe gastrointestinal illness caused by the consumption of shellfish contaminated with diarrhetic shellfish toxins (DSTs) [1]. DSTs are a group of phycotoxins that include okadaic acid (OA) and dinophysistoxin (DTX) analogues [2,3]. OA, dinophysistoxin-1 (DTX1), and dinophysistoxin-2 (DTX2) are the most important DSTs because they cause severe diarrhea. These toxins have been shown to be potent protein-phosphatase inhibitors [4], a property that can cause inflammation of the intestinal tract and diarrhea [5], possibly leading to tumor promotion [6]. Okadaic acid analogues are metabolized to the esterified toxin in many bivalve species including Japanese scallops [7], and they are collectively called dinophysistoxin-3 (DTX3). In Japan, screening and quantification of DSTs are carried out on bivalves in accordance with the guidelines based on the official instrumental method [8] in production areas and markets. However, the Japanese guidelines do not provide detailed information on the distribution of DSTs between individual bivalves and have not established an appropriate sample size due to the lack of such data obtained by accurate analytical methods [9].

The Japanese scallop *Patinopecten yessoensis* (*Mizuhopecten yessoensis*), a major and important cultured species in Japan [10], has unique characteristics, including the metabolic transformation of lipophilic toxins [11]. In the present study, we analyzed the concentrations of DSTs in individuals of *P. yessoensis* and the mussel *Mytilus edulis*, and the validity of the size of sample were examined with statistical resampling analysis of the acquired DST data. Although some of our research has been presented in a previous work [12], more detailed data and novel results are provided in our present study. Furthermore, assuming conditions for investigating cultured scallops in the sea [10], estimation of the DST population-interval (interval of concentration of DST contained in population) were performed. Finally, based on our results, we consider and propose an adequate sample size.

2. Results

2.1. Concentrations and Distribution of DSTs

2.1.1. Anatomical Compartmentalization of DST in Scallops

The compartmentalization of DSTs in scallops collected at Nonai Station, Mutsu Bay, Aomori prefecture was investigated. From 14 to 20 individual scallops, the digestive gland, gonad, mantle, gill, and adductor muscle were separately dissected. The pieces were then grouped together by the body part (Table 1).

Table 1. Sampling information and total weight (g) of each scallop tissue.

2014	26 May	2 June	9 June	30 June	14 July	22 July	28 July
Number of Individuals	**16**	**18**	**17**	**18**	**15**	**20**	**14**
Digestive gland	72.90	72.87	72.97	70.80	60.80	75.16	58.56
Gonad	42.39	39.99	40.79	44.22	48.05	54.46	39.83
Mantle	155.01	151.37	163.48	175.80	163.66	213.96	169.30
Gill	95.31	93.43	106.28	92.20	87.08	116.42	85.49
Adductor muscle	301.69	315.19	311.42	355.14	318.80	434.35	340.26

The concentration of OA and DTX1 in each part was quantified by LC/MS/MS after hydrolysis.

The dominant toxin in the scallops was DTX1, the highest concentration of which was found on 30 June, corresponding to about half of the regulation value of 0.16 mg/kg of whole meat (Figure 1).

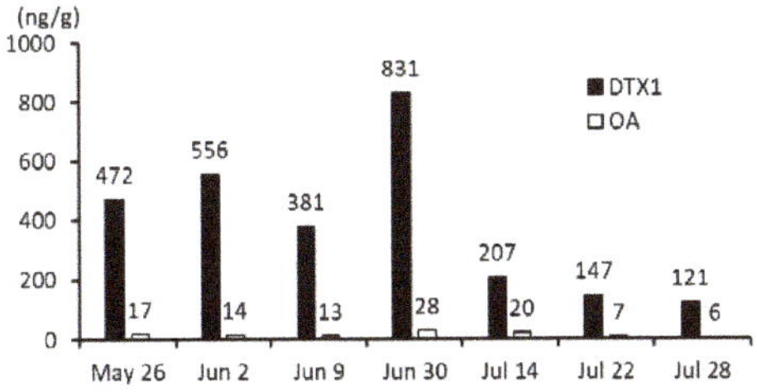

Figure 1. Concentrations of DTX1 and OA in the digestive glands of scallops. Fourteen to twenty individuals were combined into each sample set used for analysis. Black bars and white bars represent DTX1 and OA, respectively. The concentrations of toxins in the samples are shown on the vertical axis.

The proportion of the DTX1 quantity corresponding to each tissue are shown in Figure 2.

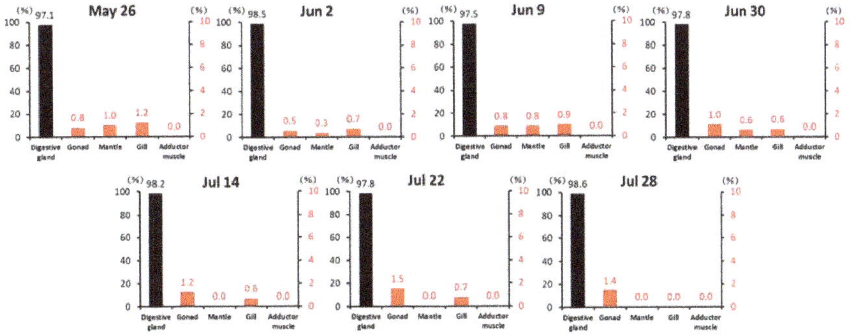

Figure 2. Percentage (%) of DTX1 in each scallop tissue.

2.1.2. DST Analysis of 30 Individual Scallops and Mussels

The concentrations of DTX1 in the digestive glands of 30 scallops or mussels collected at the Nonai Station were quantified for each individual (Figure 3 and Table 2).

The concentration of OA was not described due to the overall low concentrations found in the individual samples. The mean values of DTX1 differed even for the same date for both mussels and scallops, and the DTX1 values of the mussels were higher than those of the scallops (Figure 3). The distributions of the scallops and mussels were close to the normal distributions.

Table 2. Sampling information and mean weight (g) of the digestive glands of 30 scallops or mussels. The mean values of 30 samples ± population standard deviation (σ).

2014	26 May	2 June	9 June	16 June	7 July	8 August
Scallop (Digestive gland/Whole meat %)	3.87 ± 1.07 (10.14%)	3.62 ± 0.81 (10.56%)	3.70 ± 0.98 (8.78%)	3.81 ± 0.72 (9.18%)	-	-
Mussel (Digestive gland/Whole meat %)	-	1.69 ± 0.45 (14.72%)	-	-	1.40 ± 0.46 (14.89%)	1.51 ± 0.45 (12.90%)

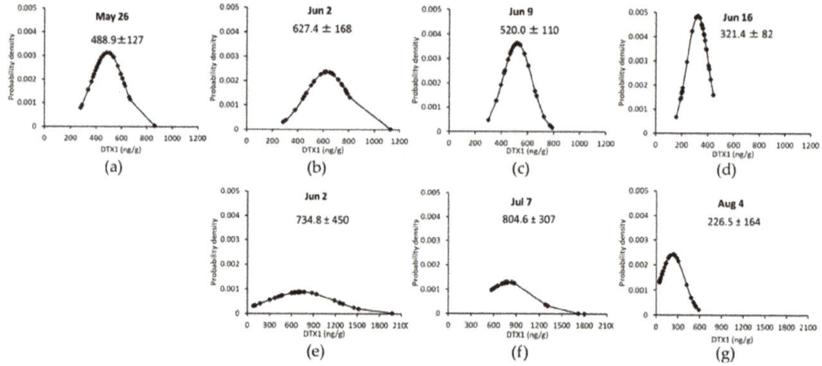

Figure 3. The 30 individual distributions, means ± σ of DTX1 in scallops and mussels. Panels (**a–d**) show the results for scallops and (**e–g**) show those for mussels.

2.1.3. Analysis of DST Concentration in Scallop Samples from Different Water Depths

The DST concentrations of scallop digestive glands collected at different depths at Yakumo Station, in the western part of Funka Bay, Hokkaido prefecture, were investigated. Sampling information about the scallops is shown in Table 3.

Table 3. Sampling information and mean weight (g) of scallop digestive glands. The mean value of digestive glands ± σ at each depth.

2016	18 May	28 June	11 August
Number of Individuals	**10**	**15**	**15**
5 m	6.45 ± 1.24	4.77 ± 0.82	1.40 ± 0.36
10 m	6.16 ± 0.91	5.18 ± 1.33	1.38 ± 0.26
15 m	5.30 ± 0.45	4.22 ± 0.75	1.46 ± 0.42

The vertical gradient of DTX1 distribution (maximum at 5 m, minimum at 15 m) was reversed over the investigation period (Figure 4). Maximum levels of about half of the regulation value (corresponding to 0.16 mg/kg of whole meat) were found at 15 m on 11 August.

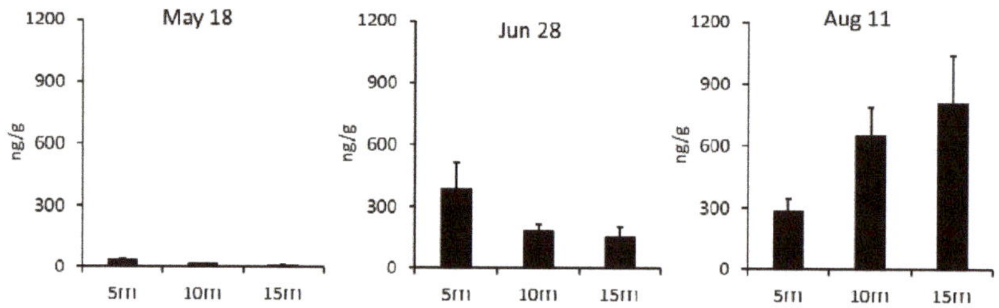

Figure 4. Vertical distribution of DTX1 and σ in scallop digestive glands.

The distributions of scallops on 28 June and 11 August were close to the normal distribution (Figure 5).

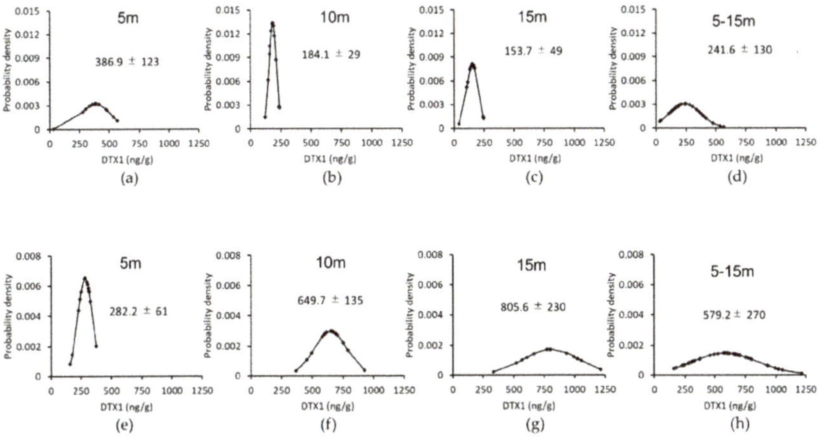

Figure 5. The distributions of scallop at each depth on 28 June and 11 August. The mean concentrations of DTX1 ± σ are shown for (**a**–**d**) 28 June and (**e**–**h**) 11 August.

Environmental conditions and vertical distribution of *Dinophysis* at Yakumo Station are represented in Table 4 and Figure 6, respectively.

Table 4. Data on environmental conditions and densities of DST producing species at Yakumo Station.

Transparency (m)	Date (2016)	Depth (m)	Water Temperature (°C)	Salinity (psu)	*D. fortii* (Cells/L)	*D. acuminate* (Cells/L)	Other *Dinophysis* (Cells/L)	
	18 May	0	11.2	30.84	0	30	0	
		5	9.7	31.98	0	60	0	
5.0		10	9.2	32.03	0	100	0	
		15	8.1	32.32	0	80	0	
		20	7.8	32.59	0	30	0	
		25	7.4	32.67	0	90	0	
		30	7.3	32.70	0	150	0	
	28 June	0	16.6	29.58	0	1120	0	
		5	14.8	31.15	30	650	60	Dt60
4.0		10	13.7	31.94	180	740	190	Dn150, Dt40
		15	13.4	32.09	30	490	80	Dn60, Dr20
		20	13.0	32.18	40	300	10	Dr10
		25	12.8	32.22	0	70	10	Dn10
		30	12.3	32.33	0	50	10	Dn10
	11 August	0	22.6	31.14	0	0	0	
		5	20.7	31.67	0	0	50	Dt50
10.5		10	16.9	32.37	0	10	30	Dt30
		15	12.7	32.64	0	0	30	Dt20, Dr10
		20	10.8	32.95	10	0	0	
		25	8.6	32.95	50	0	10	Dt10
		30	7.9	33.02	90	20	0	

Dinophysis tripos (Dt); *Dinophysis norvegica* (Dn); *Dinophysis rotundata* (Dr).

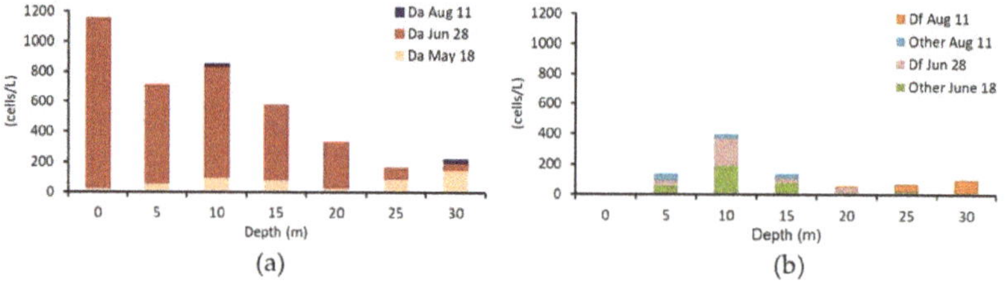

Figure 6. Vertical distributions of *Dinophysis species*. (**a**) *D. acuminata*; (**b**) *D. fortii* and other *Dinophysis species*.

D. acuminata was assumed to be main causative agent of the DST events. This species reached its maximal density on 28 June and declined on 11 August (Table 4). Other *Dinophysis* species were predominant from 10 m to the surface, and there was no clear relationship between the distribution of cells and reversal of the vertical distribution of DTX1 in scallops on 11 August (Figures 4 and 6).

2.2. Statistical Analysis

2.2.1. Statistical Resampling Analysis of DSTs in Scallops and Mussels

The number of individuals necessary to correctly reflect the DST contents of collected samples was estimated by resampling analysis. For this purpose, we used a data set collected for 30 individual scallops and 30 individual mussels at Aomori on 2 June (Figure 3). Both values were highly variable. The means of 5–25 samples were calculated with random sampling and allowing or not allowing (bootstrap method) replacement. The sample means were converted to percentages as compared with those of 30 samples (Table 5).

Table 5. Resampling analysis of scallops and mussels without replacement and with the bootstrap method. The left half of the table is a resampling analysis without replacement, while the right half shows the data using the bootstrap method. The n columns represent 5–25 samples. 1 to 99 represent percentiles. Percentage: each percentile columns represents the mean value of a data set for each mean of the 30 individuals. >±*30*; <±30; <±**20**; <±**10**.

	Scallop				Mussel					Scallop				Mussel			
n	1	5	95	99	1	5	95	99	n	1	5	95	99	1	5	95	99
5	75.6	82.1	119.0	126.3	49.5	60.4	144.4	163.7	5	72.5	80.7	120.7	130.3	44.3	58.2	149.8	172.0
6	77.7	84.0	117.0	123.7	52.0	63.9	139.4	155.8	6	75.6	82.3	118.8	127.2	48.8	61.3	144.6	164.2
7	80.0	85.4	114.9	120.4	56.2	66.9	134.8	148.8	7	76.6	83.5	116.8	124.4	51.3	63.8	139.8	157.2
8	81.1	86.5	113.9	119.0	58.5	69.5	132.6	144.4	8	78.4	84.7	115.7	122.9	54.9	66.5	137.3	154.3
9	82.9	87.6	112.9	117.6	61.9	71.8	129.8	140.3	9	79.2	85.5	114.3	121.1	56.5	67.8	133.9	150.0
10	84.4	88.5	111.6	116.0	64.1	73.7	126.9	138.6	10	80.7	86.3	114.0	120.1	59.4	69.8	132.6	147.9
11	85.5	89.3	111.0	114.7	67.0	75.9	124.8	135.4	11	81.4	86.8	113.3	119.1	60.6	70.4	131.4	145.4
12	86.1	89.8	110.4	114.1	69.4	77.4	123.7	132.1	12	82.4	87.4	112.9	118.8	62.5	72.0	130.7	144.1
13	87.4	90.7	109.4	112.9	70.6	78.5	121.6	129.7	13	82.9	87.9	112.2	117.6	63.5	73.0	128.8	140.9
14	87.8	91.2	108.6	112.1	72.5	79.7	119.9	127.7	14	83.6	88.5	112.1	117.4	65.3	74.2	128.7	140.8
15	88.7	91.7	108.0	111.1	74.2	81.2	118.9	126.3	15	84.5	88.9	111.6	116.3	65.6	75.1	126.8	137.8
16	89.7	92.5	107.6	110.3	75.0	82.2	117.5	124.2	16	84.6	89.2	111.0	115.6	66.8	75.9	126.0	136.9
17	90.0	92.8	107.1	109.7	77.6	83.7	116.5	122.4	17	85.1	89.5	110.7	115.1	67.2	76.6	124.9	136.2
18	90.8	93.2	106.5	109.1	78.5	84.8	115.1	120.4	18	85.8	89.8	110.6	115.2	68.9	77.2	124.3	135.3
19	91.4	93.6	106.2	108.4	80.0	85.6	113.8	119.2	19	86.0	90.0	110.2	114.7	69.9	77.5	123.9	134.4
20	92.0	94.0	105.8	107.8	81.1	86.7	112.9	117.3	20	85.8	90.2	109.9	114.0	69.5	78.0	123.2	133.6
21	92.6	94.5	105.2	107.2	82.2	87.4	111.9	116.0	21	86.8	90.6	109.6	113.9	70.5	78.8	122.6	132.3
22	93.1	94.9	104.9	106.6	83.7	88.4	110.8	114.5	22	87.1	90.8	109.4	113.6	71.0	79.2	122.0	132.7
23	93.5	95.2	104.5	106.3	84.7	89.2	110.1	113.5	23	87.2	91.0	109.3	113.2	72.0	79.8	121.6	131.1
24	94.1	95.7	104.0	105.5	86.1	90.2	108.8	111.7	24	87.4	91.0	109.2	113.0	72.3	79.9	121.3	130.5
25	94.6	96.1	103.6	105.0	87.3	91.1	107.9	110.3	25	88.0	91.3	109.1	113.1	73.3	80.5	121.1	130.4

In the resampling analysis without replacement, using ≥8 and ≥17 scallops fell within ±20% and 10% of the means of 30 individuals, respectively, with a probability of 98%. In the case of mussels, means of ≥13 and ≥19 individuals fell within ±30% and 20% of the means of 30 individuals, respectively, and with 98% probability (Table 5, underlined numbers in the left half). In the bootstrap method, only 11 scallops fell within ±20% of the mean value of 30 individuals with a probability of

98% (Table 5, double-underlined numbers in the right half), whereas the number of mussels was not obtained from 25 individuals.

2.2.2. Estimating the Mean Concentration of the Population (Cultured Scallops) When the Individual Concentration of a Sample Is Defined

In the former subsection, the ratio of the sample mean to the 30-individual population DST mean was analyzed using specific individual samples. Here, the mean DST concentration of the population (cultured scallops) was estimated using the sample mean concentration. Estimation of the standard normal distribution population mean with the confidence interval (CI, 95% = 100 (1 − α)%) is represented by the following equation [13]:

$$\overline{X} - 1.96 \times \sqrt{\mathrm{Var}(\overline{X})} \leq \hat{\mu} \leq \overline{X} + 1.96 \times \sqrt{\mathrm{Var}(\overline{X})} \quad (1)$$

By the central limit theorem, variance $\mathrm{Var}(\overline{X}) = \frac{\sigma^2}{n}$ [13].

$$\overline{X} - 1.96 \times \sqrt{\frac{\sigma^2}{n}} \leq \hat{\mu} \leq \overline{X} + 1.96 \times \sqrt{\frac{\sigma^2}{n}} \quad (2)$$

The unknown-population standard deviation σ can be replaced with the sample standard deviation s calculated from the sample data. Moreover, 1.96 = $t_{0.05}(\infty)$ and hence is generalized with $t_\alpha(\nu)$.

$$\overline{X} - t_\alpha(\nu) \times s/\sqrt{n} \leq \hat{\mu} \leq \overline{X} + t_\alpha(\nu) \times s/\sqrt{n} \quad (3)$$

In Equation (3), $t_\alpha(\nu) \times s/\sqrt{n}$ (CI of the population mean concentration) was estimated when s was 200 at [α = 0.05] using 10 samples. In accordance with n and α, $t_{0.05}(9)$ = 2.2622 from the Student's t-distribution in Table 6 was assigned in Equation (3).

$$t_\alpha(\nu) \times s/\sqrt{n} = 2.2622 \times 200/\sqrt{10} = 143.1 \quad (4)$$

Table 6. Student's t distribution.

ν	Two-Tailed Probability	
	0.10	**0.05**
2	2.9200	4.3027
3	2.3534	3.1824
4	2.1318	2.7764
5	2.0150	2.5706
6	1.9432	2.4469
7	1.8946	2.3646
8	1.8595	2.3060
9	1.8331	2.2622
10	1.8125	2.2281
11	1.7959	2.2010
12	1.7823	2.1788
13	1.7709	2.1604
14	1.7613	2.1448
15	1.7531	2.1314

Table 6. *Cont.*

v	Two-Tailed Probability	
	0.10	0.05
16	1.7459	2.1199
17	1.7396	2.1098
18	1.7341	2.1009
19	1.7291	2.0930
20	1.7247	2.0860
21	1.7207	2.0796
22	1.7171	2.0739
23	1.7139	2.0687
24	1.7109	2.0639
25	1.7081	2.0595
26	1.7056	2.0555
27	1.7033	2.0518
28	1.7011	2.0484
29	1.6991	2.0452
30	1.6973	2.0423
50	1.6759	2.0086
100	1.6602	1.9840
∞	1.6449	1.9600

The two-tailed probability is 0.10 or 0.05.

At $\alpha = 0.05$ and 0.10, the interval estimations (±OA group ng/g) of μ with sample sizes of 3–20 and s of 100–650 were calculated and are presented in Tables 7 and 8.

Table 7. Interval estimation (±OA group ng/g digestive gland) of μ in $\alpha = 0.05$. The n columns represent sample size 3–20 samples. Rows from 100 to 650 represent the s values.

n	t ($\alpha = 0.05$)	Sample Standard Deviation (s)											
		100	150	200	250	300	350	400	450	500	550	600	650
3	4.3027	248.4	372.6	496.8	621.0	745.2	869.5	993.7	1117.9	1242.1	1366.3	1490.5	1614.7
4	3.1825	159.1	238.7	318.3	397.8	477.4	556.9	636.5	716.1	795.6	875.2	954.8	1034.3
5	2.7764	124.2	186.2	248.3	310.4	372.5	434.6	496.7	558.7	620.8	682.9	745.0	807.1
6	2.5706	104.9	157.4	209.9	262.4	314.8	367.3	419.8	472.2	524.7	577.2	629.7	682.1
7	2.4469	92.5	138.7	185.0	231.2	277.5	323.7	369.9	416.2	462.4	508.7	554.9	601.1
8	2.3646	83.6	125.4	167.2	209.0	250.8	292.6	334.4	376.2	418.0	459.8	501.6	543.4
9	2.3060	76.9	115.3	153.7	192.2	230.6	269.0	307.5	345.9	384.3	422.8	461.2	499.6
10	2.2622	71.5	107.3	143.1	178.8	214.6	250.4	286.1	321.9	357.7	393.5	429.2	465.0
11	2.2281	67.2	100.8	134.4	167.9	201.5	235.1	268.7	302.3	335.9	369.5	403.1	436.7
12	2.2010	63.5	95.3	127.1	158.8	190.6	222.4	254.1	285.9	317.7	349.5	381.2	413.0
13	2.1788	60.4	90.6	120.9	151.1	181.3	211.5	241.7	271.9	302.1	332.4	362.6	392.8
14	2.1604	57.7	86.6	115.5	144.3	173.2	202.1	231.0	259.8	288.7	317.6	346.4	375.3
15	2.1448	55.4	83.1	110.8	138.4	166.1	193.8	221.5	249.2	276.9	304.6	332.3	360.0
16	2.1315	53.3	79.9	106.6	133.2	159.9	186.5	213.2	239.8	266.4	293.1	319.7	346.4
17	2.1199	51.4	77.1	102.8	128.5	154.2	180.0	205.7	231.4	257.1	282.8	308.5	334.2
18	2.1098	49.7	74.6	99.5	124.3	149.2	174.0	198.9	223.8	248.6	273.5	298.4	323.2
19	2.1009	48.2	72.3	96.4	120.5	144.6	168.7	192.8	216.9	241.0	265.1	289.2	313.3
20	2.0930	46.8	70.2	93.6	117.0	140.4	163.8	187.2	210.6	234.0	257.4	280.8	304.2

Table 8. Interval estimation (±OA group ng/g digestive gland) of μ in α = 0.10. The n columns represent sample size 3–20. Rows 100 to 650 represent the s values.

n	t (α = 0.10)	Sample Standard Deviation (s)											
		100	150	200	250	300	350	400	450	500	550	600	650
3	2.9200	168.6	252.9	337.2	421.5	505.8	590.1	674.3	758.6	842.9	927.2	1011.5	1095.8
4	2.3534	117.7	176.5	235.3	294.2	353.0	411.8	470.7	529.5	588.4	647.2	706.0	764.9
5	2.1318	95.3	143.0	190.7	238.3	286.0	333.7	381.3	429.0	476.7	524.4	572.0	619.7
6	2.0150	82.3	123.4	164.5	205.7	246.8	287.9	329.0	370.2	411.3	452.4	493.6	534.7
7	1.9432	73.4	110.2	146.9	183.6	220.3	257.1	293.8	330.5	367.2	404.0	440.7	477.4
8	1.8946	67.0	100.5	134.0	167.5	201.0	234.4	267.9	301.4	334.9	368.4	401.9	435.4
9	1.8595	62.0	93.0	124.0	155.0	186.0	216.9	247.9	278.9	309.9	340.9	371.9	402.9
10	1.8331	58.0	87.0	115.9	144.9	173.9	202.9	231.9	260.9	289.8	318.8	347.8	376.8
11	1.8125	54.6	82.0	109.3	136.6	163.9	191.3	218.6	245.9	273.2	300.6	327.9	355.2
12	1.7959	51.8	77.8	103.7	129.6	155.5	181.5	207.4	233.3	259.2	285.1	311.1	337.0
13	1.7823	49.4	74.1	98.9	123.6	148.3	173.0	197.7	222.4	247.2	271.9	296.6	321.3
14	1.7709	47.3	71.0	94.7	118.3	142.0	165.7	189.3	213.0	236.6	260.3	284.0	307.6
15	1.7613	45.5	68.2	91.0	113.7	136.4	159.2	181.9	204.6	227.4	250.1	272.9	295.6
16	1.7530	43.8	65.7	87.7	109.6	131.5	153.4	175.3	197.2	219.1	241.0	263.0	284.9
17	1.7459	42.3	63.5	84.7	105.9	127.0	148.2	169.4	190.5	211.7	232.9	254.1	275.2
18	1.7396	41.0	61.5	82.0	102.5	123.0	143.5	164.0	184.5	205.0	225.5	246.0	266.5
19	1.7341	39.8	59.7	79.6	99.5	119.3	139.2	159.1	179.0	198.9	218.8	238.7	258.6
20	1.7291	38.7	58.0	77.3	96.7	116.0	135.3	154.7	174.0	193.3	212.7	232.0	251.3

From Tables 7 and 8, it is possible to estimate the confidence interval of the μ when s is 100–650 for 3–20 samples, when the individual concentration data of the sample are acquired.

From Equation (5), derived from Equation (3), the s value can be calculated to estimate the mean density of μ within interval ±160 ng/g (one-tenth of the digestive gland regulatory limit).

$$t_{\alpha}(v) \times s/\sqrt{n} \leq 160 \quad (5)$$

$$s \leq 160/t_{\alpha}(v) \times \sqrt{n}. \quad (6)$$

In Equation (5), the s was estimated using $t_{0.05}(9)$ = 2.2622 from Student's t-distribution table.

$$s \leq 160/t_{\alpha}(v) \times \sqrt{n} = 160/2.2622 \times 3.1622 = 223.7 \quad (7)$$

At α = 0.05 and 0.10, the estimation of s with the mean density of μ within interval ±160 ng/g with sample sizes of 3–20 were calculated and are presented in Figure 7.

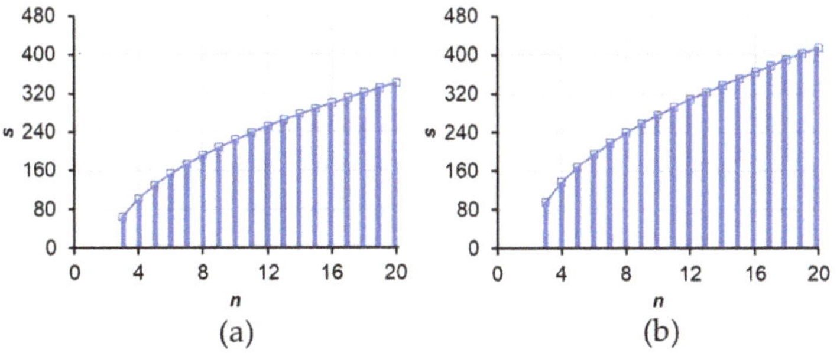

Figure 7. Estimation of s with the mean density of μ within interval ±160 ng/g at (**a**) 95% or (**b**) 90% confidence. The X axis n represents a sample size of 3–20.

For an actual sample, when the calculated **s** is less than or equal to the graph value (striped zone of Figure 7), it is considered that the mean concentration of μ can be estimated with an interval of ±160 ng/g and 90% or 95% confidence.

2.2.3. Adequacy of Sample Size Based on the t-Value and Confidence Interval

The values in Tables 7 and 8 and in Figure 7 are derived by equations with a t-value as a coefficient. n is a natural number, and the statistical degrees of freedom (ν) is a linear function. On the other hand, the t-value is defined by Equation (6) [14,15], and the upper cumulative probability (1/2 α) of the t distribution is derived from Equation (7).

$$f(t) = \frac{\Gamma\left(\frac{\nu+1}{2}\right)}{\sqrt{\nu\pi}\Gamma\left(\frac{\nu}{2}\right)}\left(1+\frac{t^2}{\nu}\right)^{-\frac{\nu+1}{2}} \quad (\Gamma \text{ is Gamma function}) \tag{8}$$

$$1/2\alpha = \int_x^\infty f(t,\ \upsilon)dt \tag{9}$$

In Equation (7), although the t-value (x) is determined by the degrees of freedom ν and significance level α, it is inversely correlated with the ν and α, and the t-value (x) gradually approaches infinite degrees of freedom at each significance level. Figure 8 represents the t-value of α = 0.10 or 0.05 with ν = 2–30. The t-value increases as the confidence value becomes greater, without intersection.

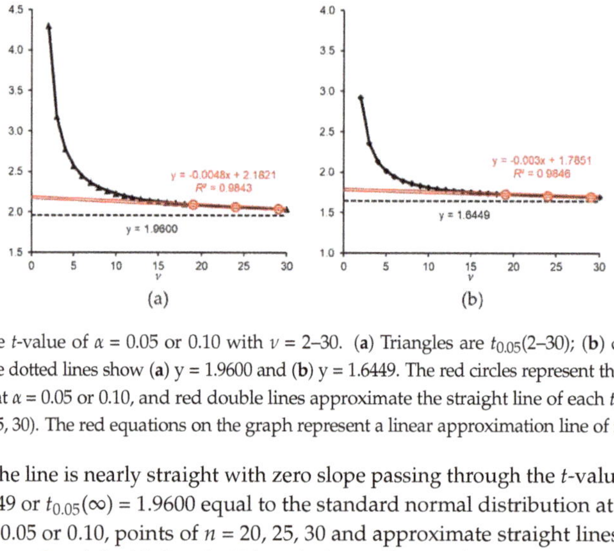

Figure 8. The t-value of α = 0.05 or 0.10 with ν = 2–30. (**a**) Triangles are $t_{0.05}$(2–30); (**b**) diamonds are $t_{0.10}$(2–30). The dotted lines show (**a**) y = 1.9600 and (**b**) y = 1.6449. The red circles represent the t-values of n = (20, 25, 30) at α = 0.05 or 0.10, and red double lines approximate the straight line of each $t_{0.05}$(20, 25, 30) and $t_{0.10}$(20, 25, 30). The red equations on the graph represent a linear approximation line of t-values.

Ultimately the line is nearly straight with zero slope passing through the t-value at each infinity ν ($t_{0.10}(\infty)$ = 1.6449 or $t_{0.05}(\infty)$ = 1.9600 equal to the standard normal distribution at each confidence level). When t = 0.05 or 0.10, points of n = 20, 25, 30 and approximate straight lines are drawn on a t-value graph (Figure 8, red double lines). Although the coefficient of approximate straight lines varies depending on the desired value and confidence, the risk of the obtained estimation value is greatly reduced as the sample size increases and the t-value approaches each linear approximation.

Both approximate straight lines start to diverge from the t-value around ν = 13 (n = 14), and the t-value increases exponentially as ν decreases. From the samples of about 14 or more, the relation between the risk of the estimated value and the size of the sample is assumed to describe a linear function. Thus, it is desirable to use a sample size of at least 14 when estimating the mean concentration of the population. When the sample size is 13 or less, the risk of the estimate value increases exponentially as the sample size decreases.

The graph of $f(t, \nu = 100)$ and the standard normal distribution $f(t, \nu = \infty)$ are almost identical (Figure 9c). The difference between $t_{0.10}(100)$ and $t_{0.10}(\infty)$ or that between $t_{0.05}(100)$ and $t_{0.05}(\infty)$ is 0.0153 or 0.024, respectively (Table 6). These levels are within a margin of error that does not matter practically. The ideal number of samples is 14 (ν = 13) or more, but considering the mathematical errors, 13 (ν = 12) or more samples is assumed to be a practical allowable range.

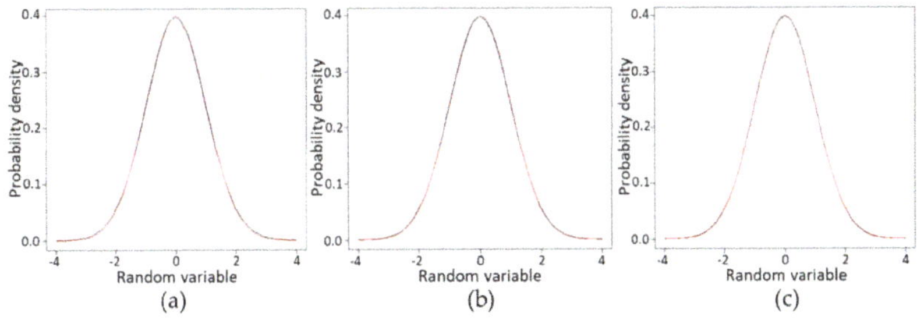

Figure 9. Overlay graphs of $f(t, \nu = 30, 50, \text{and } 100)$ red lines, and the standard normal distribution $f(t, \nu = \infty)$ black lines. (**a**) $f(t, \nu = 30)$ and $f(t, \nu = \infty)$; (**b**) $f(t, \nu = 50)$ and $f(t, \nu = \infty)$; (**c**) $f(t, \nu = 100)$ and $f(t, \nu = \infty)$.

3. Discussion

Some *Dinophysis* species in Japan produces DTX1 as the dominant toxin [7,16]. In scallops, results showing that DSTs were detected exclusively in the digestive glands and that the adductor muscles were free of DSTs agree with the results of our previous feeding experiment study [11].

In our samples, the ratio of the digestive glands to the whole meat of the mussels was about 15% (data from three groups of 30 mussel samples). Some of the mussels collected on 2 June and 7 July exceeded the regulatory level, but none of the scallop samples exceeded the regulatory level. Even though the scallops and mussels were cultured in the same spot, the amounts of accumulated DSTs and their variabilities tended to be higher in mussels than in scallops. The mussels adhered to each other via the byssus, whereas the scallops were separated from each other in the net. Ecological factors and metabolism may be involved in the magnitude of DST variability in mussels and scallops. Concentration fluctuations and DST variation determined by water depth (Figure 4) seem to reflect the vertical distribution of *Dinophysis* in the water column and the individual metabolism of scallops. The peak of *Dinophysis* species cell density was assumed to have occurred in July, but unfortunately our data did not identify this trend.

Given a sufficient sample size, it is common practice to homogenize and prepare samples, and this makes sense from the viewpoint of equalizing the samples. Generally, according to the law of large numbers, when an appropriate sample size is collected, there is no problem in obtaining the mean value of the population even if the samples are combined. However, this theorem does not present the validity of the sample size, and in fact it is a problem that convergence of mean value requires plenty of samples. Hence, there is important question as to what the pooled sample size should be. It should also be noted that valuable information on the toxin concentrations in individual shellfish flesh is lost by homogenization and cannot be used to estimate risk.

In the current DST testing of scallops or mussels, it is not feasible to collect 30 individuals, so the number of individuals necessary to reflect the mean DST content of 30 samples collected were estimated in scallops and mussels by statistical resampling analysis using the actual values. Approximately 8 or more samples were considered adequate for scallops, as the variation in DTX1 levels was less than that of mussels. In the bootstrap analysis of more highly variable mussels, 25 samples were insufficient to fall within ±30% of mean value with a probability of 98%. The sample size required changes according to the desired degree of uncertainty level, and the calculation results are restricted to those specific already-known sample data.

As mentioned above, usually a sample size of 30 is difficult to obtain for scallops or mussels. Therefore, we used statistical methods to estimate the mean value of the general population under more practical conditions. Estimation of the population by statistical processing and estimation of the size of necessary samples are basic methods that are described in some textbooks [13,17]. However, no cases have been applied to the field of shellfish toxins. To estimate the mean value of the DST populations of shellfish samples, the samples must be distributed normally in order to apply the statistical parametric test equation. From the individual data group (Figures 3 and 5), the DSTs of each sample basically have a one-peak distribution in which the histogram is almost symmetrical, and the mean and median values are almost matched. Thus, regardless of the concentration, when the variation was not extremely large, it was considered normally distributed. Moreover, it is necessary to take as random a sample as possible from the fact that the total of the depth distribution graph with 5–15 m takes a more normal distribution (Figure 5d,h).

According to the calculation results of Equations (3) and (5) (Table 7 and Figure 7), if there is individual information about the samples, the risk can be evaluated as a concrete figure for the mean concentration of the population. Even when the sample size is less than 5, the interval estimation against DST can be obtained from the value. This makes it possible to evaluate whether sampling is sufficient or not as well as the risk of estimating population concentration. Attention should be paid to the difference between σ and s in these statistical calculations. The statistical definition of σ is completely different from that of s, and s is required for estimating the value. Although in this report we did not deal directly with other shellfish toxins such as paralytic shellfish toxins (PST), the mean concentration of the population and the risk can be estimated and evaluated according to Equation (3) in the same manner.

As the sample size increases in t-value, the slope of the linear approximation decreases and the value becomes strict (Figure 8). Finally, it is a straight line with zero slope passing through the infinity t-value with the necessary reliability (ex, $y = t_{0.10}(\infty) = 1.6449$ or $y = t_{0.05}(\infty) = 1.9600$). The larger the sample size, the better, but in practice there are many cases where statistical ideals are not satisfied due to various restrictions. In the case of scallops or mussels, calculation of an approximate expression using an impractically large size of samples is irrational and not applicable to real-world conditions. Hence, the linear approximate expression at each reliability ($\alpha = 0.10$ or 0.05) was calculated using samples of 20, 25, and 30 in this study (Figure 8). Samples of about 14 or more for scallops or mussels were derived as ideal sample sizes as the result of the estimation from Figure 8. Because the graph of $f(t, \nu = 100)$ and the standard normal distribution $f(t, \nu = \infty)$ are almost identical (Figure 9), 13 or more samples are considered to be a practical preferred range including mathematical errors.

On the other hand, in an investigation or analysis that can sample from 100 to 1000 individuals, another criterion corresponding to such sample size should be applied. A small sample size such as $n = 3$ and a high risk of $\alpha = 0.10$ are presented in this report for research purposes. The desired minimum sample size is 13 or more, and it is necessary to carefully consider the risk corresponding to $\alpha = 0.10$, meaning a rejection rate of 10%.

In conclusion, our study shows that DSTs in scallops and mussels are localized in the digestive gland and the DST concentrations have a normal distribution. Statistical analysis of the normal distribution data enables estimation of DST population-interval and shows that a sample size of 13 or more individuals is desirable. Simple evaluations and calculations using tables in this article can be applied in various situations. Although it is inevitable to combine samples at the time of the actual inspection of shellfish, in research, it is desirable to try to acquire as much important individual information as possible, to obtain more accurate values, and to evaluate the risks. Those results are used as an index for risk assessment and are expected to contribute to risk management in shellfish toxins.

4. Materials and Methods

4.1. Plankton Monitoring

One liter of seawater was sampled from May to August 2016 using Van Dorn bottles at 5 m depth intervals from Yakumo Station (42°16.208′ N, 140°20.568′ E) in Uchiura Bay (Funka Bay), Hokkaido, Japan. Each 1 L sample was concentrated and resuspended to 10 mL by filtration through a 20-µm mesh plankton net sieve and fixed with 1.25% glutaraldehyde. To estimate the densities of *Dinophysis*, 1 mL of each sample was stained with 0.01% of fluorescent dye (Whitex BB, Sumitomo Chemical, Chuo-ku, Tokyo, Japan) and observed with an inverted epifluorescence microscope (IX71, Olympus,

Shinjuku-ku, Tokyo, Japan) under UV light excitation. Vertical profiles of temperature and salinity were obtained from CTD (RINKO-Profiler ASTD102, JFE Advantech, Nishinomiya, Hyogo, Japan) casts. Water transparency was recorded using the Secchi disk (30 cm in diameter, RIGO CO. LTD., Bunkyo-ku, Tokyo, Japan).

4.2. Scallops and Mussels

Scallops and mussels, several individuals grown on each lantern net [10] at the same point, were collected from Nonai Station (40°52′ N, 140°07′ E, Depth = 32 m) in Mutsu Bay, Aomori Prefecture, Japan, in 2014. The Aomori prefecture is located at the northern end of Honshu Island. Other scallops with ear-hanging [10] were harvested near Yakumo Station (42°16.558′ N, 140°20.000′ E) of Uchiura Bay, Hokkaido, Japan, in 2016. Hokkaido is the northernmost prefecture of Japan.

4.3. Extraction of DSTs and Hydrolysis of Esterified DSTs

Each dissected tissue was homogenized with 9 volumes of methanol-distilled water (9:1, v/v), and the homogenates were centrifuged at 3000 rpm for 5 min [18]. Alkaline hydrolysis of the OA group was carried out according to the EU harmonized standard operating procedure for lipophilic marine biotoxins in molluscs by LC-MS/MS, ver. 5 [19]. For hydrolysis, 125 µL of 2.5 M NaOH solution was added to a 1 mL aliquot of a methanolic extract of each sample. The mixture was kept at 80 °C for 30 min and neutralized with 125 µL of 2.5 M HCl. The hydrolyzed samples were analyzed by LC/MS/MS without further purification.

4.4. Standard Toxins

The National Metrology Institute of Japan certified reference material of okadaic acid (OA) and dinophysistoxin-1 (DTX1) [20] were dissolved in HPLC-grade methanol to prepare the calibration standards.

4.5. LC/MS/MS Analysis of DSTs

OA and DTX1 in sample extracts were analyzed and quantified by LC/MS/MS as reported previously [16,18]. Triplicate analyses were carried out for each sample extract. Multiple reaction monitoring (MRM) LC/MS/MS analysis for toxins was carried out using $[M-H]^-$ as target parent ions in Q1 and particular fragment ions of each toxin in Q3, with a dwell time of 100 ms for each analogue as follows. OA: m/z 803.5 > 255.3; DTX1: m/z 817.5 > 255.3. LoD (limit of detection) of OA and DTX1 < 0.01 mg/kg. The proportion of the DTX1 quantity corresponding to each tissue was calculated by multiplying the concentrations by the total tissue weight.

4.6. Statistical Analyses

Statistical analysis program R [21] with boot (https://CRAN.R-project.org/package=boot) and MASS (https://CRAN.R-project.org/package=MASS) packages were employed for resampling analysis and for graphing the standard normal distribution and t-distribution. The values repeatedly calculated 10,000 times with 5–25 random samplings from 30 scallops or mussels were converted to percentages as compared with the mean value of 30 scallops or mussels. This computation is a kind of bootstrap method that has been modified so as not to allow replacement. This provides an estimate of the mean distribution, and how the mean varies depending on the size of samples is presented. The bootstrap method is also applied in the same manner except to allow replacement. Since the resampling analysis without replacement picks up different random samples and the bootstrap method may pick up random samples, including the same samples, more stringent results can be obtained.

Population is parent population.

Sample size is the number of individuals within a group. Number of samples is the number of groups.

N = number of individuals in the population.
n = number of individuals in the sample.

The population mean is represented by the Greek letter *mu* (μ), and $\hat{\mu}$ represents the estimator. The x_i is an individual sample value, and the sample mean is represented by $\overline{x}$.
The population variance is denoted by σ^2.

$$\sigma^2 = \frac{1}{N}\sum_{i=1}^{N}(x_i - \mu)^2 \tag{10}$$

The population standard deviation is denoted by σ.

$$\sigma = \sqrt{\sigma^2} \tag{11}$$

The sample variance is denoted by s^2.

$$s^2 = \frac{1}{n-1}\sum_{i=1}^{n}\left(X_i - \overline{X}\right)^2 \tag{12}$$

The sample standard deviation is denoted by s.

$$s = \sqrt{s^2}. \tag{13}$$

Two-tailed significance level (α) = 0.05 or 0.10.
Confidence level = $1 - \alpha$.
Confidence interval (CI) = $100\,(1 - \alpha)\%$.
Statistical degrees of freedom = $n - 1$ = Greek letter *nu* (ν).
t is derived from Student's t-distribution table using $n - 1$ and α (Table 6).

According to the central limit theorem, regardless of the distribution of the population, if the sample number is made sufficiently large, the error between the population mean and the sample mean follows a normal distribution.

According to the law of large numbers, if the sample size is made sufficiently large, the sample mean converges to the population mean.

Author Contributions: T.S., H.O., and T.A. interpreted data and supervised the research. I.O., Y.K., and M.K. collected and prepared the samples. R.M., H.U., and R.W. analyzed the toxins. R.M. and T.S. wrote the paper.

Funding: The series of studies was conducted and supported by the Ministry of Agriculture, Forestry, and Fisheries (Regulatory Research Projects for Food Safety).

Acknowledgments: We are grateful to Hidetsugu Yoshida of the Mariculture Fisheries Research Institute, Hokkaido Research Organization, and to Daisuke Achiya of the Yakumo Town Fisheries Cooperative for their helpful assistance in the field samplings and measurement. We would like to thank Lincoln Mackenzie for assistance with English corrections and his valuable comments.

Conflicts of Interest: The authors declare no conflict of interest.

References

1. Yasumoto, T.; Oshima, Y.; Yamaguchi, M. Occurrence of a new type of shellfish poisoning in the Tohoku. *Bull. Jpn. Soc. Sci. Fish.* **1978**, *44*, 1249–1255. [CrossRef]
2. Yasumoto, T.; Murata, M.; Oshima, Y.; Sano, M.; Matsumoto, G.K.; Clardy, J. Diarrhetic shellfish toxins. *Tetrahedron* **1985**, *41*, 1019–1025. [CrossRef]
3. Yasumoto, T.; Murata, M. Marine toxins. *Chem. Rev.* **1993**, *93*, 1897–1909. [CrossRef]
4. Bialojan, C.; Takagi, A. Inhibitory effect of a marine-sponge toxin, okadaic acid, on protein phosphatases. Specificity and kinetics. *Biochem. J.* **1988**, *256*, 283–290. [CrossRef] [PubMed]

5. Terao, K.; Ito, E.; Yanagi, T.; Yasumoto, T. Histopathological studies on experimental marine toxin poisoning. I. Ultrastructural changes in the small intestine and liver of suckling mice induced by dinophysistoxin-1 and pectenotoxin-1. *Toxicon* **1986**, *24*, 1145–1151. [CrossRef]
6. Fujiki, H.; Suganuma, M.; Suguri, H.; Yoshizawa, S.; Takagi, K.; Uda, N.; Wakamatsu, K.; Yamada, K.; Murata, M.; Yasumoto, T.; et al. Diarrhetic shellfish toxin, dinophysistoxin-1, is a potent tumor promoter on mouse skin. *Jpn. J. Cancer Res.* **1988**, *79*, 1089–1093. [CrossRef] [PubMed]
7. Suzuki, T.; Ota, H.; Yamasaki, M. Direct evidence of transformation of dinophysistoxin-1 to 7-*O*-acyl-dinophysistoxin-1 (dinophysistoxin-3) in the scallop *Patinopecten yessoensis*. *Toxicon* **1999**, *37*, 187–198. [CrossRef]
8. Guidelines for Risk Management of Shellfish Toxins in Bivalves. Available online: http://www.maff.go.jp/j/syouan/tikusui/gyokai/g_kenko/busitu/pdf/150306_kaidoku_guide.pdf (accessed on 25 September 2018).
9. Standard for Liver and Raw Bivalve Molluscs (CODEX STAN 292-2008). Available online: http://www.fao.org/fao-who-codexalimentarius/sh-proxy/es/?lnk=1&url=https%253A%252F%252Fworkspace.fao.org%252Fsites%252Fcodex%252FStandards%252FCODEX%2BSTAN%2B292-2008%252FCXS_292e_2015.pdf (accessed on 25 September 2018).
10. Sandra, E.S.; Parson, J.G. *Scallops: Biology, Ecology, Aquaculture, and Fisheries*, 3rd ed.; Elsevier Science: Amsterdam, The Netherlands, 2016; Volume 40, pp. 891–936. ISBN 978-0-444-62710-0.
11. Matsushima, R.; Uchida, H.; Nagai, S.; Watanabe, R.; Kamio, M.; Nagai, H.; Kaneniwa, M.; Suzuki, T. Assimilation, accumulation and metabolism of dinophysistoxins (DTXs) and pectenotoxins (PTXs) in the Japanese scallop *Patinopecten yessoensis*. *Toxins* **2015**, *7*, 5141–5154. [CrossRef] [PubMed]
12. Matsushima, R.; Uchida, H.; Watanabe, R.; Oikawa, H.; Kosaka, Y.; Tanabe, T.; Suzuki, T. Distribution of Diarrhetic Shellfish Toxins in Mussels, Scallops, and Ascidian. *Food Saf.* **2018**, *6*, 101–106. [CrossRef]
13. Lemeshow, S.; Hosmer, D.W.; Klar, J.; Lwango, S.K. *World Health Organization. Adequacy of Sample Size in Health Studies*; John Wiley & Sons Ltd.: West Sussex, UK, 1990; pp. 36–62. ISBN 0471925179.
14. Student. The probable error of a mean. *Biometrika* **1908**, *6*, 1–25. [CrossRef]
15. Fisher, R.A. Applications of "tudent's" distribution. *Metron* **1925**, *5*, 90–104.
16. Suzuki, T.; Miyazono, A.; Baba, K.; Sugawara, R.; Kamiyama, T. LC–MS/MS analysis of okadaic acid analogues and other lipophilic toxins in single-cell isolates of several *Dinophysis* species collected in Hokkaido, Japan. *Harmful Algae* **2009**, *8*, 233–238. [CrossRef]
17. *Sampling Plans for Aflatoxin Analysis in Peanuts and Corn*; Report for FAO Technical Consultation; FAO: Rome, Italy, May 1993.
18. Suzuki, T.; Jin, T.; Shirota, Y.; Mitsuya, T.; Okumura, Y.; Kamiyama, T. Quantification of lipophilic toxins associated with diarrhetic shellfish poisoning in Japanese bivalves by liquid chromatography-mass spectrometry and comparison with mouse bioassay. *Fish. Sci.* **2005**, *71*, 1370–1378. [CrossRef]
19. EU-Harmonised Standard Operating Procedure for Determination of Lipophilic Marine Biotoxins in Molluscs by LCMS/MS Version 5. Available online: http://www.aecosan.msssi.gob.es/AECOSAN/docs/documentos/laboratorios/LNRBM/ARCHIVO2EU-Harmonised-SOP-LIPO-LCMSMS_Version5.pdf (accessed on 25 September 2018).
20. NMIJ CRM Catalog 2016–2017, National Institute of Advanced Industrial Science and Technology (AIST), National Metrology Institute of Japan (NMIJ). Available online: https://www.nmij.jp/english/service/C/CRM_Catalog_(JE)160901.pdf (accessed on 25 September 2018).
21. R: A Language and Environment for Statistical Computing. Available online: https://www.R-project.org/ (accessed on 25 September 2018).

toxins

MDPI

Article

RNA-Seq Analysis for Assessing the Early Response to DSP Toxins in *Mytilus galloprovincialis* Digestive Gland and Gill

María Verónica Prego-Faraldo, Luisa Martínez * and Josefina Méndez

Grupo Xenomar, Departamento de Bioloxía, Facultade de Ciencias and CICA (Centro de Investigacións Científicas Avanzadas), Universidade da Coruña, Campus de A Zapateira, 15071 A Coruña, Spain; veronica.prego@udc.es (M.V.P.-F.); josefina.mendez@udc.es (J.M.)

* Correspondence: m.l.martinez@udc.es; Tel.: +34-981-167000-2030; Fax: +34-981-167065

Received: 5 September 2018; Accepted: 13 October 2018; Published: 16 October 2018

Abstract: The harmful effects of diarrhetic shellfish poisoning (DSP) toxins on mammalian cell lines have been widely assessed. Studies in bivalves suggest that mussels display a resistance to the cytogenotoxic effects of DSP toxins. Further, it seems that the bigger the exposure, the more resistant mussels become. To elucidate the early genetic response of mussels against these toxins, the digestive gland and the gill transcriptomes of *Mytilus galloprovincialis* after *Prorocentrum lima* exposure (100,000 cells/L, 48 h) were de novo assembled based on the sequencing of 8 cDNA libraries obtained using an Illumina HiSeq 2000 platform. The assembly provided 95,702 contigs. A total of 2286 and 4523 differentially expressed transcripts were obtained in the digestive gland and the gill, respectively, indicating tissue-specific transcriptome responses. These transcripts were annotated and functionally enriched, showing 44 and 60 significant Pfam families in the digestive gland and the gill, respectively. Quantitative PCR (qPCR) was performed to validate the differential expression patterns of several genes related to lipid and carbohydrate metabolism, energy production, genome integrity and defense, suggesting their participation in the protective mechanism. This work provides knowledge of the early response against DSP toxins in the mussel *M. galloprovincialis* and useful information for further research on the molecular mechanisms of the bivalve resistance to these toxins.

Keywords: DSP toxins; bivalves; mussel; resistance; RNA-Seq; qPCR; metabolism; defense; immunity

Key Contribution: This work describes the transcriptome and gene expression profiles of *M. galloprovincialis* digestive gland and gill after early exposure to DSP toxins. Results showed that differentially expressed genes (DEGs) include genes involved in defense, immunity and metabolism, although some of them have been described as DEGs in response to other stimuli. This indicates that the mussel defense reaction is to some extent unspecific. This study also indicated that the expression of rpS4 and TPM genes in the digestive gland under these experimental conditions is stable and, therefore, these genes can be employed as reference genes to normalize gene expression in qPCR experiments carried out in mussels exposed to low concentrations of DSP toxins for short time periods.

---

1. Introduction

Nowadays, harmful algal blooms (HABs) constitute one of the most important sources of natural contamination in the marine environment. This term refers not only to the phenomena originated by the proliferation of harmful algae, but also the phenomena caused by proliferation of toxic algae [1]. Although there is still a considerable absence of high quality time-series data in most regions affected by HABs [2], the blooms caused by the outbreaks of diarrhetic shellfish poisoning (DSP) toxin producing species seem to be associated with most of the HABs detected in European coasts [3]. These toxins are produced by dinoflagellates of the *Dinophysis* and *Prorocentrum* genera and constitute a heterogenous group of polyethers, including okadaic acid (OA) and its analogs, the dinophysis toxins (DTXs) [3–8]. In terms of abundance and consequent toxicity, OA is considered the main DSP toxin followed by DTX1, while DTX3—a less abundant DSP toxin—has become important because of its production through metabolic transformations that occur in some bivalves [7]. DTX1 seems to have similar toxicity levels to that of OA, while DTX2, DTX3 and DTX4 are less acutely toxic. On the other hand, the acylation of the 7-hydroxyl group with a saturated fatty acid forms compounds which are approximately 20 times less toxic than OA [9]. DSP toxins have a high lipophilic character, which allows for them to be accumulated in the fatty tissues of filter-feeding organisms—mainly in bivalve mollusks—and be transferred across the food chain, causing several gastrointestinal disorders [6]. Currently, efficient monitoring programs have been established by many countries to ban the harvesting of contaminated seafood and therefore, avert human intoxications [3]. However, seafood with small quantities of DSP toxins is still commercialized.

Since the ability of OA to inhibit several types of serine/threonine protein phosphatases was discovered by Bialojan and Takai [4], numerous works have studied the harmful effects of this toxic compound on different model systems, including different mammalian cell lines [8]. However, studies that assess the effects of these toxins in their main vectors—bivalve mollusks—are scarce. Recent studies carried out by our research group showed that DSP toxins cause more severe genotoxic and cytotoxic effects in bivalve cells at low concentrations and short exposition times, while these effects decrease or disappear as exposure increases in concentration and time [5,10–12]. This suggests that these organisms may have developed a quick protection mechanism against these toxic compounds. This may be associated with the accumulation, transformation and elimination of DSP toxins. This still unknown mechanism is of great interest for predicting the time course of toxic episodes and for reducing their negative consequences. With the aim of obtaining knowledge about this early genetic response, our research group has assessed the immediate effects caused by DSP toxins in the mussel *Mytilus galloprovincialis* using different stress indicators: DNA breaks, number of apoptotic cells [12], lipid peroxidation and antioxidant enzyme activities [10]. Although these indicators constitute a good approach to assess the first harmful effects produced by these toxins, they offer just a partial view on mussel response to toxic compounds. Taking this into account, it seems necessary to carry out analyses on the transcriptome response of mussels to DSP toxins to obtain a global perspective on their defense mechanisms against these toxins. Previous works used transcriptomic techniques to determine *M. galloprovincialis* transcriptome response to several stimuli, including marine toxins and pathogens [13–19]. Transcriptomic techniques such as RNA-Seq provide a valuable contribution to determining which gene pool expression is induced or suppressed depending on its physiological role in response to different treatments [20].

Some works have determined that the accumulation and distribution of DSP toxins in mussels is tissue specific [21,22]. The digestive gland is the mussel tissue that accumulates the most DSP toxins and is considered the main site of toxin bioconversion [23]. Furthermore, gills have numerous functions related to feeding, digestion and elimination of wastes and contaminants. The large surface and thin epithelium of the mussel gill make it an efficient site for direct interaction with the environment. Thus, gills efficiently capture suspended food particles—thanks to the mucus produced by them—and mediate their transport through the mussel mouth and digestive system [24].

In this work the whole transcriptome of the mussel *M. galloprovincialis* was de novo assembled and differentially expressed genes (DEGs) in digestive gland and gill after early exposure to DSP toxin-producer *Prorocentrum lima* were identified in order to determine the first response of these bivalve mollusks to these toxins and identify transcripts which could participate in the resistance mechanisms of mussels against the harmful effects of DSP toxins. Previous studies have characterized gene expression changes related to exposition to OA in bivalve mollusks [17,18,25,26] but to our knowledge, this is the first work that uses RNA-Seq to study the early transcriptional response of the mussel *M. galloprovincialis* to DSP toxins under short exposure to low concentrations of *P. lima*.

2. Results

2.1. Toxin Accumulation

According to the High Performance Liquid Chromatography/Mass Spectrometry (HPLC/MS) analyses, the *P. lima* strain AND-A0605 had an average toxin content of 0.4 pg OA/cell. Control mussels, fed with a mixture of *Isochrysis galbana* and *Tetraselmis suecica*, did not accumulate OA (<0.1 ng/g dry weight), while OA accumulated in treated mussels—fed also with *P. lima*—was 112.12 ng/g dry weight. Based on these results, and since these levels are well below the limit allowed by the European Commission Regulation for harvesting and sale (160 μg of OA equivalent/kg dry weight), we could consider that the mussels were exposed to low microalga cell densities, similar to those at the early stages of a HAB [27].

2.2. Transcriptome Sequencing and De Novo Assembly

In order to investigate the defense mechanisms of mussels exposed to DSP toxins, eight libraries derived from the digestive gland and the gill of the mussel *M. galloprovincialis,* in the absence of and under low densities of *P. lima* exposure, were constructed and sequenced using an Illumina sequencing platform. After de novo assembly with Trinity and Oases and their subsequent clustering by homology, 95,702 transcripts were obtained. Mean transcript size was 748 bp, with lengths ranging from as small as 100 bp to as a large as 16,082 bp. About 78% of the final assemblies were >200 bp and a N50 length of 1062 bp was obtained (Table 1).

Table 1. Summary of reference transcriptome assembly for *M. galloprovincialis*.

Total number of contigs	95,702	**L25**	1682 bp
Total length	71,623.079 Kb	**N50**	21,152
Maximum contig length	16,082 Kb	**L50**	1062 bp
Minimum contig length	102 pb	**N75**	42,376
Average contig length	748 bp	**L75**	668 bp
N25	7537	**%GC**	33.20%

2.3. DEGs Among Samples

Transcriptomic analyses were performed with the aim of identifying the main molecular mechanisms involved in the response of mussels to early contamination by DSP toxins. Using a RNA-Seq experiment, we generated transcriptome profiles for the digestive gland and the gill of the mussel *M. galloprovincialis* exposed to low densities of *P. lima* (100,000 cells/L) for a short period of time (48 h) and compared these data with profiles obtained from the digestive glands and the gills of control mussels. Sequences of all DEGs obtained are listed in File S1. A Venn diagram was used to depict the overlapping of DEGs when libraries were compared (Figure 1). Regarding the digestive gland, there were a total of 2286 DEGs between treatment and control groups, from which 1198 and 1088 transcripts were up- and down-regulated, respectively. Regarding the gills, there were a total of 4523 DEGs between both groups (treatment and control), from which 2579 and 1944 transcripts were up- and down-regulated, respectively. As a complementary analysis, the comparison of treated digestive glands and gills showed a total of 27,174 DEGs; 14,985 of them were up-regulated transcripts, while 12,189 were down-regulated (File S2). Only 26 transcripts out of all DEGs obtained were detected in all comparisons, with 17 and 9 of them being up- and down-regulated, respectively. The comparison of digestive glands and gills showed a total of 253 DEGs, from which 110 and 143 transcripts were up- and down-regulated, respectively. These DEGs could be useful for discovering genes involved in the early response to DSP toxins and, thereby, for identifying putative biomarkers for monitoring in advance of contamination episodes in the marine environment.

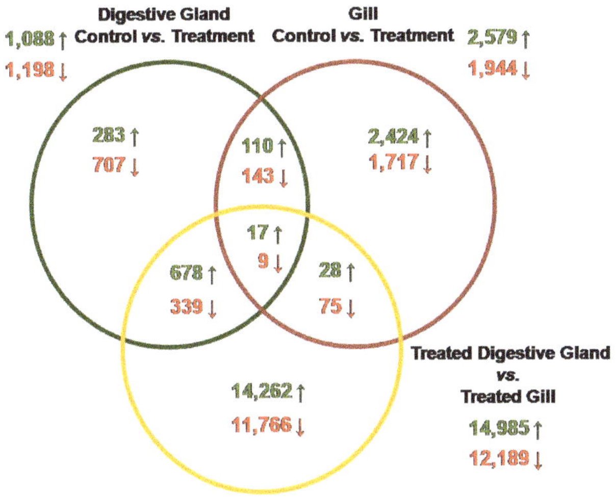

Figure 1. Venn diagram indicating the overlaping of genes significantly up-regulated (green arrows) and down-regulated (red arrows) when DEGs from different libraries were compared.

2.4. Gene Functional Annotations

Only 6% of the contigs included in the reference transcriptome showed BLAST similarity to proteins. About 20% of transcripts showed similarity to protein sequences deposited in the UniProt database and approximately 50% showed Pfam annotations. Thus, a relevant fraction of the contigs included in the reference transcriptome obtained in this work did not display any BLAST similarity or annotation.

Tables 2–5 show the 25 most significantly up- and down-regulated genes in the digestive gland and the gill after exposure to low concentrations of DSP toxins (100,000 cells/L) for a short time period (48 h). Among the top over-represented DEGs in the digestive gland are genes that encode enzymes involved in the electron transport chain or mitochondrial oxidative phosphorilation (cytochrome c oxidase), as well as genes that encode ribosomal proteins or proteolytic enzymes (ribosomal protein L23a) (Table 2). Among the infra-represented genes in this tissue are also genes that encode enzymes of the electron transport chain (NADH dehydrogenase subunit 5) and ribosomal proteins (40S ribosomal protein S10-like). On the other hand, there are genes related to apoptosis (GTPase IMAP family member 7) and genes that encode proteins involved in the formation of nacre, promoting the crystallization of calcium carbonate (Perlucin) (Table 3). Similar to the digestive gland, among the over-represented genes in the gill (Table 4) are genes that encode enzymes of the electron transport chain (NADH dehydrogenase subunit 6) and proteins that play a role in the regulation of ion transport (calcyphosin-like protein). In contrast to the results obtained in the digestive gland, a gene encoding the cytochrome c oxidase subunit I is significantly down-regulated (Table 5). Also, a gene that encodes a protein involved in lipid metabolic processes and endocytosis is down-regulated in this tissue in the early response to DSP toxins (Table 5).

Table 2. List of the 25 putative top up-regulated genes (ordered by *p*-value) in response to early concentrations of DSP toxins in the digestive gland of *M. galloprovincialis*.

Sequence ID	Description	Length (bp)	baseMean	Log2FC	FC	*p*-Value	Adjusted *p*-Value
ci∣000006456∣Bact∣Sample_MGT2∣2	cytochrome c oxidase subunit 1, partial	910	23,389.22	7.09	136.29	1.96×10^{112}	1.70×10^{-107}
ci∣000001182∣Bact∣Sample_MBT2∣2	* ATP-synt_A	578	3975.18	7.21	147.76	6.65×10^{-66}	1.92×10^{-61}
Contig39610	ribosomal protein L23a, partial	1166	2205.27	7.92	243.02	3.89×10^{-43}	6.71×10^{-39}
ci∣000005084∣Bact∣Sample_MGT2∣2	cytochrome c oxidase subunit I	1848	12,611.71	6.23	75.08	1.91×10^{-37}	2.75×10^{-33}
Contig34888	NA	529	608.03	8.47	355.72	4.04×10^{-35}	4.98×10^{-31}
ci∣000015505∣Bact∣Sample_MGT1∣2	NA	588	1046.84	5.05	33.22	9.05×10^{-35}	9.78×10^{-31}
ci∣000014133∣Bact∣Sample_MGT2∣2	* Glyco_hydro_16	949	411.92	6.95	124.04	3.09×10^{-34}	2.97×10^{-30}
Contig22742	NA	1165	944.38	6.61	97.63	4.80×10^{-33}	4.14×10^{-29}
Contig33832	Kazal-like serine protease inhibitor domain-containing protein	507	514.55	6.70	103.84	6.63×10^{-33}	5.20×10^{-29}
ci∣000004031∣Bact∣Sample_MGT1∣2	* Porin_3	1024	888.45	5.19	36.44	3.14×10^{-31}	2.09×10^{-27}
ci∣000016700∣Bact∣Sample_MGT1∣2	† COX1_MYTED	750	12,157.03	6.86	116.52	2.32×10^{-30}	1.43×10^{-26}
ci∣000022316∣Bact∣Sample_MBT1∣2	* Ribosomal_L23	340	280.82	6.68	102.35	2.26×10^{-28}	1.15×10^{-24}
Contig17884	PREDICTED: 60 kDa SS-A/Ro ribonucleoprotein	1726	227.65	5.51	45.57	6.21×10^{-25}	2.68×10^{-21}
ci∣000012420∣Bact∣Sample_MGT2∣2	NA	560	761.81	9.97	1004.61	2.04×10^{-24}	8.01×10^{-21}
ci∣000010593∣Bact∣Sample_MBC1∣2	* Ribosomal_L7Ae	458	403.47	8.29	313.91	6.26×10^{-23}	2.16×10^{-19}
ci∣000001186∣Bact∣Sample_MGT2∣2	NA	316	209.87	6.26	76.55	7.11×10^{-23}	2.36×10^{-19}
ci∣000001089∣Bact∣Sample_MGT2∣2	NA	1106	224.57	5.35	40.77	1.03×10^{-20}	3.08×10^{-17}
Contig35276	NA	420	188.91	7.45	174.32	6.35×10^{-20}	1.77×10^{-16}
Contig38903	* Myticin-prepro	506	510.91	9.28	623.48	1.02×10^{-19}	2.68×10^{-16}
ci∣000022507∣Bact∣Sample_MBT2∣2	* Ribosomal_S9	1568	918.24	5.20	36.82	3.34×10^{-19}	7.79×10^{-16}
ci∣000000480∣Bact∣Sample_MGT2∣2	* Astacin	858	563.33	6.67	101.71	4.63×10^{-19}	1.00×10^{-15}
ci∣000018470∣Bact∣Sample_MGT1∣2	* Lectin_C	633	186.73	7.90	238.40	5.47×10^{-19}	1.13×10^{-15}
ci∣000004710∣Bact∣Sample_MBC2∣2	NA	1395	219.14	6.06	66.62	1.35×10^{-18}	2.66×10^{-15}
ci∣000008308∣Bact∣Sample_MGT1∣2	NA	464	637.37	5.04	32.92	1.82×10^{-18}	3.49×10^{-15}
ci∣000004147∣Bact∣Sample_MGT2∣2	NA	622	507.89	6.81	112.02	2.47×10^{-18}	4.65×10^{-15}

FC: Fold Change. NA: No gene annotation for the transcript. * Pfam result: protein containing the specified domain. † BlastUniProt result.

Table 3. List of the 25 putative top down-regulated genes (ordered by *p*-value) in response to early concentrations of DSP toxins in the digestive gland of *M. galloprovincialis*.

Sequence ID	Description	Length (bp)	baseMean	Log2FC	FC	*p*-Value	Adjusted *p*-Value
ci|000007816|Bact|Sample_MGC1|2	NA	539	7514.26	−7.48	−178.70	1.66×10^{-82}	7.17×10^{-78}
Contig22552	NA	622	131,251.75	−6.93	−121.52	5.49×10^{-60}	1.18×10^{-55}
Contig26868	NADH dehydrogenase subunit 5, partial	719	1916.17	−6.96	−124.62	2.16×10^{-32}	1.56×10^{-28}
Contig28135	40S ribosomal protein S10-like	559	406.63	−5.12	−34.81	5.46×10^{-29}	3.14×10^{-25}
Contig30578	* DUF1082	529	3132.77	−9.97	−1005.57	2.05×10^{-28}	1.11×10^{-24}
Contig28105	* SRCR	1419	329.84	−7.74	−213.17	2.60×10^{-26}	1.25×10^{-22}
ci|000000372|Bact|Sample_MGC1|2	NA	723	851.06	−6.15	−70.81	7.19×10^{-26}	3.27×10^{-22}
ci|000009048|Bact|Sample_MBC1|2	NA	703	359.37	−8.39	−334.64	1.14×10^{-24}	4.67×10^{-21}
Contig26906	NA	530	286.75	−8.12	−279.10	1.47×10^{-23}	5.52×10^{-20}
ci|000018684|Bact|Sample_MBC2|2	* Cytochrom_B_N_2	643	2708.10	−7.79	−221.90	5.93×10^{-23}	2.13×10^{-19}
ci|000000728|Bact|Sample_MGC2|2	NA	768	510.67	−9.66	−810.78	8.67×10^{-23}	2.77×10^{-19}
Contig29976	uncharacterized protein LOC567525 isoform X1/* Fibrinogen_C	1089	167.09	−6.83	−114.10	6.31×10^{-21}	1.95×10^{-17}
ci|000000734|Bact|Sample_MGC2|2	* Zona_pellucida	1185	255.85	−9.02	−518.06	4.16×10^{-20}	1.20×10^{-16}
Contig26843	NA	984	230.17	−4.23	−18.76	7.68×10^{-20}	2.07×10^{-16}
ci|000002253|Bact|Sample_MGC2|2	PREDICTED: GTPase IMAP family member 7/* AIG1	1188	255.05	−7.83	−228.11	1.33×10^{-19}	3.37×10^{-16}
ci|000003979|Bact|Sample_MGC1|2	NA	1136	233.95	−8.88	−471.60	2.94×10^{-19}	7.25×10^{-16}
ci|000021317|Bact|Sample_MBC1|2	NA	834	1818.89	−6.97	−125.28	3.04×10^{-19}	7.29×10^{-16}
ci|000008655|Bact|Sample_MGC2|2	NA	374	1501.18	−8.07	−267.93	4.48×10^{-19}	1.00×10^{-15}
ci|000004674|Bact|Sample_MGC2|2	Perlucin	660	174.13	−5.61	−48.70	4.57×10^{-19}	1.00×10^{-15}
ci|000023153|Bact|Sample_MBT1|2	* COX1	605	4253.61	−6.85	−115.03	5.47×10^{-19}	1.13×10^{-15}
ci|000001983|Bact|Sample_MBC2|2	* KOW	607	4924.53	−2.78	−6.88	8.86×10^{-19}	1.78×10^{-15}
ci|000005149|Bact|Sample_MGC1|2	* TIG	612	148.86	−6.00	−64.19	2.90×10^{-17}	5.11×10^{-14}
ci|000009215|Bact|Sample_MGC2|2	* Glyco_hydro_10	946	136.75	−7.11	−138.62	4.08×10^{-17}	7.06×10^{-14}
Contig28020	NA	570	166.31	−8.45	−350.56	4.96×10^{-17}	8.24×10^{-14}
ci|000015516|Bact|Sample_MBT2|2	* Ribosomal_L22	1338	1356.05	−4.92	−30.37	1.19×10^{-16}	1.87×10^{-13}

FC: Fold Change. NA: No gene annotation for the transcript. * Pfam result: protein containing the specified domain.

Table 4. List of the 25 putative top up-regulated genes (ordered by *p*-value) in response to early concentrations of DSP toxins in the gill of *M. galloprovincialis*.

<table>
<tr><th>Sequence ID</th><th>Description</th><th>Length (bp)</th><th>baseMean</th><th>Log2FC</th><th>FC</th><th>p-Value</th><th>Adjusted p-Value</th></tr>
<tr><td>ci|000029194|Bact|Sample_MBT1|2</td><td>* EF-hand_1 and 7</td><td>508</td><td>3570.44</td><td>9.76</td><td>868.30</td><td>7.36×10^{-98}</td><td>6.48×10^{-93}</td></tr>
<tr><td>ci|000006043|Bact|Sample_MBT1|2</td><td>NA</td><td>471</td><td>4432.18</td><td>6.05</td><td>66.47</td><td>4.32×10^{-60}</td><td>1.90×10^{-55}</td></tr>
<tr><td>ci|000001929|Bact|Sample_MBT2|2</td><td>NA</td><td>690</td><td>803.53</td><td>7.61</td><td>195.15</td><td>4.55×10^{-49}</td><td>1.00×10^{-44}</td></tr>
<tr><td>ci|000002899|Bact|Sample_MBT1|2</td><td>NA</td><td>779</td><td>1066.24</td><td>9.48</td><td>715.09</td><td>9.38×10^{-40}</td><td>1.65×10^{-35}</td></tr>
<tr><td>Contig35833</td><td>NA</td><td>944</td><td>520.96</td><td>8.45</td><td>350.51</td><td>6.42×10^{-29}</td><td>6.28×10^{-25}</td></tr>
<tr><td>ci|000022507|Bact|Sample_MBT2|2</td><td>NADH dehydrogenase subunit 6</td><td>1568</td><td>475.01</td><td>3.90</td><td>14.88</td><td>1.10×10^{-28}</td><td>9.70×10^{-25}</td></tr>
<tr><td>ci|000017597|Bact|Sample_MBT1|2</td><td>* Antistasin</td><td>795</td><td>266.99</td><td>7.13</td><td>140.36</td><td>1.22×10^{-28}</td><td>9.79×10^{-25}</td></tr>
<tr><td>ci|000007496|Bact|Sample_MBT2|2</td><td>NA</td><td>745</td><td>425.52</td><td>6.39</td><td>84.07</td><td>4.01×10^{-28}</td><td>2.94×10^{-24}</td></tr>
<tr><td>ci|000020755|Bact|Sample_MBT2|2</td><td>† NU4M_MYTED</td><td>1483</td><td>849.56</td><td>5.15</td><td>35.44</td><td>1.44×10^{-26}</td><td>9.05×10^{-23}</td></tr>
<tr><td>ci|000025759|Bact|Sample_MBT2|2</td><td>NA</td><td>2007</td><td>257.03</td><td>7.56</td><td>188.10</td><td>1.81×10^{-26}</td><td>1.06×10^{-22}</td></tr>
<tr><td>Contig39610</td><td>* Ribosomal_L23</td><td>1166</td><td>453.85</td><td>6.46</td><td>87.80</td><td>3.94×10^{-26}</td><td>2.16×10^{-22}</td></tr>
<tr><td>Contig15942</td><td>NA</td><td>482</td><td>916.44</td><td>5.84</td><td>57.29</td><td>6.24×10^{-26}</td><td>3.23×10^{-22}</td></tr>
<tr><td>ci|000001411|Bact|Sample_MGC2|2</td><td>* HSBP1</td><td>580</td><td>421.11</td><td>4.55</td><td>23.41</td><td>1.82×10^{-25}</td><td>8.92×10^{-22}</td></tr>
<tr><td>ci|000005084|Bact|Sample_MGT2|2</td><td>* COX1</td><td>1848</td><td>3923.98</td><td>3.98</td><td>15.75</td><td>3.81×10^{-25}</td><td>1.77×10^{-21}</td></tr>
<tr><td>ci|000003417|Bact|Sample_MBT2|2</td><td>* Phospholip_A2_1</td><td>562</td><td>203.18</td><td>6.08</td><td>67.55</td><td>1.10×10^{-23}</td><td>4.05×10^{-20}</td></tr>
<tr><td>Contig20144</td><td>NA</td><td>2258</td><td>205.66</td><td>3.81</td><td>14.01</td><td>4.48×10^{-23}</td><td>1.58×10^{-19}</td></tr>
<tr><td>ci|000019916|Bact|Sample_MBT1|2</td><td>NA</td><td>768</td><td>241.64</td><td>7.15</td><td>141.88</td><td>1.42×10^{-22}</td><td>4.45×10^{-19}</td></tr>
<tr><td>ci|000001302|Bact|Sample_MBT1|2</td><td>NA</td><td>675</td><td>281.74</td><td>6.61</td><td>97.65</td><td>1.36×10^{-21}</td><td>4.00×10^{-18}</td></tr>
<tr><td>ci|000018492|Bact|Sample_MBT1|2</td><td>NA</td><td>1552</td><td>159.56</td><td>5.50</td><td>45.19</td><td>1.59×10^{-21}</td><td>4.36×10^{-18}</td></tr>
<tr><td>Contig13066</td><td>Calcyphosin-like protein</td><td>2325</td><td>853.76</td><td>3.68</td><td>12.85</td><td>2.01×10^{-21}</td><td>5.35×10^{-18}</td></tr>
<tr><td>ci|000018122|Bact|Sample_MBT2|2</td><td>* HYR and TMEM154</td><td>3321</td><td>2042.07</td><td>4.34</td><td>20.27</td><td>2.30×10^{-21}</td><td>5.95×10^{-18}</td></tr>
<tr><td>Contig12937</td><td>† RS27L_HUMAN</td><td>2183</td><td>321.15</td><td>7.71</td><td>210.04</td><td>3.66×10^{-21}</td><td>9.21×10^{-18}</td></tr>
<tr><td>ci|000000451|Bact|Sample_MGT2|2</td><td>NA</td><td>655</td><td>587.43</td><td>2.92</td><td>7.57</td><td>1.42×10^{-20}</td><td>3.38×10^{-17}</td></tr>
<tr><td>ci|000003122|Bact|Sample_MBT2|2</td><td>NA</td><td>1513</td><td>215.45</td><td>7.54</td><td>185.87</td><td>4.85×10^{-20}</td><td>1.12×10^{-16}</td></tr>
<tr><td>Contig40138</td><td>NA</td><td>584</td><td>136.63</td><td>6.17</td><td>72.15</td><td>7.64×10^{-20}</td><td>1.72×10^{-16}</td></tr>
</table>

FC: Fold Change. NA: No gene annotation for the transcript. * Pfam result: protein containing the specified domain. † Blast UniProt result.

Table 5. List of the 25 putative top down-regulated genes (ordered by *p*-value) in response to early concentrations of DSP toxins in the gill of *M. galloprovincialis*.

Sequence ID	Description	Length (bp)	baseMean	Log2FC	FC	*p*-Value	Adjusted *p*-Value
ci | 000007038 | Bact | Sample_MBC2 | 2	low-density lipoprotein receptor-related protein 8 isoform X1	689	1321.99	−9.45	−700.32	1.06×10^{-53}	3.11×10^{-49}
Contig3681	NA	895	1561.88	−10.25	−1216.97	9.98×10^{-37}	1.46×10^{-32}
Contig11592	NA	798	652.29	−9.55	−752.01	4.28×10^{-31}	5.38×10^{-27}
Contig1183	NA	581	802.66	−4.76	−27.10	9.28×10^{-30}	1.02×10^{-25}
Contig8105	NA	1717	199.06	−6.43	−86.51	3.62×10^{-27}	2.45×10^{-23}
ci | 000015242 | Bact | Sample_MGT2 | 2	NA	663	429.13	−7.24	−151.36	4.36×10^{-25}	1.92×10^{-21}
ci | 000005973 | Bact | Sample_MBC1 | 2	NA	1860	257.90	−4.59	−24.07	5.34×10^{-25}	2.24×10^{-21}
Contig10936	* Oxidored_q1	2797	18,810.53	−1.67	−3.18	3.68×10^{-24}	1.47×10^{-20}
ci | 000000312 | Bact | Sample_MBC1 | 2	NA	972	208.97	−7.32	−159.95	4.63×10^{-24}	1.77×10^{-20}
Contig6277	NA	702	2009.78	−10.35	−1303.40	6.01×10^{-23}	2.04×10^{-19}
ci | 000016192 | Bact | Sample_MBC1 | 2	* Ldl_recept_a and PRKCSH-like	946	4008.01	−2.65	−6.26	9.71×10^{-23}	3.17×10^{-19}
Contig3876	Predicted protein	536	295.82	−8.43	−344.34	5.01×10^{-22}	1.52×10^{-18}
Contig4774	neurocalcin homolog	1267	339.45	−4.83	−28.39	1.49×10^{-21}	4.22×10^{-18}
ci | 000000823 | Bact | Sample_MBC2 | 2	NA	803	325.92	−3.99	−15.91	1.06×10^{-20}	2.59×10^{-17}
Contig6059	NA	486	5331.78	−1.93	−3.82	8.13×10^{-20}	1.76×10^{-16}
Contig7283	cytochrome c oxidase subunit I	2879	132.24	−5.09	−34.06	9.51×10^{-20}	1.99×10^{-16}
ci | 000015433 | Bact | Sample_MBC1 | 2	cytochrome c oxidase subunit I	1136	17,057.57	−3.52	−11.49	3.00×10^{-19}	5.74×10^{-16}
ci | 000004320 | Bact | Sample_MBC1 | 2	* Lipoxygenase	1950	564.59	−9.46	−703.80	3.48×10^{-19}	6.24×10^{-16}
ci | 000001144 | Bact | Sample_MBC2 | 2	NA	434	221.23	−8.61	−389.88	4.06×10^{-19}	7.15×10^{-16}
ci | 000008127 | Bact | Sample_MBC2 | 2	NA	2503	364.67	−10.03	−1043.76	7.20×10^{-19}	1.22×10^{-15}
ci | 000005247 | Bact | Sample_MBC1 | 2	NA	1246	153.48	−6.35	−81.80	1.26×10^{-18}	2.09×10^{-15}
ci | 000001610 | Bact | Sample_MBC1 | 2	NA	1057	341.22	−9.94	−982.30	1.93×10^{-18}	3.11×10^{-15}
ci | 000000874 | Bact | Sample_MBC2 | 2	NA	697	153.63	−5.02	−32.42	5.21×10^{-18}	7.77×10^{-15}
ci | 000002263 | Bact | Sample_MBC1 | 2	* Pfam-B_5682	1222	151.49	−4.77	−27.37	6.23×10^{-18}	8.99×10^{-15}
ci | 000003990 | Bact | Sample_MGT2 | 2	NA	521	310.73	−9.76	−866.01	2.46×10^{-17}	3.23×10^{-14}

FC: Fold Change. NA: No gene annotation for the transcript. * Pfam result: protein containing the specified domain.

Functional enrichment studies performed using Pfam annotations obtained from the DEGs, showed 44 and 60 Pfam families significantly enriched in the digestive gland and the gill, respectively (File S3). Among these enriched domains, we found genes coding for proteins involved in GTP and calcium ion binding, transport, antibacterial activity and immune system in the digestive gland (Table 6). On the other hand, domains related to cell adhesion, cell-cell recognition, protein binding, immune system and correct folding of proteins were found in the gill (Table 7).

Table 6. Pfam families significantly enriched (False Discovery Rate (FDR) adjusted p-value < 0.1) with seven or more differentially expressed genes in digestive gland.

Category	Number of Genes	p-Value
PF04548.11//AIG1	26	0.00248912
PF01926.18//MMR_HSR1	25	0.0029543
PF00059.16//Lectin_C	21	0.01366918
PF00100.18//Zona_pellucida	16	0.00403746
PF13499.1//EF-hand_7	14	0.00221868
PF13405.1//EF-hand_6	14	0.00355134
PF00036.27//EF-hand_1	13	0.00065889
PF13202.1//EF-hand_5	13	0.02872925
PF13833.1//EF-hand_8	12	0.02032022
PF00361.15//Oxidored_q1	10	0.00489835
PF00119.15//ATP-synt_A	8	0.00023995
PF10690.4//Myticin-prepro	8	0.02237525
PF07679.11//I-set	7	0.04744078

Table 7. Pfam families significantly enriched (FDR adjusted p-value < 0.1) with seven or more differentially expressed genes in gill.

Category	Number of Genes	p-Value
PF00386.16//C1q	36	5.2×10^{-8}
PF00036.27//EF-hand_1	31	0.00035296
PF13499.1//EF-hand_7	29	0.00014495
PF13405.1//EF-hand_6	27	8.61×10^{-5}
PF00147.13//Fibrinogen_C	25	0.01665835
PF13202.1//EF-hand_5	23	0.00079724
PF13833.1//EF-hand_8	20	0.00015502
PF10690.4//Myticin-prepro	13	0.01435613
PF00361.15//Oxidored_q1	13	0.03222834
PF07679.11//I-set	9	0.00010238
PF09458.5//H_lectin	9	0.00621282
PF01607.19//CBM_14	9	0.02592731
PB002965//Pfam-B_2965	9	0.03289021
PF13895.1//Ig_2	8	0.00039907
PF00119.15//ATP-synt_A	8	0.01065053
PF13927.1//Ig_3	7	0.00090571
PF00092.23//VWA	7	0.00272518
PF07686.12//V-set	7	0.01729404
PF03281.9//Mab-21	7	0.03056683

All DEGs from each tissue were classified according to the three main Gene Ontology (GO) aspects (biological processes, molecular functions and cellular components) and subcategories within (Figures 2 and 3). Among the biological processes obtained for the digestive gland, proteolysis involved in the cellular protein catabolic process deserved special recognition for its down-regulation, while protein folding and translation are two of the most up-regulated processes. Regarding molecular functions, zinc and metal ion binding, as well as NADH dehydrogenase activity, showed considerable down-regulation in the digestive gland exposed to DSP toxins, while protein, GTP and RNA binding were up-regulated when the digestive gland responded to these toxins. The cellular components most involved in the response against DSP toxins seem to be the cytosol and the mitochondrion (cellular components up-regulated), while numerous sequences related to the extracellular exosome are down-regulated.

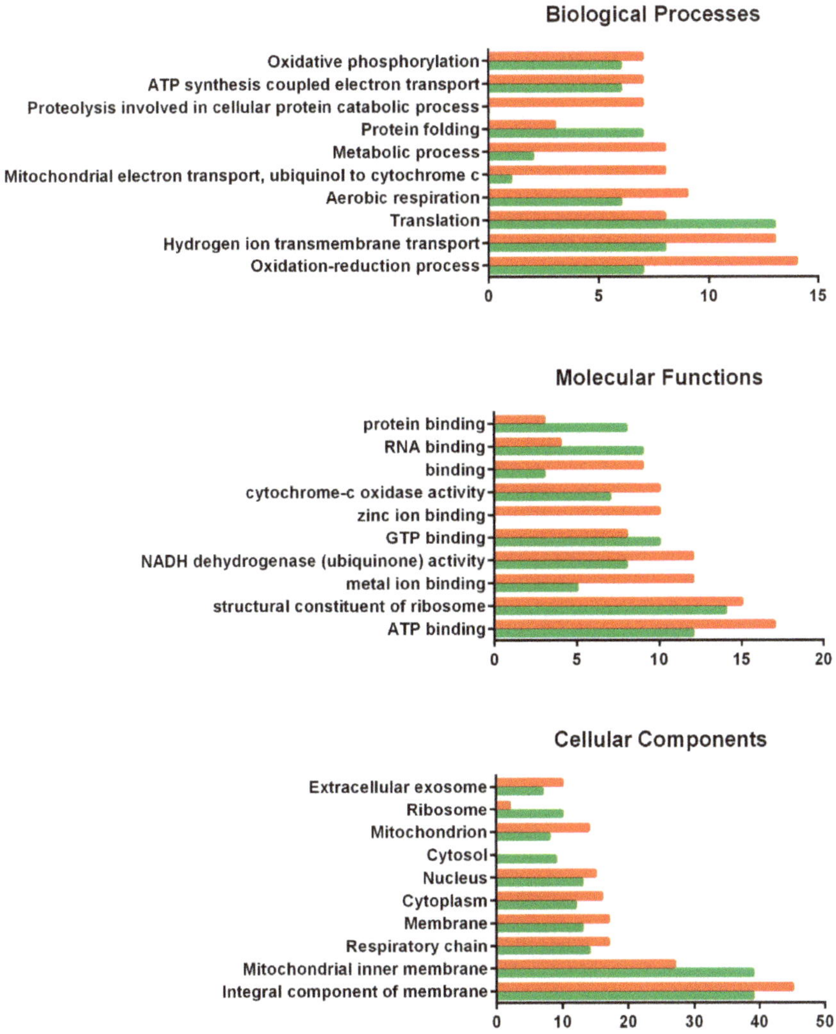

Figure 2. GO classification of DEGs from the digestive gland of the mussel *M. galloprovincialis* exposed to the DSP toxin-producing dinoflagellate *P. lima*. Overrepresented and infrarrepresented biological processes, molecular functions and cellular components are shown. Red and green bars represent the number of down- and up-regulated genes in each category, respectively. The length of the bars is determined by the number of genes identified within each subcategory.

Regarding gills, the main down-regulated biological process when this tissue is exposed to DSP toxins is apoptosis. On the contrary, processes such as translational initiation or ATP synthesis coupled proton transport are over-represented after exposure to DSP toxins. When molecular functions are considered, RNA binding and NADH dehydrogenase activity are mostly up-regulated, while iron ion binding, sequence-specific DNA binding or cytochrome c oxidase activity are mainly down-regulated in the presence of DSP toxins. In this tissue, those cellular components most involved in the response against DSP toxins seem to be the nucleolus and the mitochondrion.

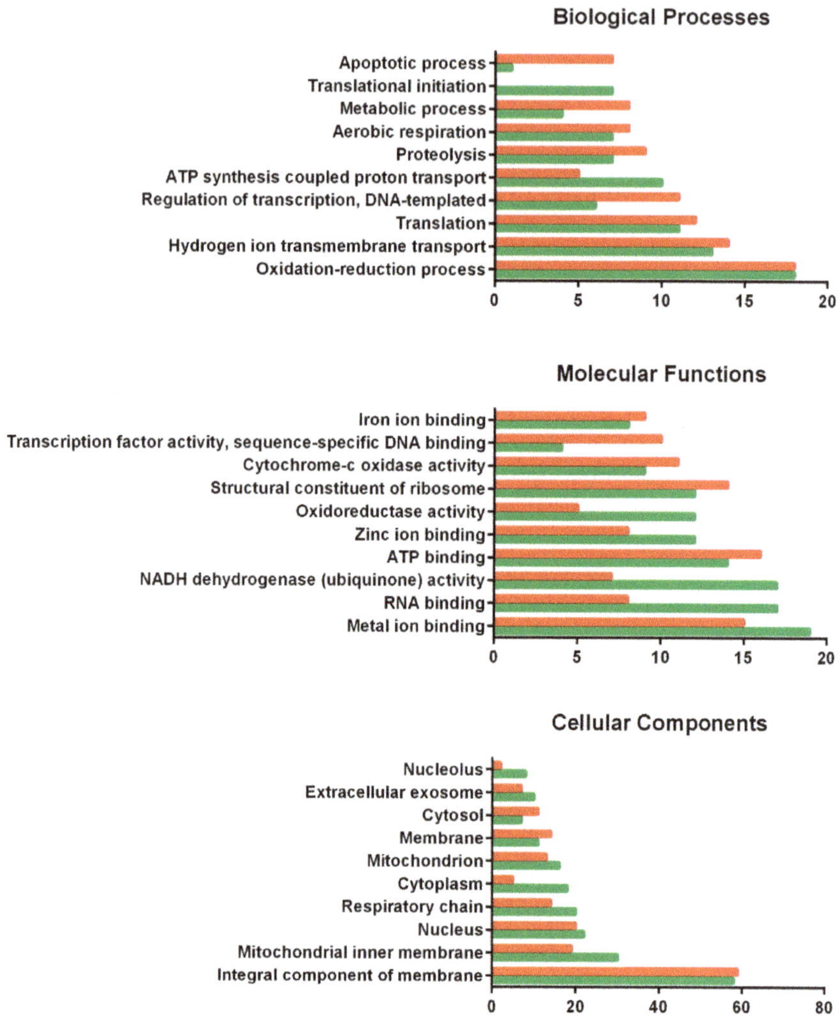

Figure 3. GO classification of DEGs from the gill of the mussel *M. galloprovincialis* exposed to the DSP toxin-producing dinoflagellate *P. lima*. The overrepresented and infrarrepresented biogical processes, molecular functions and cellular components are shown. Red and green bars represent the number of down- and up-regulated genes in each category, respectively. The length of the bars is determined by the number of genes identified within each subcategory.

2.5. Real-Time Quantitative PCR (qPCR) Validation

We selected 10 DEGs for real-time qPCR confirmation based on their functions (lipid metabolism and immunity): seven up-regulated, two down-regulated and one with no differential expression. Regarding the digestive gland, big defensin 2 (BD2), NADH dehidrogenase subunit 5 (NADH5) and KAZAL domain containing protein (KAZAL DC) were up-regulated, GIY-YIG domain containing protein (GIY-YIG DC) was down-regulated and Dynactin-subunit-6-like (DYNA) showed no expression changes. Regarding the gills, Cytosolic phospholipase A-2 like (CPLA2), Arachidonate 15-lipoxygenase B-like (ALOX15B), Alpha-L-fucosidase-like (FUCA) and H_Lectin domain containing protein (H_Lectin DC) were up-regulated, while Fibrinogen_C domain containing protein (Fibrinogen_C DC) was down-regulated.

The heatmap provided in Figure 4 illustrates the expression levels of these genes in each library.

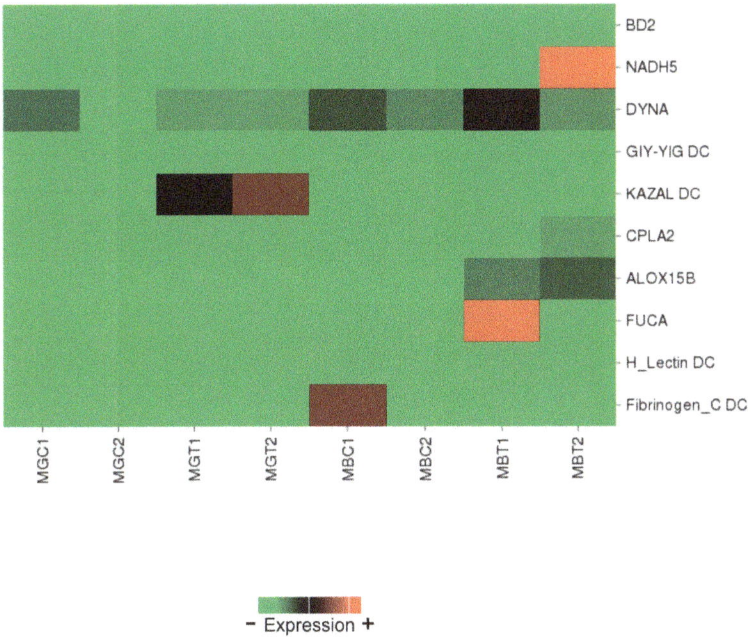

Figure 4. Heatmap showing expression levels of a set of annotated genes involved in the early response to DSP toxins in mussels and selected for qPCR validation. Columns represent one library each and cells depict gene expression levels based on the number of reads. MGC: library obtained from digestive glands of control mussels. MGT: library obtained from digestive glands of treated mussels. MBC: library obtained from gills of control mussels. MBT: library obtained from gills of treated mussels.

To confirm these patterns of expression by means of real-time qPCR, specific primers were designed. Sequences of these primers are shown in Table 8.

Table 8. Primers used in the real-time qPCR validation.

Gene Name	Abbreviation	Reference	E	Amplicon Size (bp)	Tm (°C)	Primers 5′ → 3′
Tropomyosin	TPM	ab000907.1	1.90	67	F-55.3 R-57.1	F-GATGCTGAAAATCGTGCAAC R-CGGTCTACTTCTTTTTGCAACTT
Ribosomal proteins S4	rpS4	Lozano et al. (2015)	1.83	138	F-58.8 R-60.3	F-TGGGTTATCGAGGGCGTAG R-TCCCTTAGTTTGTTGAGGACCTG
18S ribosomal RNA	18S	L33452.1	1.86	60	F-58.3 R-55.9	F-CCTGGAAAGGTCGGGTAAC R-AATTACAAGCCCCAATCCCTA
18S ribosomal RNA	18S-L33448	Cubero-Leon et al. (2012)	1.79	114	F-56.3 R-56.0	F-CATTAGTCAAGAACGAAAGTCAGAG R-GCCTGCCGAGTCATTGAAG
Glyceraldehyde 3-phosphate-dehydrogenase	GAPDH	Lozano et al. (2015)	1.92	114	F-59.4 R-58.4	F-AGGAATGGCCTTCAGGG R-TCAGATGCTGCTTTAATGGCTG
Elongation Factor 1	EF1	Suarez-Ulloa et al. (2013)	1.89	106	F-55.8 R-57.0	F-CCTCCCACCATCAAGACCTA R-GGCTGGAGCAAAGGTAACAA
Big defensin 2	BD2	Contig37896	1.83	110	F-60.3 R-59.3	F-TCTGAGCAGGGAGTATCAACAG R-TGGACAAAACAGCTACTAACAAGG
NADH dehidrogenase subunit 5	NADH5	Contig24266	1.86	90	F-53.7 R-56.5	F-GCAGTCATGCGCAAAAAG R-ACCCGGTACAAATATGGCTAAA
Dynactin-subunit-6-like	DYNA	Contig14551	1.89	60	F-58.9 R-58.9	F-AGTATTCTCAGGCATGGTTTCTG R-GGTTGTATAATTGGAGGCATGTG
GIY-YIG domain containing protein	GIY-YIG DC	ci|000000744|Bact|Sample_MBC1|2	1.83	70	F-57.6 R-55.3	F-AATCTACCAATTGCTTGTCTGTCA R-CGAAACGTAGTGTGCGAAAA
KAZAL domain containing protein	KAZAL DC	Contig33832	1.91	60	F-53.2 R-60.3	F-ATAATCGGCAGTGCAAAACA R-TTCCTTACTGAGTCAGTCG
Cytosolic phospholipase A-2 like	CPLA2	ci|000001655|Bact|Sample_MBT1|2	1.80	73	F-61.6 R-57.1	F-CCTGTACTGTGAGATTAGGTTATTGC R-CAGAAGGTTATTGACCGAAAGAA
Arachidonate 15-lipoxygenase B-like	ALOX15B	ci|000023941|Bact|Sample_MBT2|2	1.81	94	F-58.5 R-55.9	F-TGTTGTGAGTGAAGCAATAACTCTAA R-CGGAATAAATCG AGAGAACCA
Alpha-L-fucosidase-like	FUCA	ci|000010451|Bact|Sample_MBT1|2	1.87	74	F-61.0 R-55.3	F-GGAATTCCAGTAGGAATCAGTAGC R-TGGTAAATGCATACAAACCTGAA
H_Lectin domain containing protein	H_Lectin DC	Contig19341	1.85	73	F-56.5 R-55.3	F-CCCTTCTTTGCTTTAGATGCTT R-TTGATGGCCAGATTACGACA
Fibrinogen_C domain containing protein	Fibrinogen_C DC	ci|000024772|Bact|Sample_MBC1|2	1.86	67	F-57.3 R-59.4	F-AAGGTTGTCTCCAGCGTTTC R-CGGTGATGCCTCTACCAACT

E: primer efficiency; F: forward; R: reverse.

NormFinder software showed that rpS4 and TPM genes were the most stable genes and identified them as the best two-gene combination among all potential reference genes. These two genes also showed the lowest SD values when analyzed with BestKeeper. Moreover, their suitability as reference genes was supported by RefFinder results. Therefore, taking into account the combination of all results from the different analysis methods used (Table 9), TPM and rpS4 were identified as the most stable pair of reference genes in the digestive gland. These two genes were used for the normalization of gene expression in real-time qPCR.

Table 9. Rank of six candidate reference genes for real-time qPCR calculated by Normfinder and BestKeeper analyses.

Rank	Normfinder	Stability	BestKeeper	SD	*r*
1	rpS4	0.07	rpS4	0.46	0.732
2	TPM	0.17	TPM	0.50	0.448
3	GAPDH	0.20	GAPDH	0.64	0.669
4	18S	0.37	18S	0.71	0.827
5	18S-L33448	0.76	18S-L33448	1.08	
6	EF1	1.78	EF1	2.91	

SD: standard deviation; *r*: coefficient of correlation between each gene and the BestKeeper index.

The results of normalized expression (Figures 5 and 6) validated the previous observations obtained using RNA-Seq. Fibrinogen_C DC, FUCA and NADH5 qPCR analyses were carried out using three biological replicates.

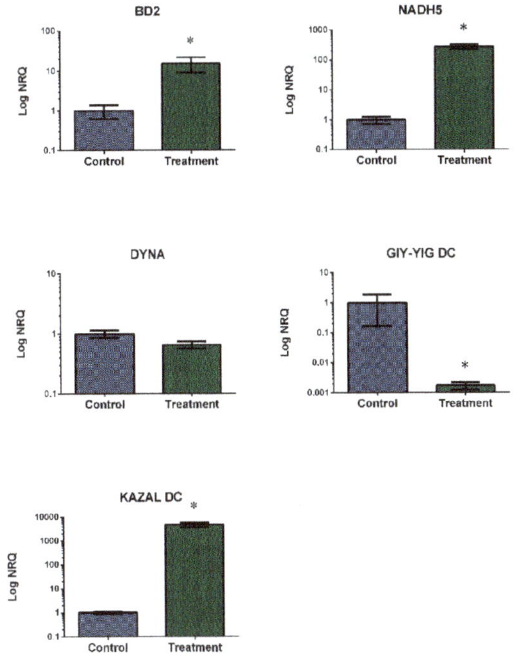

Figure 5. Relative transcript levels for each selected gene of digestive gland of the mussel *M. galloprovincialis* exposed to the DSP toxin-producing dinoflagellate *P. lima*. Blue bars: control samples. Green bars: samples treated with 100,000 cells/L for 48 h (mean ± SE). NRQ: Normalized Relative Quantification. $n = 4$. * indicates significant differences to control according to Mann-Whitney's U-test (p-value < 0.05).

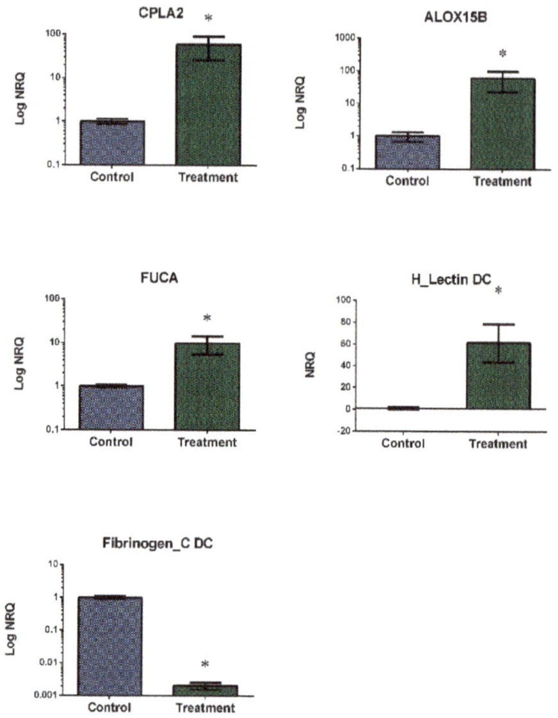

Figure 6. Relative transcript levels for each validated candidate gene of gill of the mussel *M. galloprovincialis* exposed to the DSP toxin-producing dinoflagellate *P. lima*. Blue bars: control samples. Green bars: samples treated with 100,000 cells/L for 48 h (mean ± SE). NRQ: Normalized Relative Quantification. $n = 4$. * indicates significant differences to control in Mann-Whitney's U-test (p-value < 0.05).

3. Discussion

Given the scarce knowledge of the resistance mechanisms involved in the early response of bivalve mollusks to marine toxins, the data presented in this work represent an important resource. Compared to other transcriptional works carried out in the digestive gland of the mussel *M. galloprovincialis* [13,15], a great number of DEGs were identified in the present study. This suggests a major impact of DSP toxins on gene expression regulation in the digestive gland and the gill of this species.

This study also revealed numerous transcripts assigned to Pfam families related to transport, cell adhesion, protein binding, calcium-binding proteins or immune system, among others. Many of these domains were also identified when haemolymph and digestive gland transcriptomes of mussel were analyzed in response to *Vibrio alginnolyticus* infection and domoic acid exposure [15,28,29]. Previous works carried out in bivalves exposed to marine toxins have shown significant changes in the expression levels of genes and proteins related to detoxification processes, such as cytochromes p450, ATP-binding cassette (ABC) transporters or glutathione S-transferases (GST) [12,15,30,31]. Surprisingly, although some of these genes are included among the DEGs in our results, they were not found among the most significant ones. Guo et al. [32] suggested the possible implication of p450 genes in OA metabolism in humans, generating new metabolites with less capacity to inhibit PP2A in comparison to OA. However, these transformations would not be completely effective to OA detoxification, which could explain our results.

Regarding GO, cellular organization and biogenesis, protein metabolism and modification, catabolism, response to stress and death and cell death are some of the biological processes most involved in the mussel response against toxins [33]. This is partially consistent with the main biological processes assigned in the present work when the digestive gland and the gill of mussels were exposed to DSP toxins. However, our data showed an important down-regulation of genes related to metabolic and apoptotic processes in the digestive gland and the gill, respectively, which may lay behind the first harmful effects of DSP toxins in these tissues. This result is not in agreement with the apoptosis induction observed in digestive glands when Mediterranean mussels were fed OA-contaminated nutrients [19]. Among the molecular functions involved in mussel response to toxins are protein binding, catalytic activity and transporter activity [33]. A similar result was obtained in the present work, although with important cytochrome-c oxidase and NADH dehydrogenase activities. On the other hand, the main cellular components shown in comparative transcriptomic studies of bivalves exposed to toxins were cytoplasm, nucleus, extracellular region and mitochondrion [33]. This is in agreement with some of the cellular components identified in the present work. However, our results also seem to show a key role of the extracellular exosome and respiratory chain in both mussel tissues—the digestive gland and the gill—in the early response to DSP toxins. Yamashita et al. [34] had already determined that exosomal secretion mechanisms are essential for methylmercury detoxification in the zebrafish embryo. Also, our work revealed an important participation of membrane integral components in the response to DSP toxins. This may be related to the known inhibitory effect of OA on intercellular channels in mammalian cells [35].

A large amount of contigs included in the reference transcriptome obtained in this study did not display any BLAST similarity or annotation, even with the recently sequenced *M. galloprovincialis* genome [36] or with *Crassostrea gigas* genome [37]. That was also the case for many of the top DEGs identified in this work that, despite their implication in the early response of mussel to DSP toxins, could not be identified. Similar results were obtained in a previous RNA-Seq study when digestive gland transcriptome of *M. galloprovincialis* was analyzed after exposure to the dinoflagellate *Alexandrium minutum*, a paralytic toxin producer [13]. Taking into account the length of some of these contigs as well as previous suggestions made by some authors, these sequences could be candidates to long non-coding RNA (lncRNA). lncRNA can regulate the activity of other genes by interacting with protein-coding mRNAs [38]. Milan et al. [39] observed that approximately 10% of the contigs obtained from the transcriptome of the clam *Ruditapes philippinarum* were originated by natural antisense transcription (NAT), a process that seems to be highly prevalent in bivalves.

When the data represented in the heatmap and the results obtained by qPCR were compared, a high correlation was observed between them, clear evidence that the RNA-Seq analysis conducted in this work was robust. Analyses in the digestive gland showed that the two most suitable genes for qPCR gene expression normalization were rpS4 and TPM. This result is in agreement with previous reports in which rpS4 was proposed as an optimal housekeeping gene to use under similar conditions [10,40]. To our knowledge, this is the first time that TPM is proposed and used in mussels to normalize qPCR data.

Our digestive gland data showed the up-regulation of different genes related to immune defense, including BD2, NADH5 and a KAZAL DC protein. Big defensins belong to a diverse family of peptides not only in terms of sequence, but also in terms of genomic organization and regulation of gene expression [41]. High gene expression levels of big defensin were identified in gills of the mussel *Bathymodiolus azoricus* [42]. Also, their up-regulation in haemocytes of the oyster *C. gigas* exposed to *A. minutum*—a paralytic toxin producer—has been associated with alterations in the immune system [43]. Similarly, big defensin gene expression was significantly up-regulated in haemolymph of the scallop *Argopecten irradians* when it was exposed to OA [44]. However, in a work in which the mussel *M. galloprovincialis* was exposed to the marine contaminant tris (1-choro-2-propyl) phosphate (TCPP) big defensin was down-regulated, affecting immunocompetence. Taking into account the high diversity of these genes [41] the big defensin identified in our work may correspond to a new variant of *M. galloprovincialis* related to the response to DSP toxins. On the other hand, the NADH protein family participates in transport and energy production. NADH is the third most frequently detected protein in comparative transcriptional studies that are carried out in bivalves exposed to different toxins [33]. Our results showed a significant increase in NADH5 gene expression. This is in line with an important up-regulation of NADH observed in a microarray designed based on data from normalized and suppression hybridization (SSH) libraries obtained from digestive gland and gill of the mussel *M. galloprovincialis* after exposition to sublethal concentrations of OA [17]. Our results also showed high expression levels of a putative KAZAL DC protein. Gerdol and Venier [45] have suggested that some bivalves can express Kazal-like protease inhibitors to counteract protease variants produced by invading microbes.

On the contrary, our digestive gland data showed the down-regulation of a putative GIY-YIG DC protein. This domain is present in many endonucleases involved in cellular processes such as DNA repair, the restriction of incoming foreing DNA, the movement of non-LTR retrotransposons or the maintenance of genome stability [46]. Indeed, Biscotti et al. [47] suggested that the expansion of this family in lungfish might be a genomic defense mechanism against the threat of spreading mobilome. Furthermore, Dittrich et al. [48] reported a gene which contains a GIY-YIG nuclease domain as an essential gene for proper DNA damage response in *Caenorhabditis elegans* embryos. However, mutants for this gene seem to have normal cell cycle arrest and apoptosis, which means this gene is not involved in the initial signalling process following DNA damage. This fact might partially explain the down-regulation of this transcript in the digestive gland of mussels during the early stages of DSP exposure, the situation simulated in the present study.

Our gill data showed an up-regulation of different genes related to lipid and carbohydrate metabolism, inflammatory response or immune defense, including CPLA2, ALOX15B, FUCA and a H_Lectin DC protein. CPLA2 is an enzyme that plays an important role as the primary generator of free arachidonic acid (AA)—a common precursor of a family of compounds with roles in inflammation [49]—released from membrane phospholipids. CPLA2 expression and activity are increased by reactive oxygen species (ROS) [50]. However, in a previous work, a decrease in lipid peroxidation levels was observed when mussel gills were exposed to the same DSP treatment [10]. This suggests the existence of an alternative defense mechanism. On the other hand, lipoxygenases (LOX) catalyze the generation of leukotrienes from AA producing byproducts that can function as ROS [51]. Some mussel extracts contain fatty acids with the ability to inhibit AA oxygenation by the cycloxigenase and LOX pathways, thus preventing inflammation [52]. In mammals, CPLA2 can cause membrane degradation, changes in plasma and mitochondrial membrane bioenergetics and permeability [53] and lysosomal membrane destabilization [54]. Indeed, CPLA2 is used as a stress indicator in biomonitoring programs. Some authors have also suggested that the up-regulation of genes involved in the inflammatory process, which was observed when digestive glands of the oyster *C. gigas* were exposed to *P. lima*, might represent a risk to this bivalve's integrity [55]. Heavy metals functionally alter lysosomal membranes in haemocytes of mussels [56]. Ca^{2+} dependent CPLA2 enzymes play an important role in the lysosomal membrane destabilization induced by mercury and copper in the haemolymph cells of mussels [57]. Mussel gill exposed to low DSP toxin concentration produces an inflammatory response associated with the up-regulation of CPLA2 and ALOX15B that may be partially compensated by the up-regulation of antioxidant enzymes shown in many studies [10,58].

FUCA is an enzyme located in lysosomes and involved in carbohydrate metabolism. Based on our results, this gene seems to take part in the early response of mussel gills to DSP toxins. However, FUCA did not show gene deregulation when the gill of the scallop *Nodipecten subnodosus* was exposed to *Gymnodinium catenatum*, while an up-regulation was observed in the adductor muscle [59]. A down-regulation of FUCA protein was observed when the scallop *Pecten maximus* was exposed to hypoxia at different temperatures, suggesting an energy saving strategy by reducing protein turnover [60]. Nevertheless, the restriction of carbohydrate metabolism does not seem to be an important part of the early response of mussel gill to DSP toxins. Our gill data also showed up-regulation of a putative H_Lectin DC protein. This is a common finding in this type of studies, since type C lectins are usually overrepresented in bivalve transcriptomes exposed to marine toxins [17,61].

However, there is still relatively little information available about this domain related to cell adhesion and carbohydrate binding.

On the other hand, our gill data showed the down-regulation of a putative Fibrinogen_C DC protein. A study about the immune system of the mussel *M. galloprovincialis* identified fibrinogen as one of the most abundant transcripts in the Mytibase collection [62]. More specifically, C-terminal fibrinogen-like domain has a structure that binds to the carbohydrate residues of foreing and apoptotic cells. Indeed, some fibrinogen-like domains are included in many lectins [63] and, consequently, are involved in microorganism recognition by the activation of the lectin pathway, constituting a first line of immune defense. Although fibrinogen was first associated with haemolymph, the gill together with the digestive gland were the following tissues with the highest gene expression levels when three fibrinogen-related proteins were evaluated in the mussel *M. galloprovincialis* [64]. Down-regulation of fibrinogen was also observed when haemolymph of the scallop *A. irradians* was exposed to low concentrations of OA (50 nM) for short exposure times (48 h), suggesting the potential of this toxin to inhibit the ability of scallops to recognize and remove non-self particles [65]. Gene expression levels of Fibrinogen C also decreased when bay scallop gill tissue was exposed to 500 nM of OA for 48 h [30]. Differences in gene expression of fibrinogen C were also detected in the digestive gland of the mussel *M. galloprovincialis* after exposure to domoic acid-producing *Pseudo-nitzschia* [15]. However, fibrinogen gene expression was significantly up-regulated when the haemolymph of the scallop *A. irradians* was challenged with *Listonella anguillarum* [66] or when the haemolymph of the mussel *Mytilus chilensis* was exposed to saxitoxins [58]. It is important to note that, as in the case of big defensins, proteins that contain this domain present high individual variability. Thus, different mussels usually have different gene sequences, which demonstrates the extraordinary complexity of the immune system in these organisms [62].

4. Conclusions

This work represents the first RNA-Seq approach used in the mussel *M. galloprovincialis* to analyze tissue-specific mussel transcriptome after early exposure to DSP toxins. It describes the transcriptome and gene expression profiles of *M. galloprovincialis* digestive gland and gill, therefore increasing available genomic resources for this organism.

Furthermore, results showed that DEGs in early response to DSP toxins include genes involved in defense, immunity and metabolism, shedding some light into the resistance mechanisms that these organisms have against harmful effects of DSP toxins. In the digestive gland, BD2, KAZAL DC and NADH5 genes were up-regulated while GIY-YIG DC was down-regulated and DYNA showed no expression changes. On the other hand, ALOX15B, H_Lectin DC, CPLA2 and FUCA genes were up-regulated and Fibrinogen_C DC was down-regulated in gill. Nevertheless, many of the genes that responded to these toxins have been described as DEGs in response to other stimuli, indicating that the mussel defense reaction is to some extent unspecific, which may be beneficial when faced with other potentially harmful compounds.

This study also indicated that the expression of rpS4 and TPM genes in the digestive gland under these experimental conditions is stable and, therefore, these genes can be employed as reference genes to normalize gene expression in qPCR experiments carried out in mussels exposed to low concentrations of DSP toxins for short time periods.

5. Materials and Methods

5.1. Sample Collection and Experimental Design

Adult individuals of the mussel *M. galloprovincialis* (34 ± 0.5 mm anterior-posterior shell length) were collected from a natural population in the rocky shores of O Rañal beach (43°19′40.1″ N, 8°30′45.1″ W, A Coruña, NW Spain) in April 2015. This location (used by our research group in other studies [10]) was chosen as our sampling site based on its low density of DSP toxin-producing dinoflagellates [67]. The invertebrate animal experiment was assessed by the Spanish Ministry of Economy and Competitivity (project AGL2012-30897 approved on 28 December 2012). In the laboratory, specimens were acclimated for seven days at 17 °C with constant aeration in a photoperiod chamber with a 12 h light-dark cycle and fed twice a day with a 1:1 mixture of two cultures of nontoxic microalga species, *I. galbana* (3×10^6 cells/L) and *T. suecica* (12×10^6 cells/L). After acclimatization, mussels were randomly divided into two groups (n = 30 per experimental group) (Figure 7): a control group fed only with the microalga mixture used during acclimation period, and a treatment group additionally fed with 100,000 cells/L of the DSP toxin-producing alga *P. lima*. The culture of *P. lima* (strain AND-A0605) was obtained from the Quality Control Laboratory of Fishery Resources (Huelva, Spain). The treatment group was fed, four times a day, with 100,000 cells/L of *P. lima* during 48 h. These exposure characteristics were selected based on the results obtained in previous works by our research group in which these conditions showed the most interesting response at both the cytogenotoxic and the transcriptional level [10,12]. Cell concentrations of the nontoxic microalga cultures were determined by means of a Thoma cell counting chamber (Marienfeld, Lauda-Königshofen, Germany), while that of the *P. lima* culture was estimated using the Sedgwich-Refter counting slide (Pyser-Sgi, Edenbridge, UK) after fixation with Lugol's solution. After exposure, 12 individuals from each group—control and treatment—were dissected for digestive gland and gill tissues. These tissues were frozen in liquid nitrogen and stored at −80 °C until their use for RNA extraction, while the remaining individuals were used to estimate OA—the main DSP toxin—accumulation in the mussels by means of High Performance Liquid Chromatography/Mass Spectrometry (HPLC/MS). HPLC/MS analyses were carried out by the chromatography unit at Servizos de Apoio á Investigación (SAI)-University of A Coruña, following the protocol of the European Union Reference Laboratory for Marine Biotoxins [68].

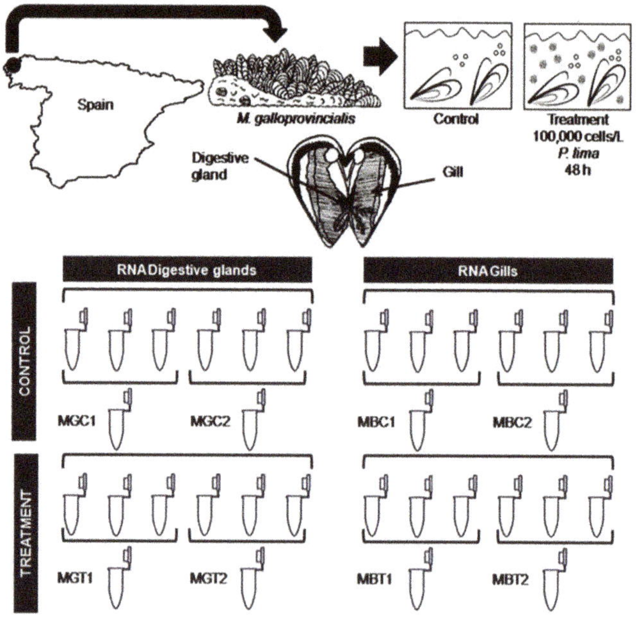

Figure 7. Experimental design diagram. Mussels from rocky shores were acclimated to laboratory conditions and subsequently exposed to 100,000 cells/L of *P. lima* for 48 h. Afterwards, gills and digestive gland were used for RNA extraction. RNA from 3 individuals was pooled for library construction and sequencing. MGC: RNA pool obtained from digestive glands of control mussels. MGT: RNA pool obtained from digestive glands of treated mussels. MBC: RNA pool obtained from gills of control mussels. MBT: RNA pool obtained from gills of treated mussels.

5.2. RNA Extraction

Total RNA of digestive gland and gill from six control and six treated mussels was individually extracted using TRIzol (Invitrogen, Carlsbad, CA, USA), according to the manufacturer's instructions (Figure 7). Isolated RNA was initially quantified using a NanoDrop 1000 spectrophotometer (Thermo Scientific, Waltham, MA, USA). With the aim of reducing inter-individual variability, these RNAs were pooled (in equal quantities) in groups of three to provide a template for Illumina libraries (Figure 7). Additionally, quantity and integrity of RNA pools were checked using a Qubit 2.0 fluorometer (Life Technologies, Saint-Aubin, France) and an Agilent 2100 Bioanalyzer (Agilent Technologies, Santa Clara, CA, USA), respectively.

5.3. Library Preparation and Sequencing

cDNA libraries were prepared and sequenced by Sistemas Genómicos (Valencia, Spain). Eight cDNA libraries were obtained from the digestive gland and the gill of mussels (two from control mussels and two from mussels exposed to *P. lima*, for each tissue, Figure 7). Poly(A)+mRNA fraction was isolated from total RNA and cDNA libraries were constructed following Illumina's recommendations. cDNA libraries were sequenced using an Illumina HiSeq 2000 sequencer (Illumina, San Diego, CA, USA) and a paired-end sequencing strategy (100 $\times$ 2 bp). Raw data are accessible from the NCBI Short Read Archive (SRA accession: SRP158485).

5.4. De Novo Assembly

A preliminary bioinformatic analysis was performed by Sistemas Genómicos (Valencia, Spain). Initially, short sequence reads were quality checked using FastQC [69] and the TrueSeq adapters were trimmed using Trim Galore software version 0.3.3 (Babraham Bioinformatics, Cambridge, UK), keeping those reads with a mean phred score >30. With the aim of obtaining a reference transcriptome, all generated results were combined in a single data set. Then, low quality reads were re-identified and removed using PrinSeq-lite software version 0.20.4 [70], while duplicate reads were then removed using FastX-Toolkit (fastx_collapser option) [71]. Subsequently, de novo transcriptome assembly was conducted with the software Oases (version 2.0.9) and Trinity (version 2.1.1). Both assemblies were correlated by combining contigs with sequence similarity (>90% homology) using cd-hit (version 4.6). Potential ORFs were predicted using TransDecoder (version 2.0) with default settings. Then, each library was mapped against the reference transcriptome obtained in the previous step using Bowtie2 (version 2.2.6) and high quality reads were selected—high mapping quality with a 1×10^{-4} error probability—to increase count expression resolution. Finally, expression inference was carried out using the counts of properly paired reads by transcript.

5.5. Differential Expression, Functional Annotation and Functional Enrichment Analysis of DEGs

The expression of each sample was normalized by library size (initial number of reads) using the R package DESeq2 version 1.8.2 [72] (R software version 3.2.3 [73]) based on a negative binomial distribution, with the aim of analyzing differential expression. Those genes with a fold change lower than -2 or higher than 2, and an adjusted p-value < 0.05 were considered differentially expressed. Additionally, the method for controlling FDR was used to calculate the adjusted p-values [74].

DEGs were initially annotated using blastx against UniProt database and blastn against the NCBI nucleotide database, using an E-value threshold of 0.01. Subsequently, sequences annotated with RNAs were identified, while sequences associated with *P. lima* were removed from further analysis. Additionally, DEGs were re-annotated by a blastx analysis (ncbi-blast/2.3.0+)—using an e-value of 1×10^{-6} as cut-off—performed through the Supercomputing Centre of Galicia (CESGA). Subsequently, to know the biological processes, molecular functions and cellular components related to DEGs, annotated sequences were analyzed using GO implemented in Blast2GO software [75,76]. A functional enrichment analysis was performed using the Pfam [77] functional information, with the aim of annotating protein domains. Additionally, a subset of annotated DEGs was selected based on their biological function and their gene expression levels were represented in a heat map using CIMminer [78].

5.6. Real-Time Quantitative PCR Validation

A subset of annotated DEGs was selected based on their biological function to validate their gene expression using real-time qPCR. Reference genes for expression quantification were selected among six potential candidate housekeeping genes, including two primers for 18S ribosomal RNA (18S) [79], ribosomal protein S4 (rpS4), glyceraldehyde 3-phosphate-dehydrogenase (GAPDH) [40], elongation factor 1 (EF1) [10] and tropomyosin (TPM). TPM primers were designed as part of this work from an annotated gene with very stable expression levels. These primers and the specific primers to amplify the selected DEGs were designed using the Universal Probe Library software [80] (Roche Diagnostics, Mannheim, Germany). Primer specificities were verified using agarose gel electrophoresis, showing one single DNA product of the expected length. Two different algorithms, Normfinder and BestKeeper, were initially used to rank candidate reference genes according to their stability in the digestive gland and to decide on the optimal number of reference genes required for accurate normalization. Normfinder was used with R version 3.0.1 [73] and BestKeeper is an Excel-based tool that uses pairwise correlations [81]. Whenever BestKeeper analysis showed genes with SD values > 1, those genes were excluded from correlation coefficient calculations. Subsequently, results were checked using RefFinder [82], a web-based tool that integrates four different algorithms (Normfinder, BesKeeper, GeNorm and Delta Ct).

RNA samples from those individuals previously used for library preparation were used for the real-time qPCR validation. Four independent biological replicates and two technical replicates were analyzed together using the sample maximization approach [83]. cDNA was synthesized using 1 μg of RNA using the First Strand cDNA Synthesis kit according to the manufacturer's instructions (Roche Diagnostics, Mannheim, Germany). qPCR amplifications were carried out using the FastStart Essential DNA Green Master kit (Roche Diagnostics, Mannheim, Germany) following the manufacturer's instructions with the following modifications. All reactions were performed in a final volume of 20 μL of master mix containing 6.4 μL H_2O, 0.8 μL of each primer (10 μM), 10 μL of the SYBR Green Mix (Roche Diagnostics, Mannheim, Germany) and 2 μL of each reverse transcribed RNA (cDNA). Reactions consisted of an initial denaturation step of 10 min at 95 °C, followed by an amplification of the target cDNA for 40 cycles (denaturation at 95 °C for 10 s, annealing at 60 °C for 10 s, elongation at 72 °C for 10 s), melting curve analysis (1 cycle at 95 °C for 5 s, 65 °C for 60 s and 95 °C for 1 s), and cooling at 40 °C for 20 s. Specificity of the qPCR product was analyzed by melting curve analysis.

Efficiency of the reaction for each mRNA was determined using LinRegPCR 2014.x software [84]. Gene relative expression levels were normalized using rpS4 and TPM as reference genes. For data analyses, Cq values were extracted with the qPCR instrument software LightCycler Software 1.5.0 (Roche Diagnostics, Mannheim, Germany). Cq values were then exported to Excel (Microsoft, Redmond, WA, USA), and differences in expression were calculated using the Pfaffl method with two reference genes [85]. Whenever a single individual sample showed a Cq value with an over five point difference to the mean Cq for the condition, that value was considered an amplification error, therefore, that sample was removed and analyses were carried out using three biological replicates instead of four. Normalized relative quantities (NRQ) for each gene were represented in bar plots (control vs. treatment) using GraphPad Prism version 6 (GraphPad Prism Software Inc., La Jolla, CA, USA). For better visualization of results some data were log transformed for graphic representation. Differences in gene expression between control and treatment samples were determined by Mann-Whitney non-parametric U test using the SPSS IBM software package version 22 (IBM, Armon, NY, USA). An additional analysis to confirm the obtained gene expression differences was conducted in REST 2009 (Qiagen, Hilden, Germany) [86].

Supplementary Materials: The following are available online at http://www.mdpi.com/2072-6651/10/10/417/s1, File S1: Nucleotide sequences—in fasta format—of all differentially expressed genes (DEGs), File S2: List of DEGs. Each spreadsheet shows DEGs from the comparison of either the same tissue under different conditions—MBT_vs_MBC_DEGs for gills and MGT_vs_MGC_DEGs for digestive gland—or two tissues under the same condition—MGT_vs_MBT_DEGs for treated digestive gland and gill. For each DEG, sequence ID, baseMean, length, Log2 Fold Change (FC), FC, *p*-value and adjusted *p*-value are given. Also, Blast_nucleotide, Blast_UniProt and Pfam columns show the best hit against Nucleotide, UniProt and Pfam databases, respectively, File S3: List of Pfam families functionally enriched. Each spreadsheet shows DEGs from the comparison of the same tissue under different conditions—MGT_vs_MGC for digestive gland and MBT_vs_MBC for gill. For each Pfam category, number of genes, *p*-value, expression patterns and gene IDs are given.

Author Contributions: M.V.P.-F. and J.M. conceived and designed the experiments; M.V.P.-F. and L.M. performed the experiments and analyzed the data; J.M. contributed reagents/materials/analysis tools; M.V.P.-F., L.M. and J.M. wrote and revised the manuscript.

Funding: This study was supported by grants from the Spanish Ministry of Economy and Competitivity (AGL2012-30897, Josefina Mendez) and M.V.P.-F. work was funded through a fellowship by Deputación da Coruña (BINV-CC/2017).

Acknowledgments: The authors would like to thank the Consello Regulador do Mexillón de Galicia for its support, Juan C. Triviño for help with bioinformatic analyses and CESGA (www.cesga.es) in Santiago de Compostela, Spain for access to computing facilities.

Conflicts of Interest: The authors declare no conflict of interest.

References

1. Anderson, D.M.; Andersen, P.; Bricelj, V.M.; Cullen, J.J.; Rensel, J.E.J. *Monitoring and Management Strategies for Harmful Algal Blooms in Coastal Waters*; Unesco: Paris, France, 2001.
2. Wells, M.L.; Trainer, V.L.; Smayda, T.J.; Karlson, B.S.O.; Trick, C.G.; Kudela, R.M.; Ishikawa, A.; Bernard, S.; Wulff, A.; Anderson, D.M.; et al. Harmful algal blooms and climate change: Learning from the past and present to forecast the future. *Harmful Algae* **2015**, *49*, 68–93. [CrossRef] [PubMed]
3. Visciano, P.; Schirone, M.; Berti, M.; Milandri, A.; Tofalo, R.; Suzzi, G. Marine biotoxins: Occurrence, toxicity, regulatory limits and reference methods. *Front. Microbiol.* **2016**, *7*, 1051. [CrossRef] [PubMed]
4. Bialojan, C.; Takai, A. Inhibitory effect of a marine-sponge toxin, okadaic acid, on protein phosphatases. Specificity and kinetics. *Biochem. J.* **1988**, *256*, 283–290. [CrossRef] [PubMed]
5. Prado-Alvarez, M.; Flórez-Barrós, F.; Sexto-Iglesias, A.; Méndez, J.; Fernandez-Tajes, J. Effects of okadaic acid on haemocytes from *Mytilus galloprovincialis*: A comparison between field and laboratory studies. *Mar. Environ. Res.* **2012**, *81*, 90–93. [CrossRef] [PubMed]
6. Prego-Faraldo, M.V.; Valdiglesias, V.; Méndez, J.; Eirín-López, J.M. Okadaic acid meet and greet: An insight into detection methods, response strategies and genotoxic effects in marine invertebrates. *Mar. Drugs* **2013**, *11*, 2829–2845. [CrossRef] [PubMed]
7. Reguera, B.; Velo-Suárez, L.; Raine, R.; Park, M.G. Harmful dinophysis species: A review. *Harmful Algae* **2012**, *14*, 87–106. [CrossRef]
8. Valdiglesias, V.; Prego-Faraldo, M.V.; Pásaro, E.; Méndez, J.; Laffon, B. Okadaic acid: More than a diarrheic toxin. *Mar. Drugs* **2013**, *11*, 4328–4349. [CrossRef] [PubMed]
9. Munday, R. Is protein phosphatase inhibition responsible for the toxic effects of okadaic acid in animals? *Toxins* **2013**, *5*, 267–285. [CrossRef] [PubMed]
10. Prego-Faraldo, M.; Vieira, L.; Eirin-Lopez, J.; Méndez, J.; Guilhermino, L. Transcriptional and biochemical analysis of antioxidant enzymes in the mussel *Mytilus galloprovincialis* during experimental exposures to the toxic dinoflagellate *Prorocentrum lima*. *Mar. Environ. Res.* **2017**, *129*, 304–315. [CrossRef] [PubMed]
11. Prego-Faraldo, M.V.; Valdiglesias, V.; Laffon, B.; Eirín-López, J.M.; Méndez, J. In vitro analysis of early genotoxic and cytotoxic effects of okadaic acid in different cell types of the mussel *Mytilus galloprovincialis*. *J. Toxicol. Environ. Health A* **2015**, *78*, 814–824. [CrossRef] [PubMed]
12. Prego-Faraldo, M.V.; Valdiglesias, V.; Laffon, B.; Mendez, J.; Eirin-Lopez, J.M. Early genotoxic and cytotoxic effects of the toxic dinoflagellate *Prorocentrum lima* in the mussel *Mytilus galloprovincialis*. *Toxins* **2016**, *8*, 159. [CrossRef] [PubMed]

13. Gerdol, M.; De Moro, G.; Manfrin, C.; Milandri, A.; Riccardi, E.; Beran, A.; Venier, P.; Pallavicini, A. RNA sequencing and *de novo* assembly of the digestive gland transcriptome in *Mytilus galloprovincialis* fed with toxinogenic and non-toxic strains of *Alexandrium minutum*. *BMC Res. Notes* **2014**, *7*, 722. [CrossRef] [PubMed]
14. Moreira, R.; Pereiro, P.; Canchaya, C.; Posada, D.; Figueras, A.; Novoa, B. RNA-Seq in *Mytilus galloprovincialis*: Comparative transcriptomics and expression profiles among different tissues. *BMC Genom.* **2015**, *16*, 728. [CrossRef] [PubMed]
15. Pazos, A.J.; Ventoso, P.; Martínez-Escauriaza, R.; Pérez-Parallé, M.L.; Blanco, J.; Triviño, J.C.; Sánchez, J.L. Transcriptional response after exposure to domoic acid-producing *Pseudo-nitzschia* in the digestive gland of the mussel *Mytilus galloprovincialis*. *Toxicon* **2017**, *140*, 60–71. [CrossRef] [PubMed]
16. Rosani, U.; Varotto, L.; Rossi, A.; Roch, P.; Novoa, B.; Figueras, A.; Pallavicini, A.; Venier, P. Massively parallel amplicon sequencing reveals isotype-specific variability of antimicrobial peptide transcripts in *Mytilus galloprovincialis*. *PLoS ONE* **2011**, *6*, e26680. [CrossRef] [PubMed]
17. Suarez-Ulloa, V.; Fernandez-Tajes, J.; Aguiar-Pulido, V.; Prego-Faraldo, M.V.; Florez-Barros, F.; Sexto-Iglesias, A.; Mendez, J.; Eirin-Lopez, J.M. Unbiased high-throughput characterization of mussel transcriptomic responses to sublethal concentrations of the biotoxin okadaic acid. *PeerJ* **2015**, *3*, e1429. [CrossRef] [PubMed]
18. Suárez-Ulloa, V.; Fernández-Tajes, J.; Aguiar-Pulido, V.; Rivera-Casas, C.; González-Romero, R.; Ausio, J.; Méndez, J.; Dorado, J.; Eirín-López, J.M. The CHROMEVALOA database: A resource for the evaluation of okadaic acid contamination in the marine environment based on the chromatin-associated transcriptome of the mussel *Mytilus galloprovincialis*. *Mar. Drugs* **2013**, *11*, 830–841. [CrossRef] [PubMed]
19. Manfrin, C.; Dreos, R.; Battistella, S.; Beran, A.; Gerdol, M.; Varotto, L.; Lanfranchi, G.; Venier, P.; Pallavicini, A. Mediterranean mussel gene expression profile induced by okadaic acid exposure. *Environ. Sci. Technol.* **2010**, *44*, 8276–8283. [CrossRef] [PubMed]
20. Wang, Z.; Gerstein, M.; Snyder, M. RNA-Seq: A revolutionary tool for transcriptomics. *Nat. Rev. Genet.* **2009**, *10*, 57. [CrossRef] [PubMed]
21. Blanco, J.; Mariño, C.; Martín, H.; Acosta, C.P. Anatomical distribution of diarrhetic shellfish poisoning (DSP) toxins in the mussel *Mytilus galloprovincialis*. *Toxicon* **2007**, *50*, 1011–1018. [CrossRef] [PubMed]
22. Moroño, A.; Arévalo, F.; Fernández, M.; Maneiro, J.; Pazos, Y.; Salgado, C.; Blanco, J. Accumulation and transformation of DSP toxins in mussels *Mytilus galloprovincialis* during a toxic episode caused by *Dinophysis acuminata*. *Aquat. Toxicol.* **2003**, *62*, 269–280. [CrossRef]
23. Manfrin, C.; De Moro, G.; Torboli, V.; Venier, P.; Pallavicini, A.; Gerdol, M. Physiological and molecular responses of bivalves to toxic dinoflagellates. *Invertebr. Surv. J.* **2012**, *9*, 184–199.
24. Beyer, J.; Green, N.W.; Brooks, S.; Allan, I.J.; Ruus, A.; Gomes, T.; Bråte, I.L.N.; Schøyen, M. Blue mussels (*Mytilus edulis* spp.) as sentinel organisms in coastal pollution monitoring: A review. *Mar. Environ. Res.* **2017**. [CrossRef] [PubMed]
25. Romero-Geraldo, R.d.J.; García-Lagunas, N.; Hernandez-Saavedra, N.Y. Effects of in vitro exposure to diarrheic toxin producer *Prorocentrum lima* on gene expressions related to cell cycle regulation and immune response in *Crassostrea gigas*. *PLoS ONE* **2014**, *9*, e97181. [CrossRef]
26. Romero-Geraldo, R.d.J.; Hernández-Saavedra, N.Y. Stress gene expression in *Crassostrea gigas* (Thunberg, 1793) in response to experimental exposure to the toxic dinoflagellate *Prorocentrum lima* (Ehrenberg) Dodge, 1975. *Aquac. Res.* **2014**, *45*, 1512–1522. [CrossRef]
27. Díaz, P.A.; Reguera, B.; Ruiz-Villarreal, M.; Pazos, Y.; Velo-Suárez, L.; Berger, H.; Sourisseau, M. Climate variability and oceanographic settings associated with interannual variability in the initiation of *Dinophysis acuminata* blooms. *Mar. Drugs* **2013**, *11*, 2964–2981. [CrossRef] [PubMed]
28. Dong, W.; Chen, Y.; Lu, W.; Wu, B.; Qi, P. Transcriptome analysis of *Mytilus coruscus* hemocytes in response to *Vibrio alginnolyficus* infection. *Fish Shellfish Immunol.* **2017**, *70*, 560–567. [CrossRef] [PubMed]
29. Ventoso, P.; Martínez-Escauriaza, R.; Sánchez, J.; Pérez-Parallé, M.; Blanco, J.; Triviño, J.; Pazos, A. In Sequencing and *de novo* assembly of the digestive gland transcriptome in *Mytilus galloprovincialis* and analysis of differentially expressed genes in response to domoic acid. In Proceedings of the International Symposium on Genetics in Aquaculture XII, Santiago de Compostela, Spain, 21–27 June 2015; p. 93, 229.
30. Chi, C.; Giri, S.; Jun, J.; Kim, S.; Kim, H.; Kang, J.; Park, S. Detoxification- and immune-related transcriptomic analysis of gills from bay scallops (*Argopecten irradians*) in response to algal toxin okadaic acid. *Toxins* **2018**, *10*, 308. [CrossRef] [PubMed]

31. Huang, L.; Zou, Y.; Weng, H.-W.; Li, H.-Y.; Liu, J.-S.; Yang, W.-D. Proteomic profile in *Perna viridis* after exposed to *Prorocentrum lima*, a dinoflagellate producing DSP toxins. *Environ. Pollut.* **2015**, *196*, 350–357. [CrossRef] [PubMed]
32. Guo, F.; An, T.; Rein, K.S. The algal hepatoxoxin okadaic acid is a substrate for human cytochromes CYP3A4 and CYP3A5. *Toxicon* **2010**, *55*, 325–332. [CrossRef] [PubMed]
33. Miao, J.; Chi, L.; Pan, L.; Song, Y. Generally detected genes in comparative transcriptomics in bivalves: Toward the identification of molecular markers of cellular stress response. *Environ. Toxicol. Pharmacol.* **2015**, *39*, 475–481. [CrossRef] [PubMed]
34. Yamashita, M.; Yamashita, Y.; Suzuki, T.; Kani, Y.; Mizusawa, N.; Imamura, S.; Takemoto, K.; Hara, T.; Hossain, M.A.; Yabu, T. Selenoneine, a novel selenium-containing compound, mediates detoxification mechanisms against methylmercury accumulation and toxicity in zebrafish embryo. *Mar. Biotechnol.* **2013**, *15*, 559–570. [CrossRef] [PubMed]
35. Creppy, E.E.; Traoré, A.; Baudrimont, I.; Cascante, M.; Carratú, M.-R. Recent advances in the study of epigenetic effects induced by the phycotoxin okadaic acid. *Toxicology* **2002**, *181*, 433–439. [CrossRef]
36. Murgarella, M.; Puiu, D.; Novoa, B.; Figueras, A.; Posada, D.; Canchaya, C. A first insight into the genome of the filter-feeder mussel *Mytilus galloprovincialis*. *PLoS ONE* **2016**, *11*, e0151561. [CrossRef]
37. Zhang, G.; Fang, X.; Guo, X.; Li, L.; Luo, R.; Xu, F.; Yang, P.; Zhang, L.; Wang, X.; Qi, H. The oyster genome reveals stress adaptation and complexity of shell formation. *Nature* **2012**, *490*, 49–54. [CrossRef] [PubMed]
38. Ilott, N.E.; Ponting, C.P. Predicting long non-coding RNAs using RNA sequencing. *Methods* **2013**, *63*, 50–59. [CrossRef] [PubMed]
39. Milan, M.; Coppe, A.; Reinhardt, R.; Cancela, L.M.; Leite, R.B.; Saavedra, C.; Ciofi, C.; Chelazzi, G.; Patarnello, T.; Bortoluzzi, S. Transcriptome sequencing and microarray development for the manila clam, *Ruditapes philippinarum*: Genomic tools for environmental monitoring. *BMC Genom.* **2011**, *12*, 234. [CrossRef] [PubMed]
40. Lozano, V.; Martínez-Escauriaza, R.; Pérez-Parallé, M.; Pazos, A.; Sánchez, J. Two novel multidrug resistance associated protein (MRP/ABCC) from the mediterranean mussel (*Mytilus galloprovincialis*): Characterization and expression patterns in detoxifying tissues. *Can. J. Zool.* **2015**, *93*, 567–578. [CrossRef]
41. Rosa, R.D.; Santini, A.; Fievet, J.; Bulet, P.; Destoumieux-Garzón, D.; Bachère, E. Big defensins, a diverse family of antimicrobial peptides that follows different patterns of expression in hemocytes of the oyster *Crassostrea gigas*. *PLoS ONE* **2011**, *6*, e25594. [CrossRef] [PubMed]
42. Bettencourt, R.; Pinheiro, M.; Egas, C.; Gomes, P.; Afonso, M.; Shank, T.; Santos, R.S. High-throughput sequencing and analysis of the gill tissue transcriptome from the deep-sea hydrothermal vent mussel *Bathymodiolus azoricus*. *BMC Genom.* **2010**, *11*, 559. [CrossRef] [PubMed]
43. Mello, D.F.; da Silva, P.M.; Barracco, M.A.; Soudant, P.; Hégaret, H. Effects of the dinoflagellate *Alexandrium minutum* and its toxin (saxitoxin) on the functional activity and gene expression of *Crassostrea gigas* hemocytes. *Harmful Algae* **2013**, *26*, 45–51. [CrossRef]
44. Chi, C.; Giri, S.S.; Jun, J.W.; Kim, H.J.; Kim, S.W.; Yun, S.; Park, S.C. Effects of algal toxin okadaic acid on the non-specific immune and antioxidant response of bay scallop (*Argopecten irradians*). *Fish Shellfish Immunol.* **2017**, *65*, 111–117. [CrossRef] [PubMed]
45. Gerdol, M.; Venier, P. An updated molecular basis for mussel immunity. *Fish Shellfish Immunol.* **2015**, *46*, 17–38. [CrossRef] [PubMed]
46. Dunin-Horkawicz, S.; Feder, M.; Bujnicki, J.M. Phylogenomic analysis of the GIY−YIG nuclease superfamily. *BMC Genom.* **2006**, *7*, 98. [CrossRef] [PubMed]
47. Biscotti, M.A.; Gerdol, M.; Canapa, A.; Forconi, M.; Olmo, E.; Pallavicini, A.; Barucca, M.; Schartl, M. The lungfish transcriptome: A glimpse into molecular evolution events at the transition from water to land. *Sci. Rep.* **2016**, *6*, 21571. [CrossRef] [PubMed]
48. Dittrich, C.M.; Kratz, K.; Sendoel, A.; Gruenbaum, Y.; Jiricny, J.; Hengartner, M.O. LEM−3–A LEM domain containing nuclease involved in the DNA damage response in *C. elegans*. *PLoS ONE* **2012**, *7*, e24555. [CrossRef] [PubMed]
49. Balsinde, J. Phospholipase A2; Cellular Regulation, Function, and Inhibition 2016. Available online: http://www.balsinde.org/publists/engplasic.pdf (accessed on 24 May 2018).
50. Korbecki, J.; Baranowska-Bosiacka, I.; Gutowska, I.; Chlubek, D. The effect of reactive oxygen species on the synthesis of prostanoids from arachidonic acid. *J. Physiol. Pharmacol.* **2013**, *64*, 409–421. [PubMed]

51. Kim, C.; Kim, J.-Y.; Kim, J.-H. Cytosolic phospholipase A_2, lipoxygenase metabolites, and reactive oxygen species. *BMB Rep.* **2008**, *41*, 555–559. [CrossRef] [PubMed]
52. Bierer, T.L.; Bui, L.M. Improvement of arthritic signs in dogs fed green-lipped mussel (*Perna canaliculus*). *J. Nutr.* **2002**, *132*, 1634S–1636S. [CrossRef] [PubMed]
53. Zhao, M.; Brunk, U.T.; Eaton, J.W. Delayed oxidant-induced cell death involves activation of phospholipase A2. *FEBS Lett.* **2001**, *509*, 399–404. [CrossRef]
54. Mukherjee, A.; Ghosal, S.; Maity, C. Lysosomal membrane stabilization by α-tocopherol against the damaging action of *Vipera russelli* venom phospholipase A2. *Cell. Mol. Life Sci.* **1997**, *53*, 152–155. [CrossRef] [PubMed]
55. Romero-Geraldo, R.d.J.; García-Lagunas, N.; Hernández-Saavedra, N.Y. *Crassostrea gigas* exposure to the dinoflagellate *Prorocentrum lima*: Histological and gene expression effects on the digestive gland. *Mar. Environ. Res.* **2016**, *120*, 93–102. [CrossRef] [PubMed]
56. Viarengo, A.; Marro, A.; Marchi, B.; Burlando, B. Single and combined effects of heavy metals and hormones on lysosomes of haemolymph cells from the mussel *Mytilus galloprovincialis*. *Mar. Biol.* **2000**, *137*, 907–912. [CrossRef]
57. Marchi, B.; Burlando, B.; Moore, M.; Viarengo, A. Mercury- and copper-induced lysosomal membrane destabilisation depends on $[Ca^{2+}]_i$ dependent phospholipase A2 activation. *Aquat. Toxicol.* **2004**, *66*, 197–204. [CrossRef] [PubMed]
58. Núñez-Acuña, G.; Aballay, A.E.; Hégaret, H.; Astuya, A.P.; Gallardo-Escárate, C. Transcriptional responses of *Mytilus chilensis* exposed in vivo to saxitoxin (STX). *J. Mollus. Stud.* **2013**, *79*, 323–331. [CrossRef]
59. Estrada, N.; de Jesús Romero, M.; Campa-Córdova, A.; Luna, A.; Ascencio, F. Effects of the toxic dinoflagellate, *Gymnodinium catenatum* on hydrolytic and antioxidant enzymes, in tissues of the giant lions-paw scallop *Nodipecten subnodosus*. *Comp. Biochem. Phys. C Toxicol. Pharmacol.* **2007**, *146*, 502–510. [CrossRef] [PubMed]
60. Artigaud, S.; Lacroix, C.; Richard, J.; Flye-Sainte-Marie, J.; Bargelloni, L.; Pichereau, V. Proteomic responses to hypoxia at different temperatures in the great scallop (*Pecten maximus*). *PeerJ* **2015**, *3*, e871. [CrossRef] [PubMed]
61. Detree, C.; Núñez-Acuña, G.; Roberts, S.; Gallardo-Escárate, C. Uncovering the complex transcriptome response of *Mytilus chilensis* against saxitoxin: Implications of harmful algal blooms on mussel populations. *PLoS ONE* **2016**, *11*, e0165231. [CrossRef] [PubMed]
62. Venier, P.; Varotto, L.; Rosani, U.; Millino, C.; Celegato, B.; Bernante, F.; Lanfranchi, G.; Novoa, B.; Roch, P.; Figueras, A. Insights into the innate immunity of the mediterranean mussel *Mytilus galloprovincialis*. *BMC Genom.* **2011**, *12*, 69. [CrossRef] [PubMed]
63. Domeneghetti, S.; Manfrin, C.; Varotto, L.; Rosani, U.; Gerdol, M.; De Moro, G.; Pallavicini, A.; Venier, P. How gene expression profiles disclose vital processes and immune responses in *Mytilus* spp. *Invertebr. Surv. J.* **2011**, *8*, 179–189.
64. Romero, A.; Dios, S.; Poisa-Beiro, L.; Costa, M.M.; Posada, D.; Figueras, A.; Novoa, B. Individual sequence variability and functional activities of fibrinogen-related proteins (FREPs) in the mediterranean mussel (*Mytilus galloprovincialis*) suggest ancient and complex immune recognition models in invertebrates. *Dev. Comp. Immunol.* **2011**, *35*, 334–344. [CrossRef] [PubMed]
65. Cheng, C. Physico-Immunological Characterizations of Exogenous Substances (Palmitoleic Acid and Okadaic Acid) in Bivalves. Ph.D. Thesis, The Graduate School of Seoul National University, Seoul, Korea, 2017.
66. Zhang, X.-J.; Qin, G.-M.; Yan, B.-L.; Xu, J.; Bi, K.-R.; Qin, L. Phenotypic and molecular characterization of pathogenic *Listonella anguillarum* isolated from half-smooth tongue sole *Cynoglossus semilaevis*. *Acta Oceanol. Sin.* **2009**, *5*, 012.
67. Intecmar, Xunta de Galicia. Available online: http://www.intecmar.gal/ (accessed on 4 January 2015).
68. EU-Harmonised Standard Operating Procedure for Determination of Lipophilic Marine Biotoxins in Molluscs by LC-MS/MS. Available online: http://www.aecosan.msssi.gob.es/CRLMB/docs/docs/metodos_analiticos_de_desarrollo/EU-Harmonised-SOP-LIPO-LCMSMS_Version5.pdf (accessed on 21 September 2018).
69. Andrews, S. FastQC: A Quality Control Tool for High throughput Sequence Data. 2010, unpublished. Available online: https://www.bioinformatics.babraham.ac.uk/projects/fastqc/ (accessed on 7 October 2015).
70. Schmieder, R.; Edwards, R. Quality control and preprocessing of metagenomic datasets. *Bioinformatics* **2011**, *27*, 863–864. [CrossRef] [PubMed]

71. Gordon, A.; Hannon, G. Fastx-Toolkit. FASTQ/A Short-Reads Preprocessing Tools. 2010, unpublished. Available online: http://hannonlab.cshl.edu/fastx_toolkit/ (accessed on 16 October 2015).
72. Love, M.I.; Huber, W.; Anders, S. Moderated estimation of fold change and dispersion for RNA-seq data with DESeq2. *Genome Biol.* **2014**, *15*, 550. [CrossRef] [PubMed]
73. Team, R. *RStudio: Integrated Development for R*; RStudio, Inc.: Boston, MA, USA, 2015. Available online: http://www.rstudio.com (accessed on 27 October 2015).
74. Benjamini, Y.; Hochberg, Y. Controlling the false discovery rate: A practical and powerful approach to multiple testing. *J. R. Stat. Soc. B Methodol.* **1995**, *57*, 289–300.
75. Conesa, A.; Götz, S.; García-Gómez, J.M.; Terol, J.; Talón, M.; Robles, M. Blast2GO: A universal tool for annotation, visualization and analysis in functional genomics research. *Bioinformatics* **2005**, *21*, 3674–3676. [CrossRef] [PubMed]
76. Götz, S.; García-Gómez, J.M.; Terol, J.; Williams, T.D.; Nagaraj, S.H.; Nueda, M.J.; Robles, M.; Talón, M.; Dopazo, J.; Conesa, A. High-throughput functional annotation and data mining with the Blast2GO suite. *Nucleic Acids Res.* **2008**, *36*, 3420–3435. [CrossRef] [PubMed]
77. Finn, R.D.; Mistry, J.; Schuster-Böckler, B.; Griffiths-Jones, S.; Hollich, V.; Lassmann, T.; Moxon, S.; Marshall, M.; Khanna, A.; Durbin, R. Pfam: Clans, web tools and services. *Nucleic Acids Res.* **2006**, *34*, D247–D251. [CrossRef] [PubMed]
78. CIMminer. Available online: http://discover.nci.nih.gov/cimminer (accessed on 19 June 2018).
79. Cubero-Leon, E.; Ciocan, C.M.; Minier, C.; Rotchell, J.M. Reference gene selection for qPCR in mussel, *Mytilus edulis*, during gametogenesis and exogenous estrogen exposure. *Environ. Sci. Pollut. Res. Int.* **2012**, *19*, 2728–2733. [CrossRef] [PubMed]
80. Universal ProbeLibrary. Available online: https://lifescience.roche.com/en_es/brands/universal-probe-library.html#assay-design-centre (accessed on 20 July 2018).
81. Pfaffl, M.W.; Tichopad, A.; Prgomet, C.; Neuvians, T.P. Determination of stable housekeeping genes, differentially regulated target genes and sample integrity: Bestkeeper–Excel-based tool using pair-wise correlations. *Biotechnol. Lett.* **2004**, *26*, 509–515. [CrossRef] [PubMed]
82. Xie, F.; Xiao, P.; Chen, D.; Xu, L.; Zhang, B. miRDeepFinder: A miRNA analysis tool for deep sequencing of plant small RNAs. *Plant Mol. Biol.* **2012**, *80*, 75–84. [CrossRef] [PubMed]
83. Hellemans, J.; Mortier, G.; De Paepe, A.; Speleman, F.; Vandesompele, J. qBase relative quantification framework and software for management and automated analysis of real-time quantitative PCR data. *Genome Biol.* **2007**, *8*, R19. [CrossRef] [PubMed]
84. Ruijter, J.; Ramakers, C.; Hoogaars, W.; Karlen, Y.; Bakker, O.; Van den Hoff, M.; Moorman, A. Amplification efficiency: Linking baseline and bias in the analysis of quantitative PRC data. *Nucleic Acids Res.* **2009**, *37*, e45. [CrossRef] [PubMed]
85. Pfaffl, M.W. A new mathematical model for relative quantification in real-time RT–PCR. *Nucleic Acids Res.* **2001**, *29*, e45. [CrossRef] [PubMed]
86. Pfaffl, M.W.; Horgan, G.W.; Dempfle, L. Relative expression software tool (REST©) for group-wise comparison and statistical analysis of relative expression results in real-time PCR. *Nucleic Acids Res.* **2002**, *30*, e36. [CrossRef] [PubMed]

toxins

MDPI

Article

Detoxification- and Immune-Related Transcriptomic Analysis of Gills from Bay Scallops (*Argopecten irradians*) in Response to Algal Toxin Okadaic Acid

Cheng Chi [1], Sib Sankar Giri [2], Jin Woo Jun [2], Sang Wha Kim [2], Hyoun Joong Kim [2], Jeong Woo Kang [2] and Se Chang Park [2,*]

1 Laboratory of Aquatic Nutrition and Ecology, College of Animal Science and Technology, Nanjing Agricultural University, Weigang Road 1, Nanjing 210095, China; chicheng0421@126.com

2 Laboratory of Aquatic Biomedicine, College of Veterinary Medicine and Research Institute for Veterinary Science, Seoul National University, Seoul 151742, Korea; giribiotek@gmail.com (S.S.G.); advancewoo@hanmail.net (J.W.J.); kasey.kim90@gmail.com (S.W.K.); hjoong1@nate.com (H.J.K.); kck90victory@naver.com (J.W.K.)

* Correspondence: parksec@snu.ac.kr; Tel.: +82-2-880-1282

Received: 29 May 2018; Accepted: 26 July 2018; Published: 28 July 2018

Abstract: To reveal the molecular mechanisms triggered by okadaic acid (OA)-exposure in the detoxification and immune system of bay scallops, we studied differentially-expressed genes (DEGs) and the transcriptomic profile in bay scallop gill tissue after 48 h exposure to 500 nM of OA using the Illumina HiSeq 4000 deep-sequencing platform. De novo assembly of paired-end reads yielded 55,876 unigenes, of which 3204 and 2620 genes were found to be significantly up- or down-regulated, respectively. Gene ontology classification and enrichment analysis of the DEGs detected in bay scallops exposed to OA revealed four ontologies with particularly high functional enrichment, which were 'cellular process' (cellular component), 'metabolic process' (biological process), 'immune system process' (biological process), and 'catalytic process' (molecular function). The DEGs revealed that cyclic AMP-responsive element-binding proteins, acid phosphatase, toll-like receptors, nuclear erythroid 2-related factor, and the NADPH2 quinone reductase-related gene were upregulated. In contrast, the expression of some genes related to glutathione S-transferase 1, C-type lectin, complement C1q tumor necrosis factor-related protein, Superoxide dismutase 2 and fibrinogen C domain-containing protein, decreased. The outcomes of this study will be a valuable resource for the study of gene expression induced by marine toxins, and will help understanding of the molecular mechanisms underlying the scallops' response to OA exposure.

Keywords: harmful algal blooms; okadaic acid; *Argopecten irradians*; transcriptomic response; deep sequencing

Key Contribution: The Illumina platform was used for the first time to analyse gene expression in the gills of bay scallop exposed to OA. Detoxification- and immune-related genes and pathway enrichment following OA exposure were detected.

---

1. Introduction

Bivalves are among the most important commercially exploited marine species in China, sharing 75–80% of the total output of aquatic products in recent years [1]. Owing to their filter-feeding and sessile habits, worldwide distribution, and diversity of aquatic environments, bivalves are widely used as marine pollution bioindicators [2]. Scallop fisheries are mainly distributed along coastal areas of Japan, Korea, and North China [3]. In addition to their economic value, bivalves have always been studied as model species in toxicological investigation and as sentinel species in environmental monitoring programmes [4].

The frequent appearance of toxin-producing harmful algal blooms (HABs) in marine environments is a well-known worldwide problem [5]. HABs are well known for their potential to induce ecological damage, risk human health, and cause adverse effects to living marine resources [6,7]. Moreover, these HABs threaten aquaculture industries and may have deleterious effects on public health [8], because their phycotoxins may cause mass mortality of cultivated animals [9]. Shellfish toxins are the main marine phycotoxin, which includes amnaesic shellfish poisoning (ASP)-, paralytic shellfish poisoning (PSP)-, neurotoxic shellfish poisoning (NSP)-, diarrhetic shellfish poisoning (DSP)-, and azaspiracid shellfish poisoning (AZP) toxins [10]. These toxins may be taken up by humans eating shellfish contaminated with them, and lead to a series of neurological and gastrointestinal syndromes [6,7]. Okadaic acid (OA), representative of the DSP toxins, can be produced by species of the genera *Dinophysis* and *Prorocentrum* [11,12], and be accumulated in the shellfish adipose tissue [13]. This is the primary cause of acute DSP intoxication of human consumers, and harvesting bans causing huge economic losses to the shellfish aquaculture industry [14]. For example, Mouratidou et al. [15] reported maximum concentrations of 36 μg OA eq/g hepatopancreas in mussels from Thermaikos Gulf, Greece. OA is capable of binding to the active sites of protein phosphatases [16], inhibiting their activity and inducing tumorigenic and apoptotic processes [14,17]. Finally, it can lead to the hyperphosphorylation of many cellular proteins, metabolic deregulation, and genotoxic and cytotoxic damage [18]. When organisms are exposed to xenobiotics, short-term responses, such as changes in their immune response, and long-term effects on other biological parameters, including growth, ingestion and reproduction rates, and other metabolic processes may be observed [19]. Earlier investigations revealed that OA or *P. lima* exposure could induce haemocyte function damage and reduced survival in *Ruditapes decussatus* [20]. Huang et al. [11] reported that OA-producing *P. lima* caused oxidative stress, disorganization of cytoskeletons, and metabolic disturbance in mussels. In a previous work, we studied the toxic effects of OA exposure, up to 48 h, in bay scallops (*Argopecten irradians*). These included changes in glutathione (GSH), reactive oxygen species (ROS), malondialdehyde (MDA), and nitric oxide (NO) contents; lysozyme, acid phosphatase (ACP), lactate dehydrogenase (LDH), alkaline phosphatase (ALP), and superoxide dismutase (SOD) activity; total haemocyte counts (THC) and haemolymph total protein levels [8,12]. Overall, our previous work demonstrated that OA exposure increased oxidative stress, disrupted metabolism, modulated the immune response, and was toxic to physiological function in *A. irradians*. There are two resistance mechanisms that may counteract the effects of DSP in shellfish: detoxification pathways for the biotransformation or elimination of phycotoxins, and antioxidant metabolism to neutralize ROS induced by DSP exposure [21–23]. However, how scallops respond to OA toxicity, and the details of their detoxification process during acute OA exposure remain unclear, particularly the integral response at the transcriptional level. An understanding of the effects of OA exposure on the bay scallop is essential to establish effective measures to estimate its toxic potential. However, owing to the constraint of related genomic resources, a better understanding of the genetic and molecular mechanisms underlying the bay scallop response to sublethal concentrations of OA is yet to be elucidated.

De novo sequencing is an effective tool to obtain whole scallop transcriptome information. In this regard, the relatively low-cost/high-output Illumina HiSeq™ 4000 sequencing platform has found increasingly widespread use [24], having been applied to a growing number of aquatic organisms, including *Oryzias melastigma* [25], *Crassostrea gigas* [26], and *Chlamys farreri* [27], to study their responses to environmental stressors. Therefore, the aim of the present study was to obtain a better understanding of the molecular response of the bay scallop after exposure to OA. We specifically focused on the gill tissue of *A. irradians*, following exposure to 500 nM of OA for up to 48 h, since our previous studies found that this toxin induced oxidative stress, modulated the immune response, and was toxic to physiological function in *A. irradians* [8,12]. The gill was chosen as the target organ because it is the first organ in contact with OA during filtration [21]. Gills act as a defence barrier, because they play a crucial role in the filtration of suspended matter. Further, the gill was previously found to be directly affected by contact with toxic algae [21], and to have a high expression of putative immune-related genes [28]. Digital gene expression (DGE) analysis was performed with the Illumina HiSeq™ 4000 sequencing system, and then quantitative real-time PCR was conducted to verify differentially expressed genes (DEGs), which were selected according to the DGE analysis. The aim of the present work was to reveal the transcript abundance to facilitate a network of bay scallop genes enriched to regulate toxicological responses to OA exposure.

2. Results

2.1. Analysis of DGE Libraries

Two DGE libraries comprising DNA from the gills of control and OA-exposed scallops were analysed using the Illumina Hiseq 4000 sequencing system. We removed adaptors from the reads, poly N, and low-quality reads from the raw data, and then generated 9.14 Gb of totally clean bases, comprising 45.92 and 45.92 Mb clean reads for control and OA-exposed cDNA libraries, respectively. The Q20 and GC percentages of the clean reads in the two cDNA libraries were 98.21% and 98.17% and 39.13% and 39.24%, for control and OA-exposed cDNA libraries, respectively (Table S1). Clean sequences from each library were assembled by the Trinity tool, thereby producing a total of 78,510 and 77,330 transcripts in the control and OA-exposed groups, respectively, which had mean sizes of 675 with N50s of 1234 for the control group and 733 bp with N50s of 1451 bp for the OA-exposed groups, respectively (Table S1). Finally, 55 876 unigenes were further merged by transcript sets from the two libraries (Table 1). The size distribution of the unigenes was as follows: 67.58% (37,759) were between 300 and 1000 bp; 20.54% (11,477) were between 1000 and 3000 bp; and 6.24% (3488) had lengths greater than 3000 bp in length, as shown in Figure 1.

Table 1. Quality metrics of unigenes.

Sample	Total Number	Total Length	Mean Length	N50	N70	N90	GC(%)
Control	51,465	41,105,722	798	1411	704	302	39.48
OA-treated	49,453	43,129,157	872	1646	803	318	39.63
All-unigene	55,876	53,465,429	956	1840	960	345	39.42

N50: a weighted median statistic within which 50% of the Total Length is contained in unigenes greater than or equal to this value. GC (%): the percentage of G and C bases in all unigenes.

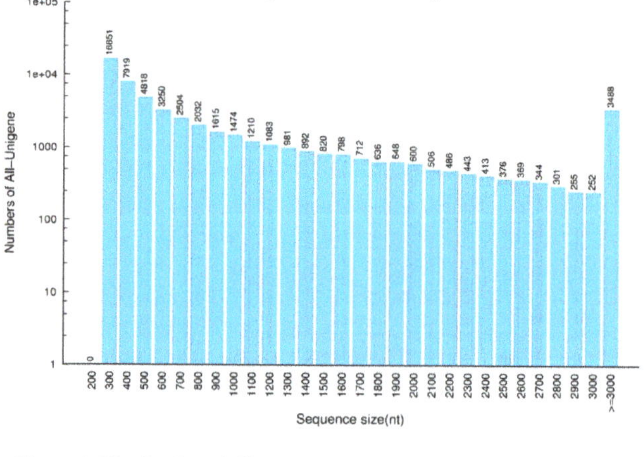

Figure 1. Distribution of all-unigenes in the bay scallop transcriptome.

2.2. Functional Annotation and Species Distribution

After assembly, functional annotation was carried out through seven functional databases for unigenes. A total of 49.31% of the total unigenes (27,555 unigenes) were annotated, of which 24,521 unigenes (43.88%) were aligned to the Nr database; 10,466 unigenes (18.73%) to Nt; 19,220 unigenes (34.40%) to Swiss-Prot, 18,523 unigenes (33.15%) to Kyoto Encyclopedia of Genes and Genomes (KEGG); 8800 (15.75%) unigenes to Clusters of Orthologous Group (COG); 18,533 (33.17%) unigenes to Interpro; and 4027 unigenes (7.21%) to Gene Ontology (GO), respectively.

The distribution of annotated species was statistically analysed with NR annotation, as shown in Figure 2. For functional classification, 15 186 unigenes were totally annotated to the COG database (Figure 3). The most frequently functional classifications were the following: 20.70% (3143) accounted for general function; 8.52% (1294) related to recombinant and repair; translation, 8.49% (1289); transcription, 6.63% (1007); post-translational-modification-related, 6.26% (950); cell-cycle-control-related, 5.64% (856), and signal-transduction-related, 5.39% (819).

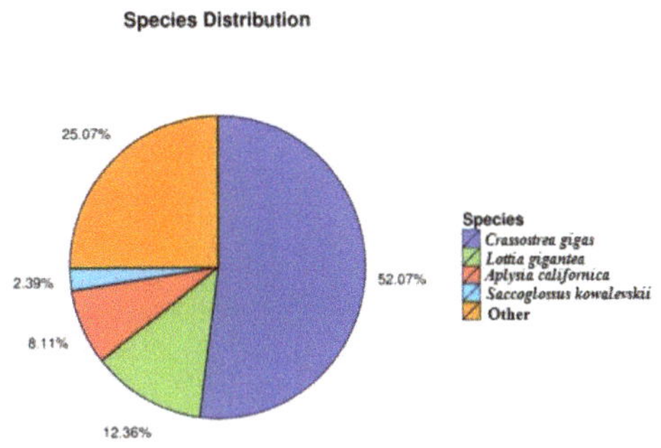

Figure 2. Annotated species and their distribution.

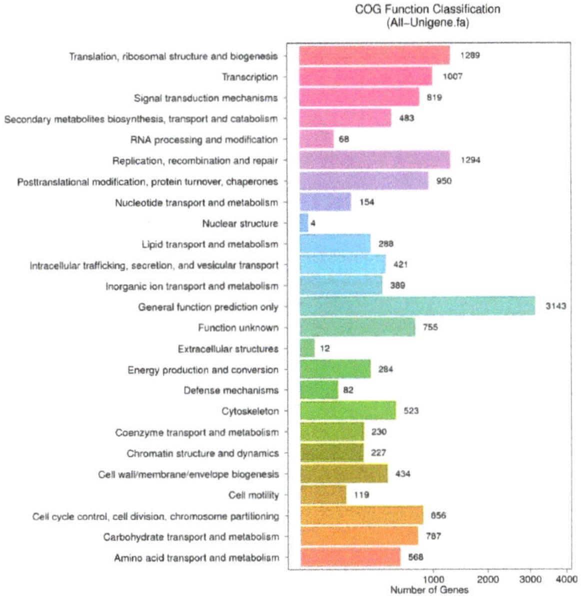

Figure 3. COG functional classification of All-unigenes.

2.3. *Differential Gene Expression Analysis*

The unigene expression levels were calculated using the Fragments Per Kilobase Million (FPKM) method (Figures 4 and 5) to identify the genes' differential expression between the control and OA-treated groups. A total of 5825 unigenes with different expression levels (with over two-fold changes, and false discovery rate (FDR) ≤ 0.001) between the control and OA-exposed groups were identified. Of these, 3204 were upregulated genes, while 2621 were downregulated genes (Table S2).

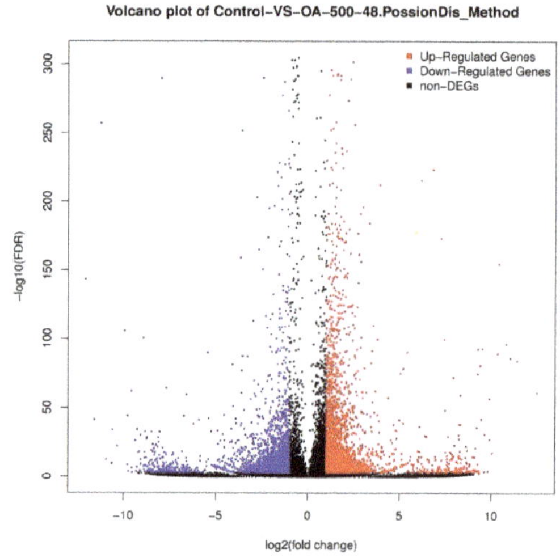

Figure 4. Gene transcription profile of the control (CN) and the OA-exposed group (OA) libraries. Blue points represent downregulated genes. Red points represent upregulated genes. Black points represent non-differential expression genes.

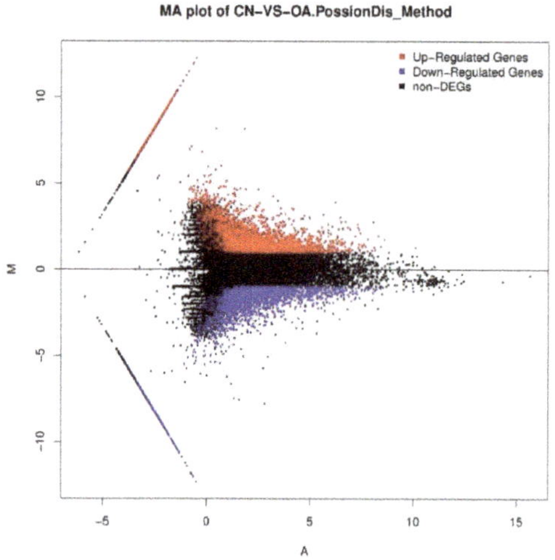

Figure 5. M (log ratio) and A (mean average) (MA) plot of DEGs of the control (CN) and the OA-exposed group (OA) libraries. X-axis represent value A (log2 mean expression level). Y-axis represents value M (log2 transformed fold change). Red points represent upregulated DEG. Blue points represent downregulated DEG. Black points represent non-DEGs.

2.4. Enrichment and Pathway Analysis

In order to identify their function, all the DEGs were mapped to the GO database. A total of 44 functional groups in the DEGs were substantially enriched compared with the genomic background (Figure 6). Genes in the OA-exposed scallop related to the terms 'metabolic process', 'cellular process', and 'catalytic activity' were dominant. Biological process and cellular components were found to be the most-represented known genes, followed by molecular function.

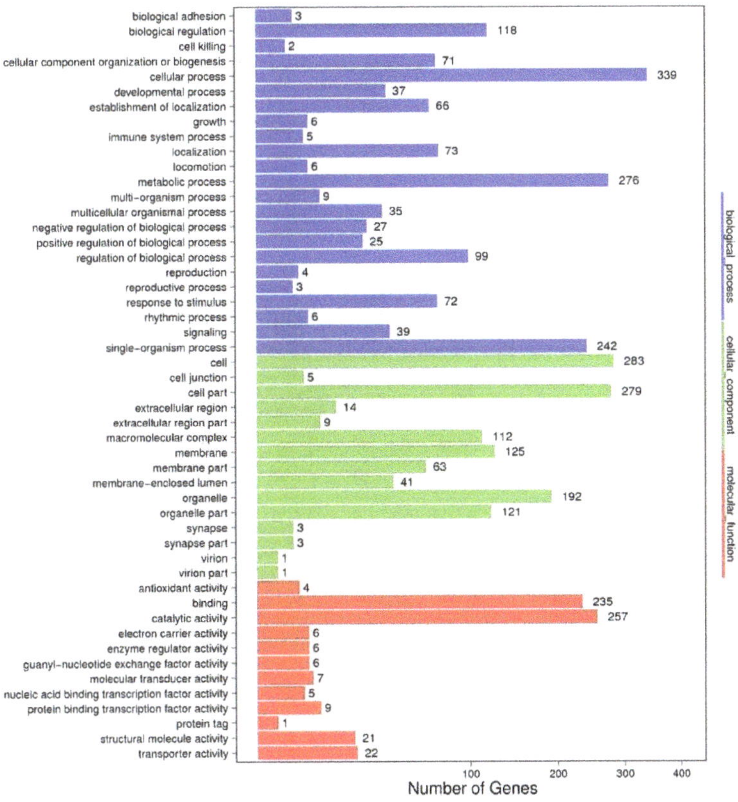

Figure 6. GO classification of differentially expressed gene (DEGs). X-axis represent the GO term.

Markedly-enriched signal transduction and metabolic pathways were identified using KEGG enrichment analysis of the DEGs. A total of 3389 DEGs were aligned at 299 pathways in the KEGG database, and 74 metabolic pathways were significantly (corrected p value < 0.05) over-represented. The pathway classification results are shown in Figure 7, and the pathway functional enrichment results in Figure 8. Among these, the expression patterns of DEGs throughout OA exposure, which involved detoxification, and immunology in mechanisms against biotoxins were further analyzed on the bases of GO and KEEG analyses. The expression of genes related to the immunology and detoxification responses such as cyclic AMP-responsive element-binding proteins, acid phosphatase, toll-like receptors, nuclear factor erythroid 2-related factor, NADPH2: quinone reductase, cytochrome P450 3A64 and 3A80 increased under exposure to OA (Table 2). In contrast, the expression of some genes related to glutathione S-transferase 1, C-type lectin, complement C1q tumor necrosis factor-related protein, Superoxide dismutase 2 and fibrinogen C domain-containing protein decreased.

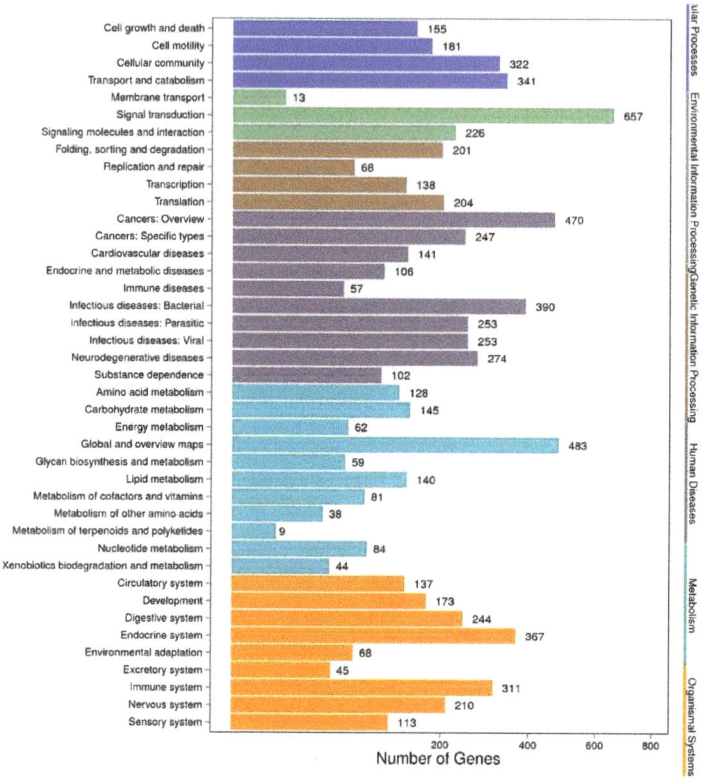

Figure 7. Pathway classification of DEGs. The *X*-axis shows the number of DEGs. The *Y*-axis shows the pathway name.

Table 2. Detoxification and immune-related differentially expressed genes (DEGs) in bay scallop gills regulated after up to 48 h exposure to 500 nM OA.

Function	Transcript	Log2 (Fold Change) (RNAseq)	Regulation
Immune system	C-type lectin superfamily 17 member A	−4.255	Down
	C-type lectin domain family 4 member E	−3.507	Down
	Complement C1q tumor necrosis factor-related protein 2	−4.791	Down
	Fibrinogen C domain-containing protein 1	−2.100	Down
	Toll-like receptor 4	2.880	Up
	Toll-like receptor 13	1.347	Up
	Acid phosphatase	2.238	Up
	NADPH oxidase 3	2.493	Up
Detoxification	ATP-binding cassette, subfamily C, member 1	1.773	Up
	ATP-binding cassette sub-family B member 10	1.165	Up
	ATP-binding cassette, sub-family C member 5	1.280	Up
	Cyclic AMP-responsive element-binding protein	1.953	Up
	Nuclear factor erythroid 2-related factor 2	1.231	Up
	NADPH2:quinone reductase	1.677	Up
	Cytochrome P450 3A80	1.207	Up
	Cytochrome P450 3A64	1.783	Up
	Cytochrome P450 1A5	−1.686	Down
	Cytochrome P450 3A24	−2.315	Down
	Superoxide dismutase Cu-Zn family	1.139	Up
	Superoxide dismutase 2	−1.126	Down
	Glutathione S-transferase 1	−1.552	Down
	Glutathione S-transferase 2	−2.511	Down
	Glutathione S-transferase omega	−1.775	Down
	Glutathione S-transferase theta-1	−1.254	Down
	Glutathione S-transferase A	−1.218	Down
	Glutathione S-transferase kappa	−2.356	Down

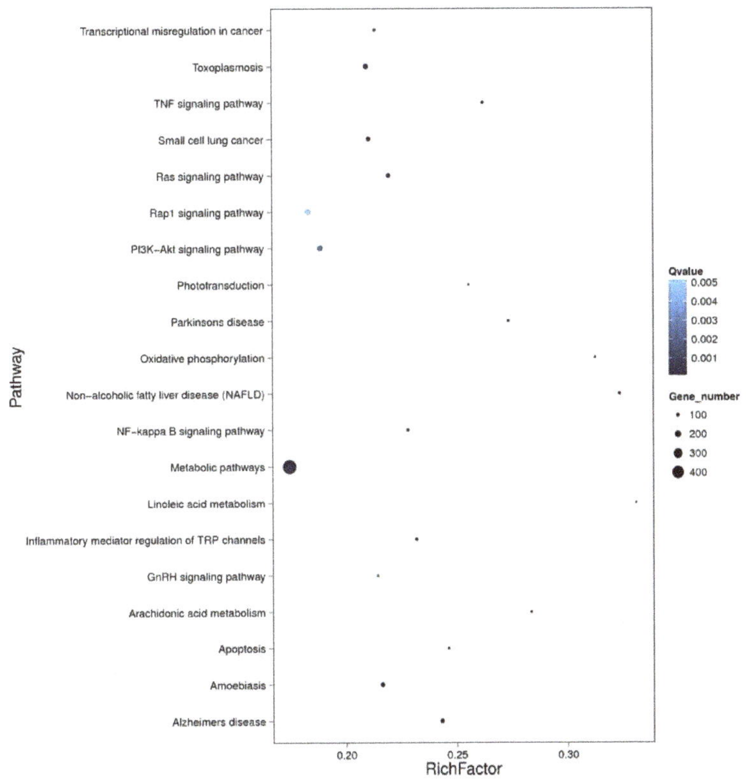

Figure 8. Enrichment of DEGs and pathways. The *X*-axis indicates enrichment factor and the *Y*-axis indicates the pathway name. Coloring indicates the *q* value (high: white, low: blue), the lower *q* value indicates the more significant enrichment. The point size indicates the DEG number (more: big, less: small).

2.5. Identification of Genes Related to OA-Induced Stress Response

The real-time quantitative PCR (qPCR) technique was used to detect the relative expression levels of nine genes, which are immunology-, detoxification- and antioxidant-ability-related genes with high expression, from the DGE libraries. Four of these genes were suppressed and the others were induced. The melting-curve analysis of each gene performed by qPCR suggested a single product. The qPCR results were compared with those from the DGE analysis. As shown in Figure 9, nine genes followed a concurrent trend between qPCR analysis and DGE library, and the correlation coefficient was calculated as 0.95 (p value < 0.001).

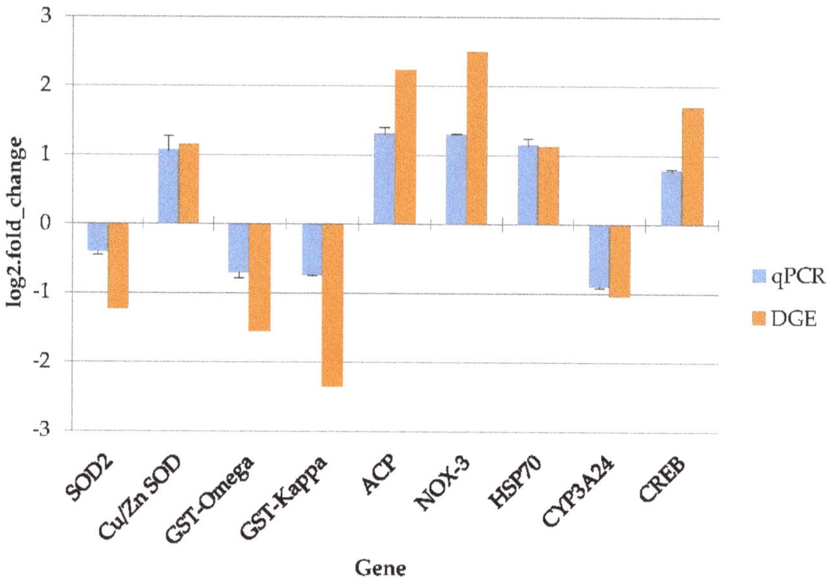

Figure 9. Results of the qPCR analysis. The *y*-axis represents the gene expressed log2 (fold change) and the *x*-axis is the gene name. *SOD2* = superoxide dismutase 2, *Cu/Zn SOD* = copper and zinc superoxide dismutase, GST = glutathione-S-transferase, ACP = acid phosphatase, *NOX-3* = NADPH oxidase 3, *HSP70* = heat shock protein 70, *CYP3A24* = cytochrome P450 3A24, *CREB* = cyclic adenosine monophosphate responsive element binding protein.

3. Discussion

Okadaic acid (OA), as a representative of DSP toxins, can accumulate in bivalves and induce diarrheic shellfish poisoning in mammals [29]. OA has been reported to be cytotoxic in several cell lines (human monocytic U-937 cells; two epithelial tumour lines, HeLa and KB; neuroblastoma cell line Neuro-2a; neuroblastoma × glioma hybrid cell line NG108-15; breast cancer cell line MCF-7) as an efficient inhibitor of serine/threonine phosphatases [30–32]. Earlier, we reported that OA exposure could affect a variety of innate immune responses (e.g., THC, total protein level, ALP, ACP, and lysozyme activities,) and physiological responses (e.g., SOD and LDH activity, ROS, NO and MDA and GSH content) in the haemolymph of scallops, and can even induce oxidative stress and disrupt metabolism in bay scallops [8,12], rendering them sensitive to OA exposure. Previous studies have demonstrated the adverse impacts of the toxin OA on other marine bivalves [11,20]; however, the molecular response of these bivalves to OA is not well characterized. In the light of our earlier studies, the results of this transcriptome information could improve the description of the acute toxicity of high concentrations of OA for some physiological and biochemical processes and provide directions and insights for future studies involving biotoxicity models in scallops. Moreover, in the present study, the calculation and normalization methods of both analyses are different, although they report transcript abundances as fold-changes relative to the control [1]. The RNA-seq expression values employ Reads Per Kilobase Million (RPKM) for calculation [33], while qPCR fold-change values employ the mean normalized expressions method and incorporated reference gene to calculate [34]. In the present investigation, both methods were used for transcript quantification. The same directions of change and a similar magnitude of the fold-change in abundance confirmed the accuracy and reliability of the DGE data. To our knowledge, the present investigation is the first to reveal the transcriptomic responses of scallops after OA exposure using deep-sequencing technology.

Highly conserved heat shock proteins (HSPs), including *HSP60*, *HSP70*, and *HSP90*, could be synthesized or secreted rapidly by cells as soon as they experience stressed [3]. Therefore, HSPs have been widely considered as effective biomarkers of exogenous stimuli or as biomonitoring tools to identify the effects of environmental pollution in aquatic animals, including bivalves [3]. Our present investigation showed that the relative expression of *HSP70*, which was validated by qPCR, was strongly increased in the gills of bay scallop up to 48 h exposure to OA. Similarly, a previous study revealed that upregulated *HSP70* expressed transcripts were identified in the mussel *Mytilus galloprovincialis* after exposure to OA stress [14]. In other investigations, the detection of *HSP70* by immunoblotting and expression analysis of *HSP70* mRNA was used to indicate marine contamination observed following exposure to heavy metals in *Dreissena polymorpha* [35], to hydrocarbon in *Crassostrea gigas* [36], to sub-lethal concentrations of quaternium-15 in *M. galloprovincialis* [37], and to cadmium in the gills of *Ostrea edulis* [38]. Therefore, in the present investigation, the upregulation of *HSP70* mRNA in the gills of bay scallops also appears to be a helpful marker for toxic effects.

The genes encoding detoxification enzymes play crucial roles in bivalves after being stimulated by a variety of exogenous stimuli, including drugs, toxicants, and chemical carcinogens [3]. Among the DEGs detected in the present study, certain detoxification-related genes were identified. The cytochrome P450 (*CYP450*) family is an essential family of enzymes related to the primary or phase I metabolism of xenobiotics, including pesticides and toxins [3,39]. Many exogenous stimuli may impact the metabolism, and then activate or suppress the activity of *CYP450* to clean exogenous stimuli [11]. A subset of cytochrome P450 enzymes, which are linked to detoxification and resistance, were involved in transforming liposoluble toxic chemicals into hydrosoluble substances that are easily eliminated [11,40]. Our results clearly showed that OA provoked the differential expression of *CYP1A5* and *CYP3A24*, which were downregulated, whereas *CYP3A4* and *CYP3A80* were upregulated. This is consistent with a previous study that reported OA-exposure-induced expression of *CYP450* mussel gills, which suggests that *CYP450* participates in the process of OA elimination [3]. Guo et al. also [41] reported that human recombinant cytochrome *CYP3A4* could eliminate OA by generating oxidized products. Accordingly, *CYP3A4* and *CYP3A80* may participate in the process of accelerating the biotransformation of OA and facilitating its excretion in bay scallops when exposed to OA. ATP-binding cassette (ABC) transporters are a family of transmembrane proteins that can transport a variety of strGSTucturally diverse substrates across biological membranes in an ATP-dependent manner [11]. In mammalian tumor cells, they are responsible for a multidrug resistance phenotype. Moreover, in aquatic organisms, they are responsible for a multixenobiotic resistance phenotype by exporting xenobiotics out of the cells or by facilitating the sequestration of toxins within specialized cells or organelles, effectively segregating them away from vulnerable protein and DNA targets [11]. In our present study, we found that *ABCB10*, *ABCC5*, and *ABCC1* were upregulated in bay scallops after 500 nM OA exposure. These results are consistent with a previous study showing that ABC transporters in mussels were upregulated after exposure to *P. lima*. Huang et al [42] also found that the expression level of a P-glycoprotein gene (*P-gp*), belonging to the family of ATP-binding cassette (ABC) transporters in the gills of *Perna viridis*, increased significantly after exposure to *P. lima*. These phenomena suggest the possible role of ABC transporters in OA detoxification.

Nicotinamide adenine dinucleotide phosphate-oxidases (NADPH-oxidases) are enzymes completely devoted to ROS production [43]. The family of NADPH-oxidases comprises trans-membrane proteins that transfer electrons across biological membranes. Owing to their involvement in ROS production, NADPH-oxidases play crucial roles in various physiological mechanisms which include host defence, gene expression, cellular signalling, apoptosis, and oxidative stress [44]. The NADPH oxidase is composed of six homologues of the cytochrome subunit (NOX1, NOX3, NOX4, NOX5, DUOX1, and DUOX2), and increased NOX activity also induces a series of pathologies [44]. Cai et al. [1] found that benzo[a]pyrene (BaP) exposure caused the upregulation of NADPH transcript in *Chlamys farreri* after three days. The findings of the present study indicated a greater abundance of *NOX-3* transcripts in the gills of scallops exposed to OA, suggesting that it induces the activation of the NADPH oxidases, thereby generating more ROS and even cell damage.

The detoxification and biotransformation of exogenous compounds also rests on Phase II and Phase III reactions [1]. Glutathione-*S*-transferase (GST), which is a kind of Phase II enzyme, could catalyse the endogenous and exogenous compounds combining with glutathione (GSH) [1,45]. Our previous field studies have shown that GSH levels in the haemolymph of *A. irradians* exposed to 500 nM OA decreased sharply at 48 hpe [12]. Consistently, in the present study, the expression of *GST* mRNAs, including *GST1*, *GST2*, *GST-A*, *GST-Theta-1*, *GST-Omeaga*, and *GST-Kappa*, in the DGE library decreased in the gills of *A. irradians* exposed to OA compared to the control group. This is consistent with previous studies showing that the expression of *GST-pi* was significantly down-regulated in the digestive gland of *M. galloprovincialis* in response to toxic dinoflagellate *Prorocentrum lima* (1000 cells/L) for 48 h [46]. These results suggest that the expression level of GST was attenuated by 500 nM OA exposure, which weakened the detoxification or antioxidant capacity of the OA-exposed scallops. SOD is a crucial gene belonging to the antioxidant defence system. It can eliminate the ROS, which can induce lipid peroxidation processes and ultimately lead to DNA damage [47]. We previously reported that *Mn SOD* expression levels in the haemolymph of OA-exposed bay scallops decreased significantly after 48 hours post-exposure [8]. These observations are in agreement with the results of the present study, verified by qPCR, showing that the *SOD2* expression levels in gills were downregulated after 48 h exposure to OA. However, we found that the expression of the *Cu/Zn SOD* mRNA was clearly induced, indicating that OA exposure could induce the expression level of *Cu/Zn SOD* in the gills when the scallops are exposed to up to 48 h 500 nM levels of OA. Additionally, it might be plausible that the downregulation of GST is partially compensated by the upregulation of *Cu/Zn SOD*, since both enzymes use the same substrate [46,48,49].

Cyclic adenosine monophosphate responsive element binding-protein (CREB) plays a pivotal role in the immune response. OA stimulation was found to enhance the levels of phosphorylated-CREB [50]. The expression of these genes is essentially regulated by the phosphorylation state of CREB, since phosphorylation is necessary for CREB to bind to the cAMP response element in the promoter of several early response genes [50]. This result is in accordance with a previous study showing that OA was able to induce CREB expression in mussels [50]. Acid phosphatase (ACP) is a kind of essential hydrolytic enzyme in phagocytic lysosomes [51]. In the present research, we found that the *ACP* mRNA expression increased in the gills of OA-exposed bay scallops. Nevertheless, in an earlier investigation, we demonstrated that OA exposure suppressed the ACP levels in the haemolymph of bay scallops, indicating that although OA could induce ACP expression, it might also affect the assembly, folding, or modification of the ACP, leading to a deficiency in the elimination of pathogens or phagocytized microorganisms in the OA-exposed gills.

In conclusion, we present here broader research into the OA-responsive genes, such as the Toll-like receptor, ATP-binding cassette, cyclic AMP-responsive element-binding protein, cytochrome P450 and Cu-Zn superoxide dismutase related genes, that show differential expression in the bay scallop, suggesting participation in the resistance to OA toxicity. These genes are related to a series of detoxification and immune processes in the response to OA. The present investigation not only reveals the transcriptional complexity of the response to OA stimulation in scallops, but also suggests the possibility of identifying the genes implicated in regulating the bivalves' tolerance or the elimination of algal toxin stress. However, it remains unclear whether these immune responses are directly stimulated by abiotic factors or whether OA exposure just facilitates the opportunistic attack of pathogens present in the scallops' microbiota [14]. Illumina next-generation sequencing technology provides a good resource to explain the immune- and detoxification-associated molecular mechanisms triggered in the bay scallop to endure the toxic effects of OA. Furthermore, it supplements and reinforces the results from our previous investigations, from which a strong cause and effect relationship between OA and the differential expression of immune- and detoxification-associated factors in the bay scallop were established. These results will be useful to develop potential countermeasures to manage the toxic effects of OA on exploited bivalve resources.

4. Materials and Methods

4.1. Maintenance of Scallops

Bay scallops *A. irradians* (weight: 46.02 ± 2.67 g; shell length: 60–70 mm) were procured in a wholesale market in Seoul, South Korea. To acclimate them to laboratory conditions, these scallops were kept for 2 weeks in 800-L tanks containing filtered and aerated seawater, with a temperature of 10 ± 1 °C and a salinity of 30 ± 0.1 psu [8]. They were fed with a commercial shellfish diet (Instant Algae®Shellfish Diet, Campbell, CA, USA) at a rate of approximately 1.2×10^{10} algae cells/scallop/day [8]. Half the seawater volume was daily renewed.

4.2. Okadaic Acid Exposure and RNA Extraction

In total, 120 scallops were divided in two groups, i.e., control and OA-exposure groups. Each group consisted of 60 scallops distributed in 3 replicate tanks with 20 scallops each. Okadaic acid (OA) (92–100% HPLC purified) was purchased from Sigma-Aldrich, USA and stored at 4 °C until use. To prepare the stock solution, OA was dissolved in 1 mL of dimethyl sulfoxide (DMSO; Sigma-Aldrich, St. Louis, MO, USA). The final concentration of OA in the OA-treated group was kept at 500 nM [8]. The scallops in the control group were treated with an equal volume of DMSO, with a final concentration of 0.0125‱DMSO in each tank [8]. After 48 h of OA exposure, six scallops were collected from each tank (i.e., 6 scallops × 3 replicates = 18 scallops per group) and maintained on ice. Scallop gills were dissected, stored in 1 mL TRIzol reagent (Invitrogen, Waltham, MA, USA), and frozen at −80 °C until use. Samples from 6 scallops were pooled for each replicate for RNA extraction [14]. Total RNA was extracted using TRIzol (Invitrogen, Waltham, MA, USA) following the manufacturer's instruction. Agarose gels (1%) electrophoresis was preformed to monitor the RNA contamination and degradation [52]. The RNA purity and contamination was checked with a NanoPhotometer® spectrophotometer (IMPLEN, Westlake Village, CA, USA) and a Qubit® RNA Assay Kit and a Qubit® 2.0 Flurometer (Life Technologies, Carlsbad, CA, USA) respectively [52]. RNA integrity was measured using the RNA Nano 6000 Assay Kit of the Agilent Bioanalyzer 2100 system (Agilent Technologies, Santa Clara, CA, USA) [52].

4.3. Library Preparation and Illumina Sequencing

After treating the total RNA extract sample with DNase I, 200 ng were purified with oligo-dT beads. In brief, total RNA and RNA Purification Beads (Illumina, San Diego, CA, USA) were incubated and resuspended in Elution Buffer (Illumina, San Diego, CA, USA). The mRNA was eluted from the beads, and then incubated to rebind the beads after adding Bead Binding Buffer (Illumina, San Diego, CA, USA). Finally, Fragment Buffer was used to fragment poly (A)-containing mRNA into small pieces. The mRNA fragments were used as templates during the cDNA synthesis. First-strand cDNA was synthesized by reverse transcription using First Strand Master Mix (Illumina, San Diego, CA, USA) and Super Script II (Invitrogen, Waltham, MA, USA). The conditions for the reverse transcription reaction were: 25 °C for 10 min; 42 °C for 50 min and 70 °C for 15 min. Next, the second-strand cDNA was synthesized at 16 °C for 1 h using Second Strand Master Mix (Illumina, San Diego, CA, USA). Then, the ds cDNA was separated from the second strand using AMPure XP beads (Agencourt, Beverly, MA, USA). The remaining overhangs were converted into blunt ends using an End Repair Mix. Next, after adding the A-Tailing Mix, the mixture was incubated at 37 °C for 30 min. The Adenylate 3′Ends DNA, RNA Index Adapter and Ligation Mix were combined and the ligate reaction incubated at 30 °C for 10 min to perform the A ligation reaction. AMPure XP Beads were used to purify the end-repaired DNA. In order to enrich the cDNA fragments, several rounds of PCR amplification were performed by adding PCR Primer Cocktail and PCR Master Mix. The AMPure XP Beads were used to purify the library fragments to select cDNA fragments of 260 bp in length. The final library quantified (qPCR) by loading 1 μL of resuspended construct on an Agilent Technologies 2100 Bioanalyzer using a DNA-specific chip (Agilent DNA 1000). For cluster generation, the qualified and quantified libraries were first amplified within the flow cell on the cBot instrument (HiSeq® 4000 PE Cluster Kit, Illumina, San Diego, CA, USA).

For paired-end sequencing, the clustered flow cell was then loaded onto the HiSeq 4000 Sequencer (HiSeq® 4000 SBS Kit, Illumina, San Diego, CA, USA) with 100 bp which was the recommended read length. The library preparation and Illumina sequencing were performed by the Beijing Genomics Institute (BGI) (Hong Kong, China).

4.4. De Novo Transcriptome Assembly

In order to remove adaptors from the reads, low-quality reads, and reads in which unknown bases (N) comprised more than 5% of the read, raw Illumina paired-end reads were filtered using the SOAPnuke software (version: v.1.5.6, Beijing Genomics Institute, Shenzhen, China, https://github.com/BGI-flexlab/SOAPnuke,). Post-filtered reads were stored in the FASTQ format [53]. To obtain unigenes, clean reads were assembled using the Trinity software (version: v2.0.6, Trinity Software, Arlington, TX, USA) [54]. The resulting sequences assembled using Trinity were referred to as transcripts. Gene family clustering was then carried out using TGICL (TIGR Gene Indices clustering tools) to obtain the final unigenes, which were classified to two categories: clusters and singletons. The former were labeled by the prefix 'CL', followed by the cluster ID. The latter were indicated by the prefix 'unigene'.

4.5. Gene Annotation and Analysis

Identification and functional annotation of all unigene sequences were carried out in seven functional databases (*e*-value < 10^{-5}): Nr, Nt, GO, COG, KEGG, Swiss-Prot, and Interpro databases. Blast (version: v2.2.23, NCBI, Bethesda, MD, USA, http://blast.ncbi.nlm.nih.gov/Blast.cgi) [55] was used to align the unigenes to NT, NR, COG, KEGG, and SwissProt to obtain annotations. Blast2GO (version: v2.5.0, BioBam, Valencia, Spain, https://www.blast2go.com) [56] used NR annotations to obtain GO annotations, and InterProScan5 (version: v5.11-51.0, EMBL-EBI, Hinxton, UK, https://code.google.com/p/interproscan/wiki/Introduction) to obtain InterPro annotations.

4.6. Differential Expression Analysis

Bowtie v2.2.5 was devoted to map the high-quality reads to the reference unigene sequences [57], and then calculate the gene expression levels, which were determined using RSEM (version: v1.2.12, http://deweylab.biostat.wisc.edu/RSEM) [58]. DEGs were detected based on a Poisson distribution using PossionDis, as described by Audic and Claverie [59]. The unigene expression level was calculated following the fragments per kilobase million (FPKM) formula. A false discovery rate (FDR) of 0.001 and a two-fold change were selected as the thresholds for significantly differential expression.

4.7. GO and KEGG Enrichment Analysis of Differentially Expressed Genes

DEGs were classified according to the official classification on the basis of the GO annotation results. Pathway functional enrichment was also carried out by the *R*-function *phyper*. The *p* value calculating formula in the hypergeometric test was as Equation (1):

$$P = 1 - \sum_{i=0}^{m-1} \frac{\binom{M}{i}\binom{N-M}{n-i}}{\binom{N}{n}} \tag{1}$$

FDR was calculated for each *p* value, and in general, the terms for which FDR did not exceed 0.001 were defined as significantly enriched.

4.8. Quantitative Real-Time PCR Validation

The expression of nine genes, which were singled out for the validation of the DGE data, was performed by qPCR. *β-actin* was used as a house-keeping gene [8]. cDNA synthesis was performed with 500 ng of DNase-treated RNA by using a PrimeScriptTM RT Reagent Kit (TaKaRa Bio, Kyoto, Japan). All qPCR reactions were carried out using SYBR Premix Ex TaqTM Perfect Real-Time Kits (TaKaRa Bio, Japan) with a QiagenRotor-Gene Q RT-PCR Detection System (Qiagen, Hilden, Germany). PCR primers, listed in Table S3, were designed using the Primer 5 software (version: v.5, PREMIER Biosoft, Palo Alto, CA, USA) based on transcriptome sequences. The reaction mixture consisted of 1 μL cDNA (50 ng), 1 μL of the forward and reverse primers (10 μM), and 6.25 μL of SYBR Premix Ex TaqTM. To ensure that the final volume of the reaction mixture was 12 μL, ultra-pure water was added. The following reaction conditions were maintained for extension: 94 °C for 2 min, followed by 40 cycles of 94 °C for 20 s, 58 °C for 30 s, and 72 °C for 40 s [8]. In order to eliminate the possibility of primer dimer formation or non-specific amplifications, a melting curve analysis was carried out after the amplification phase [8]. A standard curve was constructed from serial dilutions of the cDNA sample and drawn by plotting the natural log of the threshold cycle (Ct) against the number of molecules [8]. Standard curves for each gene were prepared in duplicate and triplicate to obtain a reliable measure of the amplification efficiency [8]. The amplification efficiencies were between 90% and 110%, and the correlation coefficients (*R*2) of all standard curves were >0.99. The relative expression ratios of the target genes were calculated using the method described by M.W. Pfaffl [60]. In all cases, PCR was carried out in triplicate. Statistical analysis was carried out using the statistical software SPSS 19.0 (version: 19.0, IBM Corp., Armonk, NY, USA, 2017). The differences were determined using the LSD test, with *p*-values < 0.05 indicating statistical significance. Values were expressed as the arithmetic mean ± standard deviation (SD).

Supplementary Materials: The following are available online at http://www.mdpi.com/2072-6651/10/8/308/s1, Table S1: Summary of sequencing reads after filtering, and quality metrics of transcripts, Table S2: The differential expression unigenes (with higher than two-fold changes, and FDR≤ 0.001) between the control and the OA-treated groups. Table S3: All primers used in the validation analysis, The accession number for our raw dataset in the GEO database is: GSE116508.

Author Contributions: C.C. and S.C.P. conceived and designed the experiments; C.C. and S.S.G. performed the experiments; C.C. and J.W.J. analyzed the data; H.J.K., S.W.K., J.W.K. contributed with reagents/materials/analysis tools; C.C. wrote the manuscript.

Funding: This research was funded by the Basic Science Research Program through the National Research Foundation of Korea (NRF) [2017R1C1B2004616] and the supportive managing project of the Center for Companion Animals Research of the Korean government [PJ013877].

Conflicts of Interest: The authors declare no conflict of interest. The funding sponsors had no role in the design of the study; in the collection, analyses, or interpretation of data; in the writing of the manuscript, or in the decision to publish the results.

References

1. Cai, Y.; Pan, L.; Hu, F.; Jin, Q.; Liu, T. Deep sequencing-based transcriptome profiling analysis of *Chlamys farreri* exposed to benzo [a] pyrene. *Gene* **2014**, *551*, 261–270. [CrossRef] [PubMed]
2. Goldberg, E.D.; Bowen, V.T.; Farrington, J.W.; Harvey, G.; Martin, J.H.; Parker, P.L.; Risebrough, R.W.; Robertson, W.; Schneider, E.; Gamble, E. The mussel watch. *Environ. Conserv.* **1978**, *5*, 101–125. [CrossRef]
3. Hu, F.; Pan, L.; Cai, Y.; Liu, T.; Jin, Q. Deep sequencing of the scallop *Chlamys farreri* transcriptome response to tetrabromobisphenol A (TBBPA) stress. *Mar. Genom.* **2015**, *19*, 31–38. [CrossRef] [PubMed]
4. Liu, N.; Pan, L.; Wang, J.; Yang, H.; Liu, D. Application of the biomarker responses in scallop (*Chlamys farreri*) to assess metals and PAHs pollution in Jiaozhou Bay, China. *Mar. Environ. Res.* **2012**, *80*, 38–45. [CrossRef] [PubMed]

5. De Jesús Romero-Geraldo, R.; García-Lagunas, N.; Hernández-Saavedra, N.Y. *Crassostrea gigas* exposure to the dinoflagellate *Prorocentrum lima*: Histological and gene expression effects on the digestive gland. *Mar. Environ. Res.* **2016**, *120*, 93–102. [CrossRef] [PubMed]
6. Zingone, A.; Enevoldsen, H.O. The diversity of harmful algal blooms: A challenge for science and management. *Ocean. Coast. Manag.* **2000**, *43*, 725–748. [CrossRef]
7. Anderson, D.M. Approaches to monitoring, control and management of harmful algal blooms (HABs). *Ocean. Coast. Manag.* **2009**, *52*, 342–347. [CrossRef] [PubMed]
8. Chi, C.; Giri, S.S.; Jun, J.W.; Kim, H.J.; Kim, S.W.; Yun, S.; Park, S.C. Effects of algal toxin okadaic acid on the non-specific immune and antioxidant response of bay scallop (*Argopecten irradians*). *Fish. Shellfish Immunol.* **2017**, *65*, 111–117. [CrossRef] [PubMed]
9. Glibert, P.M.; Anderson, D.M.; Gentien, P.; Granéli, E.; Sellner, K.G. The global, complex phenomena of harmful algal blooms. *Oceanography* **2005**, *18*, 136–147. [CrossRef]
10. Basti, L.; Hégaret, H.; Shumway, S.E. Harmful algal blooms and shellfish. In *Harmful Algal Blooms: A Compendium Desk Reference*; John Wiley & Sons, Ltd.: Hoboken, NJ, USA, 2018; pp. 135–190.
11. Huang, L.; Zou, Y.; Weng, H.W.; Li, H.Y.; Liu, J.S.; Yang, W.D. Proteomic profile in *Perna viridis* after exposed to *Prorocentrum lima*, a dinoflagellate producing DSP toxins. *Environ. Pollut.* **2015**, *196*, 350–357. [CrossRef] [PubMed]
12. Chi, C.; Giri, S.S.; Jun, J.W.; Kim, H.J.; Yun, S.; Kim, S.G.; Park, S.C. Marine Toxin Okadaic Acid Affects the Immune Function of Bay Scallop (*Argopecten irradians*). *Molecules* **2016**, *21*, 1108. [CrossRef] [PubMed]
13. Espiña, B.; Louzao, M.; Cagide, E.; Alfonso, A.; Vieytes, M.R.; Yasumoto, T.; Botana, L.M. The methyl ester of okadaic acid is more potent than okadaic acid in disrupting the actin cytoskeleton and metabolism of primary cultured hepatocytes. *Br. J. Pharmacol.* **2010**, *159*, 337–344. [CrossRef] [PubMed]
14. Suarez-Ulloa, V.; Fernandez-Tajes, J.; Aguiar-Pulido, V.; Prego-Faraldo, M.V.; Florez-Barros, F.; Sexto-Iglesias, A.; Mendez, J.; Eirin-Lopez, J.M. Unbiased high-throughput characterization of mussel transcriptomic responses to sublethal concentrations of the biotoxin okadaic acid. *PeerJ* **2015**, *3*, e1429. [CrossRef] [PubMed]
15. Mouratidou, T.; Kaniou-Grigoriadou, I.; Samara, C.; Kouimtzis, T. Detection of the marine toxin okadaic acid in mussels during a diarrhetic shellfish poisoning (DSP) episode in Thermaikos Gulf, Greece, using biological, chemical and immunological methods. *Sci. Total Environ.* **2006**, *366*, 894–904. [CrossRef] [PubMed]
16. Stonik, V.A.; Stonik, I.V. Toxins Produced by Marine Microorganisms: A Short Review. *Mar. Freshw. Toxins* **2016**, 3–21. [CrossRef]
17. Prego-Faraldo, M.V.; Valdiglesias, V.; Laffon, B.; Eirín-López, J.M.; Méndez, J. In vitro analysis of early genotoxic and cytotoxic effects of okadaic acid in different cell types of the mussel Mytilus galloprovincialis. *J. Toxicol. Environ. Health Part A* **2015**, *78*, 814–824. [CrossRef] [PubMed]
18. Mello, D.F.; Proença, L.A. d. O.; Barracco, M.A. Comparative study of various immuneparameters in three bivalve species during a natural bloom of *Dinophysis acuminata* in Santa Catarina Island, Brazil. *Toxins* **2010**, *2*, 1166–1178. [CrossRef] [PubMed]
19. Burgos-Aceves, M.A.; Faggio, C. An approach to the study of the immunity functions of bivalve haemocytes: Physiology and molecular aspects. *Fish Shellfish Immunol.* **2017**, *67*, 513–517. [CrossRef] [PubMed]
20. Prado-Alvarez, M.; Flórez-Barrós, F.; Méndez, J.; Fernandez-Tajes, J. Effect of okadaic acid on carpet shell clam (*Ruditapes decussatus*) haemocytes by in vitro exposure and harmful algal bloom simulation assays. *Cell. Biol. Toxicol.* **2013**, *29*, 189–197. [CrossRef] [PubMed]
21. Fabioux, C.; Sulistiyani, Y.; Haberkorn, H.; Hégaret, H.; Amzil, Z.; Soudant, P. Exposure to toxic *Alexandrium minutum* activates the detoxifying and antioxidant systems in gills of the oyster *Crassostrea gigas*. *Harmful Algae* **2015**, *48*, 55–62. [CrossRef] [PubMed]
22. Kim, C.S.; Lee, S.G.; Lee, C.K.; Kim, H.G.; Jung, J. Reactive oxygen species as causative agents in the ichthyotoxicity of the red tide dinoflagellate *Cochlodinium polykrikoides*. *J. Plankton Res.* **1999**, *21*, 2105–2115. [CrossRef]
23. Flores, H.S.; Wikfors, G.H.; Dam, H.G. Reactive oxygen species are linked to the toxicity of the dinoflagellate *Alexandrium spp.* to protists. *Aquat. Microb. Ecol.* **2012**, *66*, 199–209. [CrossRef]
24. Reuter, J.A.; Spacek, D.V.; Snyder, M.P. High-throughput sequencing technologies. *Mol. Cell* **2015**, *58*, 586–597. [CrossRef] [PubMed]
25. Huang, Q.; Dong, S.; Fang, C.; Wu, X.; Ye, T.; Lin, Y. Deep sequencing-based transcriptome profiling analysis of *Oryzias melastigma* exposed to PFOS. *Aquat. Toxicol.* **2012**, *120*, 54–58. [CrossRef] [PubMed]

26. Zhao, X.; Yu, H.; Kong, L.; Li, Q. Transcriptomic responses to salinity stress in the Pacific. *oyster Crassostrea gigas*. *PLoS ONE* **2012**, *7*, e46244. [CrossRef]
27. Fu, X.; Sun, Y.; Wang, J.; Xing, Q.; Zou, J.; Li, R.; Wang, Z.; Wang, S.; Hu, X.; Zhang, L. Sequencing-based gene network analysis provides a core set of gene resource for understanding thermal adaptation in Zhikong scallop *Chlamys farreri*. *Mol. Ecol. Resour.* **2014**, *14*, 184–198. [CrossRef] [PubMed]
28. Philipp, E.E.; Kraemer, L.; Melzner, F.; Poustka, A.J.; Thieme, S.; Findeisen, U.; Schreiber, S.; Rosenstiel, P. Massively parallel RNA sequencing identifies a complex immune gene repertoire in the lophotrochozoan *Mytilus edulis*. *PLoS ONE* **2012**, *7*, e33091. [CrossRef] [PubMed]
29. Svensson, S.; Särngren, A.; Förlin, L. Mussel blood cells, resistant to the cytotoxic effects of okadaic acid, do not express cell membrane p-glycoprotein activity (multixenobiotic resistance). *Aquat. Toxicol.* **2003**, *65*, 27–37. [CrossRef]
30. Ravindran, J.; Gupta, N.; Agrawal, M.; Bhaskar, A.B.; Rao, P.L. Modulation of ROS/MAPK signaling pathways by okadaic acid leads to cell death via, mitochondrial mediated caspase-dependent mechanism. *Apoptosis* **2011**, *16*, 145–161. [CrossRef] [PubMed]
31. Von Zezschwitz, C.; Vorwerk, H.; Tergau, F.; Steinfelder, H.J. Apoptosis induction by inhibitors of Ser/Thr phosphatases 1 and 2A is associated with transglutaminase activation in two different human epithelial tumour lines. *FEBS Lett.* **1997**, *413*, 147–151. [CrossRef]
32. Soliño, L.; Sureda, F.X.; Diogène, J. Evaluation of okadaic acid, dinophysistoxin-1 and dinophysistoxin-2 toxicity on Neuro-2a, NG108-15 and MCF-7 cell lines. *Toxicol. Vitro* **2015**, *29*, 59–62. [CrossRef] [PubMed]
33. Marioni, J.C.; Mason, C.E.; Mane, S.M.; Stephens, M.; Gilad, Y. RNA-seq: An assessment of technical reproducibility and comparison with gene expression arrays. *Genome Res.* **2008**, *18*, 1509–1517. [CrossRef] [PubMed]
34. Simon, P. Q-Gene: Processing quantitative real-time RT–PCR data. *Bioinformatics* **2003**, *19*, 1439–1440. [CrossRef] [PubMed]
35. Clayton, M.E.; Steinmann, R.; Fent, K. Different expression patterns of heat shock proteins hsp 60 and hsp 70 in zebra mussels (*Dreissena polymorpha*) exposed to copper and tributyltin. *Aquat. Toxicol.* **2000**, *47*, 213–226. [CrossRef]
36. Boutet, I.; Tanguy, A.; Moraga, D. Response of the Pacific oyster *Crassostrea gigas* to hydrocarbon contamination under experimental conditions. *Gene* **2004**, *329*, 147–157. [CrossRef] [PubMed]
37. Faggio, C.; Pagano, M.; Alampi, R.; Vazzana, I.; Felice, M.R. Cytotoxicity, haemolymphatic parameters, and oxidative stress following exposure to sub-lethal concentrations of quaternium-15 in *Mytilus galloprovincialis*. *Aquat. Toxicol.* **2016**, *180*, 258–265. [CrossRef] [PubMed]
38. Piano, A.; Valbonesi, P.; Fabbri, E. Expression of cytoprotective proteins, heat shock protein 70 and metallothioneins, in tissues of *Ostrea edulis* exposed to heat andheavy metals. *Cell. Stress Chaperones* **2004**, *9*, 134–142. [CrossRef] [PubMed]
39. Anzenbacher, P.; Anzenbacherová, E. Cytochromes P450 and metabolism of xenobiotics. *Cell. Mol. Life Sci.* **2001**, *58*, 737–747. [CrossRef] [PubMed]
40. Liu, D.; Pan, L.; Cai, Y.; Li, Z.; Miao, J.J. Response of detoxification gene mRNA expression and selection of molecular biomarkers in the clam *Ruditapes philippinarum* exposed to benzo[a]pyrene. *Environ. Pollut.* **2014**, *189*, 1–8. [CrossRef] [PubMed]
41. Guo, F.; An, T.; Rein, K.S. The algal hepatoxoxin okadaic acid is a substrate for human cytochromes CYP3A4 and CYP3A5. *Toxicon* **2010**, *55*, 325–332. [CrossRef] [PubMed]
42. Huang, L.; Wang, J.; Chen, W.C.; Li, H.Y.; Liu, J.S.; Jiang, T.; Yang, W.D. P-glycoprotein expression in *Perna viridis* after exposure to *Prorocentrum lima*, a dinoflagellate producing DSP toxins. *Fish Shellfish Immunol.* **2014**, *39*, 254–262. [CrossRef] [PubMed]
43. Donaghy, L.; Hong, H.K.; Jauzein, C.; Choi, K.S. The known and unknown sources of reactive oxygen and nitrogen species in haemocytes of marine bivalve molluscs. *Fish Shellfish Immunol.* **2015**, *42*, 91–97. [CrossRef] [PubMed]
44. Bedard, K.; Krause, K.H. The NOX family of ROS-generating NADPH oxidases: Physiology and pathophysiology. *Physiol. Rev.* **2007**, *87*, 245–313. [CrossRef] [PubMed]
45. Liu, D.; Pan, L.; Li, Z.; Cai, Y.; Miao, J. Metabolites analysis, metabolic enzyme activities and bioaccumulation in the clam *Ruditapes philippinarum* exposed to benzo [a] pyrene. *Ecotoxicol. Environ. Saf.* **2014**, *107*, 251–259. [CrossRef] [PubMed]

46. Prego-Faraldo, M.; Vieira, L.; Eirin-Lopez, J.; Méndez, J.; Guilhermino, L. Transcriptional and biochemical analysis of antioxidant enzymes in the mussel *Mytilus galloprovincialis* during experimental exposures to the toxic dinoflagellate *Prorocentrum lima*. *Mar. Environ. Res.* **2017**, *129*, 304–315. [CrossRef] [PubMed]
47. Jin, Q.; Pan, L.; Liu, T.; Hu, F. RNA-seq based on transcriptome reveals differ genetic expressing in *Chlamys farreri* exposed to carcinogen PAHs. *Environ. Toxicol. Pharmacol.* **2015**, *39*, 313–320. [CrossRef] [PubMed]
48. Regoli, F.; Benedetti, M.; Giuliani, M.E. Antioxidant defenses and acquisition of tolerance to chemical stress. *Toler. Environ. Contam.* **2011**, 153–173.
49. Regoli, F.; Giuliani, M.E.; Benedetti, M.; Arukwe, A. Molecular and biochemical biomarkers in environmental monitoring: A comparison of biotransformation and antioxidant defense systems in multiple tissues. *Aquat. Toxicol.* **2011**, *105*, 56–66. [CrossRef] [PubMed]
50. Manfrin, C.; Dreos, R.; Battistella, S.; Beran, A.; Gerdol, M.; Varotto, L.; Lanfranchi, G.; Venier, P.; Pallavicini, A. Mediterranean mussel gene expression profile induced by okadaic acid exposure. *Environ. Sci. Technol.* **2010**, *44*, 8276–8283. [CrossRef] [PubMed]
51. Chen, M.Y.; Yang, H.S.; Delaporte, M.; Zhao, S.J.; Xing, K. Immune responses of the scallop *Chlamys farreri* after air exposure to different temperatures. *J. Exp. Mar. Biol. Ecol.* **2007**, *345*, 52–60. [CrossRef]
52. Zhou, J.; Xiong, Q.; Chen, H.; Yang, C.; Fan, Y. Identification of the spinal expression profile of non-coding RNAs involved in neuropathic pain following spared nerve injury by sequence analysis. *Front. Mol. Neurosci.* **2017**, *10*, 91. [CrossRef] [PubMed]
53. Cock, P.J.; Fields, C.J.; Goto, N.; Heuer, M.L.; Rice, P.M. The Sanger FASTQ file format for sequences with quality scores, and the Solexa/Illumina FASTQ variants. *Nucleic Acids Res.* **2010**, *38*, 1767–1771. [CrossRef] [PubMed]
54. Grabherr, M.G.; Haas, B.J.; Yassour, M.; Levin, J.Z.; Thompson, D.A.; Amit, I.; Adiconis, X.; Fan, L.; Raychowdhury, R.; Zeng, Q. Full-length transcriptome assembly from RNA-Seq data without a reference genome. *Nat. Biotechnol.* **2011**, *29*, 644–652. [CrossRef] [PubMed]
55. Altschul, S.F.; Gish, W.; Miller, W.; Myers, E.W.; Lipman, D.J. Basic local alignment search tool. *J. Mol. Biol.* **1990**, *215*, 403–410. [CrossRef]
56. Conesa, A.; Götz, S.; García-Gómez, J.M.; Terol, J.; Talón, M.; Robles, M. Blast2GO: A universal tool for annotation, visualization and analysis in functional genomics research. *Bioinformatics* **2005**, *21*, 3674–3676. [CrossRef] [PubMed]
57. Langmead, B.; Salzberg, S.L. Fast gapped-read alignment with Bowtie 2. *Nat. Methods* **2012**, *9*, 357–359. [CrossRef] [PubMed]
58. Li, B.; Dewey, C.N. RSEM: Accurate transcript quantification from RNA-Seq data with or without a reference genome. *BMC Bioinform.* **2011**, *12*, 323. [CrossRef] [PubMed]
59. Audic, S.; Claverie, J.-M. The significance of digital gene expression profiles. *Genome Res.* **1997**, *7*, 986–995. [CrossRef] [PubMed]
60. Pfaffl, M.W. A new mathematical model for relative quantification in real-time RT–PCR. *Nucleic Acids Res.* **2001**, *29*, e45. [CrossRef] [PubMed]

toxins

MDPI

Article

Effect of Suspended Particulate Matter on the Accumulation of Dissolved Diarrhetic Shellfish Toxins by Mussels (*Mytilus galloprovincialis*) under Laboratory Conditions

Aifeng Li [1,2,*], Meihui Li [1], Jiangbing Qiu [1], Jialiang Song [1], Ying Ji [1], Yang Hu [1], Shuqin Wang [1] and Yijia Che [1]

1 College of Environmental Science and Engineering, Ocean University of China, Qingdao 266100, China; limeihui02110118@163.com (M.L.); asttl@ouc.edu.cn (J.Q.); sjl0320@163.com (J.S.); jiying2018@163.com (Y.J.); ouc_huyang@163.com (Y.H.); long052193@163.com (S.W.); cheyj0808@163.com (Y.C.)

2 Key Laboratory of Marine Environment and Ecology, Ocean University of China, Ministry of Education, Qingdao 266100, China

* Correspondence: lafouc@ouc.edu.cn; Tel.: +86-532-6678-1935

Received: 17 May 2018; Accepted: 28 June 2018; Published: 3 July 2018

Abstract: In recent years, detection of trace amounts of dissolved lipophilic phycotoxins in coastal waters has been possible using solid phase adsorption toxin tracking (SPATT) samplers. To explore the contribution of dissolved diarrhetic shellfish toxins (DST) to the accumulation of toxins by cultivated bivalves, mussels (*Mytilus galloprovincialis*) were exposed to different concentrations of purified okadaic acid (OA) and dinophysistoxin-1 (DTX1) in filtered (0.45 μm) seawater for 96 h. Accumulation and esterification of DST by mussels under different experimental conditions, including with and without the addition of the food microalga *Isochrysis galbana*, and with the addition of different size-fractions of suspended particulate matter (SPM) (<75 μm, 75–150 μm, 150–250 μm) were compared. Results showed that mussels accumulated similar amounts of OA and DTX1 from seawater with or without food microalgae present, and slightly lower amounts when SPM particles were added. Mussels preferentially accumulated OA over DTX1 in all treatments. The efficiency of the mussel's accumulation of OA and DTX1 from seawater spiked with low concentrations of toxins was higher than that in seawater with high toxin levels. A large proportion of OA (86–94%) and DTX1 (65–82%) was esterified to DTX3 by mussels in all treatments. The proportion of *I. galbana* cells cleared by mussels was markedly inhibited by dissolved OA and DTX1 (OA 9.2 μg L^{-1}, DTX1 13.2 μg L^{-1}) in seawater. Distribution of total OA and DTX1 accumulated in the mussel tissues ranked in all treatments as follows: digestive gland > gills > mantle > residual tissues. However, the percentage of total DST in the digestive gland of mussels in filtered seawater (67%) was higher than with the addition of SPM particles (75–150 μm) (51%), whereas the gills showed the opposite trend in filtered seawater with (27%) and without (14.4%) SPM particles. Results presented here will improve our understanding of the mechanisms of DST accumulation by bivalves in marine aquaculture environments.

Keywords: diarrhetic shellfish toxins (DST); *Mytilus galloprovincialis*; DST accumulation; DST esterification; suspended particulate matter (SPM)

Key Contribution: Our results confirmed that mussels could directly accumulate dissolved diarrhetic shellfish toxins (OA; DTX1) from seawater and rapidly transform them to esterified forms. Addition of suspended particulate matter did not increase but slightly hindered the mussels' toxin accumulation efficiency.

1. Introduction

Okadaic acid (OA), dinophysistoxin-1 (DTX1) and -2 (DTX2) (Figure 1) are produced by some benthic dinoflagellates of the genus *Prorocentrum*, such as *P. lima* [1], *P. concavum* [2], *P. hoffmannianum* [3], *P. rhathymum* [4] and *P. foraminosum* [5], and by planktonic dinoflagellates of the genus *Dinophysis*, including *D. acuminata*, *D. acuta*, *D. caudata*, *D. fortii*, *D. miles*, *D. norvegica*, *D. ovum*, *D. sacculus* and *D. tripos* [6]. These phycotoxins are called diarrhetic shellfish toxins (DST) because when transferred to consumers through common seafood vectors, including mussels, clams, scallops and oysters [7,8], they cause severe diarrhea due to strong inhibition of serine/threonine protein phosphatase activity leading to severe mucosal damage of the intestinal tract [9]. Diarrhetic shellfish poisoning (DSP) events are a world-wide phenomenon [10–15]. The first confirmed cases of DSP in China occurred in 2011 when more than 200 residents became ill after consuming mussels (*Mytilus galloprovincialis*) harvested from coastal waters of the East China Sea [11]. DSP has been recognized as one of the five most common illnesses caused by harmful algal bloom toxins, which also include ciguatera fish poisoning, paralytic shellfish poisoning, neurotoxic shellfish poisoning and amnesic shellfish poisoning [16].

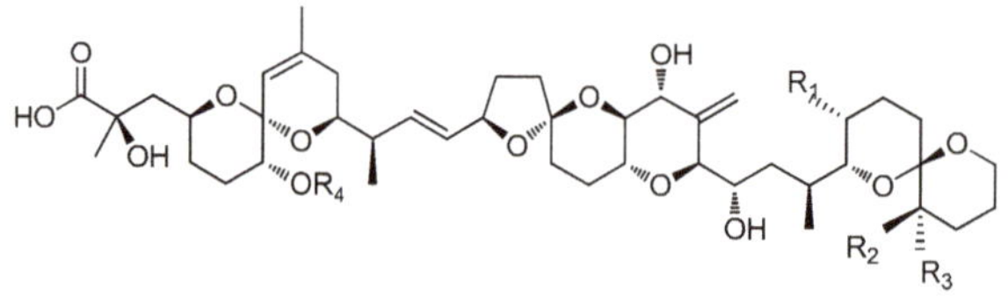

DST	R_1	R_2	R_3	R_4	Molecular Weight
OA	CH_3	H	H	H	804.5
DTX1	CH_3	CH_3	H	H	818.5
DTX2	H	H	CH_3	H	804.5
DTX3	H or CH_3	H or CH_3	H or CH_3	Acyl	1014~1082

Figure 1. Chemical structure of okadaic acid (OA) and its derivatives. DST: diarrhetic shellfish toxins.

The free forms of DST (OA, DTX1 and DTX2) produced by microalgae can be esterified in many bivalve species with different fatty acids through the –OH group at the C-7 site [11,17,18]. These 7-*O*-acyl-OA/DTX1 esters, known as dinophysistoxin-3 (DTX3) (Figure 1), with various molecular weight and fatty acid chain-lengths ranging from 12 to 22 carbons, were stored mainly in the digestive gland of scallops in a previous study [19]. Diverse DTX3 components also play important roles in the intoxication of human consumers [20,21] because they can be hydrolyzed by lipases and other enzymes to release toxins into the gastrointestinal tract [22–24]. Some other diol-esters are biosynthesized by esterification of the C-1 acid group with 4-10-carbon side chains in the dinoflagellates *P. lima* and *D. acuta* [25]. Alkaline hydrolysis is usually used to release free toxin forms from DTX3 in order to accurately quantify the potential DST levels in seafood products. Currently, a regulatory limit of 160 μg OA eq. kg^{-1} for OA and its analogues in shellfish meat is implemented by the European Union, but a more rigid control, 45 μg OA eq. kg^{-1}, is recommended by the European Food Safety Authority [26].

A great deal of effort has been devoted to forecasting toxic blooms caused by DST-producing microalgae and protecting human health. Many countries with a well-developed shellfish industry have implemented regular monitoring programs, including monitoring density of microalgae in seawater and toxin contamination of shellfish tissues, as well as detection of toxins in seawater using solid phase adsorption toxin tracking (SPATT) or solid phase extraction (SPE) methods. The SPATT technology was first adopted by MacKenzie et al. [27] to monitor dissolved lipophilic toxins in seawater and is considered an effective complementary tool for monitoring and studying algal toxin dynamics in the field and in laboratory experiments [28–30]. In addition, SPATT resins have shown many advantages in the sample preparation process [31]. Nevertheless, some SPATT-based monitoring results have not supported its value as an early warning tool for shellfish contamination with DST [32,33]. In recent years, solid phase extraction (SPE) cartridges have been used to sample dissolved lipophilic toxins in seawater. The adsorbed toxins were analyzed with highly sensitive detection technologies such as liquid chromatography-tandem mass spectrometry (LC-MS/MS), and trace amounts of DST were detected in most samples from coastal waters of Qingdao, China, since October 2012 [34,35]. This dissolved DST fraction may contribute to the accumulation of these toxins by the bivalves exposed to them.

In the present study, accumulation of dissolved DST by mussels was simulated in the laboratory and the effect of suspended particulate matter (SPM) on toxin accumulation was explored. In addition, biotransformation processes and the distribution of DST in various mussel tissues were also examined.

2. Results

2.1. Accumulation of Dissolved OA and DTX1 from Seawater by Mussels

Accumulation of dissolved OA and DTX1 by mussels was observed in all treatments. Concentrations of free and ester forms of the toxins are shown in Figure 2. Trace amounts of OA (~7–8 μg kg^{-1}) and DTX1 (~6 μg kg^{-1}) were detected in the whole soft tissue of mussels exposed to low toxin levels, and about three times more in mussels exposed to the high levels. Different accumulation efficiencies of OA and DTX1 occurred in mussels exposed to various toxin concentrations (Table 1). Similar proportions of esterified toxins were estimated for OA or DTX1 accumulated by mussels exposed to different toxin concentrations, although some slight discrepancies were noted (Table 2).

Table 1. Percentage (%) of esterified OA and DTX1 in mussels subject to different treatments.

Treatments	OA (μg L^{-1})		DTX1 (μg L^{-1})		OA:DTX1	
	0.92	9.2	1.32	13.2	Low Toxin Level	High Toxin Level
Control	53	15	9.1	2.7	5.82	5.56
Isochrysis galbana	50	15	9.2	2.9	5.43	5.17
SPM < 75 μm	36	8.8	6.1	2.4	5.90	3.67
SPM 75–150 μm	38	9.1	5.8	2.4	6.55	3.79
SPM 150–250 μm	29	7.4	4.6	2.0	6.30	3.70

Control: filtered seawater with no microalgae or suspended particulate matter (SPM) added.

Table 2. Proportions (%) of OA and DTX1 esterified by mussels under different treatments.

Treatments	OA (μg L^{-1})		DTX1 (μg L^{-1})	
	0.92	9.2	1.32	13.2
Control	93	93	80	81
Isochrysis galbana	93	94	81	82
SPM < 75 μm	91	88	72	78
SPM 75–150 μm	90	86	72	75
SPM 150–250 μm	90	89	65	80

Control: filtered seawater with no microalgae or suspended particulate matter (SPM) added.

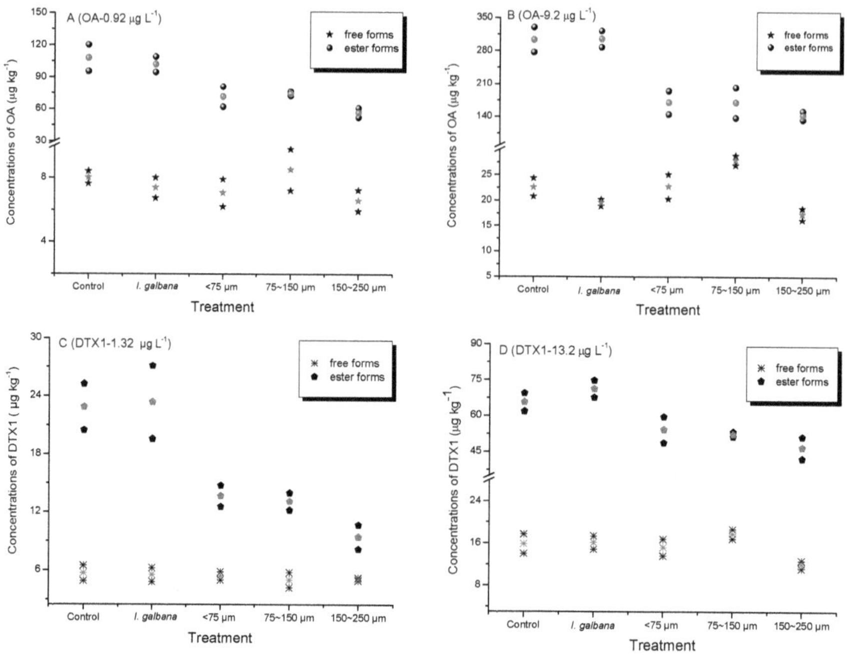

Figure 2. Concentrations of OA (**A**,**B**) and DTX1 (**C**,**D**) accumulated by mussels from seawater for treatments spiked with low (**A**,**C**) and high (**B**,**D**) toxin concentrations. Control: No microalgae or suspended particulate matter (SPM) added; either *I. galbana* or one of three different particle size-fractions of SPM (<75 μm, 75–150 μm, and 150–250 μm) were added for the treatments; red symbols indicate mean values of duplicate treatments.

2.2. Effect of OA and DTX1 on the Feeding Ability of Mussels

Although mussels were able to accumulate dissolved OA and DTX1, the toxins negatively affected their ability to feed on the microalga, *Isochrysis galbana*. The proportions of microalgae cleared by mussels subject to different treatments are shown in Figure 3.

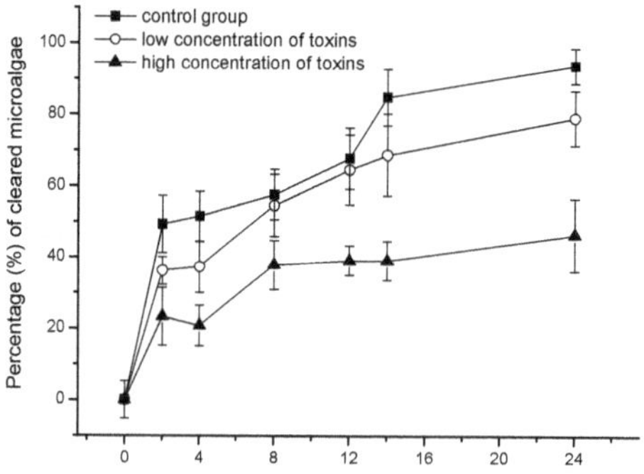

Figure 3. Percentage of microalgae cleared by mussels subject to different concentrations of dissolved toxins. Control: no toxins added; low toxin concentrations: 0.92 μg L^{-1} OA and 1.32 μg L^{-1} DTX1; high toxin concentrations: 9.2 μg L^{-1} OA and 13.2 μg L^{-1} DTX1.

2.3. Tissue Distribution of Toxins Accumulated by Mussels

Tissue distribution of OA and DTX1 accumulated by mussels with or without the addition of SPM particles were compared. Concentrations of OA and DTX1 in mantle, gills, digestive gland and residual tissues are shown in Figure 4. Relative percentages of total toxin amount distributed in the different tissues are indicated in Figure 5.

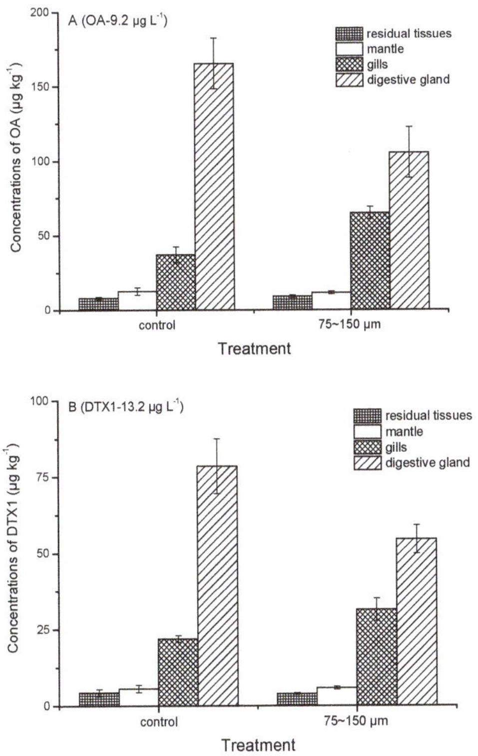

Figure 4. Distribution of OA and DTX1 toxins in different tissues of mussels exposed to high concentration of dissolved toxins (OA-9.2 μg L^{-1} (**A**) and DTX1-13.2 μg L^{-1} (**B**)) in the presence and absence of SPM particles (75–150 μm).

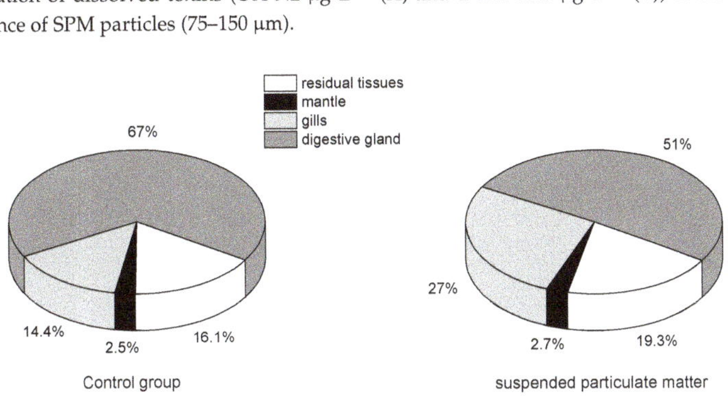

Figure 5. Percentage of toxins accumulated in different mussel tissues in the absence or presence of suspended particulate matter particles.

3. Discussion

Mean residual levels of OA ranged from 2.71 to 14.06 ng L^{-1} in seawater samples collected from Jiaozhou Bay, China, in July, August, and September 2014, but no DTX1 was detected [35]. Residual OA concentrations ranged between 1.41 and 89.52 ng L^{-1} in Qingdao coastal waters from October 2012 to September 2013 [34]. Trace amounts of OA were detected in coastal areas every month, except for elevated levels observed in August (the highest concentration = 89.52 ng L^{-1}) [34], indicating that OA degradation in seawater can occur slowly. Importantly, no blooms of *Dinophysis* or *Prorocentrum* were reported in Qingdao coastal waters during the entire year when seawater samples were collected and analyzed [34]. We hypothesize that the dissolved OA concentrations during blooms of DST-producing microalgae are higher than the residual levels reported previously [34,35]. In order to assess the contribution of dissolved DST to their accumulation by cultured bivalves, OA and DTX1 (molar ratio OA/DTX1 $\approx$ 0.71) from *P. lima* cultures were spiked into filtered (0.45 μm membrane) seawater for exposure experiments in this study. No DTX2 or DTX3 were detected in the strain of *P. lima* used here. The DST concentration used in our experiments was higher than the residual levels found in natural seawater to ensure detection of toxins accumulated by mussels after 4 days of exposure. Low levels of OA and DTX1 were set at 0.92 and 1.32 μg L^{-1}, respectively, and the high levels 10-fold more. The detection of OA and DTX1 confirmed that mussels (*M. galloprovincialis*) can accumulate dissolved OA and DTX1 from seawater under all treatment conditions. A previous study showed that blue mussels (*M. edulis*) accumulated dissolved azaspiracids (AZA) to reach concentrations above the regulatory limit [36].

To our knowledge, this is the first report confirming that bivalves are able to accumulate dissolved DST from seawater. The addition of microalgae (*I. galbana*) did not improve the accumulation of dissolved DST by mussels, and SPM particles, especially the 150–250 μm size fraction, somewhat inhibited the OA and DTX1 accumulation efficiency (Table 1). According to a previous study, the clearance and ingestion rates of scallops (*Chlamys farreri*) and clams (*Ruditapes philippinarum*) increased when the SPM particle concentration increased from 20 mg L^{-1} to 50 mg L^{-1}, and in mussels (*M. galloprovincialis*) when the concentration increased from 20 mg L^{-1} to 100 mg L^{-1} [37]. The concentration of SPM particles used here (30 mg L^{-1}) did not inhibit the clearance or ingestion rates by mussels. The lack of obvious positive effects associated with feeding on *I. galbana* demonstrated that the energy provided by non-toxic prey did not lead to improved DST accumulation nor did the microalgal cells enhance toxin accumulation via adsorptive mechanisms. In a previous study, the total amount of AZA accumulated by mussels was also virtually identical in dissolved AZA treatments with or without the addition of the non-toxic *I.* affinis *galbana* [36]. The accumulation efficiency ratios of OA to DTX1 by mussels ranged from 5.43 to 6.55 and from 3.67 to 5.56 in seawater spiked with low and high toxin levels, respectively (Table 1), which demonstrated that although only one methyl group distinguishes OA from DTX1, dissolved OA was accumulated preferentially by mussels (Figure 1). This discrepancy was also noted in our previous field experiments carried out in the coastal waters of Qingdao, China [33], in which the amount of OA adsorbed by SPATT bags was much higher than that of DTX1, although similar concentrations of OA and DTX1 were obtained by SPE cartridges. The OA content measured in scallops was also higher than for DTX1 [33]. To our knowledge, the difference in OA versus DTX1 accumulation by bivalves was not identified in previous studies due to a focus on DST accumulation by shellfish through feeding on toxic microalgae [19,38]. In the present study, the accumulation efficiencies of OA and DTX1 in mussels decreased sharply in the high toxin level treatment (Table 1). A possible explanation is that OA and DTX1 inhibited the filtration ability of mussels. That was the case in feeding experiments with an AZA-producing microalga (*Azadinium spinosum*), which had a negative effect on mussel filtration compared to non-toxic microalgal prey (*I.* aff. *galbana*) [39]. The proportion of *I. galbana* cells cleared by mussels in the current study decreased significantly over the 24 h feeding period in seawater containing dissolved DST (Figure 3). Moreover, it was confirmed that dissolved OA and DTX1 inhibited the mussel filtration ability. It can be expected that cultured bivalves exposed to blooms of DST-producing microalgae will be affected in a similar way. Although bivalves can survive DST contamination, their physiological condition and nutritional status will likely be adversely affected.

Fatty acid esters of OA and DTX1, collectively known as DTX3 and frequently found in bivalve field samples [11,13,17,18,21,40] were the predominant toxins accumulated by mussels in all treatments (Figure 2). Blue mussels (*M. edulis*) feeding on the toxic dinoflagellate *Dinophysis acuta* [38] and scallops (*P. yessoensis*) feeding on *D. fortii* [19] were also found to metabolize large proportions of OA, DTX1 and DTX1b to DTX3 under laboratory conditions. Esterification of OA and DTX1 was also observed in the present study in mussels after direct accumulation of these toxins dissolved in seawater. The DTX3 levels accumulated in mussels in the presence of SPM particles were lower than those observed for any of the other treatments (Figure 2). This discrepancy may reflect a possible negative effect of ingested SPM particles on the esterification process. SPM particles are usually retained by the gills and eliminated by the labial palps, which could affect the respiratory efficiency of filter-feeding mussels. Higher proportions of esterified OA as compared to those of DTX1 were also found in mussels (Table 2), which may explain the preferential accumulation of OA versus DTX1 during the exposure period. However, a similar pattern of DST tissue distribution occurred in mussels with or without SPM particles (75–150 μm) added (Figure 4). Total OA and DTX1 content in these mussels ranked as follows: digestive gland > gills > mantle > residual tissues. The proportion (%) of DST in the digestive gland was higher in the control group (67%) than in the seawater plus SPM treatment (51%), but the gills exhibited the opposite trend (Figure 5). This difference suggests that SPM particles do not facilitate enhanced accumulation of dissolved OA and DTX1 due to possible adsorption and transporter actions, but instead contribute to toxin retention in the gills. In a previous study of AZA uptake by mussels, the percentage of AZA accumulated in the digestive gland was highest in mussels fed with live *A. spinosum* cells, followed (in decreasing order) by those provided with lysed cells, dissolved AZA plus non-toxic cells, and dissolved toxins; however, a large proportion of toxins (42% or 46%) were stored in the gills when mussels accumulated dissolved AZA from seawater [36]. A dissolved AZA accumulation route through the gills during respiratory and filtration activities was hypothesized in the same study [36]. In the present study, it was expected that toxins adsorbed by SPM particles retained in the gills during the filtration process would contribute to the total amount of toxins retained in this tissue compartment. Yet, no enhancement in dissolved DST accumulation by mussels in the SPM treatments (regardless of size fraction) was observed.

DST-producing dinoflagellates, such as *Prorocentrum* spp. and *Dinophysis* spp., release cellular DST into the culture medium as part of their metabolism [41,42], and large amounts of DST have also been detected in the water column during *Dinophysis* blooms [27]. A range of trace amounts of OA have been measured in coastal waters of the Yellow Sea of China, although no blooms of *Dinophysis* or *Prorocentrum* were observed in the area during the study period [33–35]. Based on the new findings reported here, the persistence of trace OA concentrations in seawater will contribute to DST accumulation by bivalves. OA and DTX1 toxins accumulated by mussels and scallops feeding on toxic microalgae, except for the DTX3 stored in intracellular bodies, may be excreted into the surrounding seawater with minimal metabolic transformation [19,38]. The free forms of dissolved OA and DTX1 possibly circulated through mussels and seawater in this study. We hypothesize that DTX1 was degraded to other derivatives in the 96-h exposure period. Field investigations on lipophilic shellfish toxins in our previous study also hinted that OA in seawater was more stable than DTX1 [33]. This is consistent with the fact that OA was detected in marine sediments ranging from 0.78 to 3.34 ng g^{-1} dry weight [35]. In addition to the heterogeneous vertical distribution of *Dinophysis* cells in the water column, the accumulation of dissolved DST by mussels documented herein represents another important argument against the early warning of lipophilic shellfish toxin events based solely on dinoflagellate cell numbers [43]. Moreover, the risk of DSP outbreaks would increase if blooms of toxic *Prorocentrum* spp. occurred in marine benthic environments. We suggest that dissolved toxins should be monitored routinely and their dynamics investigated further to improve forecasting bivalve contamination with DST.

4. Conclusions

Accumulation of dissolved OA and DTX1 by mussels (*M. galloprovincialis*) was confirmed in laboratory experiments in filtered seawater with and without microalgal prey (*I. galbana*) and in the presence of different size-fractions of SPM. No positive effect of the food microalgae on DST accumulation efficiency was observed, but a slight negative effect of the SPM particles was noted. Higher accumulation efficiencies of OA as compared to DTX1 were recorded in all treatments, and the same was observed for both toxins in seawater spiked with low concentrations of the two toxins. Most of the accumulated OA and DTX1 was esterified to DTX3 in mussels in all treatments. The proportion of microalgal cells (*I. galbana*) cleared by mussels was inhibited by dissolved OA and DTX1 or by other compounds still present in the purified extract of *P. lima*. Total amount of OA and DTX1 accumulated in mussel tissues ranked as follows: digestive gland > gills > mantle > residual tissues, in all treatments. However, the proportion of total DST in the digestive gland in filtered seawater exceeded that in the presence of SPM particles (75–150 μm), but the opposite trend occurred in gills for the same conditions. The findings reported here will help us to improve the understanding of DST accumulation mechanisms by bivalves in the field.

5. Materials and Methods

5.1. Chemicals

Acetonitrile, methanol, monopotassium phosphate (KH_2PO_4) and disodium hydrogen phosphate (Na_2HPO_4) were obtained from Merck Ltd. (White-house Station, NJ, USA); formic acid, ammonium formate, sodium hydroxide, ammonium hydroxide, and hydrochloric acid (HCl) from Fisher Scientific (Fair Lawn, NJ, USA) and OA and DTX1 reference materials from the National Research Council of Canada (Halifax, NS, Canada), and Wako Pure Chemical Industries, Ltd. (Osaka, Japan), respectively. Milli-Q water (18.2 MΩ cm or better) was supplied by a Milli-Q water purification system (Millipore Ltd., Bedford, MA, USA).

5.2. Microalgae

Prorocentrum lima strain IP797 (Bigelow laboratory, National Center for Marine Algae and Microbiota, USA) was grown with filtered (0.45-μm mixed fiber membrane) and autoclaved (121 °C for 20 min) seawater (pH 8.0 ± 0.1, salinity 30 ± 1) enriched with *f*/2-Si medium [44] in conical 5000 mL flasks. Larger volumes of *P. lima* were grown in a photo-bioreactor (120 L) at 16 °C under the same light intensity of 111 μmol m^{-2} s^{-1} with a 12-h light: 12-h dark cycle. All the cultures were gently shaken or stirred twice per day at morning and night, respectively.

An axenic culture of *Isochrysis galbana* strain 3011 (Ocean University of China collection) was used as a non-toxic prey for mussels. Culture conditions were the same as those described above for *P. lima* cultures except for the temperature, which was set at 20 °C.

5.3. Toxin Extraction and Purification

Cells of *P. lima* were collected with a silk mesh (25 μm), transferred into 50 mL centrifuge tubes, centrifuged at 8000× *g* for 5 min, the supernatant was discarded and the pellet was stored at −20 °C. One g (wet weight) of cells was weighed and transferred into a 10 mL centrifuge tube, 3 mL of methanol was added and the tube was sealed before being submerged in liquid nitrogen for 15 min. Then, the cells were sonicated for 30 min at 10 °C, followed by a three-fold freeze-thaw cycle, centrifugation at 8000× *g* for 10 min and then the supernatant was transferred to a glass vial. Three mL of methanol were added into the tube and the sample was centrifuged again. This extraction process was repeated twice before the supernatants were mixed in a glass vial. The extract was filtered through a 0.22 μm membrane filter (Jinteng, Tianjin, China) and stored at −20 °C.

Salts and pigments from the toxin extracts were removed by SPE purification procedure [33]. Fifteen mL of methanol were used to activate the HLB cartridge (Oasis, 3 mL, 200 mg) and then 15 mL of 20% methanol solution was added to equilibrate the cartridge. Further 15 mL of 20% methanol solution were used to wash the cartridge after the toxin extract (3–5 mL) was loaded and 15 mL more was used to elute toxins from the SPE cartridge. The rates of the activation and equilibration steps were about 1 mL min^{-1}, and of the sample loading, washing and elution about 0.5 mL min^{-1}. The eluate was concentrated under N_2 at 30 °C and filtered through a 0.22 μm organic membrane filter (Jinteng, Tianjin, China). It was stored at −20 °C until analysis. OA and DTX1 predominated the toxin profile of the purified extract [45,46] and their concentrations were quantified using a LC-MS/MS method [47]. The toxin extract was dried under N_2 at 30 °C and the residual was re-dissolved in filtered seawater (0.45 μm) before adding to the feeding experiment.

5.4. *Preparation of Suspended Particulate Matter*

Surface sediments (<2 cm) were collected from Jiaozhou Bay (120.2573° E; 36.1796° N) and dried at room temperature (total organic carbon ~1.88%) before grinding in a mortar and sieving them through 200, 100 and 60 mesh sieves. Finally, three different size-fractions of SPM were obtained: <75 μm, 75–150 μm, and 150–250 μm, respectively [37].

5.5. *Design of Mussel Feeding Experiments*

5.5.1. Effect of Suspended Particulate Matter on the Accumulation of Toxins by Mussels

Healthy looking adult mussels (*Mytilus galloprovincialis*) were obtained from Qingdao seafood market. Natural seawater was used to carefully wash and clean the shells' surface, and the connective byssus between individuals was gently cut with scissors. Then, individual mussels were acclimated for 1 week before the experiment in filtered seawater (0.45 μm membrane, salinity 29–30, pH 8.1–8.3, temperature 15–18 °C) with continuous aeration (DO > 5 mg L^{-1}). The seawater was renewed twice per day, at morning and night respectively, with no addition of microalgal prey. Five individuals were harvested randomly to analyze their background levels of OA and DTX1 before the experiment.

The design diagram of exposure experiments is shown in Figure 6. A total of 22 glass beakers (5 L) were filled with filtered seawater (0.45 μm) and three mussels were added per beaker. Cells of *I. galbana* were collected at the exponential growth phase, and three different SPM (<75 μm, 75–150 μm, 150–250 μm) size-fractions were added to each of the four beakers, with an initial microalgal density of about 1×10^6 cells L^{-1} and a SPM concentration of 30 mg L^{-1}. Then the mixture of OA and DTX1 was added to these 16 beakers in two different concentrations of toxins (low: OA 0.92 μg L^{-1}, DTX1 1.32 μg L^{-1}; high: OA 9.2 μg L^{-1}, DTX1 13.2 μg L^{-1}) to compare the effects in duplicate treatments. Both concentration levels of toxins were also added to four controls without microalgae and SPM, in duplicate treatments. Only filtered seawater and mussels were in the other two beakers as blank control treatments. All mussels were cultured for 4 days under the same conditions before terminating the feeding experiment. The ratio of the total OA or DTX1 accumulated by mussels to the total amount of toxins added into the beaker was calculated as the accumulation efficiency of the toxins shown in Table 1. The accumulation efficiency was calculated as the ratio between the amount of toxins in the mussels and that supplied in the water.

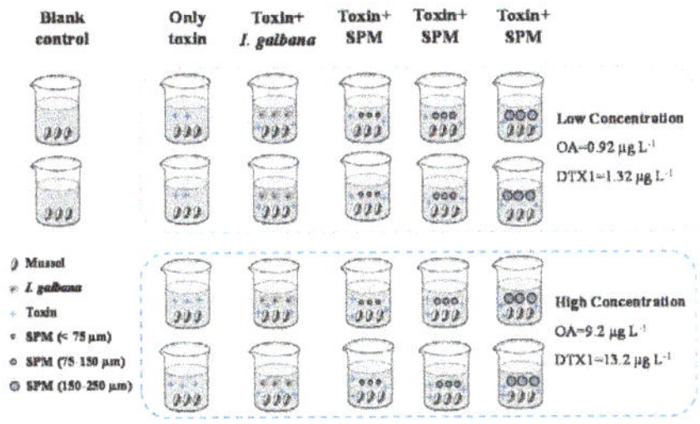

Figure 6. Design diagram of the exposure experiments (SPM = suspended particulate matter).

5.5.2. Effect of Toxins on Mussels Feeding Behaviors

A total of nine glass beakers (5 L) were filled with filtered seawater (0.45 μm) and cells of *I. galbana*, collected at the exponential growth phase. The initial density of microalgae was 1.83 × 10^6 cells L^{-1} to start the experiment. Three healthy mussels were placed in each beaker. Then two different concentrations of toxins (low: OA 0.92 μg L^{-1}, DTX1 1.32 μg L^{-1}; high: OA 9.2 μg L^{-1}, DTX1 13.2 μg L^{-1}) were added to the beakers in triplicate, respectively, and no toxins were added in the other three beakers. Microalgal density in all beakers was counted throughout the entire feeding period. The proportion of *I. galbana* cells cleared by mussels was calculated as the ratio between the number of algal cells eaten and the initial amount of microalgae added to the beakers.

5.5.3. Esterification and Distribution of OA and DTX1 in Mussels

Three healthy mussels were placed in each glass beaker (5-L) filled with filtered seawater (0.45 μm). The same density of microalgae (*I. galbana*; ~1 × 10^6 cells L^{-1}) was added to six glass beakers. OA and DTX1 toxins (OA 9.2 μg L^{-1}, DTX1 13.2 μg L^{-1}) were added into three of these beakers and no toxins were added to the other three. SPM (size-fraction 75–150 μm, 30 mg L^{-1}) was added to three glass beakers and the same concentration of toxins was also spiked. The mussels were taken out and different parts including gills, mantle, digestive gland and residual tissues were dissected after four days of feeding. Free and esterified forms of OA and DTX1 in the different mussel tissues were analyzed.

5.6. Extraction of Toxins in Mussels

Free toxin forms were extracted from mussel tissues according to Li et al. [11]. In brief, 1 g of homogenized tissue and 3 mL of methanol added to a 10-mL centrifuge tube were mixed with a vortex, the mixture centrifuged at 8000× *g* for 10 min and the supernatant was transferred to a 10-mL volumetric flask. Three mL of methanol was added and extracted twice, and all supernatants combined in the volumetric tube. Finally, the extract was made up to scale using methanol and the extraction ratio was 1 g: 10 mL. One mL of extract was filtered (0.22 μm membrane filter) and stored in sample vials at −20 °C until analysis.

The esterified forms of OA and DTX1 toxins were analyzed following [48]. One mL of the filtered (0.22 μm) extract of free toxin forms was transferred to a 4-mL glass vial, and 125 μL of 2.5 M NaOH solution was added and mixed. Then the sealed mixture was hydrolyzed at 76 °C for 40 min, neutralized with 125 μL of 2.5 M HCl and kept at room temperature. One mL of chloroform was used for a liquid-liquid extraction for the hydrolyzed extract, and this process was repeated. Finally, the chloroform phase was dried under N_2 at 40 °C. The residual material was suspended in 1 mL of methanol, which was filtered (0.22 μm membrane filter) and stored in a sample vial at −20 °C.

5.7. LC-MS/MS Analysis of OA and DTX1 Toxins

An Agilent 6430 tandem quadrupole mass spectrometer coupled with an Agilent 1290 HPLC (Palo Alto, CA, USA) was used with an ESI interface. An X-Bridge™ C18 column (150 × 3 mm i.d, 5 mm, Waters, Milford, MA, USA) at 35 °C was used to separate OA and DTX1 toxins. The alkaline elution phase (pH = 11) was composed by mobile phases A (water) and B (90% acetonitrile) both containing 6.7 mM NH_4OH [49]. A gradient was run at 300 μL min^{-1} starting with 10% 'B' for 1 min, and increasing linearly to 90% 'B' over 9 min. The mobile phase was held at 90% 'B' for 3 min, returned to 10% 'B' over 2 min, and held for 3 min before re-equilibration for the next run. An injection volume of 5 μL was adopted here.

The atomization device press was set at 40 psi, and the capillary voltage was 4000 V. The temperature of ESI source and dry N_2 gas (flow rate 10 L min^{-1}) was set at 110 °C and 350 °C, respectively. OA and DTX1 toxins were qualified and quantified by the selective reaction monitoring mode of the negative mode, and the transition ions m/z 803.5 -> 255.2, 151.1 (OA), and m/z

817.5 -> 255.2, 151.1 (DTX1), respectively. OA and DTX1 were quantified by comparing their peak areas with those of solutions with a known concentration.

Author Contributions: A.L. conceived and designed the experiments, and wrote this paper; M.L. performed the experiments and analyzed all samples; J.Q., J.S., Y.J, Y.H., S.W. and Y.C. helped to perform the experiments and to prepare some samples.

Funding: This work was funded by the Fundamental Research Funds for the Central Universities (201841003), and the National Natural Science Foundation of China (41276103).

Acknowledgments: The authors would like to thank Beatriz Regura and Gregory Doucette for English edition before first submission and revision respectively.

Conflicts of Interest: The authors declare no conflict of interest.

References

1. Marr, J.C.; Jackson, A.E.; McLachlan, J.L. Occurrence of *Prorocentrum lima*, a DSP toxin-producing species from the Atlantic coast of Canada. *J. Appl. Phycol.* **1992**, *4*, 17–24. [CrossRef]
2. Dickey, R.W.; Bobzin, S.C.; Faulkner, D.J.; Bencsath, Z.F.A.; Andrzejewski, D. Identification of okadaic acid from a Caribbean Dinoflagellate, *Prorocentrum concayum*. *Toxicon* **1990**, *28*, 371–377. [CrossRef]
3. Morton, S.L.; Bomber, J.W.; Tindall, P.M. Environmental effects on the production of okadaic acid from *Prorocentrum hoffmannianum* Faust I. temperature, light, and salinity. *J. Exp. Mar. Biol. Ecol.* **1994**, *178*, 67–77. [CrossRef]
4. An, T.; Winshell, J.; Scorzetti, G.; Fell, J.W.; Rein, K.S. Identification of okadaic acid production in the marine dinoflagellate *Prorocentrum rhathymum* from Florida Bay. *Toxicon* **2010**, *55*, 653–657. [CrossRef] [PubMed]
5. Kameneva, P.A.; Efimova, K.V.; Rybin, V.G.; Orlova, T.Y. Detection of dinophysistoxin-1 in clonal culture of marine dinoflagellate *Prorocentrum foraminosum* (Faust M.A., 1993) from the Sea of Japan. *Toxins* **2015**, *7*, 3947–3959. [CrossRef] [PubMed]
6. Reguera, B.; Velo-Suárez, L.; Raine, R.; Park, M.G. Harmful *Dinophysis* species: A review. *Harmful Algae* **2012**, *14*, 87–106. [CrossRef]
7. James, K.J.; Carey, B.; O'Halloran, J.; Van Pelt, F.N.A.M.; Škrabáková, Z. Shellfish toxicity: Human health implications of marine algal toxins. *Epidemiol. Infect.* **2010**, *138*, 927–940. [CrossRef] [PubMed]
8. Valdiglesias, V.; Laffon, B.; Pásaro, E.; Méndez, J. Okadaic acid induces morphological changes, apoptosis and cell cycle alterations in different human cell types. *J. Environ. Monit.* **2011**, *13*, 1831–1840. [CrossRef] [PubMed]
9. Terao, K.; Ito, E.; Yanagi, T.; Yasumoto, T. Histopathological studies on experimental marine toxin poisoning. I. Ultrastructural changes in the small intestine and liver of suckling mice induced by dinophysistoxin-1 and pectenotoxin-1. *Toxicon* **1986**, *24*, 1145–1151. [CrossRef]
10. Yasumoto, T.; Oshima, Y.; Yamaguchi, M. Occurrence of a new type of toxic shellfish poisoning in the Tohoku district. *Bull. Jpn. Soc. Sci. Fish* **1978**, *44*, 1249–1255. [CrossRef]
11. Li, A.; Ma, J.; Cao, J.; McCarron, P. Toxins in mussels (*Mytilus galloprovincialis*) associated with diarrhetic shellfish poisoning episodes in China. *Toxicon* **2012**, *60*, 420–425. [CrossRef] [PubMed]
12. Trainer, V.L.; Moore, L.; Bill, B.D.; Adams, N.G.; Harrington, N.; Borchert, J.; da Silva, D.A.M.; Eberhart, B.T.L. Diarrhetic shellfish toxins and other polyether toxins of human health concern in Washington State. *Mar. Drugs* **2013**, *11*, 1815–1835. [CrossRef] [PubMed]
13. Taylor, M.; McIntyre, L.; Ritson, M.; Stone, J.; Bronson, R.; Bitzikos, O.; Rourke, W.; Galanis, E. Outbreak Investigation Team. Outbreak of diarrhetic shellfish poisoning associated with mussels, British Columbia, Canada. *Mar. Drugs* **2013**, *11*, 1669–1676. [CrossRef] [PubMed]
14. MacKenzie, L.; Holland, P.; McNabb, P.; Beuzenberg, V.; Selwood, A.; Suzuki, T. Complex toxin profiles in phytoplankton and Greenshell mussels (*Perna canaliculus*), revealed by LC-MS/MS analysis. *Toxicon* **2002**, *40*, 1321–1330. [CrossRef]
15. Hinder, S.L.; Hays, G.C.; Brooks, C.J.; Davies, A.P.; Edwards, M.; Walne, A.W.; Gravenor, M.B. Toxic marine microalgae and shellfish poisoning in the British Isles: History, review of epidemiology, and future implications. *Environ. Health* **2011**, *10*, 54–65. [CrossRef] [PubMed]

16. Grattan, L.M.; Holobaugh, S.; Morris, J.G., Jr. Harmful algal blooms and public health. *Harmful Algae* **2016**, *57*, 2–8. [CrossRef] [PubMed]
17. Torgersen, T.; Wilkins, A.L.; Rundberget, T.; Miles, C.O. Characterization of fatty acid esters of okadaic acid and related toxins in blue mussels (*Mytilus edulis*) from Norway. *Rapid Commun. Mass Spectrom.* **2008**, *22*, 1127–1136. [CrossRef] [PubMed]
18. Turner, A.D.; Goya, A.B. Occurrence and profiles of lipophilic toxins in shellfish harvested from Argentina. *Toxicon* **2015**, *102*, 32–42. [CrossRef] [PubMed]
19. Matsushima, R.; Uchida, H.; Nagai, S.; Watanabe, R.; Kamio, M.; Nagai, H.; Kaneniwa, M.; Suzuki, T. Assimilation, accumulation, and metabolism of dinophysistoxins (DTXs) and pectenotoxins (PTXs) in the several tissues of Japanese scallop *Patinopecten yessoensis*. *Toxins* **2015**, *7*, 5141–5154. [CrossRef] [PubMed]
20. Vale, P.; Sampayo, M.A.M. First conformation of human diarrhoeic poisonings by okadaic acid esters ingestion of razor clams (*Solen marginatus*) and green crabs (*Carcinus maenas*) in Aveiro lagoon, Portugal and detection of okadaic acid esters in phytoplankton. *Toxicon* **2002**, *40*, 989–996. [CrossRef]
21. Jørgensen, K.; Scanlon, S.; Jensen, L.B. Diarrhetic shellfish poisoning toxin esters in Danish blue mussels and surf clams. *Food Addit. Contam.* **2005**, *22*, 743–751. [CrossRef] [PubMed]
22. García, C.; Truan, D.; Lagos, M.; Santelices, J.P.; Diaz, J.C.; Lagos, N. Metabolic transformation of dinophysistoxin-3 into dinophysistoxin-1 causes human intoxication by consumption of *O*-acyl-derivates dinophysistoxins contaminated shellfish. *J. Toxicol. Sci.* **2005**, *30*, 287–296. [CrossRef] [PubMed]
23. Doucet, E.; Ross, N.N.; Quilliam, M.A. Enzymatic hydrolysis of esterified diarrhetic shellfish poisoning toxins and pectenotoxins. *Anal. Bioanal. Chem.* **2007**, *389*, 335–342. [CrossRef] [PubMed]
24. Braga, A.C.; Alves, R.N.; Maulvault, A.L.; Barbosa, V.; Marques, A.; Costa, P.R. In vitro bioaccessibility of the marine biotoxin okadaic acid in shellfish. *Food Chem. Toxicol.* **2016**, *89*, 54–59. [CrossRef] [PubMed]
25. Torgersen, T.; Miles, C.O.; Rundberget, T.; Wilkins, A.L. New esters of okadaic acid in seawater and blue mussels (*Mytilus edulis*). *J. Agric. Food Chem.* **2008**, *56*, 9628–9635. [CrossRef] [PubMed]
26. European Food Safety Authority (EFSA). Scientific Opinion of the Panel on Contaminants in the Food Chain on a request from the European Commission on Marine Biotoxins in Shellfish—Summary on regulated marine biotoxins. *EFSA J.* **2009**, *1306*, 1–23.
27. MacKenzie, L.; Beuzenberg, V.; Holland, P.; McNabb, P.; Selwood, A. Solid phase adsorption toxin tracking (SPATT): A new monitoring tool that simulates the biotoxin contamination of filter feeding bivalves. *Toxicon* **2004**, *44*, 901–918. [CrossRef] [PubMed]
28. Rundberget, T.; Gustad, E.; Samdal, I.A.; Sandvik, M.; Miles, C.O. A convenient and cost-effective method for monitoring marine algal toxins with passive samplers. *Toxicon* **2009**, *53*, 543–550. [CrossRef] [PubMed]
29. Fux, E.; Bire, R.; Hess, P. Comparative accumulation and composition of lipophilic marine biotoxins in passive samplers and in mussels (*M. edulis*) on the West Coast of Ireland. *Harmful Algae* **2009**, *8*, 523–537. [CrossRef]
30. Li, Z.; Guo, M.; Yang, S.; Wang, Q.; Tan, Z. Investigation of pectenotoxin profiles in the Yellow Sea (China) using passive sampling technique. *Mar. Drugs* **2010**, *8*, 1263–1272. [CrossRef] [PubMed]
31. MacKenzie, L. In situ passive solid-phase adsorption of micro-algal biotoxins as a monitoring tool. *Curr. Opin. Biotechnol.* **2010**, *21*, 326–331. [CrossRef] [PubMed]
32. Pizarro, G.; Moroño, Á.; Paz, B.; Franco, J.M.; Pazos, Y.; Reguera, B. Evaluation of passive samplers as a monitoring tool for early warning of *Dinophysis* toxins in shellfish. *Mar. Drugs* **2013**, *11*, 3823–3845. [CrossRef] [PubMed]
33. Li, M.; Sun, G.; Qiu, J.; Li, A. Occurrence and variation of lipophilic shellfish toxins in phytoplankton, shellfish and seawater samples from the aquaculture zone in the Yellow Sea, China. *Toxicon* **2017**, *127*, 1–10. [CrossRef] [PubMed]
34. Li, X.; Li, Z.; Chen, J.; Shi, Q.; Zhang, R.; Wang, S.; Wang, X. Detection, occurrence and monthly variations of typical lipophilic marine toxins associated with diarrhetic shellfish poisoning in the coastal seawater of Qingdao City, China. *Chemosphere* **2014**, *111*, 560–567. [CrossRef] [PubMed]
35. Chen, J.; Li, X.; Wang, S.; Chen, F.; Cao, W.; Sun, C.; Zheng, L.; Wang, X. Screening of lipophilic marine toxins in marine aquaculture environment using liquid chromatography-mass spectrometry. *Chemosphere* **2017**, *168*, 32–40. [CrossRef] [PubMed]
36. Jauffrais, T.; Kilcoyne, J.; Herrenknecht, C.; Truquet, P.; Séchet, V.; Miles, C.O.; Hess, P. Dissolved azaspiracids are absorbed and metabolized by blue mussels (*Mytilus edulis*). *Toxicon* **2013**, *65*, 81–89. [CrossRef] [PubMed]

37. Song, Q.; Fang, J.G.; Liu, H.; Zhang, J.H.; Wang, L.L.; Wang, W. Studies on the effects of suspended sediment on the feeding physiology of three suspension-feeding bivalves. *Mar. Fish. Res.* **2006**, *27*, 21–28. (In Chinese)
38. Nielsen, L.T.; Hansen, P.J.; Krock, B.; Vismann, B. Accumulation, transformation and breakdown of DSP toxins from the toxic dinoflagellate *Dinophysis acuta* in blue mussels, *Mytilus edulis*. *Toxicon* **2016**, *117*, 84–93. [CrossRef] [PubMed]
39. Jauffrais, T.; Contreras, A.; Herrenknecht, C.; Truquet, P.; Séchet, V.; Tillmann, U.; Hess, P. Effect of *Azadinium spinosum* on the feeding behaviour and azaspiracid accumulation of *Mytilus edulis*. *Aquat. Toxicol.* **2012**, *124–125*, 179–187. [CrossRef] [PubMed]
40. Kameneva, P.A.; Imbs, A.B.; Orlova, T.Y. Distribution of DTX-3 in edible and non-edible parts of *Crenomytilus grayanus* from the Sea of Japan. *Toxicon* **2015**, *98*, 1–3. [CrossRef] [PubMed]
41. Nagai, S.; Suzuki, T.; Nishikawa, T.; Kamiyama, T. Differences in the production and excretion kinetics of okadaic acid, dinophysistoxin-1, and pectenotoxin-2 between cultures of *Dinophysis acuminata* and *Dinophysis fortii* isolated from western Japan. *J. Phycol.* **2011**, *47*, 1326–1337. [CrossRef] [PubMed]
42. Smith, J.L.; Tong, M.; Fux, E.; Anderson, D.M. Toxin production, retention, and extracellular release by *Dinophysis acuminata* during extended stationary phase and culture decline. *Harmful Algae* **2012**, *19*, 125–132. [CrossRef]
43. Alves-de-Souza, C.; Varela, D.; Contreras, C.; LaIglesia, P.; Fernández, P.; Hipp, B.; Hernández, C.; Riobó, P.; Reguera, B.; Franco, J.M.; et al. Seasonal variability of *Dinophysis* spp. and *Protoceratium reticulatum* associated to lipophilic shellfish toxins in a strongly stratified Chilean fjord. *Deep Sea Res. Part II* **2014**, *101*, 152–162. [CrossRef]
44. Guillard, R.R.L.; Hargraves, P.E. *Stichochrysis immobilis* is a diatom, not a chrysophyte. *Phycologia* **1993**, *32*, 234–236. [CrossRef]
45. Li, A.; Ma, F.; Song, X.; Yu, R. Dynamic adsorption of diarrhetic shellfish poisoning (DSP) toxins in passive sampling relates to pore size distribution of aromatic adsorbent. *J. Chromatogr. A* **2011**, *1218*, 1437–1442. [CrossRef] [PubMed]
46. Fan, L.; Sun, G.; Qiu, J.; Ma, Q.; Hess, P.; Li, A. Effect of seawater salinity on pore-size distribution on a poly(styrene)-based HP20 resin and its adsorption of diarrhetic shellfish toxins. *J. Chromatogr. A* **2014**, *1373*, 1–8. [CrossRef] [PubMed]
47. Li, A.; Chen, H.; Qiu, J.; Lin, H.; Gu, H. Determination of multiple toxins in whelk and clam samples collected from the Chukchi and Bering seas. *Toxicon* **2016**, *109*, 84–93. [CrossRef] [PubMed]
48. Suzukia, T.; Otab, H.; Yamasakia, M. Direct evidence of transformation of dinophysistoxin-1 to 7-*O*-acyl-dinophysistoxin-1 (dinophysistoxin-3) in the scallop *Patinopecten yessoensis*. *Toxicon* **1999**, *37*, 187–198. [CrossRef]
49. Gerssen, A.; Mulder, P.P.J.; McElhinney, M.A.; Boer, J. Liquid chromatography-tandem mass spectrometry method for the detection of marine lipophilic toxins under alkaline conditions. *J. Chromatogr. A* **2009**, *1216*, 1421–1430. [CrossRef] [PubMed]

toxins

MDPI

Article

Accumulation and Biotransformation of *Dinophysis* Toxins by the Surf Clam *Mesodesma donacium*

Juan Blanco [1,*], Gonzalo Álvarez [2,3,*], José Rengel [2], Rosario Díaz [2], Carmen Mariño [1], Helena Martín [1] and Eduardo Uribe [2]

1 Centro de Investigacións Mariñas, Xunta de Galicia, Pedras de Corón S/N, 36620 Vilanova de Arousa, Spain; maria.carmen.marino.cadarso@xunta.gal (C.M.); helena.martin.sanchez@xunta.gal (H.M.)
2 Departamento de Acuicultura, Universidad Católica del Norte, Larrondo 1281, Coquimbo, Chile; jrengel@unc.cl (J.R.); rdiaz@ucn.cl (R.D.); euribe@ucn.cl (E.U.)
3 Centro de Investigación y Desarrollo Tecnológico en Algas (CIDTA), Facultad de Ciencias del Mar, Larrondo 1281, Universidad Católica del Norte, Coquimbo, Chile
* Correspondence: juan.carlos.blanco.perez@xunta.gal (J.B.); gmalvarez@ucn.cl (G.Á.)

Received: 31 May 2018; Accepted: 27 July 2018; Published: 4 August 2018

Abstract: Surf clams, *Mesodesma donacium*, were shown to accumulate toxins from *Dinophysis acuminata* blooms. Only pectenotoxin 2 (PTX2) and some of its derivatives were found, and no toxins from the okadaic acid group were detected. PTX2 seems to be transformed to PTX2 seco-acid (PTX2sa), which was found in concentrations more than ten-fold those of PTX2. The seco-acid was transformed to acyl-derivatives by esterification with different fatty acids. The estimated amount of these derivatives in the mollusks was much higher than that of PTX2. Most esters were originated by even carbon chain fatty acids, but some originated by odd carbon number were also found in noticeable concentrations. Some peaks of toxin in the bivalves did not coincide with those of *Dinophysis* abundance, suggesting that there were large differences in toxin content per cell among the populations that developed throughout the year. The observed depuration (from the digestive gland) was fast (more than 0.2 day^{-1}), and was faster for PTX2 than for PTX2sa, which in turn was faster than that of esters of PTX2sa. PTX2 and PTX2sa were distributed nearly equally between the digestive gland and the remaining tissues, but less than 5% of the palmytoyl-esters were found outside the digestive gland.

Keywords: pectenotoxins; surf clam; accumulation; biotransformation; depuration

Key Contribution: *Mesodesma donacium* accumulates only PTX2, and no other pectenotoxin or toxin of the okadaic acid group from *Dinophysis acuminata* blooms in northern Chile, suggesting that only this toxin is produced by *D. acuminata* from the area. This compound is quickly transformed to PTX2sa and to acyl-ester, and also depurates quickly.

1. Introduction

Toxins produced by the dinoflagellate genus *Dinophysis* frequently accumulate in bivalves making them unsafe for human consumption and leading to closures of fisheries or marketing of aquaculture products. The impacts of these toxins are widely distributed across the oceans, but some areas are particularly affected, as is the case in Southern Chile and North-Western Spain [1–8].

Species of the genus *Dinophysis* are known to produce two different groups of toxic compounds: toxins of the okadaic acid (OA) group and pectenotoxins (PTX) [7]. The production of one or both types of toxins is known to be species-specific, but important strain variation exists. Some species produce only pectenotoxins (Figure 1) while others usually produce toxins of both groups, although in some cases, with a low relative proportion of pectenotoxins [7]. While the toxins of the OA group have caused numerous intoxications [9], there is no evidence that PTXs are toxic for humans by oral exposure [10]. However, due to their toxicity by intraperitoneal injection (and some contradictory results about the effects of oral administration) in mice and rats, some regulatory systems, such as the European one, still maintain quarantine levels for these compounds [11,12], with a noticeable incidence for products that target these markets.

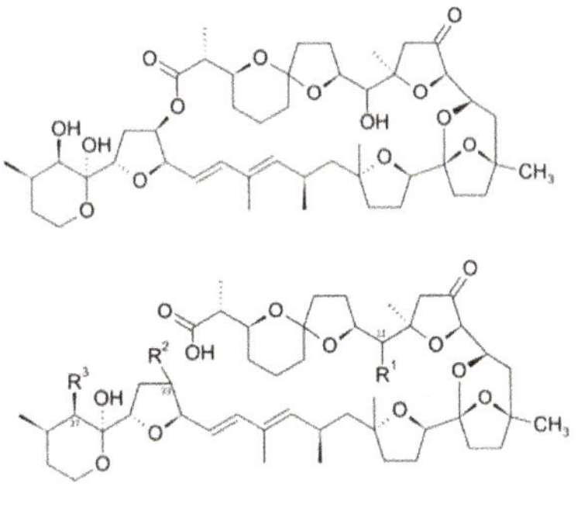

Compound(s)	R1	R2	R3
PTX2sa	OH	OH	OH
PTX2sa 11-*O*-acyl esters	O-acyl	OH	OH
PTX2sa 33-*O*-acyl esters	OH	O-acyl	OH
PTX2sa 37-*O*-acyl esters	OH	OH	O-acyl

Figure 1. PTX2 (upper structure) and PTX2 seco-acid (PTX2sa) and its acyl esters (lower structure).

In many bivalves, the accumulated toxins of the okadaic acid (OA) group are transformed to 7-*O*-acyl derivatives (generically known as DTX3) by esterification with fatty acids of different carbon chain length [13–15]. Very likely this is the main route for the elimination of those compounds from the bivalves. Less information exists for pectenotoxins, but it is known that they can be enzymatically transformed to their corresponding seco-acid (by opening the macro-ring of the molecule) in the digestive system of some mollusks [16]. These seco-acids can be esterified by fatty acids (as in the case of the toxins of the OA group) at least in the mussel *Mytilus edulis* [17] and in an Australian clam (probably *Plebidonax deltoids*) [14], suggesting that this can also be a depuration route.

In the northern region of Chile, the impact of the toxins produced by *Dinophysis* is less than in the south, but some closures, mostly of the economically important aquaculture of the pectinid *Argopecten purpuratus*, have taken place, as happened in 2005 due to a bloom of *Dinophysis acuminata* [18]. In that case *D. acuminata* was shown to have an atypical toxin profile, producing only pectenotoxins, without traces of toxins of the okadaic acid group. *D. acuminata* had been shown to be present in the north of Chile many years earlier [19–21], and could be assumed to be persistent in the area. DSP harvesting closures in the area, notwithstanding, were not needed until October 2005 [18], suggesting that toxin production was low, or that the toxins produced were quickly degraded or depurated from the bivalves in the area.

In this work, we studied *D. acuminata* populations, and the accumulation in the surf clam *Mesodesma donacium* of the toxins produced by this species in Coquimbo Bay, a significant fishing area for this economically important species. The objectives of the study were: (a) to obtain the profile of accumulated toxins; (b) to check if the accumulated toxin follows the *D. acuminata* cell abundance; (c) to obtain an estimate of the depuration rate of the toxins involved; and d), to gather knowledge about the possible transformations that take place in the bivalve.

2. Results

2.1. Abundance and Composition of Dinophysis Populations

Dinophysis populations were always present in the area and were dominated by *Dinophysis acuminata*. Its abundance was generally low, with cell concentrations below 300 cells L^{-1} in 75% of the sampled weeks. However, some blooms, with abundances over 900 cells L^{-1} were recorded in April 2009, and in January and February 2010, reaching a maximum of 2100 cells L^{-1}. On some occasions, *Dinophysis caudata* and *D. tripos* were detected but only in net samples (with very low concentrations) and their populations could not be quantified. The cells of *Dinophysis acuminata* were almost oval in shape with the left sulcal list well developed and extending about one-half to two-thirds of the cell length (Figure 2). The thecal plates that constitute the hypotheca were covered with circular areolae. The antapex of the cells was rounded, and in some cells two to four small knob-shaped posterior protrusions were found. The length (L) of the cell was 47.61 ± 3.87 µm and the dorso-ventral width (W) was 34.69 ± 3.47 µm, while the L/W ratio was 1.38.

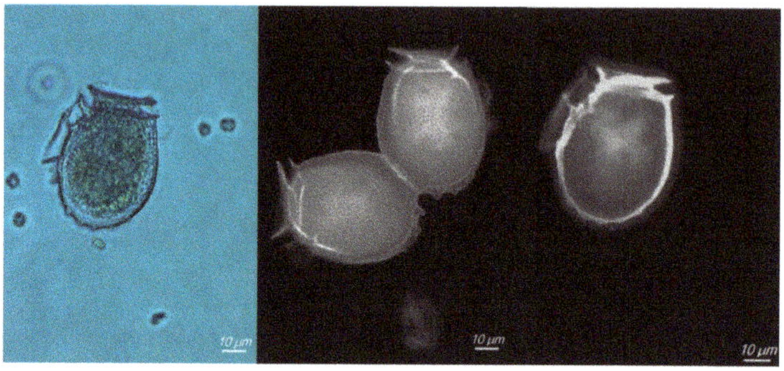

Figure 2. Phase contrast (**left**) and fluorescence photomicrographs of Calcofluor stained (**right**) *Dinophysis acuminata* cells from samples of the study.

2.2. Toxin Profiles

OA, DTX1 or DTX2 were not detected in either the raw or the hydrolyzed samples, in this study. The only PTX found was PTX2, which was accompanied by its seco-acid and by acyl-esters of its seco-acid (Figures 3 and 4). None of the other monitored PTX compounds (Table 1) were found. The main esters of PTX2-sa found were produced by esterification with palmitic acid (C16), but other esters—from fatty acids with even carbon numbers (mainly C16:1, C14:0, C18:0, C18:1, C10:5) and with odd carbon numbers (mainly, C15:0, C17:0 and C17:1)—were also found (Figure 4). The detected acyl-esters seem to be mostly products of the esterification of the hydroxyl groups at C33 and/or C37, as their fragmentation pattern presented relevant peaks at m/z 823, which is typical of these types of esters (Figure 5). Additional small peaks also appeared when the product m/z 1061.5 was monitored, probably due to the presence of C11 esters. A regression of the signals of m/z 823 and 1061 in all measured samples gave an R^2 of 0.999, indicating that the contribution of the C11 esters (associated with m/z 1061 but not with m/z 823) was very small.

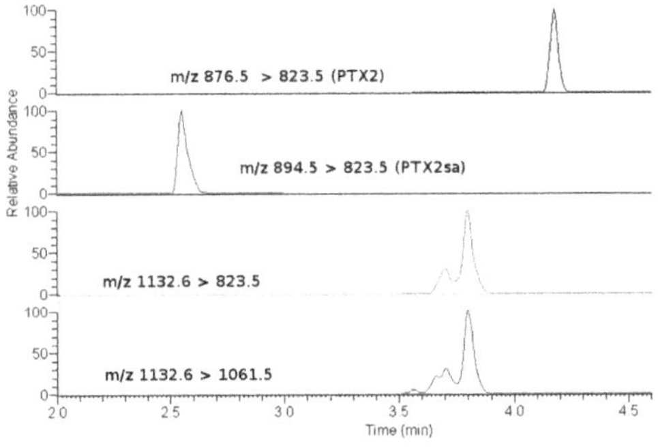

Figure 3. Chromatograms of the main pectenotoxin (PTX) analogs detected (sample of the digestive gland on 12 August 2009). The two lower chromatograms correspond to transitions of palmytoyl-esters of PTX2sa. The upper one of these is more affected by C33 and C37 esters and the lower one of these is also affected by C11 esters.

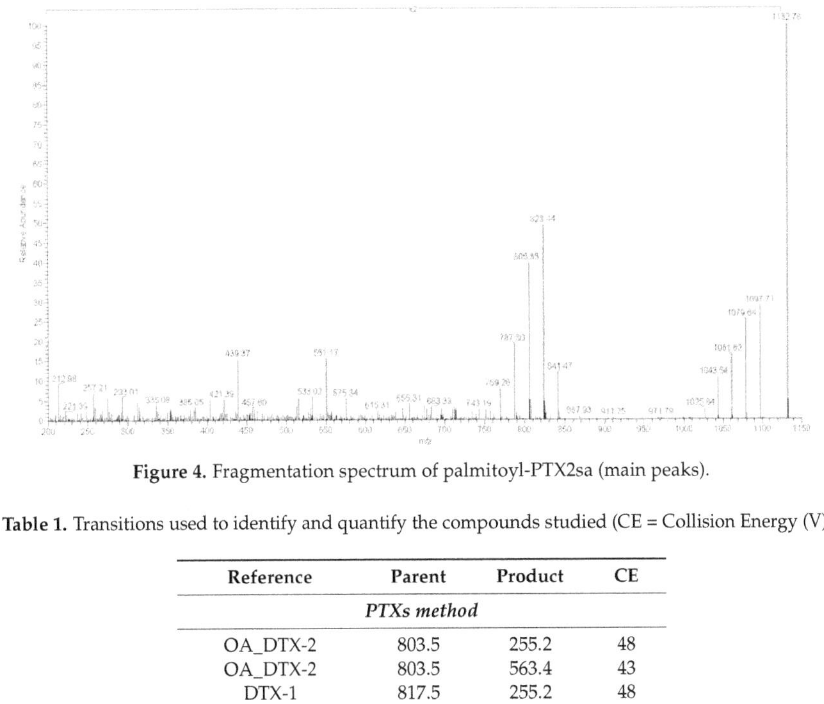

Figure 4. Fragmentation spectrum of palmitoyl-PTX2sa (main peaks).

Table 1. Transitions used to identify and quantify the compounds studied (CE = Collision Energy (V)).

Reference	Parent	Product	CE
	PTXs method		
OA_DTX-2	803.5	255.2	48
OA_DTX-2	803.5	563.4	43
DTX-1	817.5	255.2	48
DTX-1	817.5	563.5	43
PTX-2	876.5	805.5	23
PTX-2	876.5	823.5	21
PTX1	892.5	839.5	23
PTX6	906.5	853.5	23
PTX12	874.5	821.5	23
PTX2sa	894.5	823.5	21
PTX2sa	894.5	805.5	21
PTX11sa	910.5	179.2	50
PTX11sa	910.5	137.2	50
C16-PTX2sa $C_{33,37}$	1132.6	823.5	23
C16-PTX2sa C_{11}	1132.6	1061.5	23

Table 1. *Cont.*

Reference	Parent	Product	CE
Acyl derivatives method			
C14:0-PTX2sa	1104.6	823.5	23
C15:0-PTX2sa	1118.6	823.5	23
C16:1-PTX2sa	1130.6	823.5	23
C16:0-PTX2sa	1132.6	823.5	23
C17:1-PTX2sa	1144.6	823.5	23
C17:0-PTX2sa	1146.6	823.5	23
C18:5-PTX2sa	1150.6	823.5	23
C18:4-PTX2sa	1152.6	823.5	23
C18:3-PTX2sa	1154.6	823.5	23
C18:2-PTX2sa	1156.6	823.5	23
C18:1-PTX2sa	1158.6	823.5	23
C18:0-PTX2sa	1160.6	823.5	23
C20:5-PTX2sa	1178.6	823.5	23
C20:4-PTX2sa	1180.6	823.5	23
C20:2-PTX2sa	1184.6	823.5	23
C20:1-PTX2sa	1186.6	823.5	23
C20:0-PTX2sa	1188.6	823.5	23
C22:6-PTX2sa	1204.6	823.5	23

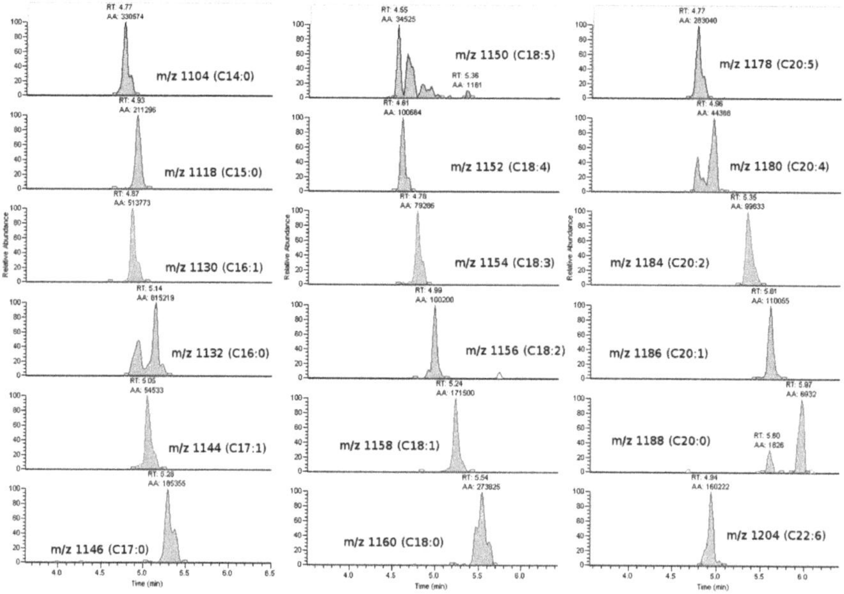

Figure 5. Chromatograms of the main acyl-derivatives of PTX2sa in the sample corresponding to the digestive gland of the *Mesodesma donacium* taken on 12 August 2009. m/z numbers are the parent masses (product m/z = 823) corresponding to esters of PTX2sa with fatty acids of the indicated chain.

Several esters, and perhaps several conformational isomers of them, for each fatty acid may be involved as they were not resolved as a unique chromatographic peak, as shown for the esters with palmitic acid (Figure 3).

PTX2 seco-acid (PTX2sa) concentrations were much higher than those of PTX2. Even though the precise contribution of PTX2sa could not be determined because of the lack of reference solutions, the response in our method (estimated by means of a biotransformation experiment not reported here) was approximately one-third that of PTX2. Taking this into account, the PTX2sa concentrations found were on average nearly 20-fold and 10-fold those of PTX2, in the digestive gland and in the remaining tissues, respectively.

Assuming that the response of the palmitoyl-esters of PTX2sa detected in the mass spectrometer was the same as that of the unesterified compound, esters (even when only those of palmitic acid were quantified) had, on average, half the concentration of PTX2sa in the digestive gland and were nearly absent from the remaining tissues (Figure 6).

The relationship between the pectenotoxins concentration and those of its derivatives was linear and statistically significant, both, in the digestive gland and in the remaining tissues (Supplementary Material).

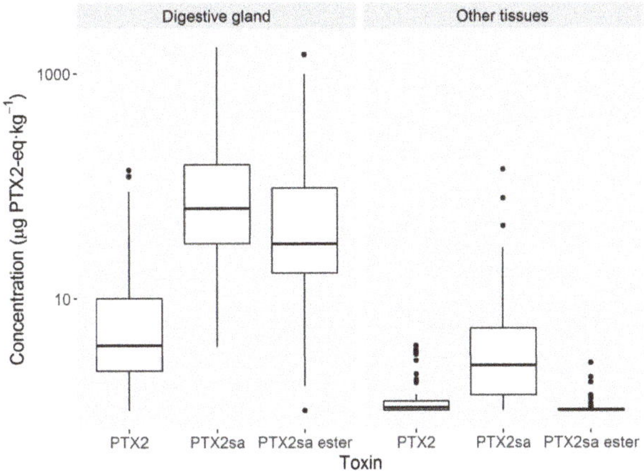

Figure 6. Concentration of the studied toxins in digestive gland and remaining tissues of *Mesodesma donacium* (PTX2sa ester = palmytoyl-PTX2sa). The limits of each box correspond to the 75% and 25% quartiles. The central horizontal line inside the box is the median. The extremes of the vertical lines are the extreme observations excluding the outliers and the isolated dots are outliers.

2.3. Anatomical Distribution of Toxins

The concentrations of all toxins studied were much higher in the digestive gland than in the remaining tissues (Figure 7a). The concentrations of PTX2 and PTX2sa in the digestive gland were approximately 10-fold those in other tissues, but the difference was even more important for esters which were more than 300-fold more concentrated in the digestive gland (Figure 7a).

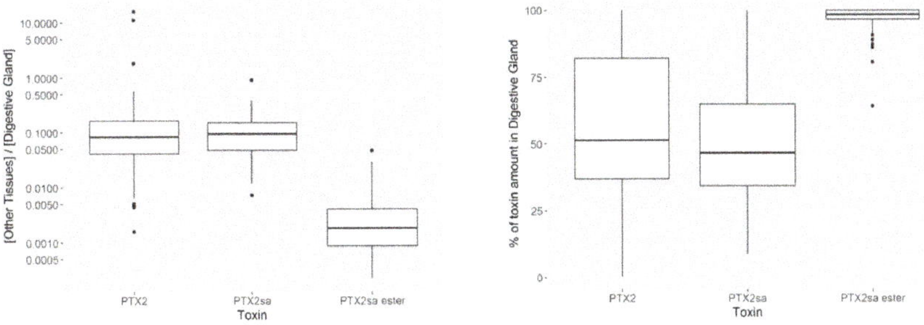

(a) (b)

Figure 7. (**a**) Ratio between concentration of the toxins in digestive gland and other tissues (left panel) and (**b**) percentage of the total toxin burden in the digestive gland (right panel).

The amounts of PTX2 and PTX2sa were evenly distributed between the digestive gland and the remaining tissues (with slightly less PTX2sa in the remaining tissues) (Figure 7b), but nearly all esters were located in the digestive gland (with significant differences between esters and the other two toxins, but not between PTX2 and PTX2sa).

2.4. *Dinophysis* Abundance and Toxin Concentration

Dinophysis abundance was generally low, exceeding 500 cells L^{-1} on only a few occasions. The maximum weekly mean of cell concentration attained was 1825 cells L^{-1} (Figure 8). The time-course of toxin concentration of *M. donacium* in the digestive gland showed three main peaks, which took place at the same time for the PTX1, PTX2sa and PTX2sa esters. In general (when records of both, toxins and cells were available) the peaks of *D. acuminata* abundance and toxin concentration in surf clams did not coincide.

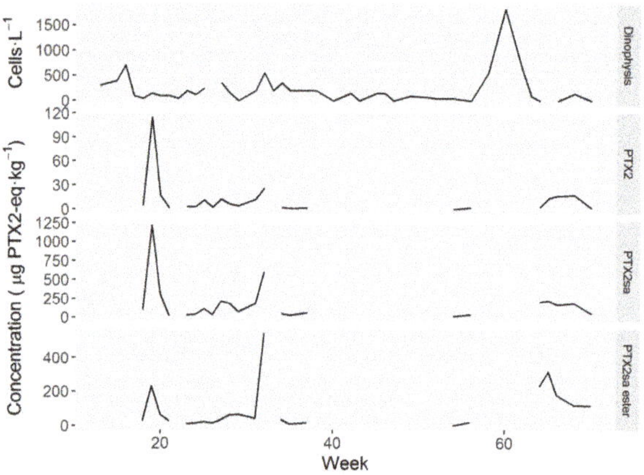

Figure 8. *Dinophysis acuminata* abundance and average weekly toxin concentrations in *M. donacium* in samples from Bahía Coquimbo. Periods not connected by lines correspond to weeks in which samples could not be obtained.

2.5. Depuration Rates

The estimated depuration rates (Figure 9) were higher for PTX2 than for PTX2-sa and PTX2-sa esters. The average values were high at 0.3, 0.23 and 0.2 day^{-1}, respectively.

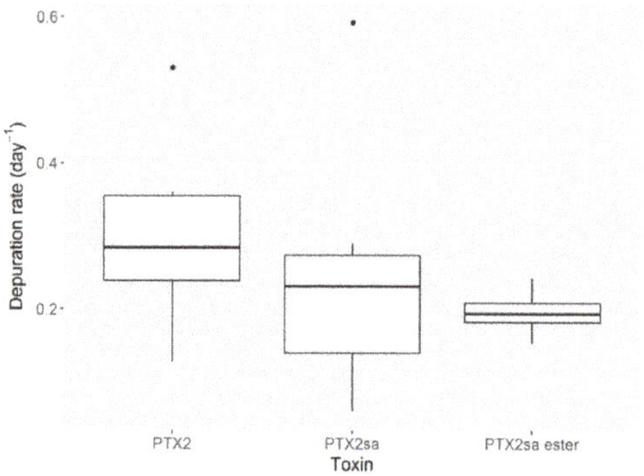

Figure 9. Estimated depuration rates for PTX2 and its derivatives.

3. Discussion

In Chile, the presence of *Dinophysis acuminata* has been described in several distinct geographical locations. In northern Chile this species has been described between 18 °S and 33 °S [18–22]. The taxonomic examination of specimens from phytoplankton net samples revealed that the main morphological features correspond to descriptions of this species given by Faust and Gulledge [23]. In relation to cell size, the length is consistent with measures given by Faust and Gulledge [23] (38–58 μm), Lebour [24] (38–51 μm), Dodge and Hart-Jones [25] (38–58 μm), Olenina et al. [26] (38–58 μm) and Reguera [27] (44–58 μm). However, our cells were larger than those reported by Sar et al. [28] (31.5–38 μm). In relation to cell width, our measures are consistent with the values reported by Olenina et al. [26] (30–38 μm), Faust and Gulledge [23] (30–40 μm) and Reguera [27] (24–43 μm).

Dinophysis acuminata was found to be persistent in the area, but without attaining high cell concentrations. This finding seems to be consistent with observations that the species is common in Northern Chile [18–21], but that it seldom results in market closures of fisheries or aquaculture products [18].

The toxin profiles observed in *M. donacium*, with a complete absence of toxins of the okadaic acid group, suggest that the lack of these toxins in *D. acuminata* from the area found in a bloom in 2005 by Blanco, Alvarez and Uribe [18], was not a special case but rather a general characteristic of this species in the area. The diversity of toxins and derivatives of the PTX group was very limited. Only PTX2 and some of its derivatives in the form of seco-acid and seco-acid esters were found, suggesting that the *Dinophysis* populations contain only PTX2, as PTX2-sa (as also seems to be the case on the Argentinian coast [29]) and its esters are formed by the action of the bivalve [16,17,30–32]. Apart from *Mytilus edulis* [14,17] and an "Australian clam" (cited by Doucet et al. [14] without specifying the species, but which was probably *Plebidonax deltoides* as high accumulations of PTX2sa had been found in this species in the area [7,33]), *Mesodesma donacium* is the first species in which esters of PTX2sa have been found, suggesting that this transformation could be general in molluscs. In other bivalve species, such as *Patinopecten yessoensis*, PTX2 undergoes an oxidation that yields PTX6 as the final product and PTX1 as intermediate one [34,35], but neither PTX6 nor PTX1 have been found in *M. donacium* which means that that oxidation route that generates these derivatives is not active in the species.

The fact that the observed peaks of cell abundance did not produce equivalent peaks of pectenotoxins in *M. donacium* suggests that there were substantial differences in toxin/cell among the different *D. acuminata* populations that developed throughout the sampled year. Other causes, such as differences in the availability of the toxic cells to the infaunal populations of the mollusks cannot be discarded. However, downwelling in the area (computed from the wind data of a meteorological station on-shore, data not shown)—the main process that could potentially regulate this availability—was not related to the toxin peaks in the clams.

The presence in *M. donacium* of PTX2, PTX2sa and PTX2sa esters suggests that PTX2 is transformed to PTX2sa and then to PTX2sa esters. The first step (PTX2 to PTX2sa) could take place in the gut, during = the process of extracellular digestion of the ingested phytoplankton, as demonstrated by MacKenzie, Selwood and Marshall [16] for *Perna canaliculus* but it is possible that the transformation continues once PTX2 is inside the digestive cells as it has also been observed in vitro by treating PTX2 with homogenates [30–32] (or even in cells of other tissues). Esters of PTX2sa should be generated inside the cells as happens with other toxins, such as those of the OA group [13,36,37], brevetoxins [38], spirolides [39], gymnodimines [40], and other lipophilic compounds such as esteroids [41,42]. Very likely the mechanism is a transesterification similar to that found in OA [36,43]. It is clear that this process, in the case of *M. donacium*, only takes place in the digestive gland and not in other tissues, as their content in esters is marginal.

The fact that the apparent depuration rates from the digestive gland are lower as the compound required more transformation steps (PTX2 > PTX2-sa > PTX2-sa esters) can be explained in multiple ways. One possibility is that there were differences in the actual depuration rate of the compounds. A second possibility, which seems more likely, is that the biotransformations altered the estimated depuration rates because the losses by depuration of the transformed compound are increased by the amount of compound that is transformed, while those corresponding to the product compound are decreased by the same reason. A combination of the two processes could also take place. A more detailed study involving the analysis of these possibilities would be required to elucidate the precise cause of the observed differences.

The observed depuration rates, even though they are likely to be underestimates (because the cells rarely disappeared from the water), are relatively high in comparison with those of other lipophylic toxins as those in the OA group [44,45]. *Mesodesma donacium* seems to depurate PTXs much faster than Norwegian mussels and oysters, [46] with estimates of $t_{1/2}$ (semidepuration time) of 6–13 days for PTX2 in mussels *Mytilus edulis* and oysters, while in this study they ranged from 2.3 to 3.1 days, for PTX2 and palmytoyl-PTX2sa, respectively. Notwithstanding this, in a previous study, the estimated depuration rates for PTX2 and PTX2sa from another mussel (*Mytilus galloprovincialis*), and the cockle *Cerastoderma edule*, were much higher, ranging from 0.6 to 1.1 and from 1 to 3 day^{-1}, respectively ($t_{1/2}$ 1.2–0.6 days and 0.7–0.2 days) [47]. Okadaic acid in the same studies was found to depurate from the bivalves at substantially lower rates [46,47].

These high depuration rates indicate that most of the accumulated toxins are likely to have been recently incorporated, and that the levels of these kinds of toxins in *M. donacium* are strongly dependent on the precise nature of the causative organisms.

4. Materials and Methods

4.1. Area of Study, Phytoplankton Sampling, Quantification and Taxonomic Analyses

Phytoplankton samples were collected periodically (weekly when possible) in Bahía Coquimbo (29°51′ S, 71°16′ W) from 1 May 2009 to 28 April 2010, by means of vertical net hauls (20 µm mesh) and a 10 m hose, in order to obtain integrated samples of the entire water column. Bahía Coquimbo is a wide bay with a mean depth of 25 m, and is very dynamic, with typical surficial tidal currents of around 10 $cm{\cdot}s^{-1}$ and bottom currents between 4 and 13 $cm{\cdot}s^{-1}$ [48]. The bottom sediment is mostly sand and is sorted by depth, with the finest particles in the deepest locations [49], indicating a high dynamism in the shallow areas. A thermocline sometimes exists, at a depth of 10 m. The phytoplankton samples were obtained from the same location as those of *Mesodesma donacium*. Two aliquots were preserved—one with formaldehyde 4% (net hauls) and another with Lugol's iodine (hose)—for taxonomic and quantitative analyses, respectively. Phytoplankton composition, including *D. acuminata* cells, were routinely identified using an Olympus IX71 epifluorescence inverted microscope and the method describe by Fritz and Triemer [50]. Phytoplankton and *D. acuminata* cells were quantified using the Utermöhl method, described by Hasle [51], using 10-mL sedimentation chambers with an Olympus IX71 inverted microscope.

4.2. Shellfish Sampling, Toxin Extraction and Hydrolysis

Shellfish samples were collected from 1 May 2009 to 28 April 2010 at the same station as the phytoplankton samples, from 10 to 15 m deep, by means of hookah diving. When possible, a weekly periodicity was maintained. Samples were homogenized and extracted with methanol 100% at a ratio of 1:4 (weight:volume). Extracts were clarified by centrifugation (10,000× *g*, 15 min) and then filtered through 0.20 µm Clarinert nylon syringe filters (13 mm diameter) (Agela technologies).

In order to check the presence of derivatives of toxins of the okadaic acid group some extracts, selected because of their high PTX2 levels (which could be expected to be correlated with toxins of the OA group), were subjected to alkaline hydrolysis following the standard procedure of the EU Reference Laboratory for Marine Biotoxins [52].

4.3. Toxin Detection and Quantification

The toxins contained in the extracts were determined by HPLC-MS/MS, with a Thermo Accela chromatographic system (UHPLC) coupled to a Thermo TSQ Quantum Access Max by means of a HESI-II electrospray interface.

Basically, the chromatographic method by Regueiro et al. 2010 [53] was used, but modified in order to use a shorter column and to allow enough time for the elution, not only of the free toxins, but also of their acylated derivatives. Two chromatographic phases were used: A = 6.7 mM NH_4OH in MilliQ water (Millipore); and B = 90% ACN with 6.7 mM NH_4OH. First, the sample was injected into an online solid phase extraction (SPE) column (Phenomenex Security Guard 4 × 2 mm with phase Gemini-NX C18 (AJO-8367) in an isocratic flow of 90% A and 10% B, while the chromatographic column was kept at 80% A. After 1.5 min the system flow was switched (with a Rheodyne 2-position 6-way valve) and the content of the SPE column started to elute to the chromatographic column (Phenomenex Gemini-NX C18 50 × 2 mm 3 μm). The phase B percentage was raised in a linear manner until reaching 90% at min 3.85 and maintained at that concentration until min 8.25 when the initial conditions were put in place again and maintained until min 10.5. At min 7.5 the Rheodyne valve was switched again in order to equilibrate the SPE column for the next injection. For detailed analysis of PTX2sa acyl-derivatives the chromatographic gradient was modified by extending it for 3 additional minutes.

The mass spectrometer was operated in positive and negative ionization mode using the following settings: Spray Voltage Positive 3500 V, Negative 3000 V, Sheath Gas Pressure 50, Aux Gas Flow: 5; Vaporizer Temperature: 110; Capillary Temperature 360; Collision Gas Pressure (mTorr): 1.5. For identification and quantification, the transitions given in Table 1 were used.

The toxin concentration in the extracts was quantified by comparing the area or the peaks obtained in the chromatograms with those of certified reference materials obtained from Laboratorio CIFGA, Spain and the NCR, Canada. When those materials were not available—as was the case for PTX2 seco-acid and esters of PTX2 seco-acid—a relative quantification was carried out using the signal of PTX2 as reference.

4.4. Estimation of Depuration Rates

Rough estimates of depuration rates were obtained by using concentration values in two consecutive weeks based on the following selection criteria: (a) that the first observation had a high concentration value; (b) that the *D. acuminata* abundance in the following week was low; and (c) there was no substantial increase of toxin concentration in the third week. This approach would yield underestimated values of the depuration rate as some toxin uptake had taken place during the period for which depuration was estimated. It was assumed that depuration followed an exponential decrease, and the rate for each period was computed as $\mathrm{Ln}[\mathrm{Tox}]_{\mathrm{week0}} - [\mathrm{Tox}]_{\mathrm{week1}})/7$ days and was expressed as day^{-1}.

4.5. Statistical Analysis

Regression, correlation and ANOVA analyses were carried out with *R* [54]. Descriptive statistical plots were built with the ggplot2 package [55].

Supplementary Materials: The following are available online at http://www.mdpi.com/2072-6651/10/8/314/s1, Raw data of toxin concentration in the extract. Raw data of *Dinophysis acuminata* cell counts. Figure S1: Relationships between the PTX2 derivatives.

Author Contributions: Conceptualization: J.B., G.Á., E.U. Formal analysis: J.B. Funding acquisition: G.Á., E.U., J.B. Investigation: G.Á., J.R., E.U., R.D., C.M., H.M. Visualization: J.B., G.Á. Writing-original draft: J.B., G.Á. Writing-review and editing: J.B., G.Á., J.R., E.U.

Funding: This research was funded by the "CONICYT + FONDEF/PRIMER CONCURSO INVESTIGACIÓN TECNOLÓGICA TEMATICO EN SISTEMAS PESQUERO ACUICOLAS FRENTE A FLORECIMIENTOS

ALGALES NOCIVOS FANS IDeA DEL FONDO DE FOMENTO AL DESARROLLO CIENTÍFICO Y TECNOLÓGICO, FONDEF/CONICYT 2017, IT17F10002" and by CIMA (Xunta de Galicia). Gonzalo Álvarez was funded by the CHILEAN NATIONAL COMMISSION FOR SCIENTIFIC AND TECHNOLOGICAL RESEARCH (CONICYT+ PAI/CONCURSO NACIONAL INSERCION EN LA ACADEMIA CONVOCATORIA 2015, 79150008).

Acknowledgments: We would like to thank the Asociación Gremial de Pescadores Artesanales de Caleta Peñuelas A.G., and the Asociación Gremial de Pescadores y Buzos Mariscadores Caleta San Pedro La Serena A.G. for their support.

Conflicts of Interest: The authors declare no conflicts of interest.

References

1. Guzmán, L.; Campodonico, I. Marea roja en la región de Magallanes. *Pub. Inst. Patagon. Ser. Monogr.* **1975**, *9*, 44.
2. Lembeye, G.; Yasumoto, Y.; Zhao, J.; Fernández, R. DSP outbreak in Chilean fjords. In *Toxic Phytoplankton Blooms in the Sea*; Smayda, T.J., Shimizu, Y., Eds.; Elservier: Amsterdam, The Netherlands, 1993; pp. 525–529.
3. Zhao, J.; Lembeye, G.; Cenci, G.; Wall, B.; Yasumoto, T. Determination of okadaic acid and dinophysistoxin-1 in mussels from Chile, Italy and Ireland. In *Toxic Phytoplankton Blooms in the Sea*; Smayda, T.J., Shimizu, Y., Eds.; Elsevier: Amsterdam, The Netherlands, 1993; pp. 587–592.
4. IOC. *Second IOC Regional Science Planning Workshop on Harmful Algal Blooms in South America*; IOC: Mar del Plata, Argentina, 1995; p. 75.
5. Uribe, J.C.; García, C.; Rivas, M.; Lagos, N. First report of diarrhetic shellfish toxins in Magellanic fjord, Southern Chile. *J. Shellfish Res.* **2001**, *20*, 69–74.
6. Villarroel, O. Detección de toxina paralizante, diarreica y amnésica en mariscos de la XI región por Cromatografía de Alta Resolución (HPLC) y bioensayo de ratón. *Ciencia y Tecnologia del Mar* **2004**, *27*, 33–42.
7. Reguera, B.; Riobó, P.; Rodríguez, F.; Díaz, P.; Pizarro, G.; Paz, B.; Franco, J.; Blanco, J. Dinophysis Toxins: Causative Organisms, Distribution and Fate in Shellfish. *Mar. Drugs* **2014**, *12*, 394–461. [CrossRef] [PubMed]
8. Blanco, J.; Correa, J.; Muñíz, S.; Mariño, C.; Martín, H.; Arévalo, F. Evaluación del impacto de los métodos y niveles utilizados para el control de toxinas en el mejillón. *Revista Galega dos Recursos Mariños* **2013**, *3*, 1–55. Available online: https://www.researchgate.net/publication/236842103_Evaluacion_del_impacto_de_los_metodos_y_niveles_utilizados_para_el_control_de_toxinas_en_el_mejillon (accessed on 24 June 2018).
9. Gestal Otero, J.J. Epidemiology of marine toxins. In *Seafood and Freshwater Toxins. Physiology, Pharmacology and Detection*, 3rd ed.; Botana, L.M., Ed.; CRC Press, Taylor and Francis Group: Boca Ratón, FL, USA, 2014; pp. 123–195.
10. Munday, R. Toxicology of seafood toxins: A critical review. In *Seafood and Freshwater Toxins: Pharmacology, Physiology, and Detection*; CRC Press, Taylor and Francis Group: Boca Ratón, FL, USA, 2014; pp. 197–290.
11. EFSA Panel on Contaminants in the Food Chain. Marine biotoxins in shellfish—Pectenotoxin group: Marine biotoxins in shellfish—Pectenotoxin group. *EFSA J.* **2009**, *7*. [CrossRef]
12. EFSA Panel on Contaminants in the Food Chain. Scientific Opinion of the Panel on Contaminants in the Food Chain on a request from the European Commission on Marine Biotoxins in Shellfish—Summary on regulated marine biotoxins. *EFSA J.* **2009**, *1306*, 1–23.
13. Suzuki, T.; Ota, H.; Yamasaki, M. Direct evidence of transformation of dinophysistoxin-1 to 7-*O*-acyl-dinophysistoxin-1 (dinophysistoxin-3) in the scallop *Patinopecten yessoensis*. *Toxicon* **1999**, *37*, 187–198. [CrossRef]
14. Doucet, E.; Ross, N.N.; Quilliam, M.A. Enzymatic hydrolysis of esterified diarrhetic shellfish poisoning toxins and pectenotoxins. *Anal. Bioanal. Chem.* **2007**, *389*, 335–342. [CrossRef] [PubMed]
15. Torgersen, T.; Sandvik, M.; Lundve, B.; Lindegarth, S. Profiles and levels of fatty acid esters of okadaic acid group toxins and pectenotoxins during toxin depuration. Part II: Blue mussels (*Mytilus edulis*) and flat oyster (*Ostrea edulis*). *Toxicon* **2008**, *52*, 418–427. [CrossRef] [PubMed]
16. MacKenzie, L.A.; Selwood, A.I.; Marshall, C. Isolation and characterization of an enzyme from the Greenshell (TM) mussel *Perna canaliculus* that hydrolyses pectenotoxins and esters of okadaic acid. *Toxicon* **2012**, *60*, 406–419. [CrossRef] [PubMed]
17. Wilkins, A.L.; Rehmann, N.; Torgersen, T.; Rundberget, T.; Keogh, M.; Petersen, D.; Hess, P.; Rise, F.; Miles, C.O. Identification of fatty acid esters of pectenotoxin-2 seco acid in blue mussels (*Mytilus edulis*) from Ireland. *J. Agric. Food Chem.* **2006**, *54*, 5672–5678. [CrossRef] [PubMed]

18. Blanco, J.; Alvarez, G.; Uribe, E. Identification of pectenotoxins in plankton, filter feeders, and isolated cells of a *Dinophysis acuminata* with an atypical toxin profile, from Chile. *Toxicon* **2007**, *49*, 710–716. [CrossRef] [PubMed]
19. Avaria, S.; Muñoz, P. Composición y biomasa del fitoplancton marino del norte de Chile en mayo de 1981 (operación oceanográfica MarChile XII-ERFEN III). *Ciencia y Tecnología del Mar CONA* **1983**, *7*, 109–140.
20. Avaria, S.; Muñoz, P. Efectos del fenómeno "El Niño" sobre el fitoplancton marino del norte de Chile en diciembre de 1982. *Ciencia y Tecnologia del Mar* **1985**, *9*, 3–30.
21. Avaria, S.; Muñoz, P.; Uribe, E. Composición y biomasa del fitoplancton marino del norte de Chile en Diciembre de 1980 (Operación oceanográfica MARCHILE XI-ERFEN II). *Ciencia y Tecología del Mar CONA* **1982**, *6*, 5–36.
22. Santander, E.; Herrera, L.; Merino, C. Fluctuación diaria del fitoplancton en la capa superficial del océano durante la primavera de 1997 en el norte de Chile (20 18 S): II. Composición específica y abundancia celular. *Revista de Biología Marina y Oceanografía* **2003**, *38*, 13–25. [CrossRef]
23. Faust, M.A.; Gulledge, R.A. Identifying harmful marine dinoflagellates. *Contrib. USA Natl. Herb.* **2002**, *42*, 1–144.
24. Lebour, M.V. *The Dinoflagellates of Northern Seas*; Marine Biological Association of the United Kingdom: Plymouth, UK, 1925; Volume 250.
25. Dodge, J.D.; Hart-Jones, B. *Marine Dinoflagellates of the British Isles*; Her Majesty's Stationery Office (HMSO): London, UK, 1982.
26. Olenina, I.; Hajdu, S.; Edler, L.; Andersson, A.; Wasmund, N.; Busch, S.; Göbel, J.; Gromisz, S.; Huseby, S.; Huttunen, M.; et al. *Biovolumes and Size-Classes of Phytoplankton in the Baltic Sea*; Baltic Marine Environment Protection Commission: Helsinki, Filand, 2006.
27. Reguera, B. Biología, Autoecología y Toxinología de las Principales Especies del Género" Dinophysis" Asociadas a Episodios de Intoxicación Diarreogénica por Bivalvos (DSP). Ph.D. Thesis, Universidad de Barcelona, Barcelona, Spain, 2003.
28. Sar, E.A.; Sunesen, I.; Lavigne, A.; Goya, A. *Dinophysis* spp. asociadas a detección de toxinas diarreicas (DSTs) en moluscos y a intoxicación diarreica en humanos (Provincia de Buenos Aires, Argentina). *Revista de Biología Marina y Oceanografía* **2010**, *45*, 451–460. [CrossRef]
29. Fabro, E.; Almandoz, G.O.; Ferrario, M.; Tillmann, U.; Cembella, A.; Krock, B. Distribution of Dinophysis species and their association with lipophilic phycotoxins in plankton from the Argentine Sea. *Harmful Algae* **2016**, *59*, 31–41. [CrossRef] [PubMed]
30. Suzuki, T.; Mackenzie, L.; Stirling, D.; Adamson, J. Pectenotoxin-2 seco acid: A toxin converted from pectenotoxin-2 by the New Zealand Greenshell mussel, *Perna canaliculus*. *Toxicon* **2001**, *39*, 507–514. [CrossRef]
31. Suzuki, T.; Mackenzie, L.; Stirling, D.; Adamson, J. Conversion of pectenotoxin-2 to pectenotoxin-2 seco acid in the New Zealand scallop, *Pecten novaezelandiae*. *Fish. Sci.* **2001**, *67*, 506–510. [CrossRef]
32. Miles, C.O.; Wilkins, A.L.; Munday, R.; Dines, M.H.; Hawkes, A.D.; Briggs, L.R.; Sandvik, M.; Jensen, D.J.; Cooney, J.M.; Holland, P.T.; et al. Isolation of Pectenotoxin-2 From *Dinophysis acuta* and Its Conversion to Pectenotoxin-2 Seco Acid, and Preliminary Assessment of Their Acute Toxicities. *Toxicon* **2004**, *43*, 1–9. [CrossRef] [PubMed]
33. Burgess, V.; Shaw, G. *Investigations into the Toxicology of Pectenotoxin-2-Seco Acid and 7-Epi Pectenotoxin 2-Seco Acid to Aid in a Health Risk Assessment for the Consumption of Shellfish Contaminated with These Shellfish Toxins in Australia*; Report on Project No. 2001/258; Fisheries Research and Development Corporation: Canberra, Australia, 2003; ISBN 0975025910.
34. Suzuki, T.; Mitsuya, T.; Matsubara, H.; Yamasaki, M. Determination of pectenotoxin-2 after solid-phase extraction from seawater and from the dinoflagellate *Dinophysis fortii* by liquid chromatography with electrospray mass spectrometry and ultraviolet detection. Evidence of oxidation of pectenotoxin-2 to pectenotoxin-6 in scallops. *J. Chromatogr. A* **1998**, *815*, 155–160. [CrossRef] [PubMed]
35. Suzuki, T. Chemistry and Detection of Okadaic Acid/Dinophysistoxins, Pectenotoxins and Yessotoxins. In *Toxins and Biologically Active Compound from Microalgae. Vol 1 Origin, Chemistry and Detection*; Rossini, G.P., Ed.; CRC Press: Boca Raton, FL, USA, 2014; pp. 99–152.
36. Rossignoli, A.E.; Fernandez, D.; Regueiro, J.; Marino, C.; Blanco, J. Esterification of okadaic acid in the mussel *Mytilus galloprovincialis*. *Toxicon* **2011**, *57*, 712–720. [CrossRef] [PubMed]

37. Marr, J.C.; Hu, T.; Pleasance, S.; Quilliam, M.A.; Wright, J.L.C. Detection of new 7-*O*-acyl derivatives of diarrhetic shellfish poisoning toxins by liquid chromatography-mass spectrometry. *Toxicon* **1992**, *30*, 1621–1630. [CrossRef]
38. Morohashi, A.; Satake, M.; Murata, K.; Naoki, H.; Kaspar, H.F.; Yasumoto, T. Brevetoxin B3, a new brevetoxin analog isolated from the greenshell mussel *Perna canaliculus* involved in neurotoxic shellfish poisoning in new zealand. *Tetrahedron Lett.* **1995**, *36*, 8995–8998. [CrossRef]
39. Aasen, J.A.; Hardstaff, W.; Aune, T.; Quilliam, M.A. Discovery of fatty acid ester metabolites of spirolide toxins in mussels from Norway using liquid chromatography/tandem mass spectrometry. *Rapid Commun. Mass Spectrom* **2006**, *20*, 1531–1537. [CrossRef] [PubMed]
40. De la Iglesia, P.; McCarron, P.; Diogene, J.; Quilliam, M.A. Discovery of gymnodimine fatty acid ester metabolites in shellfish using liquid chromatography/mass spectrometry. *Rapid Commun. Mass Spectrom.* **2013**, *27*, 643–653. [CrossRef] [PubMed]
41. Janer, G.; Lavado, R.; Thibaut, R.; Porte, C. Effects of 17β-estradiol exposure in the mussel *Mytilus galloprovincialis*: A possible regulating role for steroid acyltransferases. *Aquat. Toxicol.* **2005**, *75*, 32–42. [CrossRef] [PubMed]
42. Janer, G.; Mesia-Vela, S.; Porte, C.; Kauffman, F.C. Esterification of vertebrate-type steroids in the Eastern oyster (*Crassostrea virginica*). *Steroids* **2004**, *69*, 129–136. [CrossRef] [PubMed]
43. Furumochi, S.; Onoda, T.; Cho, Y.; Fuwa, H.; Sasaki, M.; Yotsu-Yamashita, M.; Konoki, K. Effect of carbon chain length in acyl coenzyme A on the efficiency of enzymatic transformation of okadaic acid to 7-*O*-acyl okadaic acid. *Bioorg. Med. Chem. Lett.* **2016**, *26*, 2992–2996. [CrossRef] [PubMed]
44. Blanco, J.; Fernández, M.L.; Míguez, A.; Moroño, A. Okadaic acid depuration in the mussel *Mytilus galloprovincialis*: One- and two-compartment models and the effect of environmental conditions. *Mar. Ecol. Prog. Ser.* **1999**, *176*, 153–163. [CrossRef]
45. Moroño, A.; Arévalo, F.; Fernández, M.L.; Maneiro, J.; Pazos, Y.; Salgado, C.; Blanco, J. Accumulation and transformation of DSP toxins in mussels *Mytilus galloprovincialis* LMK during a toxic episode caused by *Dinophysis acuminata*. *Aquat. Toxicol.* **2003**, *62*, 269–280. [CrossRef]
46. Lindegarth, S.; Torgersen, T.; Lundve, B.; Sandvik, M. Differential Retention of okadaic acid (OA) group toxins and pectenotoxins (PTX) in the blue mussel, *Mytilus edulis* (L.), and european glat oyster, *Ostrea edulis* (L.). *J. Shellfish Res.* **2009**, *28*, 313–323. [CrossRef]
47. Vale, P. Differential Dynamics of Dinophysistoxins and Pectenotoxins Between Blue Mussel and Common Cockle: A Phenomenon Originating From the Complex Toxin Profile of *Dinophysis acuta*. *Toxicon* **2004**, *44*, 123–134. [CrossRef] [PubMed]
48. Valle-Levinson, A.; Moraga, J.; Olivares, J.; Blanco, J.L. Tidal and residual circulation in a semi-arid bay: Coquimbo Bay, Chile. *Cont. Shelf Res.* **2000**, *20*, 2009–2028. [CrossRef]
49. Berríos, M.; Olivares, J. Caracterización granulométrica y contenido de carbono orgánico de los sedimentos marinos superficiales, en el sistema de bahías de la IV Región. *Coquimbo. Cienc. Tecnol. Mar.* **1996**, *19*, 37–45.
50. Fritz, L.; Triemer, R.E. A rapid simple technique utilizing calcofluor white M2R for the visualization of dinoflagellate thecal plates. *J. Phycol.* **1985**, *21*, 662–664. [CrossRef]
51. Hasle, R.G. The inverted microscope method. In *Phytoplankton Manual*; UNESCO: Paris, France, 1978; pp. 88–96.
52. EURLMB. EU-Harmonised Standard Operating Procedure for Determination of Lipophilic Marine Biotoxins in Molluscs by LC-MS/MS. Version 5. Available online: http://aesan.msssi.gob.es/CRLMB/docs/docs/metodos_analiticos_de_desarrollo/EU-Harmonised-SOP-LIPO-LCMSMS_Version5.pdf (accessed on 30 June 2015).
53. Regueiro, J.; Rossignoli, A.E.; Alvarez, G.; Blanco, J. Automated on-line solid-phase extraction coupled to liquid chromatography tandem mass spectrometry for determination of lipophilic marine toxins in shellfish. *Food Chem.* **2011**, *129*, 533–540. [CrossRef]
54. R Core Team. *R: A Language and Environment for Statistical Computing*; R Foundation for Statistical Computing: Vienna, Austria, 2014.
55. Wickham, H. *Ggplot2: Elegant Graphics for Data Analysis*; Springer: New York, NY, USA, 2016.

toxins

Review

Accumulation of *Dinophysis* Toxins in Bivalve Molluscs

Juan Blanco

Centro de Investigacións Mariñas, Pedras de Corón s/n, 36620 Vilanova de Arousa, Spain; juan.carlos.blanco.perez@xunta.gal; Tel.: +34-886-206-340

Received: 25 September 2018; Accepted: 23 October 2018; Published: 2 November 2018

Abstract: Several species of the dinoflagellate genus *Dinophysis* produce toxins that accumulate in bivalves when they feed on populations of these organisms. The accumulated toxins can lead to intoxication in consumers of the affected bivalves. The risk of intoxication depends on the amount and toxic power of accumulated toxins. In this review, current knowledge on the main processes involved in toxin accumulation were compiled, including the mechanisms and regulation of toxin acquisition, digestion, biotransformation, compartmentalization, and toxin depuration. Finally, accumulation kinetics, some models to describe it, and some implications were also considered.

Keywords: okadaic acid; pectenotoxins; *Dinophysis* toxins; accumulation; digestion; biotransformation; compartmentalization; depuration; kinetics

Key Contribution: The main aspects of the process of *Dinophysis* toxins accumulation are summarized and analyzed.

1. Introduction

1.1. *Dinophysis*-Produced Toxins

Some dinoflagellates of the genus *Dinophysis* produce toxins belonging to the okadaic acid group (okadaic acid and dinophysistoxins, OA and DTXs, respectively) and/or to pectenotoxins (PTXs). Both groups of toxins are polyethers having a linear structure in the OA group and a macrocyclic lactone in pectenotoxins. The compounds in the OA group have a terminal carboxylic function, which in some cases, esterifies diols or other compounds, and a hydroxyl in C-7 that is frequently esterified with fatty acids to yield the group of derivatives generically known as "DTX3" (Figure 1). The macrolactone cycle of PTXs could be opened to produce seco-acids that in turn can be esterified with fatty acids (Figure 7).

Dinophysistoxin-1 (DTX1) was identified in 1982 as the substance responsible for a toxic syndrome (Diarrhetic Shellfish Poisoning, DSP) [1,2], which affected more than 1600 people in Japan [3]. This toxin is a 35-R-Methyl derivative of okadaic acid, a compound that had previously been isolated from two sponges of the genus *Halichondria* (*H. okadai* and *H. melanodocia*) [4], and which since then, has been associated with numerous DSP outbreaks occurring all over the world [5–9]. The allowable levels in shellfish of this toxin and other toxins or derivatives of the same group have been regulated in many countries. In Europe and other areas, the established regulatory threshold is 160 µg OA-eq/Kg of edible product (quantified together with pectenotoxins) [10–12].

Pectenotoxins have never been linked to any human intoxication [13], but they were discovered because they co-elute with the toxins of the okadaic group and are lethal to mice by intraperitoneal injection in the bioassays typically used to monitor DSP toxins. The regulatory level in Europe is the same as the one for the toxins of the OA group (quantified jointly) [11].

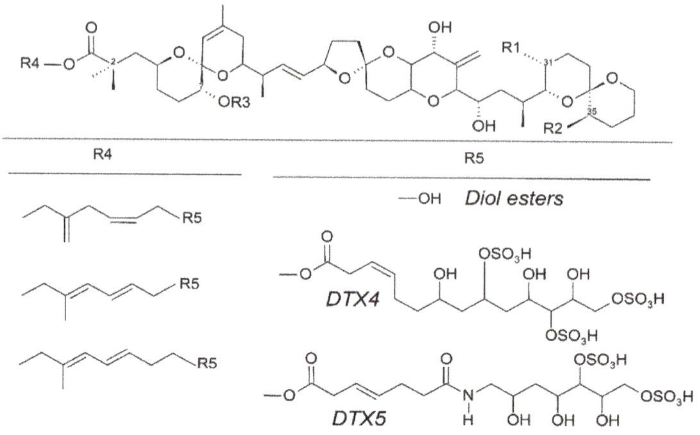

	R1	R2	R3	R4	R5
Okadaic acid	CH_3	H	H	-	-
DTX2	H	CH_3	H	-	-
DTX1	CH_3	CH_3	H	-	-
"DTX3"			-Acyl	-	-
Diol esters			H	-diol-	OH
"DTX4", "DTX5"			H	-diol-	figure
Hybrid esters 1			-Acyl	-diol-	OH
Hybrid esters 2			H	-diol-	-Acyl

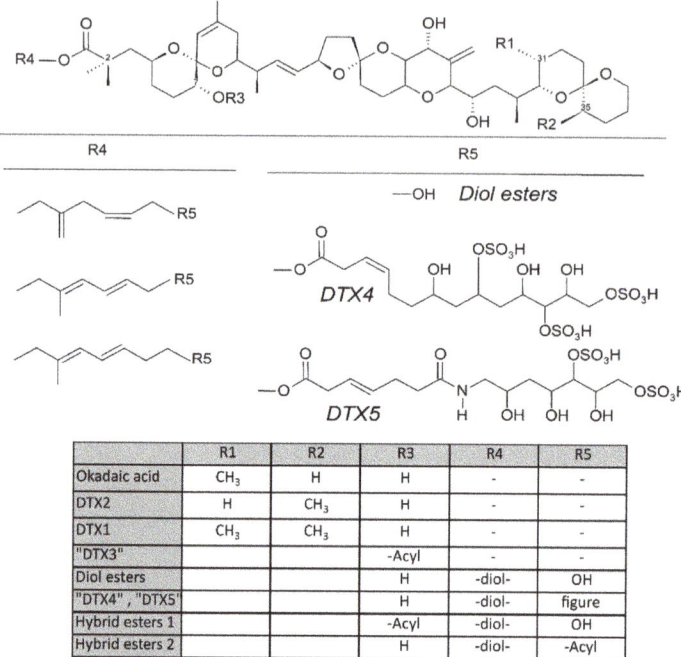

Figure 1. Structure of the toxins of the okadaic acid group. R4 and R5 are some examples of structures which may be more complex.

The threat that these toxins pose to human health makes it mandatory to implement monitoring systems. Legal/regulatory strategies must allow for the proper management of marine resources (including aquaculture) to preserve public health and minimize the economic losses of fishermen and farmers [14]. Both monitoring and management have costs and these can be high, depending on the importance and value of the resources and means of commercialization [15].

Bivalves, retain, ingest, and digest *Dinophysis* cells, bioaccumulate the toxins they contain and biotransform them into derivatives that could have different toxicities than their parent toxins. Understanding these processes is essential to developing predictive capability of the intensity and duration of toxic episodes of *Dinophysis*, and consequently, using the abundance of its populations as a warning in monitoring systems and designing mechanisms to mitigate their impact by means of the acceleration of the depuration process or the reduction of toxin uptake.

1.2. Toxins in Phytoplankton

Different species (or strains) of *Dinophysis* produce different toxins. Phytoplanktonic populations usually contain free toxins (the main toxin structure without esterifying or being esterified with any other compound). Thus, okadaic acid, DTX1, DTX2, and PTX2 (PTX11 and 12 to a lesser extent) are the main toxins found.

Okadaic acid is present in many *Dinophysis* species and is dominant in European waters. In Japan, Chile, and the U.S., DTX1 appeared more frequently [16–19]. DTX2 seems to be practically restricted (with the exception of a few samples from Baja California, Mexico [20]) to the Atlantic coast of Europe (Ireland [21] (where it was first identified), Spain [22,23], Portugal [24], Southern Norway [25], Great Britain [26]), Northern Africa (Morocco [27], Tunisia [28]), and the Mediterranean Sea [29],) and is mostly (or exclusively) associated with *Dinophysis acuta* [21,30,31].

Derivatives of the free toxins in which the carboxylic function esterifies diols (diol esters), triols, or more complex molecules (DTX4, DTX5) (Figure 1) have been described from certain OA-producer *Prorocentrum* species [32–39]. In some species of the genus *Dinophysis*, such as *D. acuta* [40–42], diol esters have been found and their presence is suspected in others like *D. ovum* and *D. acuminata*, in view of the increase in free OA produced by the alkaline hydrolysis of the extracts of a bloom [43,44]. Some other species, such as *D. fortii* [40], and probably some strains of the cited ones, do not seem to contain these kinds of compounds.

Pectenotoxins—mainly PTX2, but sometimes also PTX11 and 12 [42,45,46]—are produced by several *Dinophysis* species [45,47–60]. Frequently their detection is concurrent with that of toxins of the OA group, but in some cases, only pectenotoxins seem to be produced [17,61,62].

2. Ingestion

Toxins can be acquired by bivalves in two ways: (1) Directly from the dissolved phase, and (2) from the cells or particulate matter that contain them.

The uptake of okadaic acid by bivalves from the dissolved phase has been demonstrated [63,64]. The capability of this toxin to pass through lipid bilayers by forming aggregates [65] or dimers [66] had been previously shown. Other lipophilic toxins—the azaspiracids—for which this capability has not been demonstrated, could also be acquired by mussels in a similar way [67]. Li et al. [63], observed that the concentration of OA in bivalves exposed to dissolved toxin exceeded the levels that could be expected in view of concentrations in the water, suggesting that an active uptake mechanism could exist, at least in the digestive gland.

Most toxins, notwithstanding, are retained by bivalves together with the cells that produce them. Bivalves pump water, with the particles suspended in it, through the gill and retain them in a proportion which depends, among other factors, on their size. The feeding process comprises water pumping and filtration, pre-ingestive particle selection, ingestion, post-ingestive selection, and food amount regulation (reviewed in Dame [68] and Gosling [69]). Most bivalves retain particles larger that 5–7 μm with efficiencies of 100% [70–73], and consequently, can retain *Dinophysis* cells (mostly between 45 and 85 μm [74]) with high efficiency. Therefore, practically all particles pumped through the gill are filtered and retained. The pumping rate depends mostly on the species, size of the individuals, and concentration, as well as the quality of the particles suspended in water (seston). In general, filtration is low at low seston concentrations, maximum at intermediate levels, and submaximal when the concentration is high (reviewed in Gosling [69]), as is the case, for example, of the cockle *Cerastoderma edule* in most conditions [75] (Figure 2).

When the filtration efficiency is close to 100%, the filtration rate and clearance rate (the rate at which particles are withdrawn from water) are equivalent.

Filtration rate is a species-specific characteristic that can explain, at least in part, the differences in the accumulation of *Dinophysis*-produced toxins between species. Oysters, for example, accumulate fewer toxins than mussels [76–79], and their maximum filtration rate is, in general, lower [80,81]. Filtration rate is dependent on the gill area, and consequently, proportional to (approximately) the square of the body length (L^2), and also approximately to body weight ($W^{2/3}$) (reviewed by Cranford et al. [82] and Gossling [69], which means that smaller individuals of the same species filtrate more cells or particles in relation to their body weight than larger ones.

The phytoplankton species may also affect filtration and clearance rates, as has been demonstrated for some PSP producing species of *Alexandrium* [83] and some *Pseudo-nitzschia* (whether or not they produce domoic acid) [84], but there is no evidence of these kinds of effects being caused by any natural population of *Dinophysis*. Two species of scallops, *Patinopecten yessoensis* and *Mimachlamys nobilis*, were shown to be affected by cultures of a PTX2-producer, *Dinophysis acuta*, but to a degree that was not dependent on the toxin quota of the cultured cells [85]. Another okadaic acid-producing species, *Prorocentrum lima*, has been shown to reduce the filtration rate of mussels [86], and recently, Li et al. [63]

also found a reduced clearance rate in mussels exposed to okadaic acid isolated from the same species. In none of these cases can the possible contribution of other biologically active substances be ruled out.

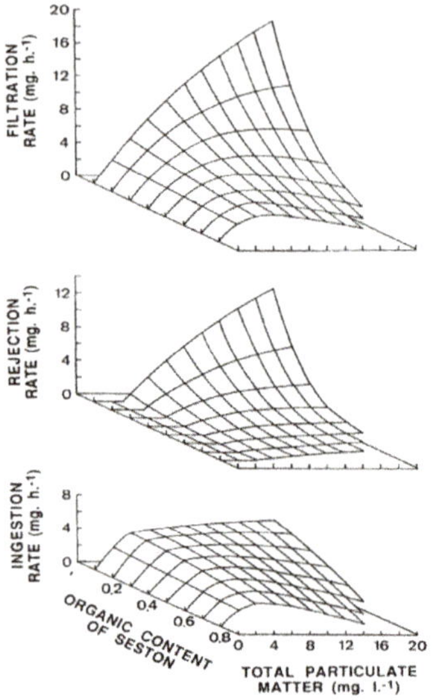

Figure 2. Filtration, ingestion, and rejection of seston by the cockle *Cerastoderma edule* as a function of organic content and seston concentration. Reproduced with permission from Iglesias et al. [75], published by Elsevier 1996.

In some cases, a proportion of the cleared particles is rejected, in a degree that is dependent, at the very least, on the seston concentration and on its organic content, with maximum rejection levels at high concentrations of inorganic particulate matter. *Dinophysis* blooms are associated with a wide range of particulate matter concentrations, ranging from very low (in cases where hardly any other phytoplankton species are present) to very high (in cases where *Dinophysis* are only minor accompanying species). Therefore, a constant response of bivalves, in terms of rejection, would not be expected. Sampayo et al. [87] and Haamer [88] found that the toxicity degree of bivalves exposed to *Dinophysis* populations was lower when the abundance of accompanying species was low, which, among other causes, could be due to increased rejection under these conditions.

Not all particles that are retained by the gill are ingested afterwards. Some particles are negatively selected and rejected through the production of pseudofaeces [75,89–92] or other mechanisms [93,94]. In general, particles with a high organic content, which include phytoplankton, and therefore *Dinophysis* cells, are preferentially ingested [90]. Size may also play an important role in particle selection. Inorganic particles, with the same shape, larger than the threshold size (depending on the species) were found to be rejected preferentially [95]. Mafra et al. [84] also found that the oyster *Crassostrea virginica* preferentially rejects large cells of *Pseudo-nitzschia multiseries*—a diatom producer of the ASP toxin domoic acid—an occurrence which they associated with the fact that the large cells exceeded the width of the principal filament aperture (approx. 68 μm). Even when *Dinophysis* cells are above that size threshold, there is no evidence that they (or other organic particles) are rejected preferentially. Contrarily, it seems that the mussel *Mytilus galloprovincialis* can ingest *Dinophysis* cells preferentially over other phytoplanktonic species, in view of the gut remains [96].

Intraspecific differences in OA accumulation during the early stages of a *Dinophysis* bloom (therefore, probably related to cell ingestion) have also been found in mussels. These differences would have a genetic basis, as a heritability greater than 30% was estimated [97].

3. Post-Ingestive Selection and Regulation of Food Processing

Once ingested, the *Dinophysis* cells, jointly with other particles go through the esophagus to the stomach and the crystalline stylus sac where they are broken down [98] into fine fragments, before being transferred to the digestive tubules. The walls of the stomach of the bivalves have a complex network of ciliated folds that are believed to act by sorting particles [99]. If the number of particles ingested is low, a high proportion of the large particles are recurrently sent to the crystalline style sac for additional processing, and another proportion is directly rejected and sent to the intestine. If the amount of food ingested is high, a larger proportion of the ingested cells is diverted unprocessed to the intestine and eliminated with feces (Figure 3). The higher the volume of ingested material, the shorter the time it will stay in the digestive system (gut passage time, GPT), and it will consequently go through less processing and digestion, leading to a lower absorption efficiency of the organic matter [100,101]—including the toxins [102,103]—it contains. These processes could help explain why the bivalves exposed to *Dinophysis* populations acquire less toxicity when the accompanying populations of other phytoplankton species are abundant [87,88].

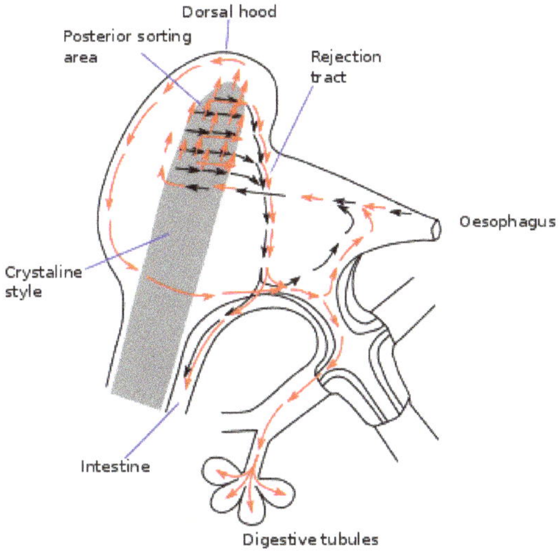

Figure 3. Schematic representation of the particle flow through the digestive system of a bivalve (redrawn and simplified from Owen [98]). Black arrows represent large particles and red arrows small particles.

The ingested particles could be selectively diverted to the intestine and eliminated with feces without further processing by post-ingestive selection, which has been documented for several species and types of particles [92,104–106]. This kind of selection has not been demonstrated for *Dinophysis*, but it was shown for another okadaic acid producer [107,108], *Prorocentrum lima*, where this mechanism was hypothesized as being a way to reduce the accumulation of the toxin and avoid its possible effects [108].

4. Digestion and Uptake

Digestion in bivalves has two components: one is extracellular, which takes place mostly in the stomach and crystalline style sac, and the other is intracellular, which takes place mostly in the cells of the digestive tubules (Figure 4). In the first step, the ingested particles, including *Dinophysis* and other phytoplankton cells, are broken down and consequently, the released substances are subjected to the action of both the autolytic enzymes of the ingested phytoplankton and the digestive enzymes secreted by the bivalve. The pH of the digestive system is also different from the one in seawater but it is not extreme, with its minimum value being around 6. Neither the enzymatic activity nor the pH levels seem to degrade or transform the main *Dinophysis*-produced toxins [64,109], as the amounts of toxin ingested and excreted have been found to be approximately the same. At least some of their derivatives, notwithstanding, could be hydrolyzed to the main toxins or to other (simpler) derivatives. The enzymes of the diatom *Thalassiosira weissflogii*, for example, were shown to quickly convert DTX4 and DTX5 to diol-esters, and those, at a lower rate, to the main toxins [110]. The same processes are known to take place with autolytic enzymes of the OA producer *Prorocentrum lima*, as shown by the fact that the cell concentrates must be boiled to inactivate enzymes to obtain these compounds [36,111,112]. It can be expected that enzymes of this kind will be released into the stomach after cell breakage and catalyze the hydrolysis as discussed earlier. The digestive enzymes of the bivalves also play a role in transformations of this type as these compounds are quickly hydrolyzed by esterases [34] and bivalves secrete enzymes of this group [69,113]. Some studies of the time-course of OA, DTX2 (and their conjugated forms) depuration in the mussel *Mytilus galloprovincialis* showed a quick decrease in conjugated forms just after *Dinophysis* ingestion stopped, which was interpreted as corresponding to the hydrolysis of the conjugated forms acquired from the *Dinophysis* cells [44,114]. Mackenzie et al. [115] isolated a digestive esterase from the green mussel *Perna canaliculus*, which has the capability of hydrolyzing diol-esters, as well as 7-O-acyl esters, of OA (which may also be also present in seston after OA is biotransformed by *Dinophysis* consumers). It is possible that not all diol-esters are hydrolyzed at the same rate, as the activity of the enzyme varies noticeably with the chain length of several 4-nitrophenyl esters tested [115].

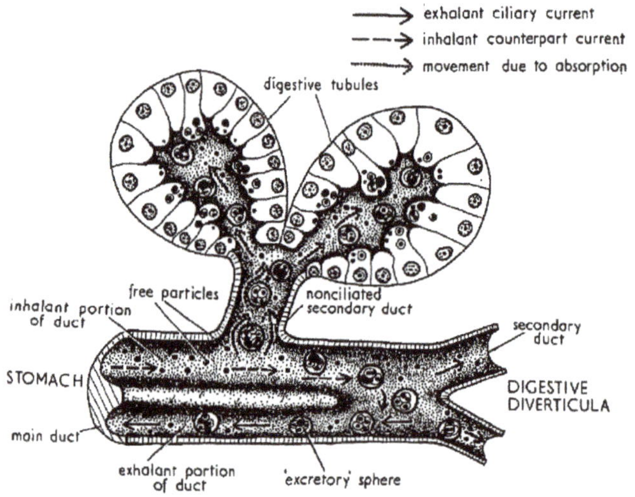

Figure 4. Structure of the digestive tubules and diverticula, showing incoming particles and outgoing excretory spheres (rejection bodies). Reproduced with permission from Owen [98], published by Company of Biologists 1955.

Much less information is available on pectenotoxins. The main change induced by digestive processes is the opening of the macrolactone ring to produce a secoic acid. As discussed earlier, the esterase isolated from *P. viridis* catalyzes this transformation of some, but not all, pectenotoxins. PTX2 and PTX1, for example, are readily hydrolyzed while PTX11, PTX2c, and other analogues are not affected. Additionally, at least the latter two compounds act as competitive inhibitors of PTX2 hydrolysis [115], which may also be true of equivalent enzymes of other bivalve species.

From the stomach, the partially digested material is diverted to the digestive tubules where extracellular digestion is completed, and where intracellular digestion takes place [69,113]. The uptake of the toxins of the OA group by digestive cells has been the object of very few studies, but there are several mechanisms that could be involved. Rossignoli [64] found that OA was taken up by fragments of digestive gland much faster when supplied in dissolved form than in an emulsion of oil droplets. Moreover, it was recently found that dissolved OA and DTX1 can be taken out by different tissues of the mussel *Mytilus galloprovincialis* [63], but especially by the digestive gland. Even when, at the pH levels found in the digestive gland, the main toxins of the OA group are ionized, in view of their pKa [116], they were shown to be able to self-assemble [66] or to form aggregates of several molecules [65] in a way that hides the charged parts of the molecule, allowing them to pass through the lipid bilayers (as cell membranes). Diol-esters are less polar than their corresponding main toxins and the carboxylic function, being combined with a diol, cannot be charged. Hence, they could be taken up more easily than the free toxins. It would be expected that the toxins taken up by this mechanism are initially stored in the cytosol, as was found for OA by Rossignoli and Blanco [117] and by Guéguen et al. (mostly) [118].

Some endocytic mechanisms, such as phagocytosis or pinocytosis that are involved in the uptake of different components of food by digestive cells, do not require the toxins to be uncharged because they do not need to pass through the cellular membrane (Figure 5). Dissolved OA could be absorbed mainly by means of phagocytosis when associated with debris of *Dinophysis* cells, or by pinocytosis, in addition to diffusion through the membrane, when it is in solution. In both cases, the toxins would enter the cell inside endosomes that would be progressively converted into lysosomes. Guéguen et al. [118] found a noticeable proportion of the cellular okadaic acid to be located in lysosomes, which means that this route of uptake could also be important. Phagocytosis has been suggested for highly lipophilic xenobiotics [119], with an octanol-water partition coefficient ≥ 4 (log P), because they are mostly associated (adsorbed or dissolved into them) with organic particles or lipid droplets [120].

Phytoplanktonic pectenotoxins, which have a polarity similar to that of OA, and which are not ionized at a pH below 8, are expected to share the same uptake routes.

The dominance of one route or another is probably a complex mixture of the distribution of toxins in the lumen of the digestive tubules, the concentration of free toxins in the cytosol of the cells and the rates of diffusion (passive or facilitated) or phagocytosis.

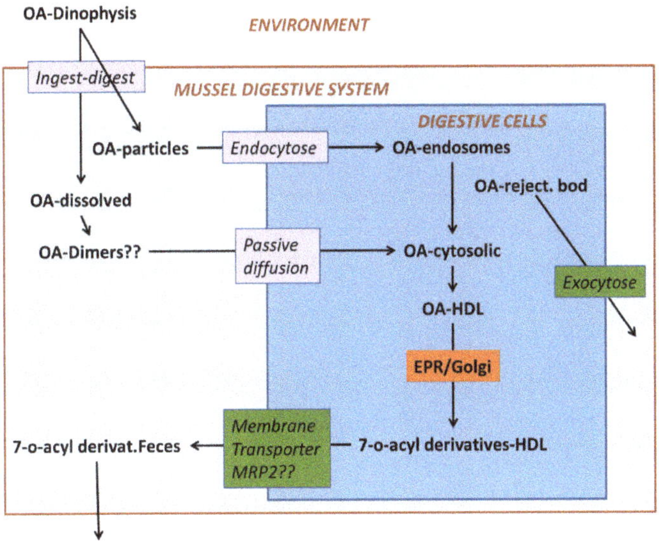

Figure 5. Hypothetical steps involved in the accumulation of toxins in the okadaic acid (OA) group.

5. Compartmentalization

When the toxins enter the digestive gland cells, they are distributed heterogeneously between the different types and the different parts of the cells. Okadaic acid was shown to be stored preferentially in the digestive cells of *M. galloprovincialis* rather than the secretory cells [121] (the two main cellular types that integrate the digestive tubules) [113,122]. The structure and function of each cellular type could explain this preferential storage, as secretory cells present less surface to tubule lumen than digestive cells, and their function as secretory cells does not include endocytic processes.

Once inside the cells, okadaic is mostly located in the cytosol and bounded to (or dissolved into) high-density lipoprotein(s) (HDL) [117] (the same was observed for acyl-derivatives of OA, unpublished information), but in some cases, a noticeable proportion of OA could be also found in lysosomes or similar cellular structures [118]. It seems very likely that the toxin contained in the lysosomes entered the cell by means of an endocytic mechanism and in the cytosolic fraction it entered the cell in dissolved form and/or was transferred to the cytosol from the lysosomes.

The association with HDLs probably has a transport function, since this group of proteins is strongly linked to the transport of lipophilic substances in the organism. In humans, for example, HDLs in association with ABC membrane transporters are responsible for removing excess cholesterol from cells and transporting it to the liver and other steroidogenic tissues to be metabolized and excreted [123].

There is no information available on the cellular or subcellular distribution of pectenotoxins, but it would seem likely that they share this with other compounds of similar polarity, such as OA or cholesterol.

Anatomically, both pectenotoxins and toxins of the OA group are heterogeneously distributed among organs and/or tissues. Okadaic acid has been shown to be concentrated especially in the digestive gland of the mussels *Mytilus galloprovincialis* [124], *M. edulis* [86,125–127], and in the scallop *Argopecten irradians* [108]. It also appears to be the case with two Australian scallop species, *Pecten fumatus* [128] and *P. maximus* [129], the clams *Spisula solida* and *Donax trunculus* [130], and the razor clam *Pinna bicolor* [128]. Notwithstanding, recently in *Crenomytilus grayanus*, it was found that the acyl-esters of OA were more abundant in other organs than in the digestive gland (quantified by means of ELISA assay) [131].

Little information is available on pectenotoxins, even though it is generally admitted that the digestive gland is the main accumulator of this group of toxins, and this organ was used to isolate pectenotoxins as a step prior to their purification (e.g., Daiguji et al. [48]). In the Chilean surf clam *Mesodesma donacium* PTX2 and PTX2sa were 10-fold more concentrated in the digestive gland than in the remaining tissues, and the esters were nearly absent outside the digestive gland (approx. 300 times less concentrated) [132]

It is highly likely that compartmentalization influences depuration. As the main organs involved in excretion in bivalves are the kidney and digestive gland, the toxins located in other body tissues would probably be transported to these organs before starting depuration, which would slow down the process.

6. Transformation

The toxins produced by *Dinophysis* undergo transformations during the extracellular digestive process, as is the case of the hydrolysis of conjugated forms of the toxins in the OA group (Figure 6), and the formation of secoic acids of the pectenotoxins (Figure 7). Thereafter, they are partially transformed inside the cells of the bivalves. The main transformation route is the esterification with fatty acids of different chain lengths. In the toxins of the OA group, the hydroxyl group in C7 is frequently esterified with fatty acids, forming 7-O-acyl derivatives, generically known as DTX3 [133].

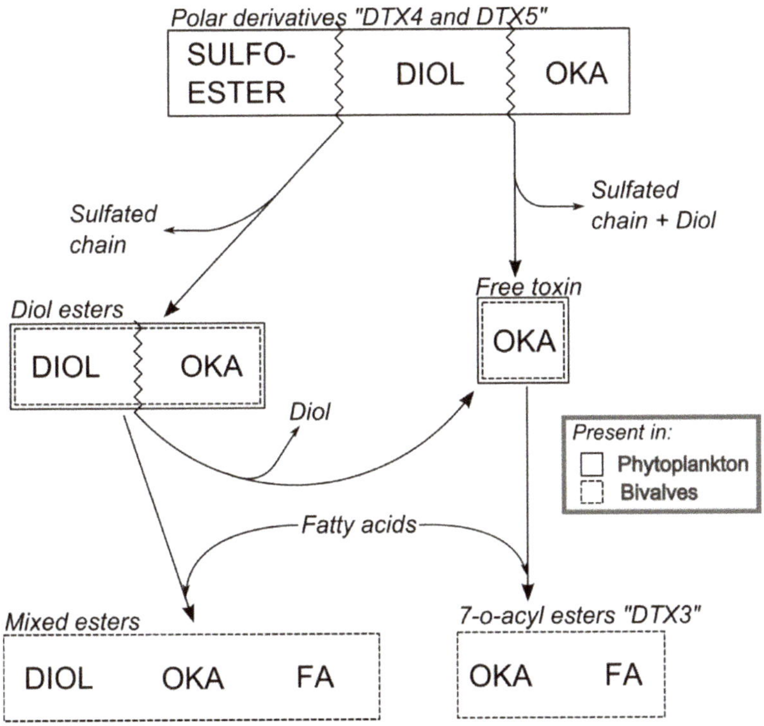

Figure 6. Main transformations of the toxins of the okadaic acid group. Labels inside the boxes indicate the moieties that constitute the molecule. Zigzag lines indicate the bonds that are broken to generate other compounds. The line(s) of each box indicate whether the compounds are found in phytoplankton or in bivalves. From Reguera et al. [74].

The free toxins undergo an esterification with fatty acids [134,135], where the microsomal fraction of the digestive gland cells—probably originating from the endoplasmic reticulum—is involved [134]. In some cases it seems that diol- or triol-esters which may not be partially hydrolyzed during the digestion process, are also esterified yielding mixed (or hybrid) esters, where the carboxylic function of the OA (or other analogues) is esterifying a diol or triol and a hydroxyl (in C7 of the OA or in any location of the diol/triol) is esterified with a fatty acid [38]. The proportion of the different fatty acids involved in the formation of the esters is variable, depending mainly on the bivalve species. Linear fatty acids with an even number of carbon atoms are frequent in all molluscs [136–141], and the esters of OA and PTX are usually formed with these fatty acids. Nevertheless, some infaunal species like cockles and clams, seem to have a noticeable proportion of odd-chain and branched-chain fatty acids involved in the esterification of the toxins [136], which Vale [142] hypothesized as possibly being caused by bacterial action.

Not all bivalve species have the same esterification capability and not all toxins are esterified at the same rate. In most of the studied bivalve species, the esterification is fast, reaching nearly 100% soon after the supply of free toxins is interrupted. This is the case, for example, of the cockle *Cerastoderma edule*, the peppery furrow shell *Scrobicularia plana*, the carpet shell *Venerupis pullastra*, the Pacific oyster *Crassostrea japonica* (*Magallana gigas*), the razor clams *Ensis* spp., *Ruditapes decussatus* [143,144], the European flat oyster *Ostrea edulis* [26,144,145], the surf clam *Spisula* [146], the littleneck clam *Leukoma staminea* [143], the scallop *Patinopecten yessoensis* [147,148], the Manila clam *Ruditapes philippinarum* (unpublished data), and some Chilean mussels (the blue mussel *M. chilensis* and the ribbed mussel *Aulacomya ater* [149]). In other mussels, such as *Mytilus edulis* [144],

M. galloprovincialis [44,114,130,134,148,150–152], *M. coruscus* [139], and *Crenomytilus grayanus* [131]), as well as in some other species, like the clam *Donax trunculus* [136] or the variegated scallop *Aequipecten opercularis* (unpublished observation), the proportion of esterified toxins is usually much lower than 100%.

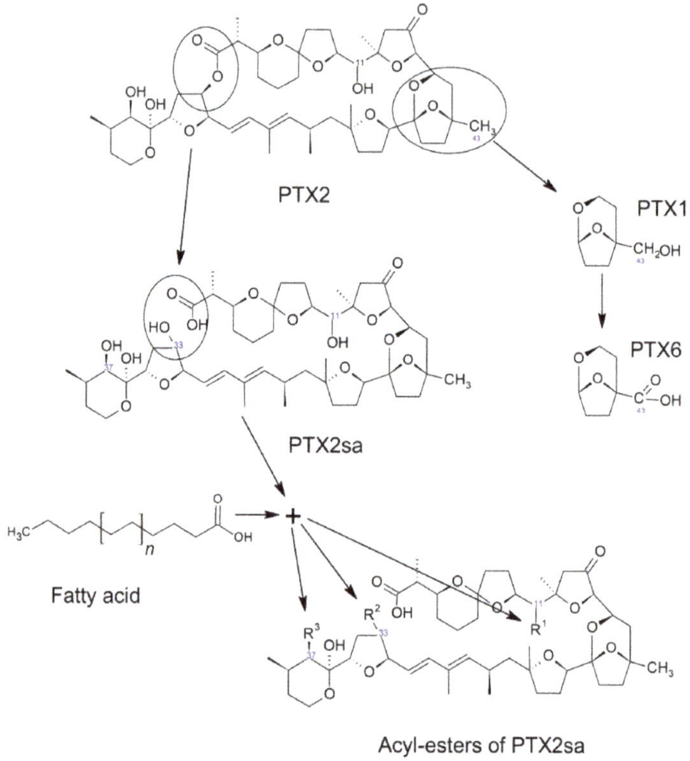

Figure 7. Transformations of PTX2 in bivalves.

Different toxins could be differentially esterified, depending on the species. In general, it seems that the species that readily esterify OA (most infaunal species and oysters) do not show important differences between toxins, whilst other species, such as *Mytilus galloprovincialis* or *M. edulis*, for example, where OA is only partially esterified, esterify other toxins of the same group much less efficiently. In Norway [144], the flat oyster *Ostrea edulis*, was shown to contain a high proportion of esterified OA (86%) and also high proportions of esterified DTX1 and DTX2 (93 and 83%, respectively), whilst the blue mussel *Mytilus edulis*, with only 41% of the OA esterified, contained substantially lower proportions of esterified DTX1 and DTX2 (27 and 21%, respectively). The same pattern was found in an intoxication experiment with the same species and toxins involved [145], and in the early work of Marr et al. [141]. In Portugal, Vale and Sampayo [150] found no difference in the esterification of OA and DTX2, in most clams, cockle, and oyster, which esterified these compounds almost completely. However, they did find a substantially lower percentage of esterified DTX2 than OA in mussels, where the proportion of esterified OA was less than 50%. The same pattern was also observed in Galicia (NW Spain) [153].

Pectenotoxins are also transformed inside bivalves. The most frequent transformation seems to be the opening of the macrolactone ring to produce the seco-acids corresponding to each toxin [46,48,52,59–61,130,132,145,152,154–159]. It is very likely that this transformation takes place during digestion, as found by MacKenzie et al. [115] in *Perna canaliculus* and other species.

Notwithstanding, the transformation from pectenotoxins to their corresponding seco-acids is a species- and toxin- dependent process. The Japanese scallop *Patinopecten yessoensis*, for example, does not hydrolyze the macrolactone ring of PTX2, and consequently it does not generate seco-acids [49,160,161]. There are other bivalve species which have been found to be unable to transform PTX2 into its seco-acid when this toxin was incubated with homogenates of their hepatopancreas or other organs [115]. While the enzyme isolated from *Perna canaliculus* can hydrolyze PTX2 and PTX1, it does not have the same capability for some of their stereoisomers, such as PTX2b and c, and with other compounds of the same group, as PTX6 and PTX11 [45]. PTX12 seco-acids also seem to be less readily formed than those of PTX2 in blue mussels from Norway, but not in the cockle *Cerastoderma edule* from the same location (at least in some cases) [46].

Patinopecten yessoensis transforms pectenotoxins in a significantly different way (Figure 7). This species performs a series of successive oxidations of C-43. From PTX2, its hydroxy (PTX1), its aldehyde (PTX3), and finally its carboxylic derivative (PTX6) are formed [49,162]. As far as we know, this sequential oxidation route of PTX2 has only be found in *Patinopecten yessoensis*, and it has the additional peculiarity that it does not take place *in vitro* by incubation with digestive gland extracts [162]. However, the possibility that this process could take place in other bivalve species cannot be ruled out.

The seco-acid of PTX2, at least in some bivalves, undergoes an esterification with fatty acids, as happens with other lipophilic compounds, like okadaic acid and dinophysistoxins 1 and 2 [134] or steroids [163,164]. Three types of esters have been described, depending on the position of the esterified hydroxyl group: C-11, C-37, and C-33 [165]. These esterified forms could be found in some bivalves in a noticeable proportion in relation to PTX2 and PTX2sa [132]. Like the 7-O-acyl esters of the okadaic acid group, several fatty acids may be involved and the mechanism could also be a trans-esterification in which Coenzyme A is involved. In the digestive gland of mussels (*M. galloprovincialis*), an overexpression of genes related to the Coenzyme A activity has been found after exposure to the OA-producing organism *Prorocentrum lima* [166].

7. Depuration

Lipophilic toxins do not remain in bivalves indefinitely. They are eliminated from their organs (depurated) at rates that are species- and toxin-dependent. During the intoxication phase, toxins are stored into two main compartments: (a) The outer part of the digestive system (stomach, gut, digestive diverticula), and (b) inside the cells of different organs, mainly the digestive gland. During the depuration phase, shortly after the supply of toxic organisms ceased, the first compartment loses most of its importance, because it includes only the toxins that are being released with feces. Obviously, the mechanisms involved in the elimination of the toxins from each of these two compartments would be completely different. In the case of the first compartment, depuration consists only (or almost only) of the evacuation of the toxins and/or of the particles containing them from the lumen of the digestive organs. In this case, the velocity of the depuration would be related to the rate of renewal of the digestive system, and therefore to the gut passage time, which in turn, is related to the volume of the ingested material. Neither the renewal rate nor the forms in which the toxins are present are expected to be the same in the digestive diverticula and the remaining parts of the digestive system. The digestive diverticula receive material that have already been processed in the stomach and which have been subjected to post-ingestive selection. On the contrary, the stomach and gut contain materials that are unprocessed, are being processed, or have been negatively selected due to their characteristics and/or because of an excess amount of food to be processed. Typically, gut content is renewed within hours, but renewing the diverticula content takes days.

Once the toxins are inside the cells, the depuration mechanisms involved are not very well known. In the okadaic acid group at least, the degradation of the main toxin structural backbone does not seem to be important in light of the existing mass balance studies [64]. As far as we know, no mass balance of the pectenotoxins in the bivalves has been carried out, in part because of the methodological difficulties entailed in quantifying seco-acid esters. Hence, the possibility of the degradation of these toxins cannot be ruled out. In fact, the formation of seco-acids could be considered a degradation of the toxin as the structure is substantially modified by opening the macrolactone cycle and its toxicity is lost.

Therefore, it seems that efflux from the cells would be the main process involved in depuration. Efflux by means of passive diffusion is unlikely because, if that mechanism were important, no accumulation of the toxins would take place. Thus, active efflux through the plasma membrane would take place. This can be done by means of protein membrane transporters or by vesicular transport. In the first case, a number of transporters may be involved, but only a few have been studied. Martínez-Escauriaza [167] and Lozano [168] found in mussels exposed to okadaic acid, an overexpression of genes that codify for membrane transporters, more precisely for a Multidrug Resistance Protein (MDR1, P-glycoprotein) and a Multidrug Resistance-Related Protein (MRP2), both of the ATP-Binding Cassette (ABC) type, which, as commented above, are related to the transport of excess cholesterol and involved in the elimination of multiple xenobiotics from bivalve cells [169–176]. Huang et al. [177] found that the genes that codify for a p-glycoprotein (MDR type) were overexpressed in the mussel *Perna viridis* after its exposure to the OA-producing dinoflagellate *Prorocentrum lima*. Notwithstanding, some specific inhibitors of the activity of the equivalent protein in humans did not increase the amount of OA accumulated by the mussels, which led the authors to suggest that MRP-type proteins could be involved in the efflux of OA. It should be taken into account that inhibitors, known to be effective in human transporter proteins, might be ineffective in their bivalve homologues [170].

The acylation of the molecules of the OA group seems to be an important step in depuration (with the exception of short-term depuration), as most toxins found in bivalve feces are conjugated with fatty acids [64] (+additional unpublished information). This depuration route holds true even for species with a relatively low acylation capability for these toxins, such as the mussel *Mytilus galloprovincialis*, and suggests that the main route for depuration is selective enough to exclude the free forms of the toxins, which suggests that it includes a selective transporter. In fact, from that mussel, DTX2 which esterifies to a lower percentage than OA, depurates more slowly [114,130,145,152].

Vesicular transport could also contribute to depuration. The formation of excretion spheres is a common mechanism of digestive cells to eliminate unassimilated substances (Figures 4 and 8), and we have observed that feeding toxic mussels with substances which bind OA and that cannot be easily digested, like Diaion HP-20 (a synthetic resin) or Olestra (a polyester of sucrose with fatty acids, from Procter and Gamble) substantially accelerated the depuration velocity [64] (Figure 9).

Suárez-Ulloa et al. [166] found that genes related to vesicle-mediated transport are overexpressed in the mussel digestive gland after exposure to the OA producer dinoflagellate *Prorocentrum lima*, which could also support our findings with Diaion and Olestra.

The depuration rates of these toxins are also dependent on the bivalve species and the toxin. It is difficult to extract reliable depuration rates from the literature because they have been obtained in different ways, and in many cases, do not consider all the processes that could affect the amount of a particular toxin in the bivalve body, for instance: (a) In some cases, the change in the toxin burden of the bivalves was used to estimate the rates; however, in many other instances, toxin concentration was used, which means that the estimates are affected by changes in body weight. (b) The whole body was used in some cases, and the digestive gland alone in others. (c) The total amount of a toxin or a particular form of the toxins has also been used. In the former case, the estimated depuration rate is the real depuration rate, but if a particular form of a toxin (free form, for example) is used, then the depuration rate obtained is only apparent because the actual rate is increased by the loss of that form of the toxin—not only by depuration but also by transformation to other forms (for example to acyl-derivatives). Moreover, it is decreased by the transformation of other forms to it (for example from diol-esters to OA) (see some examples in Figure 8, in which some forms of the toxins that do not depurate in the model, have "apparent" depuration rates higher than the forms that are actually depurated). (d) In the cases in which depuration was estimated from bioassay or immunoassay data, the estimates are affected by the toxin profile and its changes. The following data should therefore be considered rough approximations.

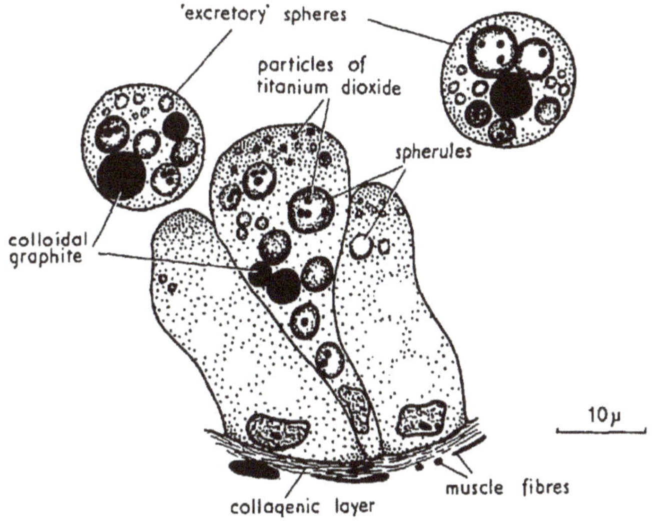

Figure 8. Cells of a digestive tubule after being fed with particles of titanium oxide and colloidal graphite showing the formation and expulsion of excretory spheres containing these materials. Reproduced with permission from Owen [98], published by Company of Biologists 1955.

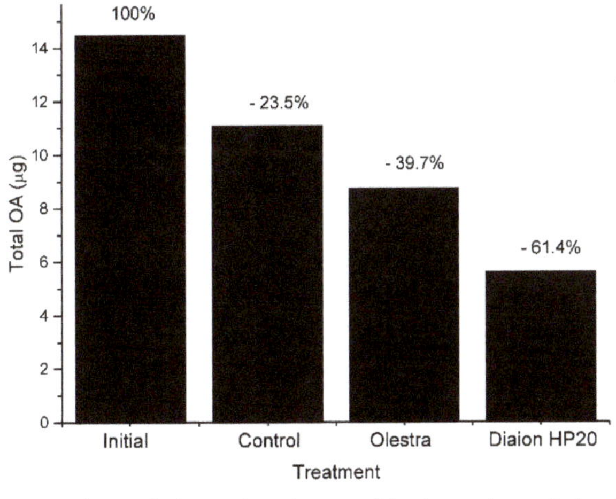

Figure 9. Content in okadaic acid of mussels at the start of the depuration period and after one week. Initial = start of the experiment. Control, Olestra, and Diaion HP20 = after one week being fed with *Tetraselmis suecica* (control), supplemented with Olestra and Diaion HP20.

In general, the elimination of OA, usually estimated by fitting a first-order exponential decay, is relatively fast in all molluscs. In cultured Galician mussels *Mytilus galloprovincialis*, average depuration rates were around 0.17 to 0.07 day^{-1} or even less at the final part of the depuration phase [44,114,178,179]; 0.19 in *M. galloprovincialis* in the Adriatic sea [180]; and 0.13 in Portugal [130]; approx. 0.13 for Briton and Mediterranean mussels, respectively [181]; 0.05 for *M. edulis* from Norway [145] and 0.13 from Denmark [182]; between 0.07 and 0.17 for *Donax trunculus* [130,183], 0.22 for *Spisula solida* [130], and 0.23 for *Perna viridis* [184].

In general, the estimates of the depuration rates for DTX1 and DTX2 are equal to or lower than for OA [114,145,152]. In *Mytilus galloprovincialis* and *Donax trunculus*—species with low esterification rates—DTX1 and DTX2 are depurated more slowly than OA, which also seems to be true for species with a moderate esterification capability, such as the European oyster *Ostrea edulis* [145]. In several species with high esterification rates, like the cockle *Cardium edule* and others, OA and DTX2 appear to be depurated at similar rates [130,152]. The most likely reason is that these toxins are mostly (after the first steps) depurated as esters, and considering that depuration is proportional to the concentration of the toxin to be depurated, a lower proportion of esters leads to a lower depuration rate.

Very few studies have examined the depuration of esters. Vale [130,152] estimated the depuration rates of OA and DTX2 esters to be higher than those of their free form counterparts, but the opposite was found by Lindegarth et al. [145]. This could be explained because the number of accumulated esters is determined by the balance between esterification and depuration, and consequently, the estimated depuration is only "apparent" and not the real one.

The estimation of the depuration of pectenotoxins is even more inaccurate than that of the toxins of the okadaic acid group because it is impossible to measure the total toxin. In toxins of the OA group, it is possible to transform all chemical forms into free toxins by hydrolysis, but this is not possible with pectenotoxins due to their instability under extreme pH conditions. For example, the estimates of the depuration of PTX2 are overestimated because it is simultaneously depurated and transformed into PTX2sa. The estimates corresponding to PTX2sa are on the one hand, overestimated because it is transformed into PTX2sa-acyl esters, and on the other, underestimated because it derives from PTX2. Even if all these steps are combined in a model, it would be difficult to obtain a correct estimate because it is not possible to quantify all PTX2-acyl esters due to the huge number of possible combinations of fatty acids and locations in the molecule of the esterified hydroxyls.

The "apparent" depuration rate of PTX2 was estimated to be 0.09 day^{-1} for the Norwegian blue mussel *Mytilus edulis* and the flat oyster *Ostrea edulis* [145]. In another mussel, *M. galloprovincialis*, in Portugal, the estimated rate was much higher (0.6–1.1 day^{-1}), as was the case of the cockle *Cerastoderma edule* (1–3 day^{-1}) [152] and the Chilean surf clam *Mesodesma donacium* [132]. In the Norwegian and Portuguese species, the "apparent" depuration rates of PTX2 were higher than those of OA.

The "apparent" depuration rate of PTX2sa in the flat oyster and *M. edulis* from Norway were similar to that of PTX2 (0.1 and 0.09 day^{-1}, respectively) [145]. In the two species studied in Portugal, *C. edule* depurated at a slower rate (0.38 day^{-1}) and *M. galloprovincialis* at a similar rate (1.04 day^{-1}) [152]. In *Mesodesma donacium* the "apparent" depuration rate showed a decreasing trend with the degree of biotransformation, ranging from 0.3 day^{-1} for PTX2 to 0.2 day^{-1} for palmytoyl-PTX2sa, with an intermediate value of 0.23 day^{-1} for PTX2sa [132].

8. Accumulation Kinetics and Modeling

Different models have been used to describe the accumulation kinetics of lipophilic and hydrophilic toxins [185]. For toxin acquisition, the simplest approach assumes a constant feeding rate (K), and a toxin uptake that depends on the feeding rate, the toxin content of the water (TCW), and the absorption efficiency

$$\mathrm{dTox/dt = K \cdot TCW \cdot (AE)} \quad (1)$$

where TCW can be computed by multiplying the toxic cell concentration in water ($\mathrm{Cell_{water}}$) by the toxin content per cell ($\mathrm{Tox_{cell}}$)

$$\mathrm{dTox/dt = K \cdot Cell_{water} \cdot Tox_{cell} \cdot AE} \quad (2)$$

When, after entering the digestive gland, toxins are distributed to other organs or tissues, a multicompartment (usually a two-compartment) model could be used, where the main compartment

(compartment 1) acquires the toxin and then it loses a part to the second compartment. In such a case, losses are usually assumed to be proportional to the amount or concentration of toxin

$$dTox_1/dt = K \cdot Cell_{water} \cdot Tox_{cell} \cdot AE - TR_{1\text{-}2} \cdot Tox_1 \quad (3)$$

$$dTox_2/dt = + TR_{1\text{-}2} \cdot Tox_1 \quad (4)$$

where subindices refer to the compartment and TR is the Transfer Rate between compartments.

When large differences are found in cell concentration in the water, then it might be necessary to express AE (absorption efficiency) as a function of the available cell (or particle) volume which determines the gut passage time (GPT), and consequently the AE, and even to express the feeding rate K as a function of the cell or seston concentration (see Sections 2 and 3).

When several toxins or toxin derivatives are present, including biotransformations in the kinetic models is mandatory. For example, if diol-esters or sulphated OA or DTXs derivatives (okadaates) are present in *Dinophysis* cells, the free toxins are going to be released and the time course of their abundance cannot be correctly described without transformations. This could explain the anomalies in the accumulation kinetics found by Svensson [186]. Fernández et al. [114] and Moroño et al. [44] included the transformation of these kinds of toxins into free forms, thus improving the model fitting and obtaining what appears to be more realistic estimates of different rates in the model. In OA and Okadaates, the equations would be:

$$dOA = K \cdot Cell_{water} \cdot OA_{cell} \cdot AE + HR \cdot Okadaates \quad (5)$$

$$dOkadaates/dt = K \cdot Cell_{water} \cdot Okadaates_{cell} \cdot AE - HR \cdot Okadaates \quad (6)$$

where OA_{cell} and $Okadaates_{cell}$ are the concentrations of OA and Okadaates in the cells, and HR is the rate of hydrolysis of Okadaates into OA.

Needless to say, several toxins, derivatives, and compartments could be included.

After the first steps of toxin acquisition, toxin losses due to depuration and/or metabolic transformations of the compounds start to be quantitatively important and should be included in the models. Both biotransformations (formation of 7-O-acyl derivatives ("DTX3"), for example) and depuration are usually assumed to be dependent on the amount (or concentration) of the accumulated toxin. The system of Equations (5) and (6) should be modified to include these two components. Assuming that only 7-O-acyl esters are eliminated, the equation system would be the following:

$$dOA = K \cdot Cell_{water} \cdot OA_{cell} \cdot AE + HR \cdot Okadaates - AR \cdot OA \quad (7)$$

$$dOkadaates/dt = K \cdot Cell_{water} \cdot Okadaates_{cell} \cdot AE - HR \cdot Okadaates \quad (8)$$

$$dDTX3 = + AR \cdot OA - DR \cdot DTX3 \quad (9)$$

where DR is the depuration rate of "DTX3".

It is clearly necessary to know the toxin forms that are depurated to correctly formulate a model. In the toxins of the OA group, the 7-O-acyl esters appear to be the main toxin form that is depurated, but in the case of pectenotoxins no information is available. Noticeable differences in the kinetics could derive from the routes modeled, as can be observed in some examples in Figure 10.

In the initial steps of depuration, when the undigested toxin stored in the digestive system is quantitatively important, it could be necessary to include an additional compartment and reformulate the models to fit its kinetics. Some possible approaches have been suggested (for particulate matter) by Penry [187].

The build-up of biomass can also be included in the models, thus allowing in this way to describe and predict the allometric changes during the time-course of toxin accumulation.

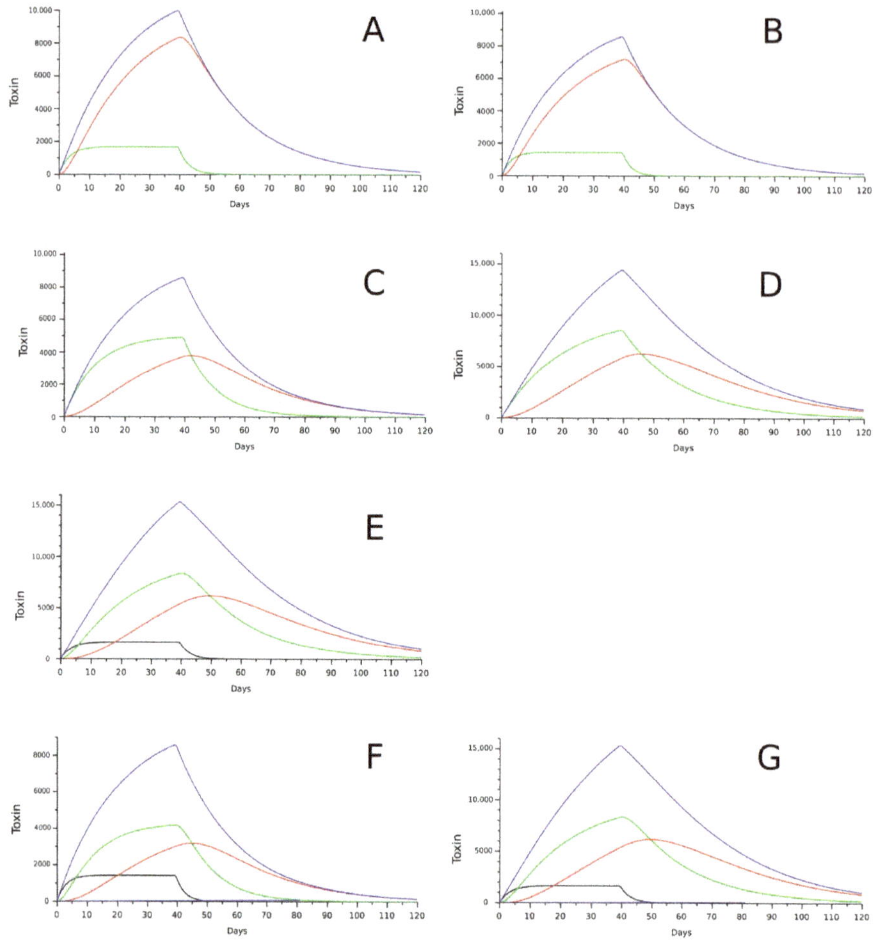

Figure 10. Models of the kinetics of OA and "DTX3" (**A–D**), the previous ones plus "DTX5" (**E**), and PTX2, PTX2sa and its esters (**F,G**), after 40 days of intoxication (with constant cell abundance in the environment) and 80 days of depuration. The blue line represents total toxin, black is "DTX5" or PTX2, green shows OA or PTX2sa and red, DTX3 or PTX2sa esters. Kinetics with high acylation rate (=0.3 day^{-1}) with only DTX3 depuration (**A**), and with OA and DTX3 depuration at the same rate (**B**). Kinetics with low acylation rate (0.05 day-1) with only DTX3 depuration (**C**), and with OA and DTX3 depuration at the same rate as in A and B (**D**). Same as C with input of OA and "DTX5" (50%) (**E**). With depuration of the three forms of PTX2 (**F**) and with depuration of only PTX2sa esters (**G**).

Recently, a DEB (Dynamic Energy Budgets) model was developed for PSP toxins in the Pacific oyster [188]. Models of this kind include the main metabolic processes of bivalves (including spawning) and would be especially useful when long-term simulations are needed.

9. Perspectives

Many areas still need considerable efforts to gather the knowledge that would facilitate the understanding and prediction of the accumulation of toxins produced by *Dinophysis* in bivalve molluscs. When dealing with toxin acquisition, it is necessary to evaluate the effects of *Dinophysis* populations on filtration and on the efficiencies of pre- and post-ingestive selection, as well as the precise mechanism involved in the toxin uptake by the bivalve cells. The mechanisms of depuration for the different toxins, and their interconnection with biotransformation, should also be studied in depth. The use of transcriptomic methodology is promising, but currently, the complexity of the results obtained, together with the lack of knowledge of the precise functions of proteins with or without mammal homologues, makes it difficult to obtain solid and interpretable results. Linking molluscan genes (especially those that codify for membrane transporters) to their actual function would lead to a considerable advance in the elucidation of the depuration mechanisms. It is also important to know which forms of the toxins are eliminated from the bivalves, since they condition not only the possible depuration mechanisms, but also the correct kinetics that should be modeled to obtain a good prediction capability.

In addition to allowing for the development of more precise predictive models, a good knowledge of the mechanisms involved in the accumulation of toxins from *Dinophysis*, would make it easier to develop genetic selection programs, to obtain bivalves with a reduced ability to acquire toxins or with an increased ability to eliminate them. It would also allow development of effective depuration treatments for bivalve species with high commercial value.

Funding: This research received no external funding.

Acknowledgments: I acknowledge Ángeles Moroño for critically reviewing the manuscript.

Conflicts of Interest: The authors declare no conflict of interest.

References

1. Yasumoto, T.; Oshima, Y.; Yamaguchi, M. Occurrence of a new type of shellfish poisoning in the Tohoku district. *Bull. Jpn. Soc. Sci. Fish.* **1978**, *44*, 1249–1255. [CrossRef]
2. Yasumoto, T.; Oshima, Y.; Yamaguchi, M. Occurrence of a new type of toxic shellfish in Japan and chemical properties of the toxin. In *Toxic Dinoflagellate Blooms*; Taylor, D.L., Seliger, H.W., Eds.; Elsevier: New York, NY, USA, 1979; pp. 395–398.
3. Murata, M.; Shimatani, M.; Sugitani, H.; Oshima, Y.; Yasumoto, T. Isolation and structural elucidation of the causative toxin of diarrhetic shellfish poisoning. *Bull. Jpn. Soc. Sci. Fish.* **1982**, *48*, 549–552. [CrossRef]
4. Tachibana, K.; Scheuer, P.; Tsukitani, Y.; Kikuchi, H.; Enden, V.; Clardy, J.; Gopichand, Y.; Schmitz, F. Okadaic acid, a cytotoxic polyether from two marine sponges of the genus *Halichondria*. *J. Am. Chem. Soc.* **1981**, *103*, 2469–2471. [CrossRef]
5. Tangen, K. Shellfish poisoning and the ocurrence of potentially toxic dinoflagellates in Norwegian waters. *Sarsia* **1983**, *68*, 1–7. [CrossRef]
6. Kat, M. Diarrhetic mussel poisoning in the Netherlands related to the dinoflagellate *Dinophysis acuminata*. *Antonie Van Leeuenhoek* **1983**, *49*, 417–427.
7. Kumagai, M.; Yanagi, T.; Murata, M.; Yasumoto, T.; Kat, M.; Lassus, P.; Rodriguez-Vázquez, J.A. Okadaic acid as the causative toxin of Diarrhetic Shellfish Poisoning in Europe. *Agric. Biol. Chem.* **1986**, *50*, 2853–2857.
8. Van Egmond, H.P.; Aune, T.; Lassus, P.; Speijers, G.J.A.; Waldock, M. Paralytic and diarrhoeic shellfish poisons: Occurrence in Europe, toxicity, analysis and regulation. *J. Nat. Toxins* **1993**, *2*, 41–82.
9. James, K.J.; Carey, B.; O'Halloran, J.; van Pelt, F.N.A.M.; Skrabakova, Z. Shellfish toxicity: Human health implications of marine algal toxins. *Epidemiol. Infect.* **2010**, *138*, 927–940. [CrossRef] [PubMed]
10. EFSA Panel on Contaminants in the Food Chain. Opinion of the Scientific Panel on Contaminants in the Food chain on a request from the European Commission on marine biotoxins in shellfish okadaic acid and analogues. *EFSA J.* **2008**, *589*, 1–62.
11. EFSA Panel on Contaminants in the Food Chain. Scientific Opinion of the Panel on Contaminants in the Food Chain on a request from the European Commission on Marine Biotoxins in Shellfish—Summary on regulated marine biotoxins. *EFSA J.* **2009**, *1306*, 1–23.
12. Anonymous. Commission Regulation (EU) No 15/2011. Amending Regulation (EC) No 2074/2005 as Regards Recognised Testing Methods for Detecting Marine Biotoxins in Live Bivalve Molluscs. Available online: https://eur-lex.europa.eu/LexUriServ/LexUriServ.do?uri=OJ:L:2011:006:0003:0006:EN:PDF (accessed on 24 October 2018).

13. EFSA Panel on Contaminants in the Food Chain. Marine biotoxins in shellfish—Pectenotoxin group: Marine biotoxins in shellfish—Pectenotoxin group. *EFSA J.* **2009**, *7*, 1109.
14. Fernández, M.L.; Shumway, S.E.; Blanco, J. Management of shellfish resources. In *Manual on Harmful Marine Microalgae*; Hallegraeff, G.M., Anderson, A.D., Anderson, D.M., Eds.; UNESCO Publishing: Paris, France, 2003; pp. 657–692.
15. Blanco, J.; Correa, J.; Muñíz, S.; Mariño, C.; Martín, H.; Arévalo, F. Evaluación del impacto de los métodos y niveles utilizados para el control de toxinas en el mejillón. *Revista Galega dos Recursos Mariños* **2013**, *3*, 1–55.
16. Lee, J.S.; Igarashi, T.; Fraga, S.; Dahl, E.; Hovgaard, P.; Yasumoto, T. Determination of diarrhetic shellfish toxins in various dinoflagellate species. *J. Appl. Phycol.* **1989**, *1*, 147–152. [CrossRef]
17. Fux, E.; Smith, J.L.; Tong, M.; Guzmán, L.; Anderson, D.M. Toxin profiles of five geographical isolates of *Dinophysis* spp. from North and South America. *Toxicon* **2011**, *57*, 275–287. [CrossRef] [PubMed]
18. Uribe, J.C.; García, C.; Rivas, M.; Lagos, N. First report of diarrhetic shellfish toxins in Magellanic fjord, Southern Chile. *J. Shellfish Res.* **2001**, *20*, 69–74.
19. Taylor, M.; McIntyre, L.; Ritson, M.; Stone, J.; Bronson, R.; Bitzikos, O.; Rourke, W.; Galanis, E.; Team, O. Outbreak of Diarrhetic Shellfish Poisoning Associated with Mussels, British Columbia, Canada. *Mar. Drugs* **2013**, *11*, 1669–1676. [CrossRef] [PubMed]
20. García-Mendoza, E.; Sánchez-Bravo, Y.A.; Turner, A.; Blanco, J.; O'Neil, A.; Mancera-Flores, J.; Pérez-Brunius, P.; Rivas, D.; Almazán-Becerril, A.; Peña-Manjarrez, J.L. Lipophilic toxins in Mediterranean Mussels from the northwest coast of Baja California, México. *Toxicon* **2014**, *90*, 111–123. [CrossRef] [PubMed]
21. Carmody, E.P.; James, K.J.; Kelly, S.S. Dinophysistoxin-2: The predominant diarrhetic shellfish toxin in Ireland. *Toxicon* **1996**, *34*, 351–359. [CrossRef]
22. Blanco, J.; Fernández, M.L.; Mariño, J.; Reguera, B.; Miguez, A.; Maneiro, J.; Cacho, E.; Martínez, A. From *Dinophysis* spp. toxicity to DSP outbreaks: Apreliminary model of toxin accumulation in mussels. In *Harmful Marine Algal Blooms*; Lassus, P., Arzul, G., Erard-Le Denn, E., Gentien, P., Marcaillou-Le Baut, C., Eds.; Lavoisier: Paris, France, 1995; pp. 777–782.
23. Gago, A.; Rodriguez-Vázquez, J.A.; Thibault, P.; Quilliam, M.A. Simultaneus occurrence of diarrhetic and paralytic shellfish poisoning toxins in Spanish mussels in 1993. *Nat. Toxins* **1996**, *4*, 72–79. [CrossRef]
24. Vale, P.; Sampayo, M.A. DTX-2 in Portuguese bivalves. In *Harmful and Toxic Algal Blooms*; Yasumoto, T., Oshima, Y., Fukuyo, Y., Eds.; IOC of UNESCO: Sendai, Japan, 1996; pp. 539–542.
25. Aune, T.; Larsen, S.; Aasen, J.A.B.; Rehmann, N.; Satake, M.; Hess, P. Relative Toxicity of Dinophysistoxin-2 (DTX-2) Compared With Okadaic Acid, Based on Acute Intraperitoneal Toxicity in Mice. *Toxicon* **2007**, *49*, 1–7. [CrossRef] [PubMed]
26. Dhanji-Rapkova, M.; O'Neill, A.; Maskrey, B.H.; Coates, L.; Teixeira Alves, M.; Kelly, R.J.; Hatfield, R.G.; Rowland-Pilgrim, S.J.; Lewis, A.M.; Algoet, M.; et al. Variability and profiles of lipophilic toxins in bivalves from Great Britain during five and a half years of monitoring: Okadaic acid, dinophysis toxins and pectenotoxins. *Harmful Algae* **2018**, *77*, 66–80. [CrossRef] [PubMed]
27. Elgarch, A.; Vale, P.; Rifai, S.; Fassouane, A. Detection of Diarrheic Shellfish Poisoning and Azaspiracid Toxins in Moroccan Mussels: Comparison of the LC-MS Method with the Commercial Immunoassay Kit. *Mar. Drugs* **2008**, *6*, 587–594. [CrossRef] [PubMed]
28. Armi, Z.; Turki, S.; Trabelsi, E.; Ceredi, A.; Riccardi, E.; Milandri, A. Occurrence of diarrhetic shellfish poisoning (DSP) toxins in clams (*Ruditapes decussatus*) from Tunis north lagoon. *Environ. Monit. Assess.* **2012**, *184*, 5085–5095. [CrossRef] [PubMed]
29. Pavela-Vrancic, M.; Mestrovic, V.; Marasovic, I.; Gillman, M.; Furey, A.; James, K.J. DSP toxin profile in the coastal waters of the central Adriatic Sea. *Toxicon* **2002**, *40*, 1601–1607. [CrossRef]
30. Vale, P.; Sampayo, M.A. Dinophysistoxin-2: A rare diarrhoeic toxin associated with *Dinophysis acuta*. *Toxicon* **2000**, *38*, 1599–1606. [CrossRef]
31. Draisci, R.; Giannetti, L.; Lucentini, L.; Marchiafava, C.; James, K.J.; Bishop, A.G.; Healy, B.M.; Kelly, S.S. Isolation of a new okadaic acid analog from phytoplankton implicated in diarrhetic shellfish poisoning. *J. Chromatogr.* **1998**, *798*, 137–145. [CrossRef]
32. Hu, T.; Doyle, J.; Jackson, D.M.; Marr, J.; Nixon, E.; Pleasance, S.; Quilliam, M.A.; Walter, J.A.; Wright, J.L.C. Isolation of a new diarrhetic shellfish poison from Irish mussels. *J. Chem. Soc. Chem. Commun.* **1992**, *40*, 39–41. [CrossRef]

33. Hu, T.; Marr, J.; de Freitas, A.S.W.; Quilliam, M.A.; Walter, J.A.; Wright, J.L.C.; Pleasance, S. New diol esters isolated from cultures of *Prorocentrum lima* and *Prorocentrum concavum*. *J. Nat. Prod.* **1992**, *55*, 1631–1637. [CrossRef]
34. Hu, T.; Curtis, J.M.; Walter, J.A.; McLachlan, J.L.; Wright, J.L.C. Two new water-soluble dsp toxin derivatives from the dinoflagellate *Prorocentrum maculosum*: Possible storage and excretion products. *Tetrahedron Lett.* **1995**, *36*, 9273–9276. [CrossRef]
35. Hu, T.; Curtis, J.M.; Walter, J.A.; Wright, J.L.C. Identification of DTX-4, A New water-soluble phosphatase inhibitor from the toxic dinoflagellate *Prorocentrum lima*. *J. Chem. Soc. Chem. Commun.* **1995**, *5*, 597–599. [CrossRef]
36. Hu, T.M.; LeBlanc, P.; Burton, I.W.; Walter, J.A.; McCarron, P.; Melanson, J.E.; Strangman, W.K.; Wright, J.L.C. Sulfated diesters of okadaic acid and DTX-1: Self-protective precursors of diarrhetic shellfish poisoning (DSP) toxins. *Harmful Algae* **2017**, *63*, 85–93. [CrossRef] [PubMed]
37. Pan, L.; Chen, J.H.; Shen, H.H.; He, X.P.; Li, G.J.; Song, X.C.; Zhou, D.S.; Sun, C.J. Profiling of Extracellular Toxins Associated with Diarrhetic Shellfish Poison in *Prorocentrum lima* Culture Medium by High-Performance Liquid Chromatography Coupled with Mass Spectrometry. *Toxins* **2017**, *9*, 308. [CrossRef] [PubMed]
38. Torgersen, T.; Miles, C.O.; Rundberget, T.; Wilkins, A.L. New Esters of Okadaic Acid in Seawater and Blue Mussels (*Mytilus edulis*). *J. Agric. Food Chem.* **2008**, *56*, 9628–9635. [CrossRef] [PubMed]
39. Cruz, P.G.; Daranas, A.H.; Fernandez, J.J.; Souto, M.L.; Norte, M. DTX5c, a new OA sulphate ester derivative from cultures of *Prorocentrum belizeanum*. *Toxicon* **2006**, *47*, 920–924. [CrossRef] [PubMed]
40. Suzuki, H.; Beuzenberg, V.; MacKenzie, A.L.; Quilliam, M.A. Discovery of okadaic acid esters in the toxic dinoflagellate *Dinophysis acuta* from New Zealand using liquid chromatography/tandem mass spectrometry. *Rapid Commun. Mass Spectrom.* **2004**, *18*, 1131–1138. [CrossRef] [PubMed]
41. Miles, C.O.; Wilkins, A.L.; Hawkes, A.D.; Jensen, D.J.; Cooney, J.M.; Larsen, K.; Petersen, D.; Rise, F.; Beuzenberg, V.; MacKenzie, A.L. Isolation and identification of a cis-C-8-diol-ester of okadaic acid from Dinophysis acuta in New Zealand. *Toxicon* **2006**, *48*, 195–203. [CrossRef] [PubMed]
42. Pizarro, G.; Paz, B.; Franco, J.; Suzuki, T.; Reguera, B. First detection of Pectenotoxin-11 and confirmation of OA-D8 diol-ester in *Dinophysis acuta* from European waters by LC-MS/MS. *Toxicon* **2008**, *52*, 889–896. [CrossRef] [PubMed]
43. Campbell, L.; Olson, R.; Sosik, H.M.; Abraham, A.; Henrichs, D.W.; Hyatt, C.; Buskey, E.J. First harmful *Dinophysis* (Dinophyceae, Dinophysiales) bloom in the U.S. is revealed by automated imaging flow cytometry. *J. Phycol.* **2010**, *46*, 66–75. [CrossRef]
44. Moroño, A.; Arevalo, F.; Fernandez, M.; Maneiro, J.; Pazos, Y.; Salgado, C.; Blanco, J. Accumulation and transformation of DSP toxins in mussels *Mytilus galloprovincialis* during a toxic episode caused by *Dinophysis acuminata*. *Aquat. Toxicol.* **2003**, *62*, 269–280. [CrossRef]
45. Suzuki, T.; Walter, J.A.; LeBlanc, P.; MacKinnon, S.; Miles, C.O.; Wilkins, A.L.; Munday, R.; Beuzenberg, V.; MacKenzie, L.; Jensen, D.J.; et al. Identification of Pectenotoxin-11 as 34S-Hydroxypectenotoxin-2, a New Pectenotoxin Analogue in the Toxic Dinoflagellate *Dinophysis acuta* from New Zealand. *Chem. Res. Toxicol.* **2006**, *19*, 310–318. [CrossRef] [PubMed]
46. Miles, C.O.; Wilkins, A.L.; Samdal, I.A.; Sandvik, M.; Petersen, D.; Quilliam, M.A.; Naustvoll, L.J.; Jensen, D.J.; Cooney, J.M. A novel pectenotoxin, PTX-12, in *Dinophysis* spp. and shellfish from Norway. *Chem. Res. Toxicol.* **2004**, *17*, 1423–1433. [CrossRef] [PubMed]
47. Draisci, R.; Lucentini, L.; Giannetti, L.; Boria, P.; Poletti, R. First report of pectenotoxin-2 (PTX-2) in algae (*Dinophysis fortii*) related to seafood poisoning in Europe. *Toxicon* **1996**, *34*, 923–935. [CrossRef]
48. Daiguji, M.; Satake, M.; James, K.J.; Bishop, A.; MacKenzie, L.; Naoki, H.; Yasumoto, T. Structures of new pectenotoxin analogs, pectenotoxin-2 seco acid and 7-epi-pectenotoxin-2 seco acid, isolated from a dinoflagellate and greenshell mussels. *Chem. Lett.* **1998**, *7*, 653–654. [CrossRef]
49. Suzuki, T.; Mitsuya, T.; Matsubara, H.; Yamasaki, M. Determination of pectenotoxin-2 after solid-phase extraction from seawater and from the dinoflagellate *Dinophysis fortii* by liquid chromatography with electrospray mass spectrometry and ultraviolet detection. Evidence of oxidation of pectenotoxin-2 to pectenotoxin-6 in scallop. *J Chomatogr. A* **1998**, *815*, 155–160.

50. Suzuki, T.; Miyazono, A.; Baba, K.; Sugawara, R.; Kamiyama, T. LC-MS/MS analysis of okadaic acid analogues and other lipophilic toxins in single-cell isolates of several *Dinophysis* species collected in Hokkaido, Japan. *Harmful Algae* **2009**, *8*, 233–238. [CrossRef]
51. Suzuki, T.; Miyazono, A.; Okumura, Y.; Kamiyama, T. LC-MS/MS Analysis of Lipophilic Toxins in Japanese *Dinophysis* Species. Available online: http://www.pices.int/publications/presentations/PICES_15/Ann15_W4/W4_Suzuki.pdf (accessed on 20 October 2018).
52. James, K.J.; Bishop, A.G.; Draisci, R.; Palleschi, L.; Marchiafava, C.; Ferretti, E.; Satake, M.; Yasumoto, T. Liquid chromatographic methods for the isolation and identification of new pectenotoxin-2 analogues from marine phytoplankton and shellfish. *J. Chromatogr.* **1999**, *844*, 53–65. [CrossRef]
53. Sasaki, K.; Takizawa, A.; Tubaro, A.; Sidari, L.; Loggia, R.D.; Yasumoto, T. Fluorometric analysis of pectenotoxin-2 in microalgal samples by high performance liquid chromatography. *Nat. Toxins* **1999**, *7*, 241–246. [CrossRef]
54. Fernández, M.L.; Reguera, B.; González-Gil, S.; Míguez, A. Pectenotoxin-2 in single-cell isolates of *Dinophysis caudata* and *Dinophysis acuta* from the Galician Rías (NW Spain). *Toxicon* **2006**, *48*, 477–490. [CrossRef] [PubMed]
55. Kamiyama, T.; Suzuki, T. Production of dinophysistoxin-1 and pectenotoxin-2 by a culture of *Dinophysis acuminata* (Dinophyceae). *Harmful Algae* **2009**, *8*, 312–317. [CrossRef]
56. Nagai, S.; Suzuki, T.; Nishikawa, T.; Kamiyama, T. Differences in the production and excretion kinetics of okadaic acid, dinophysistoxin-1, and pectenotoxin-2 between cultures of *Dinophysis acuminata* and *Dinophysis fortii* isolated from western Japan. *J. Phycol.* **2011**, *47*, 1326–1337. [CrossRef] [PubMed]
57. MacKenzie, L.; Beuzenberg, V.; Holland, P.; McNabb, P.; Suzuki, T.; Selwood, A. Pectenotoxin and okadaic acid-based toxin profiles in *Dinophysis acuta* and *Dinophysis acuminata* from New Zealand. *Harmful Algae* **2005**, *4*, 75–85. [CrossRef]
58. Fabro, E.; Almandoz, G.O.; Ferrari, M.E.; Hoffmeyer, M.S.; Pettigrosso, R.E.; Uibrig, R.; Krock, B. Co-occurrence of Dinophysis tripos and pectenotoxins in Argentinean shelf waters. *Harmful Algae* **2015**, *42*, 25–33. [CrossRef]
59. Vale, P.; Sampayo, M.A. Pectenotoxin-2 seco acid, 7-epi-pectenotoxin-2 seco acid and pectenotoxin-2 in shellfish and plankton from Portugal. *Toxicon* **2002**, *40*, 979–987. [CrossRef]
60. Fernández-Puente, P.; Fidalgo Sáez, M.J.; Hamilton, B.; Furey, A.; James, K.J. Studies of polyether toxins in the marine phytoplankton, *Dinophysis acuta*, in Ireland using multiple tandem mass spectrometry. *Toxicon* **2004**, *44*, 919–926. [CrossRef] [PubMed]
61. Blanco, J.; Álvarez, G.; Uribe, E. Identification of pectenotoxins in plankton, filter feeders, and isolated cells of a *Dinophysis acuminata* with an atypical toxin profile from Chile. *Toxicon* **2007**, *49*, 710–716. [CrossRef] [PubMed]
62. Nielsen, L.T.; Krock, B.; Hansen, P.J. Effects of light and food availability on toxin production, growth and photosynthesis in *Dinophysis acuminata*. *Mar. Ecol. Prog. Ser.* **2012**, *471*, 37–50. [CrossRef]
63. Li, A.; Li, M.; Qiu, J.; Song, J.; Ji, Y.; Hu, Y.; Wang, S.; Che, Y. Effect of Suspended Particulate Matter on the Accumulation of Dissolved Diarrhetic Shellfish Toxins by Mussels (*Mytilus galloprovincialis*) under Laboratory Conditions. *Toxins* **2018**, *10*, 273. [CrossRef] [PubMed]
64. Rossignoli, A.E. Acumulación de Toxinas DSP en el mejillón *Mytilus galloprovincialis*. Ph.D. Thesis, University of Santiago de Compostela, Santiago de Compostela, Spain, 2011.
65. Nam, K.Y.; Hiro, M.; Kimura, S.; Fujiki, H.; Imanishi, Y. Permeability of a non-TPA-type tumor promoter, okadaic acid, through lipid bilayer membrane. *Carcinogenesis* **1990**, *11*, 1171–1174. [CrossRef] [PubMed]
66. Daranas, A.H.; Cruz, P.G.; Creus, A.H.; Norte, M.; Fernández, J.J. Self-assembly of okadaic acid as a pathway to the cell. *Org. Lett.* **2007**, *9*, 4191–4194. [CrossRef] [PubMed]
67. Jauffrais, T.; Kilcoyne, J.; Herrenknecht, C.; Truquet, P.; Sechet, V.; Miles, C.O.; Hess, P. Dissolved azaspiracids are absorbed and metabolized by blue mussels (*Mytilus edulis*). *Toxicon* **2013**, *65*, 81–89. [CrossRef] [PubMed]
68. Dame, R.F. *Bivalve Filter Feeders: In Estuarine and Coastal Ecosystem Processes*; Springer-Verlag: Berlin/Heidelberg, Germany, 2013; Volume 33.
69. Gosling, E. *Marine Bivalve Molluscs*; John Wiley & Sons: Hoboken, NJ, USA, 2015.
70. Møhlenberg, F.; Riisgård, H.U. Efficiency of particle retention in 13 species of suspension feeding bivalves. *Ophelia* **1978**, *17*, 239–246. [CrossRef]

71. Riisgård, H.U. Efficiency of particle retention and filtration rate in 6 species of Northeast American bivalves. *Mar. Ecol. Prog. Ser.* **1988**, *45*, 217–223. [CrossRef]
72. Vahl, O. Particle retention and relation between water transport and oxygen uptake in *Chlamys opercularis* (L.) (Bivalvia). *Ophelia* **1972**, *10*, 67–74. [CrossRef]
73. Sobral, P.; Widdows, J. Effects of increasing current velocity, turbidity and particle-size selection on the feeding activity and scope for growth of Ruditapes decussatus from Ria Formosa, southern Portugal. *J. Exp. Mar.Biol. Ecol.* **2000**, *245*, 111–125. [CrossRef]
74. Reguera, B.; Riobó, P.; Rodríguez, F.; Díaz, P.; Pizarro, G.; Paz, B.; Franco, J.; Blanco, J. Dinophysis Toxins: Causative Organisms, Distribution and Fate in Shellfish. *Mar. Drugs* **2014**, *12*, 394–461. [CrossRef] [PubMed]
75. Iglesias, J.I.P.; Urrutia, M.B.; Navarro, E.; Alvarez-Jorna, P.; Larretxea, X.; Bougrier, S.; Heral, M. Variability of feeding processes in the cockle *Cerastoderma edule* (L.) in response to changes in seston concentration and composition. *J. Exp. Mar.Biol. Ecol.* **1996**, *197*, 121–143. [CrossRef]
76. Pitcher, G.C.; Krock, B.; Cembella, A.D. Accumulation of diarrhetic shellfish poisoning toxins in the oyster *Crassostrea gigas* and the mussel *Choromytilus meridionalis* in the southern Benguela ecosystem. *Afr. J. Mar. Sci.* **2011**, *33*, 273–281. [CrossRef]
77. García-Altares, M.; Casanova, A.; Fernández-Tejedor, M.; Diogène, J.; De La Iglesia, P. Bloom of *Dinophysis* spp. dominated by *D. sacculus* and its related diarrhetic shellfish poisoning (DSP) outbreak in Alfacs Bay (Catalonia, NW Mediterranean Sea): Identification of DSP toxins in phytoplankton, shellfish and passive samplers. *Reg. Stud. Mar. Sci.* **2016**, *6*, 19–28. [CrossRef]
78. Kim, J.H.; Lee, K.J.; Suzuki, T.; Kang, Y.S.; Ho Kim, P.; Song, K.C.; Lee, T.S. Seasonal Variability of Lipophilic Shellfish Toxins in Bivalves and Waters, and Abundance of *Dinophysis* spp. in Jinhae Bay, Korea. *J. Shellfish Res.* **2010**, *29*, 1061–1067. [CrossRef]
79. Kacem, I.; Bouaïcha, N.; Hajjem, B. Comparison of okadaic acid profiles in mussels and oysters collected in Mediterranean lagoon, Tunisia. *Int.J. Biol.* **2010**, *2*, 238–245. [CrossRef]
80. Comeau, L.A.; Pernet, F.; Tremblay, R.; Bates, S.S.; LeBlanc, A. Comparison of eastern oyster (*Crassostrea virginica*) and blue mussel (*Mytilus edulis*) filtration rates at low temperatures. *Can. Tech. Rep. Fish. Aquat. Sci.* **2008**, *2810*, 1–17.
81. McFarland, K.; Donaghy, L.; Volety, A.K. Effect of acute salinity changes on hemolymph osmolality and clearance rate of the non-native mussel, *Perna viridis*, and the native oyster, Crassostrea virginica, in Southwest Florida. *Aquat. Invasions* **2013**, *8*, 299–310. [CrossRef]
82. Cranford, P.J.; Ward, J.E.; Shumway, S.E. Bivalve filter feeding: Variability and limits of the aquaculture biofilter. In *Shellfish Aquaculture and the Environment*; Shumway, S.E., Ed.; John Wiley & Sons: Hoboken, NJ, USA, 2011; pp. 81–124.
83. Bricelj, V.M.; Lee, J.H.; Cembella, A.D. Influence of dinoflagellate cell toxicity on uptake and loss of paralytic shellfish toxins in the northern quahog *Mercenaria mercenaria*. *Mar. Ecol. Prog. Ser.* **1991**, *74*, 33–46. [CrossRef]
84. Mafra, L., Jr.; Bricelj, V.; Ouellette, C.; Léger, C.; Bates, S. Mechanisms contributing to low domoic acid uptake by oysters feeding on *Pseudo-nitzschia* cells. I. Filtration and pseudofeces production. *Aquat. Biol.* **2009**, *6*, 201–212. [CrossRef]
85. Basti, L.; Uchida, H.; Kanamori, M.; Matsushima, R.; Suzuki, T.; Nagai, S. Mortality and pathology of Japanese scallop, *Patinopecten* (*Mizuhopecten*) *yessoensis*, and noble scallop, *Mimachlamys nobilis*, fed monoclonal culture of PTX-producer, *Dinophysis caudata*. In *Marine and Freshwater Harmful Algae, Proceedings of the 16th International Conference on Harmful Algae, Wellington, New Zealand, Wellington, New Zealand, 27–31 October 2014*; Cawthron Institute and International Society for the Study of Harmful Algae (ISSHA): Nelson, New Zealand, 2014; pp. 27–30.
86. Pillet, S.; Houvenaghel, G. Influence of experimental toxification by DSP producing microalgae, *Prorocentrum lima*, on clearance rate in blue mussels *Mytilus edulis*. In *Harmful Marine Algal Blooms*; Lassus, P., Arzul, G., Erard, E., Gentien, P., Marcaillou, C., Eds.; Lavoisier Publishing/Intercept Ltd.: Paris, France, 1995; pp. 481–486.
87. Sampayo, M.A.; Alvito, P.; Franca, S.; Sousa, I. *Dinophysis* spp. toxicity and relation to accompanying species. In *Toxic Marine Phytoplankton*; Granéli, E., Sundström, B., Edler, L., Anderson, D.M., Eds.; Elsevier: New York, NY, USA, 1990; pp. 215–220.
88. Haamer, J. Presence of the phycotoxin okadaic acid in mussel (*Mytilus edulis*) in relation to nutrient composition in a Swedish coastal water. *J. Shellfish Res.* **1995**, *14*, 209–216.

89. Jorgensen, C.B. *Bivalve Filter Feeding: Hydrodynamics, Bioenergetics, Physiology and Ecology*; Olsen & Olsen: Fredensborg, Denmark, 1990.
90. Iglesias, J.I.P.; Navarro, E.; Alvarez Jorna, P.; Armentia, I. Feeding, particle selection and absorption in cockles *Cerastoderma edule* (L.) exposed to variable conditions of food concentration and quality. *J. Exp. Mar. Biol. Ecol.* **1992**, *162*, 177–198. [CrossRef]
91. Shumway, S.E.; Cucci, T.L.; Lesser, M.P.; Bourne, N.; Bunting, B. Particle clearance and selection in three species of juvenile scallops. *Aquac. Int.* **1997**, *5*, 89–99. [CrossRef]
92. Shumway, S.E.; Cucci, T.L.; Newell, R.C.; Yentsch, C.M. Particle selection, ingestion, and absorption in filter-feeding bivalves. *J. Exp. Mar. Biol. Ecol.* **1985**, *9*, 77–92. [CrossRef]
93. Ward, J.E.; Shumway, S.E. Separating the grain from the chaff: Particle selection in suspension- and deposit-feeding bivalves. *J. Exp. Mar.Biol. Ecol.* **2004**, *300*, 83–130. [CrossRef]
94. Bricelj, V.M.; Ward, J.E.; Cembella, A.D.; MacDonald, B.A. Application of video-endoscopy to the study of bivalve feeding on toxic dinoflagellates. In *Harmful Algae*; Reguera, B., Blanco, J., Fernández, M.L., Wyatt, T., Eds.; Xunta de Galicia and IOC of UNESCO: Santiago de Compostela, Spain, 1998; pp. 453–456.
95. Defossez, J.M.; Hawkins, A.J.S. Selective feeding in shellfish: Size-dependent rejection of large particles within pseudofaeces from *Mytilus edulis*, *Ruditapes philippinarum* and *Tapes decussatus*. *Mar. Biol.* **1997**, *129*, 139–147. [CrossRef]
96. Sidari, L.; Nichetto, P.; Cok, S.; Sosa, S.; Tubaro, A.; Honsell, G.; DellaLoggia, R. Phytoplankton selection by mussels, and diarrhetic shellfish poisoning. *Mar. Biol.* **1998**, *131*, 103–111. [CrossRef]
97. Pino-Querido, A.; Alvarez-Castro, J.M.; Guerra-Varela, J.; Toro, M.A.; Vera, M.; Pardo, B.G.; Fuentes, J.; Blanco, J.; Martinez, P. Heritability estimation for okadaic acid algal toxin accumulation, mantle color and growth traits in Mediterranean mussel (*Mytilus galloprovincialis*). *Aquaculture* **2015**, *440*, 32–39. [CrossRef]
98. Owen, G. Observations on the Stomach and Digestive Diverticula of the Lamellibranchia: I. The Anisomyaria and Eulamellibranchia. *Q. J. Microsc. Sci.* **1955**, *s3-96*, 517–537.
99. Purchon, R.D. The stomach in the bivalvia. *Philos. Trans. R. Soc. Lond.* **1987**, *316*, 183. [CrossRef]
100. Hawkins, A.J.S.; Navarro, E.; Iglesias, J.I.P. Comparative allometries of gut-passage time, gut content and metabolic faecal loss in *Mytilus edulis* and *Cerastoderma edule*. *Mar. Biol.* **1990**, *105*, 197–204. [CrossRef]
101. Navarro, E.; Iglesias, J.I.P. Infaunal Filter-Feeding Bivalves and the Physiological Response to Short-Term Fluctuations in Food Availability and Composition. In *Bivalve Filter Feeders*; Dame, R.F., Ed.; Springer-Verlag: Berlin/Heidelberg, Germany, 1993; pp. 25–56.
102. Moroño, A.; Franco, J.; Miranda, M.; Reyero, M.I.; Blanco, J. The effect of mussel size, temperature, seston volume, food quality and volume-specific toxin concentration on the uptake rate of PSP toxins by mussels (*Mytilus galloprovincialis* LmK). *J. Exp. Mar. Biol. Ecol.* **2001**, *257*, 117–132. [CrossRef]
103. Guéguen, M.; Lassus, P.; Laabir, M.; Bardouil, M.; Baron, R.; Séchet, V.; Truquet, P.; Amzil, Z.; Barillé, L. Gut passage times in two bivalve molluscs fed toxic microalgae: *Alexandrium minutum, A. catenella* and *Pseudo-nitzschia calliantha*. *Aquat. Living Res.* **2008**, *21*, 21–29. [CrossRef]
104. Brillant, M.G.; MacDonald, B.A. Postingestive selection in the sea scallop, *Placopecten magellanicus* (Gmelin): the role of particle size and density. *J. Exp. Mar. Biol. Ecol.* **2000**, *253*, 211–227. [CrossRef]
105. Bricelj, V.M.; Bass, A.E.; Lopez, G.R. Absorption and gut passage time of microalgae in a suspension feeder: an evaluation of the 51Cr: 14C twin tracer technique. *Mar. Ecol. Prog. Ser.* **1984**, *17*, 57–63. [CrossRef]
106. Bayne, B.L. Feeding physiology of bivalves: Time-dependence and compensation for changes in food availability. In *Bivalve Filter Feeders*; Springer-Verlag: Berlin/Heidelberg, Germany, 1993; pp. 1–24.
107. Bauder, A.G.; Cembella, A.D. Viability of the toxic dinoflagellate *Prorocentrum lima* following ingestion and gut passage in the bay scallop *Argopecten irradians*. *J. Shellfish Res.* **2000**, *19*, 321–324.
108. Bauder, A.G.; Cembella, A.D.; Bricelj, V.M.; Quilliam, M.A. Uptake and fate of diarrhetic shellfish poisoning toxins from the dinoflagellate *Prorocentrum lima* in the bay scallop *Argopecten irradians*. *Mar. Ecol. Prog. Ser.* **2001**, *213*, 39–52. [CrossRef]
109. Rossignoli, A.E.; Fernández, D.; Acosta, C.P.; Blanco, J. Microencapsulation of okadaic acid as a tool for studying the accumulation of DSP toxins in mussels. *Mar. Environ. Res.* **2011**, *71*, 91–93. [CrossRef] [PubMed]
110. Windust, A.J.; Hu, T.M.; Wright, J.L.C.; Quilliam, M.A.; McLachlan, J.L. Oxidative metabolism by *Thalassiosira weissflogii* (Bacillariophyceae) of a diol-ester of okadaic acid, the diarrhetic shellfish poisoning. *J. Phycol.* **2000**, *36*, 342–350. [CrossRef]

111. Quilliam, M.A.; Hardstaff, W.R.; Ishida, N.; McLachlan, J.L.; Reeves, A.R.; Ross, N.W.; Windust, A.J. Production of diarrhetic shellfish poisoning (DSP) toxins by *Prorocentrum lima* in culture and development of analytical methods. In *Harmful and Toxic Algal Blooms*; Yasumoto, T., Oshima, Y., Fukuyo, Y., Eds.; IOC of UNESCO: Sendai, Japan, 1996; pp. 289–292.
112. Quilliam, M.A.; Ishida, N.; McLachlan, J.L.; Ross, N.W.; Windust, A.J. Analytical Methods for Diarrhetic Shellfish Poisoning (DSP) Toxins and A Study of Toxin Production by Prorocentrum lima in Culture. UJNR Technical Report No. 24 1996; pp. 101–106. Available online: https://repository.library.noaa.gov/view/noaa/12555/noaa_12555_DS1.pdf?#page=101 (accessed on 18 May 2018).
113. Morton, B. Feeding and digestion in Bivalvia. In *The Mollusca. Physiology Part 2*; Saleuddin, A.S.M., Wilbur, K.M., Eds.; Academic Press: New York, NY, USA, 1983; pp. 65–147.
114. Fernández, M.L.; Miguez, A.; Moroño, A.; Cacho, E.; Martínez, A.; Blanco, J. Detoxification of low polarity toxins (DTX3) from mussels *Mytilus galloprovincialis* in Spain. In *Harmful Algae*; Reguera, B., Blanco, J., Fernández, M.L., Wyatt, T., Eds.; Xunta de Galicia & Intergovernmental Oceanografic Comission of UNESCO: Santiago de Compostela, Spain, 1998; pp. 449–452.
115. MacKenzie, L.A.; Selwood, A.I.; Marshall, C. Isolation and characterization of an enzyme from the Greenshell (TM) mussel *Perna canaliculus* that hydrolyses pectenotoxins and esters of okadaic acid. *Toxicon* **2012**, *60*, 406–419. [CrossRef] [PubMed]
116. Fux, E. Development and Evaluation of Passive Sampling and LC-MS Based Techniques for the Detection and Monitoring of Lipophilic Marine Toxins in Mesocosm and Field Studies. Ph.D. Thesis, The Marine Institute, School of Chemical and Pharmaceutical Sciences, Dublin, Germany, 2008.
117. Rossignoli, A.E.; Blanco, J. Subcellular distribution of okadaic acid in the digestive gland of *Mytilus galloprovincialis*: First evidences of lipoprotein binding to okadaic acid. *Toxicon* **2010**, *55*, 221–226. [CrossRef] [PubMed]
118. Guéguen, M.; Duinker, A.; Marcaillou, C. A first approach to localizing biotoxins in mussel digestive glands. In Proceedings of the 7th International Conference on Molluscan Shellfish Safety, Nantes, France, 14–19 June 2009.
119. Moore, M.N.; Willows, R.I. A model for cellular uptake and intracellular behaviour of particulate-bound micropollutants. *Mar. Environ. Res.* **1998**, *46*, 509–514. [CrossRef]
120. Smedes, F. Sampling and partitioning of neutral organic contaminants in surface waters with regard to legislation, environmental quality and flux estimations. *Int. J. Environ. Anal. Chem.* **1994**, *57*, 215–229. [CrossRef]
121. Rossignoli, A.; Blanco, J. Cellular distribution of okadaic acid in the digestive gland of *Mytilus galloprovincialis* (Lamarck, 1819). *Toxicon* **2008**, *52*, 957–959. [CrossRef] [PubMed]
122. Weinstein, J.E. Fine structure of the digestive tubule of the eastern oyster, *Crassostrea virginica* (Gmelin, 1791). *J. Shellfish Res.* **1995**, *14*, 97–104.
123. Jonas, A. Lipoprotein structure. In *Biochemistry of Lipids, Lipoproteins and Membranes*, 4th ed.; Vance, D.E., Vance, J.E., Eds.; Elsevier: New York, NY, USA, 2002; pp. 483–504.
124. Blanco, J.; Mariño, C.; Martín, H.; Acosta, C.P. Anatomical distribution of Diarrhetic Shellfish Poisoning (DSP) toxins in the mussel *Mytilus galloprovincialis*. *Toxicon* **2007**, *50*, 1011–1018. [CrossRef] [PubMed]
125. Marcaillou, C.; Haure, J.; Mondeguer, F.; Courcoux, A.; Dupuy, B.; Penisson, C. Effect of food supply on the detoxification in the blue mussel, *Mytilus edulis*, contaminated by diarrhetic shellfish toxins. *Aquat. Living Resour.* **2010**, *23*, 255–266. [CrossRef]
126. Edebo, L.; Lange, S.; Li, X.P.; Allenmark, S.; Lindgren, K.; Thompson, R. Seasonal, geographic and individual variation of okadaic acid content in cultivated mussels in Sweden. *Apmis* **1988**, *96*, 1036–1042. [CrossRef] [PubMed]
127. McCarron, P.; Kilcoyne, J.; Hess, P. Effects of cooking and heat treatment on concentration and tissue distribution of okadaic acid and dinophysistoxin-2 in mussels (*Mytilus edulis*). *Toxicon* **2008**, *51*, 1081–1089. [CrossRef] [PubMed]
128. Madigan, T.L.; Lee, K.G.; Padula, D.J.; McNabb, P.; Pointon, A.M. Diarrhetic shellfish poisoning (DSP) toxins in South Australian shellfish. *Harmful Algae* **2006**, *5*, 119–123. [CrossRef]

129. Hess, P.; McMahon, T.; Slattery, D.; Swords, D.; Dowling, G.; McCarron, M.; Clarke, D.; Gibbons, W.; Silke, W.; O'Cinneide, M. Use of LC-MS testing to identify lipophilic toxins, to stablish local trends and interspecies differences and to test the comparability of LC-MS testing with mouse bioassay: An example from the Irish Biotoxin Monitoring Programme 2001. In *Molluscan Shellfish Safety, Proceedings of the 4th International Conference on Molluscan Shellfish Safety, Xunta De Galicia, Spain, 4–8 June 2002*; Villalba, A., Reguera, B., Romalde, J.L., Beiras, R., Eds.; Consellería de Pesca e Asuntos Marítimos, Xunta de Galicia and IOC of UNESCO: Santiago de Compostela, Spain, 2003; pp. 57–66.
130. Vale, P. Differential Dynamics of Dinophysistoxins and Pectenotoxins, Part II: Offshore Bivalve Species. *Toxicon* **2006**, *47*, 163–173. [CrossRef] [PubMed]
131. Kameneva, P.A.; Krasheninina, E.A.; Slobodskova, V.V.; Kukla, S.P.; Orlova, T.Y. Accumulation and Tissue Distribution of Dinophysitoxin-1 and Dinophysitoxin-3 in the Mussel *Crenomytilus grayanus* Feeding on the Benthic Dinoflagellate *Prorocentrum foraminosum*. *Mar. Drugs* **2017**, *15*, 330. [CrossRef] [PubMed]
132. Blanco, J.; Álvarez, G.; Rengel, J.; Díaz, R.; Mariño, C.; Martín, H.; Uribe, E. Accumulation and Biotransformation of *Dinophysis* Toxins by the Surf Clam *Mesodesma donacium*. *Toxins* **2018**, *10*, 314. [CrossRef] [PubMed]
133. Suzuki, T.; Ota, H.; Yamasaki, M. Direct evidence of transformation of dinophysistoxin-1 to 7-O-acyl-dinophysistoxin-1 (Dinophysis-3) in the scallop *Patinopecten yessoensis*. *Toxicon* **1999**, *37*, 187–198. [CrossRef]
134. Rossignoli, A.E.; Fernández, D.; Regueiro, J.; Mariño, C.; Blanco, J. Esterification of okadaic acid in the mussel *Mytilus galloprovincialis*. *Toxicon* **2011**, *57*, 712–720. [CrossRef] [PubMed]
135. Konoki, K.; Onoda, T.; Watanabe, R.; Cho, Y.; Kaga, S.; Suzuki, T.; Yotsu-Yamashita, M. In Vitro Acylation of Okadaic Acid in the Presence of Various Bivalves' Extracts. *Mar. Drugs* **2013**, *11*, 300–315. [CrossRef] [PubMed]
136. Vale, P. Detailed profiles of 7-O-acyl esters in plankton and shellfish from the Portuguese coast. *J. Chomatogr. A* **2006**, *1128*, 181–188. [CrossRef] [PubMed]
137. Quilliam, M.A.; Vale, P.; Sampayo, M.A.M. Direct detection of acyl esters of okadaic acid and dinophysistoxin-2 in Portuguese shellfish by LC-MS. In *Molluscan Shellfish Safety*; Villalba, A., Reguera, B., Romalde, J., Beiras, R., Eds.; Consellería de Pesca e Asuntos Marıtimos da Xunta de Galicia and IOC of UNESCO: Santiago de Compostela, Spain, 2003; pp. 67–73.
138. Iglesia, P.; Fonollosa, E.; Diogène, J. Assessment of acylation routes and structural characterisation by liquid chromatography/tandem mass spectrometry of semi-synthetic acyl ester analogues of lipophilic marine toxins. *Rapid Commun. Mass Spectrom.* **2014**, *28*, 2605–2616. [CrossRef] [PubMed]
139. Suzuki, T.; Kamiyama, T.; Okumura, Y.; Ishihara, K.; Matsushima, R.; Kaneniwa, M. Liquid-chromatographic hybrid triple–quadrupole linear-ion-trap MS/MS analysis of fatty-acid esters of dinophysistoxin-1 in bivalves and toxic dinoflagellates in Japan. *Fish. Sci.* **2009**, *75*, 1039–1048. [CrossRef]
140. Torgersen, T.; Wilkins, A.L.; Rundberget, T.; Miles, C.O. Characterization of fatty acid esters of okadaic acid and related toxins in blue mussels (*Mytilus edulis*) from Norway. *Rapid Commun. Mass Spectrom.* **2008**, *22*, 1127–1136. [CrossRef] [PubMed]
141. Marr, J.; Hu, T.; Pleasance, S.; Quilliam, M.A.; Wright, J.L.C. Detection of new 7-*O*-acyl derivatives of diarrhetic shellfish poisoning toxins by liquid chromatography- mass spectometry. *Toxicon* **1992**, *30*, 1621–1630. [CrossRef]
142. Vale, P. Profiles of fatty acids and 7-O-acyl okadaic acid esters in bivalves: Can bacteria be involved in acyl esterification of okadaic acid? *Comp. Biochem. Physiol. C Toxicol. Pharmacol.* **2010**, *151*, 18–24. [CrossRef] [PubMed]
143. Trainer, V.L.; Moore, L.; Bill, B.; Adams, N.; Harrington, N.; Borchert, J.; da Silva, D.; Eberhart, B. Diarrhetic Shellfish Toxins and Other Lipophilic Toxins of Human Health Concern in Washington State. *Mar. Drugs* **2013**, *11*, 1815–1835. [CrossRef] [PubMed]
144. Torgersen, T.; Sandvik, M.; Lundve, B.; Lindegarth, S. Profiles and levels of fatty acid esters of okadaic acid group toxins and pectenotoxins during toxin depuration. Part II: Blue mussels (*Mytilus edulis*) and flat oyster (*Ostrea edulis*). *Toxicon* **2008**, *52*, 418–427. [CrossRef] [PubMed]
145. Lindegarth, S.; Torgersen, T.; Lundve, B.; Sandvik, M. Differential retention of Okadaic Acid (OA) group toxins and Pectenotoxins (PTX) in the blue mussel, *Mytilus edulis* (L.), and european flat oyster, *Ostrea edulis* (L.). *J. Shellfish Res.* **2009**, *28*, 313–323. [CrossRef]

146. Jorgensen, K.; Scanlon, S.; Jensen, L.B. Diarrhetic Shellfish Poisoning Toxin Esters in Danish Blue Mussels and Surf Clams. *Food Addit. Contam.* **2005**, *22*, 743–751. [CrossRef] [PubMed]
147. Suzuki, T.; Quilliam, M.A. LC-MS/MS Analysis of Diarrhetic Shellfish Poisoning (DSP) Toxins, Okadaic Acid and Dinophysistoxin Analogues, and Other Lipophilic Toxins. *Anal. Sci.* **2011**, *27*, 571–584. [CrossRef] [PubMed]
148. Suzuki, T.; Mitsuya, T. Comparison of dinophysistoxin-1 and esterified dinophysistoxin-1 (dinophysistoxin-3) contents in the scallop *Patinopecten yessoensis* and the mussel *Mytilus galloprovincialis*. *Toxicon* **2001**, *39*, 905–908. [CrossRef]
149. Garcia, C.; Pruzzo, M.; Rodriguez-Unda, M.; Contreras, C.; Lagos, N. First evidence of Okadaic acid acyl-derivative and Dinophysistoxin-3 in mussel samples collected in Chiloe Island, Southern Chile. *J. Toxicol. Sci.* **2010**, *35*, 335–344. [CrossRef] [PubMed]
150. Vale, P.; Sampayo, M.A. Esterification of DSP toxins by Portuguese bivalves from the northwest coast determined by LC-MS-a widespread phenomenon. *Toxicon* **2002**, *40*, 33–42. [CrossRef]
151. Blanco, J.; Moroño, A.; Fernández, M.L. Toxic episodes in shellfish, produced by lipophilic phycotoxins: an overview. *Revista Galega dos Recursos Mariños* **2005**, *1*, 1–70.
152. Vale, P. Differential Dynamics of Dinophysistoxins and Pectenotoxins Between Blue Mussel and Common Cockle: A Phenomenon Originating From the Complex Toxin Profile of Dinophysis acuta. *Toxicon* **2004**, *44*, 123–134. [CrossRef] [PubMed]
153. Villar-González, A.; Rodríguez-Velasco, M.L.; Ben-Gigirey, B.; Botana, L.M. Lipophilic toxin profile in Galicia (Spain): 2005 toxic episode. *Toxicon* **2007**, *49*, 1129–1134. [CrossRef] [PubMed]
154. Suzuki, T.; Mackenzie, L.; Stirling, D.; Adamson, J. Conversion of pectenotoxin-2 to pectenotoxin-2 seco acid in the New Zealand scallop, *Pecten novaezelandiae*. *Fish. Sci.* **2001**, *67*, 506–510. [CrossRef]
155. Suzuki, T.; MacKenzie, L.; Stirling, D.; Adamson, J. Pectenotoxin-2 seco acid: A toxin converted from pectenotoxin-2 by the New Zealand Greenshell mussels, *Perna canaliculus*. *Toxicon* **2001**, *39*, 507–514. [CrossRef]
156. Miles, C.O.; Wilkins, A.L.; Munday, R.; Dines, M.H.; Hawkes, A.D.; Briggs, L.R.; Sandvik, M.; Jensen, D.J.; Cooney, J.M.; Holland, P.T.; et al. Isolation of pectenotoxin-2 from *Dinophysis acuta* and its conversion to pectenotoxin-2 seco acid, and preliminary assessment of their acute toxicities. *Toxicon* **2004**, *43*, 1–9. [CrossRef] [PubMed]
157. MacKenzie, L.; Holland, P.; McNabb, P.; Beuzenberg, V.; Selwood, A.; Suzuki, T. Complex toxin profiles in phytoplankton and Greenshell mussels (*Perna canaliculus*), revealed by LC–MS/MS analysis. *Toxicon* **2002**, *40*, 1321–1330. [CrossRef]
158. Fernández, M.L.; Míguez, A.; Martínez, A.; Moroño, A.; Arévalo, F.; Pazos, Y.; Salgado, C.; Correa, J.; Blanco, J.; González-Gil, S.; et al. First report of Pectenotoxin-2 in phytoplankton net-hauls and mussels from the Galician Rías Baixas (NW Spain) during proliferations of *Dinophysis acuta* and *Dinophysis caudata*. In *Molluscan Shellfish Safety*; Villalba, A., Reguera, B., Romalde, J., Beiras, R., Eds.; Consellería de Pesca e Asuntos Marítimos da Xunta de Galicia and Intergovernmental Oceanographic Commission of UNESCO: Santiago de Compostela, Spain, 2003; pp. 75–83.
159. Amzil, Z.; Sibat, M.; Royer, F.; Masson, N.; Abadie, E. Report on the First Detection of Pectenotoxin-2, Spirolide-A and Their Derivatives in French Shellfish. *Mar. Drugs* **2007**, *5*, 168–179. [CrossRef] [PubMed]
160. Suzuki, T.; Jin, T.; Shirota, Y.; Mitsuya, T.; Okumura, Y.; Kamiyama, T. Quantification of Lipophilic Toxins Associated With Diarrhetic Shellfish Poisoning in Japanese Bivalves by Liquid Chromatography-Mass Spectrometry and Comparison With Mouse Bioassay. *Fish. Sci.* **2005**, *71*, 1370–1378. [CrossRef]
161. Suzuki, T.; Igarashi, T.; Ichimi, K.; Watai, M.; Suzuki, M.; Ogiso, E.; Yasumoto, T. Kinetics of Diarrhetic Shellfish Poisoning Toxins, Okadaic Acid, Dinophysistoxin-1, Pectenotoxin-6 and Yessotoxin in Scallops *Patinopecten yessoensis*. *Fish. Sci.* **2005**, *71*, 948–955. [CrossRef]
162. Suzuki, T. Lipophilic Toxins, Pectenotoxins, and Yessotoxins: Chemistry, Metabolism, and Detection. In *Seafood and Freshwater Toxins: Pharmacology, Physiology, and Detection*; Botana, L.M., Ed.; CRC Press: Boca Ratón, FL, USA, 2014; pp. 627–656.
163. Janer, G.; Lavado, R.; Thibaut, R.; Porte, C. Effects of 17β-estradiol exposure in the mussel *Mytilus galloprovincialis*: A possible regulating role for steroid acyltransferases. *Aquat. Toxicol.* **2005**, *75*, 32–42. [CrossRef] [PubMed]

164. Janer, G.; Mesia-Vela, S.; Porte, C.; Kauffman, F.C. Esterification of vertebrate-type steroids in the Eastern oyster (*Crassostrea virginica*). *Steroids* **2004**, *69*, 129–136. [CrossRef] [PubMed]
165. Wilkins, A.L.; Rehmann, N.; Torgersen, T.; Rundberget, T.; Keogh, M.; Petersen, D.; Hess, P.; Rise, F.; Miles, C.O. Identification of fatty acid esters of pectenotoxin-2 seco acid in blue mussels (*Mytilus edulis*) from Ireland. *J. Agric. Food Chem.* **2006**, *54*, 5672–5678. [CrossRef] [PubMed]
166. Suarez-Ulloa, V.; Fernandez-Tajes, J.; Aguiar-Pulido, V.; Prego-Faraldo, M.V.; Florez-Barros, F.; Sexto-Iglesias, A.; Mendez, J.; Eirin-Lopez, J.M. Unbiased high-throughput characterization of mussel transcriptomic responses to sublethal concentrations of the biotoxin okadaic acid. *PeerJ* **2015**, *3*, e1429. [CrossRef] [PubMed]
167. Martínez-Escauriaza, R. Identificación de genes implicados en la eliminación de biotoxinas en el mejillón *Mytilus galloprovincialis* Lmk.: clonación y expresion de los cDNA que codifican para dos proteinas transportadoras ABC de la subfamilia B (proteínas MDR). Ph.D. Thesis, Universidade de Santiago de Compostela, Santiago de Compostela, Spain, 2013.
168. Lozano, V. Identificación de genes implicados en la eliminación de biotoxinas en el mejillón *Mytilus galloprovincialis* Lmk.: clonación y expresion de los cDNA que codifican para tres proteinas transportadoras ABC pertenecientes a las subfamilias C (proteínas MRP) y G. Ph.D. Thesis, Universidade de Santiago de Compostela, Santiago de Compostela, Spain, 2013.
169. Luedeking, A.; Koehler, A. Regulation of expression of multixenobiotic resistance (MXR) genes by environmental factors in the blue mussel *Mytilus edulis*. *Aquat. Toxicol.* **2004**, *69*, 1–10. [CrossRef] [PubMed]
170. Luedeking, A.; Van Noorden, C.J.F.; Koehler, A. Identification and characterisation of a multidrug resistance-related protein mRNA in the blue mussel *Mytilus edulis*. *Mar. Ecol. Prog. Ser.* **2005**, *286*, 167–175. [CrossRef]
171. Eufemia, N.; Epel, D. Induction of the multixenobiotic defense mechanism (MXR), P-glycoprotein, in the mussel *Mytilus californianus* as a general cellular response to environmental stresses. *Aquat. Toxicol.* **2000**, *49*, 89–100. [CrossRef]
172. Feldstein, T.; Nelson, N.; Mokady, O. Cloning and expression of MDR transporters from marine bivalves, and their potential use in biomonitoring. *Mar. Environ. Res.* **2006**, *62*, 118. [CrossRef] [PubMed]
173. Kingtong, S.; Chitramvong, Y.; Janvilisri, T. ATP-Binding Cassette Multidrug Transporters in Indian-Rock Oyster Saccostrea Forskali and Their Role in the Export of an Environmental Organic Pollutant Tributyltin. *Aquat. Toxicol.* **2007**, *85*, 124–132. [CrossRef] [PubMed]
174. Kurelec, B. The multixenobiotic resistance mechanism in aquatic organisms. *Crit. Rev. Toxicol.* **1992**, *22*, 23–43. [CrossRef] [PubMed]
175. Luckenbach, T.; Epel, D. ABCB-and ABCC-type transporters confer multixenobiotic resistance and form an environment-tissue barrier in bivalve gills. *Am. J. Physiol. Regul. Integr. Comp. Physiol.* **2008**, *294*, R1919–R1929. [CrossRef] [PubMed]
176. Faria, M.; Navarro, A.; Luckenbach, T.; Piña, B.; Barata, C. Characterization of the multixenobiotic resistance (MXR) mechanism in embryos and larvae of the zebra mussel (*Dreissena polymorpha*) and studies on its role in tolerance to single and mixture combinations of toxicants. *Aquat. Toxicol.* **2011**, *101*, 78–87. [CrossRef] [PubMed]
177. Huang, L.; Wang, J.; Chen, W.C.; Li, H.Y.; Liu, J.S.; Jiang, T.; Yang, W.D. P-glycoprotein expression in *Perna viridis* after exposure to *Prorocentrum lima*, a dinoflagellate producing DSP toxins. *Fish Shellfish Immunol.* **2014**, *39*, 254–262. [CrossRef] [PubMed]
178. Blanco, J.; Fernández, M.L.; Míguez, A.; Moroño, A. Okadaic acid depuration in the mussel *Mytilus galloprovincialis*: One- and two-compartment models and the effect of environmental conditions. *Mar. Ecol. Prog. Ser.* **1999**, *176*, 153–163. [CrossRef]
179. Moroño, A.; Fernández, M.L.; Franco, J.M.; Martínez, A.; Reyero, I.; Míguez, A.; Cacho, E.; Blanco, J. PSP and DSP detoxification kinetics in mussel, *Mytilus galloprovincialis*: Effect of environmental parameters and body weight. In *Harmful Algae*; Reguera, B., Blanco, J., Fernández, M.L., Wyatt, T., Eds.; Xunta de Galicia and IOC of UNESCO: Santiago de Compostela, Spain, 1998; pp. 445–448.
180. Poletti, R.; Viviani, R.; Casadei, C.; Lucentini, L.; Giannetti, L.; Funari, E.; Draisci, R. Decontamination dynamics of mussels naturally contaminated with diarrhetic toxins relocated to a basin of the Adriatic Sea. In *Harmful and Toxic Algal Blooms*; Yasumoto, T., Oshima, Y., Fukuyo, Y., Eds.; IOC of UNESCO: Paris, France, 1996; pp. 429–432.

181. Marcaillou-Le Baut, C.; Bardin, B.; Bardouil, M.; Bohec, M.; Le Denn, E.; Masselin, P.; Truquet, P. DSP depuration rates of mussels reared in a laboratory and an aquaculture pond. In *Toxic Phytoplankton Blooms in the Sea*; Smayda, T.J., Shimizu, Y., Eds.; Elsevier: Amsterdam, The Netherlands, 1993; pp. 531–535.
182. Nielsen, L.T.; Hansen, P.J.; Krock, B.; Vismann, B. Accumulation, transformation and breakdown of DSP toxins from the toxic dinoflagellate *Dinophysis acuta* in blue mussels, *Mytilus edulis*. *Toxicon* **2016**, *117*, 84–93. [CrossRef] [PubMed]
183. Botelho, M.J.; Vale, C.; Joaquim, S.; Costa, S.T.; Soares, F.; Roque, C.; Matias, D. Combined effect of temperature and nutritional regime on the elimination of the lipophilic toxin okadaic acid in the naturally contaminated wedge shell *Donax trunculus*. *Chemosphere* **2018**, *190*, 166–173. [CrossRef] [PubMed]
184. Holmes, M.; Teo, S.; Lee, F.; Khoo, H. Persistent low concentratrions of diarrhetic shellfish toxins in green mussels *Perna viridis* from the Johor Strait, Singapure: First record of diarrhetic shellfish toxins from South-East Asia. *Mar. Ecol. Prog. Ser.* **1999**, *181*, 257–268. [CrossRef]
185. Blanco, J. Modelling as a mitigation strategy for harmful algal blooms. In *Shellfish Safety and Quality*; Shumway, S.E., Rodrick, G.E., Eds.; Woodhead Publishing: Cambridge, MA, USA, 2009; pp. 200–227.
186. Svensson, S. Depuration of Okadaic acid (Diarrhetic Shellfish Toxin) in mussels, *Mytilus edulis* (Linnaeus), feeding on different quantities of nontoxic algae. *Aquaculture* **2003**, *218*, 277–291. [CrossRef]
187. Penry, D.L. Digestive kinematics of suspension-feeding bivalves: Modeling and measuring particle-processing in the gut of *Potamocorbula amurensis*. *Mar. Ecol. Prog. Ser.* **2000**, *197*, 181–192. [CrossRef]
188. Pousse, É.; Flye-Sainte-Marie, J.; Alunno-Bruscia, M.; Hégaret, H.; Rannou, É.; Pecquerie, L.; Marques, G.M.; Thomas, Y.; Castrec, J.; Fabioux, C. Modelling paralytic shellfish toxins (PST) accumulation in *Crassostrea gigas* by using Dynamic Energy Budgets (DEB). *J. Sea Res.* **2018**. [CrossRef]

MDPI
St. Alban-Anlage 66
4052 Basel
Switzerland
Tel. +41 61 683 77 34
Fax +41 61 302 89 18
www.mdpi.com

Toxins Editorial Office
E-mail: toxins@mdpi.com
www.mdpi.com/journal/toxins

www.ingramcontent.com/pod-product-compliance
Lightning Source LLC
LaVergne TN
LVHW071443100526
838202LV00088B/6620
* 9 7 8 3 0 3 9 2 1 3 6 3 4 *